D0811355

PRESTON POLYTECHNIC LIBRARY

Chorley Campus	Tel.	5811	☐
Lancaster Campus	Tel.	68121	☐
Marshall House, Preston	Tel.	23111	☐
Poulton Campus	Tel.	884651	☐
Preston Campus	Tel.	51831	☑

FOR REFERENCE ONLY

616.025 EME   A/C 140471

30107   000 690 849

EMERGENCIES IN
MEDICAL PRACTICE

Emergencies in
Medical Practice

EDITED BY

C. ALLAN BIRCH
M.D., F.R.C.P.

Honorary Consulting Physician,
Chase Farm Hospital, Enfield,
Middlesex

TENTH EDITION

CHURCHILL LIVINGSTONE
EDINBURGH LONDON AND NEW YORK
1976

CHURCHILL LIVINGSTONE
Medical Division of Longman Group Limited

Distributed in the United States of America by
Longman Inc., 19 West 44th Street, New York,
N.Y. 10036 and by associated companies, branches
and representatives throughout the world.

© LONGMAN GROUP LIMITED, 1976

*All rights reserved. No part of this publication
may be reproduced, stored in a retrieval system, or
transmitted in any form or by any means, electronic,
mechanical, photocopying, recording or otherwise,
without the prior permission of the publishers
(Churchill Livingstone, 23 Ravelston Terrace,
Edinburgh, EH4 3TL).*

ISBN 0 443 01169 9

Library of Congress Catalog Card Number 74-33160

First edition	-	1948
Second edition	-	1950
Third edition	-	1952
Fourth edition	-	1954
Fifth edition	-	1956
German translation	-	1956
Spanish translation	-	1956
Sixth edition	-	1960
Seventh edition	-	1963
Eighth edition	-	1967
Ninth edition	-	1971
Tenth edition	-	1976

Library of Congress Cataloging in Publication Data

Birch, Charles Allan, ed.
    Emergencies in medical practice.

    Includes bibliographies and index.
    1. Medical emergencies.   I. Title.   [DNLM:
1. Emergencies. WB100 E515]
RC87.B57 1975   616'.025   74-33160

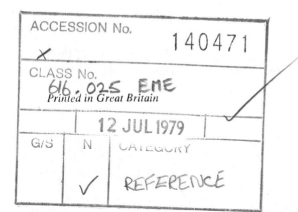

ACCESSION No. 140471

CLASS No.
616.025 EME

Printed in Great Britain

12 JUL 1979

G/S   N   CATEGORY

✓   REFERENCE

Preface to the Tenth Edition

REVISION for this tenth edition has been a continuous process since the ninth appeared. The arrangement of chapters remains the same but much pruning has been needed to accommodate new material. Twelve of the 32 contributors are new. Only three of the original 19 authors of 1948 remain (Birch, Cheetham and Avery Jones). Retirement and change of interest, but death in only one case, has caused changes in the authorship of seven chapters. Dr Wilkinson's account of 'Emergencies in Blood Diseases' has been taken over by Dr John MacIver, also of Manchester. Surgeon Captain Peter Preston, Professor of Naval Medicine, fills the gap caused by the death of Surgeon Captain J. M. Cliff. Professor G. M. Bull, because his contact with renal disease has lessened, has handed his chapter to Dr J. M. Goldsmith of the Urological Centre in Liverpool. David Pyke continues from King's College Hospital the authoritative account of diabetic emergencies originally written by Wilfrid Oakley. Dr Bertram Mandelbrote of Oxford gives an account of psychiatric emergencies previously written by Denis Leigh. Roger Williams and Martin Smith, who have made liver disease one of the growing points of medicine, contribute a section on hepatic coma. Gillian Hanson from her wide experience of intensive care at Whipps Cross Hospital writes on 'Resuscitation' in place of Sherwood Jones and has helped me to bring the account of postoperative emergencies up-to-date. Thelwall Jones in retirement has been replaced by Professor Schilling and J. M. Harrington. Dr R. E. Irvine and Dr Theodore Strouthidis, from their experience at St Helen's Hospital, Hastings, and the country's newest geriatric unit at Bexhill, emphasise special aspects of medical emergencies in old people.

This is one of the few medical textbooks which has survived for over 25 years and its success is very gratifying. Of the many doctors who have helped me to produce this tenth edition I must first record my grateful thanks to Bobbie Irvine, the clinical tutor at Hastings, for his kindness in allowing me to maintain contact with clinical medicine in two acute hospitals and the Postgraduate Centre. Other Hastings doctors who have helped me include Gwyn Roberts, M.S., F.R.C.S. (surgeon and my former H.P.); Duncan Lawrie (cardiologist); Harry Middleton and Stephen Bramwell (anaesthetists); Kathleen J. Harrison (haematologist) and Eurwen Innes (rheumatologist), as well as many registrars. In addition I have corresponded with many professional people, particularly Dr A. S. R. Peffers of the Air Corporations Joint Medical Service; Mr S. R. Speller, O.B.E., LL.B., Ph.D., late Secretary and Director of Education of the Institute of Hospital Administrators; David Maclean, F.R.C.S., of the Surgical Unit of the London Hospital and Robert Sells, F.R.C.S., of Liverpool. Lord Platt and Dr John Surtees of Eastbourne have given valuable advice. Mr D. B. Mathieson, Chief Pharmacist at The Royal East Sussex Hospital, Hastings, has willingly answered many queries. All contributors have been very patient with my editorial actions in some of which they have shared.

Many of the lists in the appendices of earlier editions are now unnecessary and have been deleted. The temptation to flood the text with references has been resisted without, it is hoped, making the statements too dogmatic. I have not sought to include detailed descriptions of all emergency procedures, feeling that hospital doctors should seek instruction by colleagues where necessary.

Tables and figures have been numbered by chapter and not serially. The words intravenous, intravenously and intramuscular appear so often in the text that they have been replaced by i v and i m. I am grateful to many doctors who have written advice and criticism. I will be glad to have correspondence about this edition. It will be carefully considered by Colin Ogilvie who I hope will become editor as well as remaining a contributor next time.

Although medicine is my main interest my wife has seen to it that I have continued with other pursuits and I have not neglected my bees entirely. Secretarial work has been managed personally at Salter's Corner with some professional help from Mrs Marion Packer. Messrs Churchill Livingstone have been very patient with my efforts to produce a perfect edition.

SALTER'S CORNER,

HASTINGS, May 1976.

C. Allan Birch

From the Preface to the First Edition

A MEDICAL emergency is any condition or circumstance of a patient which calls for immediate action other than surgery. Just what conditions might be included in this definition is a matter of opinion and the doctor's list, consisting mostly of absolute emergencies, will be shorter than the patient's which includes the relative ones.

Our methods for dealing with urgent and non-urgent illnesses differ. In the latter it is not very important whether the diagnosis is made to-day or to-morrow and so there is time to consider every detail. In the urgent case, however, a diagnosis must be made at once. We must recognise what matters at the moment and there is rarely time to appeal to special diagnostic methods.

When events are moving fast, it is the physician who is deeply versed in the natural history of disease who is likely to be of the greatest service to the patient in peril of his life. In the words of Professor J. A. Ryle, ' Eyes without the microscope, ears without the stethoscope, wits without the help of chemistry and radiology, not that we should deny ourselves the proper use of these, can often carry us a long way.' In an emergency they may have to carry us the whole way.

Another important aspect of emergencies which it behoves us to remember is the anxiety of the patient and his relatives. When summoned we should go at once, preserving the equanimity which Osler taught us to cultivate, yet avoiding the bustle and bounce against which Trotter warned us. Our attitude should be one of alertness in diagnosis, safety in treatment and care in what we say.

With these principles in mind I started some years ago to prepare statements on the treatment of the acute and urgent illnesses which came my way. I had found that clear and concise instructions on what to do in these emergencies were scattered amongst the sections on general therapeutics in medical text books.

When I reviewed my notes with a view to publication it was apparent that I could not hope to deal adequately with all aspects of the subject. I therefore sought the help of colleagues in the various fields of medicine. Our aim has been to provide information as accurate and explicit as possible for the practitioner and hospital physician faced with an acutely ill patient or a critical situation. As a mere list of treatments would be dull, some discussion has been included on diagnosis and the principles on which treatment is based. Details are given of important practical points such as where the rarer drugs may be obtained, and the telephone numbers which might be needed in an emergency. References to original work have been included only in a few special instances.

LONDON, 1948   C. ALLAN BIRCH

Acknowledgement

THE illustration, 'Colours for Medical Gas Cylinders', which appears facing page 68, is reproduced from BS 1319 : 1955 by permission of the British Standards Institution, 2 Park Street, London WIA 2BS.

Note on SI Units

TRADITIONAL and SI units are given in the text, since this edition appears when the change over to SI units is not completed everywhere. It is hoped that the period when both units are in use will be short, but to help the reader who may be uncomfortable with SI units and also to facilitate the reading of articles written before 1975 conversion factors are given in the table reproduced, slightly altered, by kind permission, from *Practical Paediatric Problems,* 4th edition, 1975, by Professor J. H. Hutchison, CBE, MD, London: Lloyd-Luke. Alternatively nomograms can be used.

The SI system (*Système International d'Unités*) was recommended in 1960 by the General Conference of Weights and Measures. It is based on seven fundamental units: metre, kilogram, second, ampère, kelvin, candela and mole. In it the new unit for chemical measurement is the mole (mol). Strictly this is the amount of a substance which contains as many atoms as 0.012 kg of carbon 12. In practice

$$a \ mole = \frac{Weight \ in \ grams}{Molecular \ weight \ (MW)}$$

The unit of volume in SI units is the cubic metre but as this is so large the litre or cubic decimetre is used in clinical chemistry. The old term 'mg per 100 ml' (often erroneously stated as 'mg per cent') becomes mg/dl.

For many measurements the amounts will be expressed in millimoles per litre (mmol/l). For convenience other fractions or multiples of the basic unit have been defined.

Factor	Name	Symbol
10^{12}	tera-	T
10^{9}	giga-	G
10^{6}	mega-	M
10^{3}	kilo-	k
10^{2}	hecto-	h
10^{1}	deca-	da
10^{-1}	deci-	d
10^{-2}	centi-	c
10^{-3}	milli-	m
10^{-6}	micro	μ
10^{-9}	nano	n
10^{-12}	pico	p
10^{-15}	femto	f
10^{-18}	atto	a

Measurements of plasma electrolytes are already expressed in SI units, for example, plasma sodium 140 mmol/l, and these will not alter but because the molecular weight of glucose is 180 a blood glucose of 180 mg/100 ml becomes 10 mmol/l. For bilirubin it is assumed that it is unconjugated and has a MW of 585 but as, by convention, it is desirable to use units resulting in numerical values between 0.1 and $1\,000$ the micromol is used instead of the mmol to produce a normal range of about $1-20\mu$mol/l.

Although there is a recommendation to express haemoglobin in SI units it will probably remain g/dl, with red cells as 10^{12}/l (instead of 10^{3}/mm^3), conversion factor 10^{6}. PCV (haematocrit) is no longer given as a percentage but as a ratio of two measurements. Thus 40 per cent becomes 0.40 (conversion factor 0.01).

For the present, column measurements (BP and CVP) will continue to be stated in mmHg and cm water. When conversion is required 1 mmHg equals 133 pascals and 1 cm water equals 98 pascals.

pH is not excluded by the SI system and since it is on a logarithmic scale it cannot be simply converted by a factor to hydrogen ion concentration in litres of solution. It may be retained until it is decided to adopt reporting H ion concentration in mmol/l.

The reporting of enzyme activity is not altered by the adoption of SI units. The recommended convention at present is units/l.

Drugs are prescribed in mass units but when estimated in body fluids in the laboratory the result is generally expressed in SI units although the precise convention is not completely agreed.

Proteins and materials of uncertain molecular weight are expressed as mass concentrations per litre, i.e. g/l (not mg/100 ml). To convert mg/100 ml to mmol/l we divide by the molecular weight and multiply by 10.

Some easily remembered approximate factors to convert SI units back to traditional units are:

    urea, multiply by 6
    calcium, multiply by 4
    glucose, multiply by 18.

For other conversions the table should be consulted or a pocket converter such as the one issued by St Thomas' Hospital or used by Ciba Laboratories.

Conversion Factors for SI Units

	MW	FROM SI UNITS	TO SI UNITS
mino-acid			
nitrogen	14·01		
Plasma		mmol/l × 1·401 = mg/dl	mg/dl × 0·714 = mmol/l
Urine		mmol/24 hr × 14·01 = mg/24 hr	mg/24 hr × 0·0714 = mmol/24 hr
mmonium	17·03	μmol/l × 1·703 = μg/dl	μg/dl × 0·587 = μmol/l
arbiturate	184·2	μmol/l × 0·0184 = mg/dl	mg/dl × 54·29 = μmol/l
ilirubin	584·7	μmol/l × 0·0585 = mg/dl	mg/dl × 17·1 = μmol/l
alcium	40·08		
Plasma		mmol/l × 4·008 = mg/dl	mg/dl × 0·250 = mmol/l
Urine		mmol/24 hr × 40·08 = mg/24 hr	mg/24 hr × 0·0250 = mmol/24 hr
atecholamines			
(Urine)	183·2	μmol/24 hr × 183 = μg/24 hr	μg/24 hr × 0·00546 = μmol/24 hr
holesterol	386·7	mmol/l × 38·7 = mg/dl	mg/dl × 0·0259 = mmol/l
opper	63·54		
Plasma		μmol/l × 6·35 = μg/dl	μg/dl × 0·157 = μmol/l
Urine		μmol/24 hr × 63·5 = μg/24 hr	μg/24 hr × 0·0157 = μmol/24 hr
ortisol	362·5	nmol/l × 0·0362 = μg/dl	μgdl/ × 27·6 = nmol/24 hr
reatinine	113·1		
Plasma		μmol/l × 0·0113 = mg/dl	mg/dl × 88·4 = μmol/l
Urine		mmol/24 hr × 0·113 = g/24 hr	g/24 hr × 8·84 = mmol/24 hr
thanol (Alcohol)	46·07	mmol/l × 4·607 = mg/dl	mg/dl × 0·217 = mmol/l
at (Faecal) (as			
stearic acid)	284·5	mmol/24 hr × 0·284 = g/24 hr	g/24 hr × 3·52 = mmol/24 hr
brinogen	Uncertain	g/l × 100 = mg/dl	mg/dl × 0·01 = g/l
lucose	180·2		
Blood or Plasma		mmol/l × 18·02 = mg/dl	mg/dl × 0·0555 = mmol/l
Urine		mmol/l × 0·0180 = g/dl	g/dl × 55·5 = mmol/l
CSF		as for blood or plasma	as for blood or plasma
MMA (or VMA)			
(Urine)	198·2	μmol/24 hr × 0·198 = mg/24 hr	mg/24 hr × 5·05 = μmol/24 hr
ydroxyproline			
(Urine)	131·1	mmol/24 hr × 131·1 = mg/24 hr	mg/24 hr × 0·00763 = mmol/24 hr

Conversion Factors for SI Units—contd.

	MW	FROM SI UNITS	TO SI UNITS
Iron and TIBC (Total Iron Binding Capacity)	55·85	μmol/l $\times$ 5·59 = μg/dl	μg/dl $\times$ 0·179 = μmol/l
Lead	207·2		
Blood		μmol/l $\times$ 20·7 = μg/dl	μg/dl $\times$ 0·0483 = μmol/l
Urine		μmol/24 hr $\times$ 207 = μg/24 hr	μg/24 hr $\times$ 0·00483 = μmol/24 hr
Magnesium	24·31		
Plasma		mmol/l $\times$ 2·43 = mg/dl	mg/dl $\times$ 0·411 = mmol/l
Urine		mmol/24 hr $\times$ 24·3 = mg/24 hr	mg/24 hr $\times$ 0·0411 = mmol/24 hr
Oestriol (Urine)	288·4	μmol/24 hr $\times$ 0·288 = mg/24 hr	mg/24 hr $\times$ 3·47 = μmol/24 hr
Phenylalanine	165·2	μmol/l $\times$ 0·0165 = mg/dl	mg/dl $\times$ 60·5 = μmol/l
Phosphate	30·97		
Serum		mmol/l $\times$ 3·10 = mg/dl	mg/dl $\times$ 0·323 = mmol/l
Urine		mmol/24 hr $\times$ 0·0310 = g/24 hr	g/24 hr $\times$ 32·3 = mmol/24 hr
Pregnanediol (Urine)	320·5	μmol/24 hr $\times$ 0·320 = mg/24 hr	mg/24 hr $\times$ 3·12 = μmol/24 hr
Pregnanetriol (Urine)	336·5	μmol/24 hr $\times$ 0·336 = mg/24 hr	mg/24 hr $\times$ 2·97 = μmol/24 hr
Protein	Uncertain	g/l $\times$ 0·1 = g/dl	g/dl $\times$ 10 = g/l
Serum			
Albumin	Uncertain	g/l $\times$ 0·1 = g/dl	g/dl $\times$ 10 = g/l
CSF Protein	Uncertain	g/l $\times$ 100 = mg/dl	mg/dl $\times$ 0·01 = g/l
Protein-bound Iodine	126·9	nmol/l $\times$ 0·0127 = μg/dl	μg/dl/78·8 = nmol/l
Salicylate	138·1	mmol/l $\times$ 13·81 = mg/dl	mg/dl $\times$ 0·0724 = mmol/l
17-Ketosteroids (Urine) (as de-hydroepiandrosterone)	288·4	μmol/24 hr $\times$ 0·288 = mg/24 hr	mg/24 hr $\times$ 3·47 = μmol/24 hr
Thyroxine	776·9	nmol/l $\times$ 0·0777 = μg/dl	μg/dl $\times$ 12·87 = nmol/l
Triiodothyronine	651·01	nmol/l $\times$ 0·651 = ng/dl	ng/dl $\times$ 1·54 = nmol/l
Triglyceride (as triolein)	885·4	mmol/l $\times$ 88·5 = mg/dl	mg/dl $\times$ 0·0113 = mmol/l
Urate (uric acid)			
Plasma	168·1	mmol/l $\times$ 16·81 = mg/dl	mg/dl $\times$ 0·0595 = mmol/l
Urea	60·06	mmol/l $\times$ 6·01 = mg/dl	mg/dl $\times$ 0·166 = mmol/l
Po$_2$, Pco$_2$	—	kPa $\times$ 7·52 = mmHg	mmHg $\times$ 0·133 = kPa

Contributors

THOMAS H. BEWLEY, M.A., M.D.(Dublin), F.R.C.P.(Ireland), Consultant Psychiatrist, Drug Dependence Treatment Units, St George's, St Thomas's and Tooting Bec Hospital Groups.

DRUG DEPENDENCE

C. ALLAN BIRCH, M.D.(L'pool), F.R.C.P.(Lond.), D.P.H., D.C.H. Honorary Consulting Physician, Chase Farm Hospital, Enfield, Middlesex.

ACUTE POISONING
THE HAZARDS OF MEDICAL PROCEDURES
ACUTE (NON-SURGICAL) ABDOMINAL CATASTROPHES
OTHER (NON-SURGICAL) ABDOMINAL EMERGENCIES
FITS, FAINTS AND UNCONSCIOUSNESS
BITES AND STINGS AND MISCELLANEOUS
    EMERGENCIES
MEDICO-LEGAL AND OTHER NON-CLINICAL
    EMERGENCIES
POST-OPERATIVE MEDICAL EMERGENCIES
    (with Gillian C. Hanson)
SOME PRACTICAL PROCEDURES

J. W. CHEETHAM, O.B.E., M.D.(L'pool), M.R.C.S.(Eng.), L.R.C.P.(Lond.). General Practitioner, Widnes, Merseyside.

THE EMERGENCY BAG AND CUPBOARD

LEWIS CITRON, M.B., B.S.(London), D.L.O., F.R.C.S.(Eng.). Consultant Oto-laryngologist, Enfield District Hospital, Enfield, Middlesex; late Scientific Assistant, Otological Research Unit, Medical Research Council, National Hospital, Queen Square, London.

EMERGENCIES IN EAR, NOSE AND THROAT DISEASE

GEOFFREY DIXON, M.B., B.S.(London), Ph.D.(London), F.R.C.P.(Ed.), F.R.C.O.G. Professor of Obstetrics and Gynaecology, University of Bristol.

MEDICAL EMERGENCIES IN OBSTETRICS AND
GYNAECOLOGY

xiii

J. H. DOBREE, M.S.(Lond.), F.R.C.S.(Eng.), D.O.(Oxon.).
Surgeon to the Eye Department, St Bartholomew's Hospital, London, and to the North Middlesex Hospital, Edmonton, London.
OPHTHALMIC EMERGENCIES

DAVID FERRIMAN, D.M.(Oxon.),, F.R.C.P.(Lond.).
Physician, Regional Endocrine Centre, North Middlesex and Prince of Wales' Hospitals, London.
MEDICAL EMERGENCIES IN OTHER ENDOCRINE DISORDERS

H. J. GOLDSMITH, M.D.(Lond.), M.D.(New York), F.R.C.P.
Consultant Physician, United Liverpool Hospitals; Nephrologist, Liverpool Regional Urological Centre, Sefton General Hospital, Liverpool.
MEDICAL EMERGENCIES IN RENAL DISEASE

J. F. GOODWIN, M.D.(Lond.), F.R.C.P., F.A.C.C.
Professor of Clinical Cardiology, Royal Postgraduate Medical School; Consultant Physician, Hammersmith Hospital, London.
CARDIOVASCULAR EMERGENCIES

GILLIAN C. HANSON, M.B., B.S.(Lond.), M.R.C.P.(Lond.)
Consultant Physician, Whipps Cross Hospital, Leytonstone, London.
RESUSCITATION
POST-OPERATIVE MEDICAL EMERGENCIES
(with C. Allan Birch)

J. M. HARRINGTON, M.Sc., M.B.(London), M.R.C.P.
Lecturer in Occupational Medicine, T.U.C. Centenary Institute of Occupational Health, London School of Hygiene and Tropical Medicine, Keppel Street (Gower Street), London.
EMERGENCIES IN OCCUPATIONAL MEDICINE
(with R. S. F. Schilling)

Group Captain PETER HOWARD, O.B.E., Ph.D., M.B., B.S., (London), M.R.C.P., F.R.Ae.Soc., R.A.F.
Consultant Adviser in Aviation Physiology, Royal Air Force, R.A.F. Institute of Aviation Medicine, Farnborough, Hants.
MEDICAL EMERGENCIES IN THE AIR

J. H. HUTCHISON, C.B.E., F.R.S.E., M.D., F.R.C.P.(Lond., Edin., Glasg.), F.A.C.P.(Hon.).
Samson Gemmell Professor of Child Health, The University of Glasgow; Visiting Physician, Royal Hospital for Sick Children, Glasgow; Consultant Paediatrician, Queen Mother's Hospital, Glasgow.
MEDICAL EMERGENCIES IN INFANCY AND CHILDHOOD

R. E. IRVINE, M.A., M.D.(Cantab.), F.R.C.P.(Lond.).
Consulting Physician, Geriatric Unit, Hastings.
GERIATRIC EMERGENCIES
(with Theodore Strouthidis)

D. MacG. JACKSON, M.A., M.D.(Cantab.), F.R.C.S.(Eng.).
Surgeon in Charge, Medical Research Council, Burns Unit, Birmingham Accident Hospital and Rehabilitation Centre, Bath Row, Birmingham.
BURNS

W. J. JENKINS, M.D.(Wales), F.R.C.Path., Medical Director, North East Thames Blood Transfusion Service, Brentwood, Essex.
THE HAZARDS OF BLOOD TRANSFUSIONS

Sir FRANCIS AVERY JONES, C.B.E., M.D.(Lond.), M.D.(Melbourne), F.R.C.P.(Lond.).
Consulting Physician, Department of Gastroenterology, Central Middlesex Hospital, London, N.W.10; Consultant in Gastroenterology, St Mark's Hospital, London and to the Royal Navy.
HAEMATEMESIS AND MELAENA

LEON KAUFMAN, M.D.(Edin.), F.F.A.R.C.S.
Consultant Anaesthetist to University College Hospital and St Mark's Hospital, London.
EMERGENCIES DURING ANAESTHESIA

BERTRAM M. MANDELBROTE, B.Sc., M.A.(Oxon.), M.B., Ch.B.(Capetown), F.R.C.P.(Lond.), F.R.C.Psych., D.P.M.
Physician Superintendent, Littlemore Hospital, Oxford; Consultant Psychiatrist, Oxfordshire Regional Health Authority (Teaching); Clinical Lecturer in Psychiatry, University of Oxford.
PSYCHIATRIC EMERGENCIES

JOHN E. MacIVER, M.D.(Cantab.), F.R.C.Path.
Honorary Lecturer, Department of Clinical Haematology, University of Manchester; Consultant Haematologist, United Manchester Hospitals.
EMERGENCIES IN BLOOD DISEASES

G. DONALD W. McKENDRICK, M.A., B.M.(Oxon.), F.R.C.P.
Physician, St Ann's Hospital, London and Rush Green Hospital, Essex; Lecturer in Infectious Diseases to The Middlesex Hospital, St Bartholomew's Hospital and the London School of Hygiene and Tropical Medicine.
EMERGENCIES IN INFECTIOUS DISEASES

COLIN OGILVIE, M.D.(L'pool), F.R.C.P.
Consultant Physician, The Royal Infirmary, The Regional Cardio-thoracic Surgical Centre and The Regional Cardiac Centre, Liverpool. Lecturer in Clinical Medicine, the University of Liverpool.
RESPIRATORY EMERGENCIES

Surgeon Captain P. J. PRESTON, O.B.E., F.R.C.P.(London), D.T.M.&H., R.N.
Professor of Naval Medicine, Royal Naval Hospital, Haslar, Gosport, Hants.
MEDICAL EMERGENCIES AT SEA

DAVID PYKE, M.D.(Cantab.), F.R.C.P.
Physician in Charge, Diabetic Department, King's College Hospital, London.
MEDICAL EMERGENCIES IN DIABETES

BRIAN RUSSELL, M.D.(Lond.), F.R.C.P.(Lond.), D.P.H.
Consulting Physician, The Skin Department, The London Hospital, London; Consulting Physician, St John's Hospital for Diseases of the Skin.
EMERGENCIES IN SKIN DISEASE

R. S. F. SCHILLING, C.B.E., M.D.(London), D.Sc., F.R.C.P., D.P.H., D.I.H
Professor of Occupational Health, University of London, Director of T.U.C. Centenary Institute of Occupational Health, London School of Hygiene and Tropical Medicine, Keppel Street (Gower Street), London.
EMERGENCIES IN OCCUPATIONAL MEDICINE
(with J. M. Harrington)

D. R. SEATON, M.B.(Cantab.), F.R.C.P.(Lond.), D.T.M.
Consultant Physician for Tropical Diseases, Liverpool Royal Infirmary; Consultant Physician to the Ministry of Overseas Development; Clinical Lecturer, Liverpool School of Tropical Medicine.

EMERGENCIES IN TROPICAL MEDICINE

JOHN A SIMPSON, M.D.(Glasg.), F.R.C.P.(Lond.), F.R.C.P. (Edin.), F.R.C.P. (Glasg.), F.R.S.Ed.
Professor of Neurology, University of Glasgow; Physician-in-Charge, Department of Neurology, Institute of Neurological Sciences, Southern General Hospital, Glasgow, GS1 4TF.
Consultant in Neurology, Western Infirmary, Glasgow; Consultant in Neurology to the Army in Scotland.

NEUROLOGICAL EMERGENCIES

MARGARET D. SNELLING, M.B., B.S.(Lond.), F.R.C.P.(Lond.), F.R.C.S.(Eng.), F.R.C.R.
Deputy Director of the Meyerstein Institute of Radiology, The Middlesex Hospital, London.

EMERGENCIES RESULTING FROM NUCLEAR AND ALLIED RADIATION

MARTIN SMITH, M.A., M.B.(Cantab.), M.R.C.P.
Senior Medical Registrar,* The Liver Unit, King's College Hospital, London.

HEPATIC COMA AND PRECOMA
(with Roger Williams)

THEODORE STROUTHIDIS, M.B.(Alexandria), L.M.S.S.A., M.R.C.P.(Lond.).
Consulting Physician (Geriatrics), Hastings Group Hospitals.

GERIATRIC EMERGENCIES
(with R. E. Irvine)

ROGER WILLIAMS, M.D.(London), F.R.C.P.
Director of the Liver Unit and Consultant Physician, King's College Hospital, London.

HEPATIC COMA AND PRECOMA
(with M. G. M. Smith)

* Now Consultant Physician, St Luke's Hospital, Guildford.

Contents

CHAPTER 1

The Emergency Bag and Cupboard

' Have also another bag ready to hand for journeys, simply pre-pared and handy too by method of arrangement.' Hippocrates. De decenti habitu. *Opera Medicorum Graecorum.* ed. Kühn 1825. Vol. 21, page 72.

Every practitioner who is liable to be called in an emergency should have ready for immediate use an ' emergency bag.' Whether it is a combined medical and surgical bag will depend on the doctor and his type of practice. Some doctors prefer two bags, one for common emergencies and the other to hold drugs and appliances which are only needed occasionally. Many will want a ' midder bag ' also. As experience and skill are at least as important as the contents of the bag, only the drugs and equipment with whose use he is familiar should be included (see also Identification of Tablets, p. 693). The following list was made of the drugs actually carried by several practitioners and from it a personal selection can be made. This should be checked regularly and out-of-date drugs replaced. The contents of the bag should be checked periodically. Regulation 14 of the Misuse of Drugs Regulations 1973 makes it necessary to enter in the controlled drugs register every quantity of morphine (includ-ing Cyclimorph) and pethidine obtained and every quantity supplied or administered to a patient.

DRUGS

Cardio-respiratory and diuretic

Injections

Aminophylline Injection 250 mg in 10 ml amps.
Nikethamide Injection 2·0 ml amps.
Adrenaline Injection 0·5 ml amps.
Lignocaine Hydrochloride Injection 2 per cent in 20 ml vials.
Digoxin Injection 0·5 mg in 2 ml.
Frusemide (Lasix) 20 mg in 2 ml amps.
Practolol (Eraldin) 5 ml amps of 2 mg/ml.

Tablets

Digoxin 0·25 mg.
Glyceryl trinitrate 0·5 mg.
Quinidine sulphate 200 mg.

1

Propranolol (Inderal) 40 mg.
Isoprenaline sulphate 20 mg.
Ephedrine 30 mg.
Frusemide (Lasix) 40 mg
Bendrofluazide 2·5 mg.
Ventolin (Salbutanol) inhaler.

Analgesics

Injections
Morphine Sulphate Injection 20 mg.
   or Cyclimorph 15 mg in 1 ml.
Pentazocine (Fortral) 30 mg in 1 ml.
Pethidine Injection 100 mg in 2 ml.

Tablets
Pethidine 50 mg.
Paracetamol 500 mg.

Antibiotics

Injections
Benzylpenicillin 500 000 unit vials.
Triplopen (benethamine penicillin G) single dose vials.
Ampicillin (Penbritin) 500 mg.
Erythromycin (Erythrocin i m) 100 mg in 2 ml.
Tetracycline (Tetracyn) 100 mg.

Tablets
Tetracycline (Tetracyn) 250 mg.
Erythromycin 250 mg.
Co-trimoxazole (Bactrim. Septrin).
Ampicillin (Penbritin) 250 mg capsules.
Ceporex 250 mg.

Steroids

Injections
Hydrocortisone (Efcortesol) 100 mg in 1 ml.
Corticotrophin (ACTH) 40 i u per ml × 5 ml vials.

Tablets
Prednisolone 5 mg.

Antispasmodics
Atropine Sulphate Injection 1 mg in 1 ml.

Sedatives and anticonvulsants

Injections

Paraldehyde 10 ml amps.
Phenobarbitone Injection 200 mg.
Brietal (methohexitone) 50 ml amps (500 mg).
 or Epontol (propanidid) 10 ml amps (500 mg). *These short-acting anaesthetics must only be used when there are means at hand for intubation and inflation of the lungs.*
Diazepam (Valium) 10 mg in 2 ml.
Haloperidol (Serenace) 5 mg in 1 ml.
Promazine (Sparine) 100 mg in 2 ml.

Tablets

Phenobarbitone 30 mg.
Butobarbitone (Soneryl) 100 mg.
Diazepam (Valium) 5 mg.
Chlormethiazole (Heminevrin) 0·5 g.

Anti-emetics

Injections

Promazine Injection (Sparine) 50 mg in 1 ml.
Cyclizine (Valoid) 50 mg in 1 ml.

Hypotensives

Diazoxide (Eudemine) 300 mg in 20 ml.

Vasopressors

Metaraminol (Aramine) 10 mg in 1 ml (for i m use).

Anticoagulants

Heparin Injection 5 000 units per ml.

Haemostatic

Epsikapron (aminocaproic acid) 0·4 g per ml.

Antidotes

Levallorphan Injection 5 mg in 5 ml.
Naloxone (Narcan) 0·4 mg in 1 ml.
Protamine Sulphate Injection 50 mg in 5 ml.
Phytomenadione (vitamin K) 10 mg in 1 ml.
Desferrioxamine (Desferal) 500 mg vials.
Activated carbon powder (' Carbon 315 ') (see p. 28).

Drugs for migraine and vertigo

Injections
Ergotamine Injection (Fermergin) 0·5 mg in 1 ml.
Prochlorperazine (Stemetil) 12·5 mg in 1 ml.
Suppositories
Cafergot.
Prochlorperazine (Stemetil) 5 and 25 mg.

Antihistamines

Injections
Promethazine Hydrochloride Injection (Phenergan) 25 mg in 1 ml.
Chlorpheniramine (Piriton) 10 mg in 1 ml.
Tablets
Piriton 4 mg.
Phenergan 25 mg.

For diabetes

Insulin Injection 40 units per ml.
Dextrose Injection 50 per cent 50 ml amps.
Glucagon Injection 1 mg.

Eye preparations (preferably in individual dose containers)
Amethocaine Eye-drops 1 per cent.
Homatropine Eye-drops 2 per cent.
Pilocarpine Eye-drops 1 per cent.
Betamethasone drops (Betnesol).
Gentamicin (Genticin) drops.
Fluorescein impregnated filter paper.
Chloramphenicol Eye Ointment 1 per cent.
Acetazolamide Injection (Diamox) 500 mg vial.
Acetazolamide (Diamox) tablets 250 mg.
Mydricaine (see p. 534).

Miscellaneous

Ergometrine 0·5 mg in 1 ml.
Calcium gluconate (Calcium Sandoz) 10 g/dl amps.
Micralax or similar enemas.
Bisacodyl (Dulcolax) suppositories 5 and 10 mg.
Water for Injection, 2 ml amps.

Paediatric mixtures

Chloral Elixir Paediatric, BPC.
Belladonna Mixture Paediatric, BPC.

Alupent (orciprenaline) syrup 10 mg in 5 ml.
Lomotil (diphenoxylate) liquid.
Single dose sachets of Ampicillin (125 mg) and Erythromycin (100 mg).

Anaesthetics
Lignocaine Hydrochloride Injection 1 per cent.
Ether, chloroform or vinyl ether (Vinesthene) for open inhalation.

APPLIANCES

The choice is a very personal one but most doctors will carry a stethoscope, sphygmomanometer, ophthalmoscope, auriscope and two thermometers (ordinary and low reading) in their bag. Other instruments should be in a separate bag such as catheters, stomach tubes and other instruments needed for gastric lavage. A Resusciade (p. 733) or a Brook (p. 733) or Salad (p. 733) airway should be carried as well as mediswabs, material for suturing and a variety of dressings.

THE 'MIDDER' BAG

Although in Britain the days of heroic obstetrics in the home have gone the family doctor should still carry the forceps of his choice, suturing equipment and perhaps a dextran giving set. A Blease-Simpson infant resuscitator and sucker is a wise addition. The drugs are a matter of choice but most would carry Valium (diazepam), ergometrine, pitocin and vitamin K.

Four non-medical items will on occasion prove very helpful: some 2p pieces for emergency phone calls, a street map of the district and a magnifying glass, and a four-pound hammer (to gain access to a patient collapsed in the lavatory).

THE EMERGENCY CUPBOARD

Many more drugs than those listed above will generally be kept in the emergency cupboard and 'MAY DAY' or resuscitation boxes which most hospitals maintain. They are chiefly those mentioned in Chapter 10 on Cardiovascular Emergencies and Chapter 32 on Practical Procedures. The doctor should make himself familiar with the contents of the cupboard and always leave a note in it of anything he removes. Although it is rarely necessary because of mental disorder to detain compulsorily a patient already in hospital, this can be done under Section 30 of the Mental Health Act, 1959. Form 6 for this purpose should be kept in the cupboard.

J. W. CHEETHAM

CHAPTER 2

Resuscitation

THE aim of resuscitation is to maintain in equilibrium or to restore vital physiological functions, especially those of circulation and respiration.

The emergencies calling for resuscitation are circulatory, respiratory and metabolic. Some are considered elsewhere in the book and relevant pages are indicated below.

CIRCULATORY EMERGENCIES

Cardiac arrest (see also pp. 724-730).
Shock (see also bacteraemic, endotoxic and Gram negative shock) p. 428.
anaphylactic shock p. 81.
shock from burns p. 554.
cardiogenic shock p. 238.

RESPIRATORY EMERGENCIES

Intermittent positive pressure ventilation (IPPV).

METABOLIC AND BIOCHEMICAL EMERGENCIES

Acute ionic changes.
Water depletion (p. 607).
Sodium depletion and intoxication (p. 605).
Abnormalities of acid-base balance (p. 615).
Metabolic acidosis (p. 194).
Metabolic alkalosis (p. 194).
Fluid and electrolyte disturbance (p. 602).
Potassium depletion (pp. 148, 344, 602).
Potassium intoxication (pp. 379, 605).

CIRCULATORY EMERGENCIES

Cardiac resuscitation depends on the prompt and effective management of cardiac arrest. This is the sudden cessation of effective heart action resulting in failure to maintain adequate oxygenation of the brain and other vital organs. Restoration of cardiac output is essential within four minutes (or less in already hypoxic subjects) if irreversible brain damage is to be prevented. Circulatory arrest and its step by step management is described on pp. 724 *et seq.*

Factors precipitating cardiac arrest

Many factors precipitate cardiac arrest and awareness of these may help to prevent it. They are

1. HEART DISEASE. The incidence of cardiac arrest is greater among patients who have heart disease. It is important therefore to monitor such patients when they are subject to further stress. Ventricular fibrillation is generally preceded by short bursts of arrhythmia.

2. PULMONARY EMBOLISM. See p. 241.

3. CARDIAC TAMPONADE. See p. 248.

4. MYOCARDITIS.

5. SURGERY. A third of all arrests occur during abdominal operations and a sixth during chest and heart operations. Many factors may be involved including hypotension, hypothermia, hypoxia, metabolic imbalance and the effect of the anaesthetic itself.

6. DRUGS. Certain drugs may cause arrest either through a hypersensitivity mechanism (quinidine) or by myocardial suppression through overdosage. A diseased heart may be suppressed by moderate dosage. Elimination may be impaired as in renal or hepatic failure. Digitalis, procainamide, Largactil and barbiturates all have myocardial suppressant qualities (see also p. 320). Thiazide diuretics may precipitate hypokalaemia thereby inducing digoxin toxicity. Mono-amine oxidase inhibitors (p. 565) may precipitate ventricular fibrillation when used with certain nervous stimulants, potent analgesics or after eating amine-rich food, e.g. cheese.

7. METABOLIC AND ELECTROLYTE DISTURBANCES. Calcium and potassium ions in correct intracellular and extracellular concentrations are essential for normal myocardial contractility. Rapid changes in the concentration of these ions may also precipitate cardiac arrest. Hyperkalaemia may be increased by an associated respiratory acidosis and this may be sufficient to induce cardiac arrest. Digoxin toxicity is accentuated by hypercalaemia. Calcium should never be used in resuscitation if digoxin excess is suspected (p. 88).

8. SHOCK AND TRAUMA. Shock may lead to hypoxia, poor peripheral perfusion and consequent lactic acid acidosis. Cardiac contusion may occur with chest trauma.

9. HYPOXIA. This is a common factor leading to cardiac arrest.

10. VISCERAL REFLEXES. Autonomic reflexes set off by the vagus may cause cardiac arrest. The stimulus can be external as in anal dilatation or internal as in urethral catheterisation or traction on the gall bladder. Atropine will prevent such reflexes.

ELECTROCUTION

Cardiac arrest from electrocution is usually due to faulty equipment or carelessness (pp. 648 and 726).

Table 2.1. *Measurements used in the evaluation of shock.*

FUNCTION ASSESSED	MEASUREMENT
Renal function	Urine volume per hour.
	U/P osmolality ratio prior to diuretic therapy.
	Response to i v mannitol (in the presence of oliguria and a normal central venous pressure).
Dynamic blood volume	Central venous pressure.
Cardiac output	Pulse pressure.
Peripheral circulation	Skin and rectal temperature differential.
Metabolic and respiratory status	Blood gas analysis. pH and acid-base status.
Blood coagulation	Fibrinogen titre.
	Prothrombin time.
	Kaolin partial thromboplastin time.
	Thrombin time.
	Platelet count.

SHOCK

The shock state is a complex interelated set of physiologic, haemodynamic, microcirculatory and biochemical derangements initiated by one or more events. The combination of these and the reaction of the body to stress leads to the clinical syndrome of shock. It is characterised by arterial hypotension and tachycardia with subsequent deterioration in perfusion of the vital organs and the skin (see Table 2.1).

HAEMODYNAMIC ASSESSMENT. It is essential to decide which haemodynamic components are involved. Assessment should be made of the cardiac function, the dynamic blood volume and the state of the microcirculation.

ASSESSMENT OF CARDIAC FUNCTION. Cardiogenic shock is discussed on p. 238. Non-cardiac pathology such as hypovolaemia and endotoxaemia can affect cardiac output and it is therefore important to assess myocardial function in all forms of shock. The pulse pressure reflects cardiac output; the central venous pressure (p. 751) is an indicator of the volume of blood returning to the right atrium and also reflects right ventricular function.

ASSESSMENT OF DYNAMIC BLOOD VOLUME. It is very important in the restoration of blood pressure to ensure that the dynamic blood volume is normal. A central venous pressure (CVP) line (p. 751) with the tip in the right atrium is essential in the management of severe shock (p. 12). Sequential changes in the CVP are more important than the initial reading. A CVP reading of less than 2 cm water, read at the mid-thoracic level, reflects a decreased volume of blood returning to the heart. Levels higher than 16 cm water imply cardiac failure. The CVP is used as an indicator of the ability of the cardiovascular system to handle increasing intravascular volume. When the CVP begins to rise rapidly with the administration of measured increments of fluid the limits of cardiovascular competence have been reached. Pulmonary artery pressure may increase before the CVP when left heart failure develops (Hardaway et al., 1967). Evidence of left heart failure is an indication to stop infusion whatever the CVP. For this reason, provided the systolic blood pressure is 100 mm Hg or above, it is wise to keep the CVP at 3-4 cm H_2O.

In more sophisticated conditions other measurements may be used to assess the dynamic blood volume. These include blood volume and cardiac output studies and monitoring of the pulmonary artery wedge pressure. Radio-isotope assessment of blood volume in shock is not reliable and the more elaborate monitoring systems take time to set up and analyse. Shock from whatever cause requires urgent treatment and can generally be satisfactorily managed using the simpler techniques.

ASSESSMENT OF THE MICROCIRCULATION. Temperature as measured from the medial aspect of the great toe (using a surface strap-on thermister probe) indicates the adequacy of the peripheral circulation. A rapidly falling toe temperature is a bad prognostic sign. If it is less than 27°C and the difference between toe and ambient temperature less than 2°C the likelihood of death is high (Joly and

Weil, 1969). A skin temperature widely divergent from the rectal figure also implies severe peripheral vasoconstriction. Rectal and toe temperature readings may give a serial guide as to the efficacy of peripheral vasodilator therapy (Ross *et al.*, 1969). Blood gas analysis is a guide to the state of the pulmonary microcirculation and the degree of metabolic acidosis is an indication of the severity in reduction of peripheral perfusion.

In severe shock it is essential to assess the coagulation components since poor peripheral perfusion is generally associated with hyper-coagulation. This phase may pass into one of hypocoagulability which, particularly in obstetric and endotoxic shock, may lead to fatal haemorrhage. Thrombocytopenia frequently occurs in septic shock and should not be used as the only indication of a coagulation abnormality. Other clotting indices which may be used are shown in Table 2.1.

Renal function reflects splanchnic organ flow. A deterioration in renal function generally shows as oliguria. An assessment of the urine/plasma osmolality ratio is a valuable diagnostic aid in the management of shock associated with a fall in urine volume (see Table 2.2).

Table 2.2. *Differential diagnosis of oliguria.*
(*see also p.* 372)

TEST	DEHYDRATION	POOR RENAL PERFUSION	ACUTE RENAL FAILURE
U/P osmolality ratio	2·7-4·0	2·0-1·3	1·2 or less
U/P urea ratio	20	20-14	10
IV mannitol 0·2 g/kg BW infused over 2-3 minutes			
Urine output	60 ml/hr	40-60 ml/hr	40 ml/hr

Treatment.

1. Place the patient supine.

2. Assess adequacy of ventilation. Give oxygen and if necessary use mechanical ventilation.

3. Assess electrolyte and acid-base status. Take blood for typing and cross matching. Insert a central venous pressure line.

4. Restore the circulating blood volume with the relevant plasma expander and, if possible, correct the acid-base and metabolic status.

The volume of fluid required to re-expand the plasma volume is assessed according to the pulse, blood pressure and CVP. Fluid should be infused until the CVP is within normal limits (5 to 13 cm as measured in the mid-axillary line). Should the CVP be normal and signs of shock remain a further 200 ml of relevant fluid is given over 10 minutes. If the CVP remains the same aliquots of 200 ml of fluid may be given until the CVP rises above 12 cm when the infusion should be stopped. Should shock continue in the presence of a high normal CVP suspect the onset of cardiac failure or an associated factor such as septicaemia (see also p. 751).

5. Should the patient be unconscious observe the urine output by catheterisation (p. 720). Take samples for u/p osmolality ratio and once the CVP is normal and the systolic blood pressure greater than 90 mm Hg give mannitol 0·2 g/kg body weight i v over 2-3 minutes. The u/p osmolality ratio and mannitol infusion test will give a guide as to whether acute intrinsic renal failure has developed. It is very easy to overload an oliguric patient with i v fluids.

Ventilation

Hypoxaemia characteristically occurs in shock and, should it become sufficiently severe, may lead to respiratory depression and consequent hypercarbia. Oxygen therapy should be regulated according to serial blood gas analysis. Should the PaO_2 not rise above 70 mm Hg (9·31 kPa) when oxygen is given via a face mask IPPV should be started. Pre-existing lung pathology may result in a patient having a PaO_2 normally less than 70 mm Hg (9·31 kPa). In such instances he will probably be able to tolerate lower levels of PaO_2 and the decision to ventilate will have to be taken individually.

Metabolic balance

Many patients with poor peripheral perfusion will show a metabolic acidosis. It is important not to overcorrect this since, with restoration of the circulating blood volume, the tendency towards a metabolic acidosis will diminish. Sodium bicarbonate is generally used for correction (p. 727) but if given to excess may lead to sodium overload.

It is wise to correct to a base deficit of 8 on the Astrup analysis according to the formula

(Measured base deficit − 8) × 0·3 × Kg BW = mmol of bicarbonate ions required. (Modified from Astrup, 1961.)

The sodium bicarbonate should be run in over 30 minutes. Further Astrup analyses are made according to the patient's progress, the degree of the original metabolic deficit and the respiratory status (see also p. 616).

Plasma expanders

When there is no severe blood loss or frank metabolic abnormality Dextran 70 has proved to be an excellent blood volume expander (Gruber, 1970). The maximum amount which can be infused in 24 hours is 1·5 g/kg body weight. (Blood should be taken for typing and cross matching before giving Dextran.) Blood should not be given through the same infusion set as Dextran. An extra infusion set (preferably with a warming coil in a water bath heated to 37°C) should be available so that this can be exchanged for the Dextran infusion set should blood be required. In cases of sodium depletion isosmotic sodium chloride solution should be used but it has only a short stay in the circulation. It is of value as a temporary plasma expander in haemorrhagic shock. In other types of shock there is a danger of sodium overload. PPF (plasma protein fraction, p. 796) has the advantage of being free from hepatitis antigen; has the same osmolality as plasma, and an electrolyte content of sodium, 140 to 160 mmol and potassium of 2·2 to 2·4 mmol/litre. This solution has proved to be an excellent plasma expander and will probably replace Dextran 70 except where administration of sodium ions is considered hazardous.

Haemorrhagic shock

The volume of blood lost can generally be correlated with the clinical findings (Table 2.3). Any overt source of bleeding must be controlled by pressure or ligation.

Blood should not be given unless absolutely necessary since there is still a risk of hepatitis even if the blood is Australia antigen (HB_sA_g) negative.

Blood should be as fresh as possible and infused as soon as it has been removed from the blood bank. 2·3 diphosphoglyceric acid (2·3 DPG), a glycolytic intermediate in the red cell, has a potent effect on the carriage of oxygen by haemoglobin. 2·3 DPG may be depleted in old blood and this results in an increase in the haemoglobin affinity for oxygen with consequent reduction in oxygen available for the tissues. Similar changes occur in the presence of a metabolic or respiratory alkalosis, i.e the oxy-haemoglobin dissociation curve is shifted to the left.

When the clinical picture is consistent with blood loss a drip should be set up and the BP and pulse rate recorded every 15 minutes. Blood is rarely needed in **mild shock** and the BP can be restored by Dextran 70. If bleeding continues blood should be given after a full cross match. In **severe shock** two drips should be running —one being the CVP line (which can be used for saline infusions also). In **profound shock** oxygen by a face mask is essential. Intubation and hand ventilation may be needed. Uncrossed matched Group O Rh negative blood should be given rapidly. Two doctors and one nurse are needed. One doctor maintains adequate ventilation (pulmonary aspiration is common in profound shock following gastric haemorrhage) and the other puts up the infusions. The nurse must record the volume and type of fluid infused.

Table 2.3. *Haemorrhagic shock.*

Correlation of the degree of blood loss with clinical findings.

DEGREE	BLOOD LOSS PERCENTAGE OF BLOOD VOLUME	BLOOD PRESSURE SYSTOLIC IN MM HG (BP PREVIOUSLY NORMAL)	SIGNS AND SYMPTOMS
Compensated or preshock	10-15	Normal	Dizziness Palpitation Tachycardia
Mild	15-30	Slight fall	Thirst Tachycardia Weakness Sweating
Moderate	30-35	70-80	Restlessness Pallor Oliguria
Severe	35-40	50-70	Pallor Cyanosis Collapse
Profound	40-50	50	Collapse Air hunger Anuria

Hypothermia is a hazard of rapid transfusion. Blood warming is advisable when blood is given through a central line or when large volumes are given via a peripheral vein. A disposable heat exchanging coil (Plexitron R66) should be used in a temperature controlled water bath. Another hazard is potassium intoxication and to avoid this 10 ml of 10 per cent calcium chloride should be given after every 3 000 ml of blood. Calcium ions replacing potassium ions in the plasma thereby driving potassium ions into the cells. Three packets of fresh frozen plasma should be given after every 5 000 ml of blood to replace labile coagulation factors missing in old blood. The acid-base status should be checked after every 6 000 ml of blood and a base deficit greater than 8 corrected with sodium bicarbonate.

Coagulation defects

After massive transfusion coagulation factors must be checked and relevant deficits replaced. If there is no other cause for haemorrhage other factors such as excess of anticoagulants or deficiency of vitamin K from hepatocellular failure should be considered. Rarer causes are hereditary coagulation defects, thrombocytopenia, hypofibrinogenaemia, disseminated intravascular coagulation or fibrinolysis.

Septicaemic, endotoxic and Gram negative shock are considered on page 428. Certain other aspects of treatment in shock associated with sepsis should be emphasised.

Corticosteroids

Corticosteroids may have an important place in the treatment of septic shock where hypotension, oliguria and poor peripheral perfusion persist in spite of antibiotics and adequate volume replacement. Bolus doses of methylprednisolone sodium succinate (30 mg/kg body weight) should be given i v. This can be repeated 4-6 hourly. It should be stopped once the clinical state has improved, and should not be given for more than 36 hours. Massive doses of steroids lower peripheral resistance and increase renal perfusion. CVP monitoring is essential since a fall in dynamic blood volume and/or hypokalaemia may develop. Should steroids fail to improve peripheral perfusion and the cardiac output remain low—isoprenaline may be indicated (see below).

Digitalis

This is particularly indicated when there is a sustained tachycardia. The serum potassium must be normal before it is given and the dose must be low since there is a danger of digoxin toxicity if renal function is impaired. An initial dose of 0·5 mg should be given slowly into a vein under ECG control and a further dose of 0·25 mg over the next 12 hours if indicated. Digitalis can often be stopped after 48 hours when the patient's condition has improved.

Isoprenaline

If shock persists after the use of steroids isoprenaline is the next drug of choice. It is a pure beta-mimetic drug which causes arteriolar dilatation and an increase of heart rate and stroke volume and so of cardiac output (Hermreck and Thal, 1968). Continuous ECG monitoring is mandatory to detect increased ventricular excitability. A concentration of $8\mu g/ml$ is infused in 5 per cent dextrose, the drip rate being regulated so that the pulse rate remains below 130 per minute (infusion rate approximately 2-10 $\mu g/minute$). Tachycardia, ventricular or supraventricular, can generally be reverted by stopping the infusion. A β-adrenergic blocker such as practolol (Eraldin) should be used if tachycardia persists. β-adrenergic blockers should be used with extreme caution in endotoxic shock since there is a danger of asystolic arrest. Practolol is preferable to propranolol (Inderal) because of its intrinsic sympathomimetic activity.

Haematological status

It is important in prolonged septic shock to exclude a haemorrhagic diathesis (Table 2.4).

A fall in platelet count and fibrinogen titre is common in septicaemic shock especially when due to the meningococcus. Poor peripheral perfusion secondary to endotoxic shock leads to local hypoxic vessel wall damage and subsequent intravascular coagulation (Editorial, 1968). Once intravascular coagulation arises physiological mechanisms come into play to remove the fibrin or ' decoagulate '. The decision to be made is when to use drugs preventing disseminated intravascular coagulation. Patients with evidence of excessive bleeding, a falling fibrinogen titre and platelet count, and a prolonged prothrombin time should receive fibrinogen, or three packets of fresh frozen plasma. Blood should be replaced with preferably fresh blood or a plasma expander. Should peripheral perfusion remain poor in spite of blood volume replacement, steroids and antibiotics, then anticoagulation with heparin should be considered. Give 50–100 units/kg BW as a bolus and continue this dose four hourly as a drip reducing by 25 to 50 per cent if platelets are less than $100 \times 10^9/l$. Fibrinolysis in isolation is rare and if present should be stopped by i v epsilon-amino-caproic acid (Epsikapron). Inhibitors of fibrinolysis should always be preceded by i v heparin should there be evidence of intravascular coagulation (Merskey, 1967). Should there be a source of infection which requires drainage, surgery should be considered as soon as the patient has been adequately resuscitated. On rare occasions (as in Clostridial myonecrosis) it may be necessary to operate in the presence of shock. In such circumstances it is essential to correct the blood volume and metabolic imbalance and cover the operative period with antibiotics. Steroids and digitalis may also be considered necessary.

RESPIRATORY EMERGENCIES

Adequate ventilation is essential during and after resuscitation. It is generally started as mouth-to-mouth or mouth-to-nose artificial respiration (p. 732) and is followed by oral intubation with an endotracheal tube and subsequent hand ventilation. Inflation should

Table 2.4. *Measurements which may be affected in Septicaemic Shock associated with Haemorrhagic Diathesis.*

MEASUREMENT	PRIMARY ACTIVATION OF INTRINSIC COAGULATION SYSTEM (COMMON)	PRIMARY ACTIVATION OF FIBRINOLYTIC SYSTEM (RARE)	ACTIVATION OF BOTH SYSTEMS (MODERATELY COMMON)
Fibrinogen	Reduced	Reduced	**Reduced**
Platelets	Reduced	Usually normal	**Reduced**
Prothrombin time	Prolonged	Usually normal	**Prolonged**
Fibrinolytic activity	Normal or slightly increased	Increased	Increased

be synchronised with the patient's inspiratory effort. The lungs should be inflated initially with oxygen. The indications for IPPV following resuscitation are:

1. Failure to maintain blood gases within limits considered normal for that patient.

2. Prolonged resuscitation because this is likely to be complicated by cerebral oedema. Ventilation should be continued for at least 24 hours following resuscitation, the blood gases being maintained within normal limits.

3. Exhaustion. Patients who are hypercatabolic and toxic should be ventilated after resuscitation even if spontaneous ventilation appears adequate. These patients easily become exhausted and hypoxia is a common feature.

The physiological changes associated with IPPV are discussed in detail by Nunn (1971). The intrathoracic pressure is invariably raised by IPPV unless subatmospheric pressure is used during expiration. In the healthy this does not normally affect venous return because of compensatory peripheral vasoconstriction. Impairment of venous return is likely when capacitance vessels are already fully constricted as in hypovolaemic hypotension and in patients with paralysis of the vasomotor system as in polyneuritis. The cardiac output then falls and may lead to further impairment of peripheral vascular perfusion. It is obvious that placing a resuscitated patient on a ventilator requires a working knowledge of the ventilator being used and the likely response to IPPV. The typical phase durations for the adult patients are:

Duration of inspiration -	-	1·5 seconds
Duration of expiration -	-	2·25 seconds
Total duration of cycle -	-	3·75 seconds
Respiratory frequency -	-	16 breaths per minute.

The minute volume is normally set at 8-10 litres per minute, this being altered according to serial analysis of the $PaCO_2$ The percentage of oxygen delivered to the patient is adjusted according to the PaO_2. The level is maintained between 80 and 110 mm Hg. Failure to maintain an adequate PaO_2 may necessitate the use of a positive end expiratory pressure (PEEP, see p. 601).

Drugs used for IPPV

Most patients start to breath spontaneously after being resuscitated but their respiratory drive should be eliminated by drugs. Muscle relaxants are not often used now for this purpose because they make it difficult to assess the level of consciousness. It is better to produce a neuroleptic state by a combination of a potent analgesic and a tranquilliser such as, for an adult, phenoperidine (Operidine) 2 mg i v hourly and diazepam (Valium) 10 to 20 mg i v hourly as required. When there is no pain a tranquilliser may be sufficient.

METABOLIC AND BIOCHEMICAL EMERGENCIES

Many of the emergencies related to acute ionic changes are discussed elsewhere: Hypokalaemia p. 602, Hyperkalaemia pp. 379 and 605, Hypocalcaemia p. 368, Hypomagnesaemia pp. 369 and 607.

ABNORMALITIES OF FLUID AND ELECTROLYTE BALANCE

The amount of water in different phases of body fluids is determined by the number of small particles exerting an osmotic attraction to the phase. Sodium is the dominant ion in maintaining the osmolality and hence the fluid volume in the extracellular space. Small molecule non-electrolytes such as urea and glucose may contribute to the osmolality of the extracellular fluid when their levels are above normal.

Water depletion

Clinical water depletion is usually the result of insufficient intake or excessive loss by sweating, polyuria or hyperventilation. In conscious patients the diagnosis should present no difficulty since the dominant complaint is severe thirst. The patient is apathetic and unable to give a history. Hypotension does not occur until late. The serum sodium and serum osmolality are increased. Unconscious patients who are vomiting should have water restored with glucose 5 g/dl i v. Water can also be given via a Ryle's tube to patients who are not vomiting. Water replacement should not be too rapid. In severe water depletion approximately half the estimated deficit plus the amount of water likely to be lost should be replaced over the first 24 hours.

Water intoxication is described on p. 73.

Sodium depletion

This term should be limited to those states in which sodium has actually been lost from the body and should not be used for a fall in sodium concentration. A low sodium intake does not in itself lead to a significant sodium depletion but it may aggravate losses of sodium ions from the gastrointestinal tract and in urine and sweat. Large losses of sodium from the lower bowel are found only in watery diarrhoea. The most immediate effect of sweating is predominant water depletion but if this is replaced by water alone the cumulative loss of sodium ions becomes significant. The sodium level of sweat is higher in patients with fibrocystic disease thereby making them more susceptible to sodium depletion. When sodium is lost from the body the amount of fluid which can be contained in the extracellular compartment is decreased and there is a resultant fall in blood pressure and cardiac output. The loss of interstitial fluid volume leads to loss in tissue elasticity and turgor and a fall in intraocular tension.

Treatment. In mild cases salt by mouth is adequate but in moderately severe cases isosmotic sodium chloride solution should be given i v. A metabolic acidosis should be corrected with sodium bicarbonate. In severe cases a high sodium ion concentration is essential either as double strength isosmotic chloride or hypertonic sodium bicarbonate, depending on the acid-base status.

Sodium intoxication

For calculation to avoid giving excess see p. 606.

ABNORMALITIES OF ACID-BASE BALANCE

The normal rate of production of the H ion is so considerable that slight changes can cause serious acid-base disturbances. The main normal H^+ production occurs in the cells as a result of carbo-hydrate breakdown. CO_2 is produced and once this is dissolved H^+ appears. CO_2 is eliminated via the lungs leaving water (see Table 2.5).

Acid-base balance is a reflection of hydrogen ion metabolism and can be assessed by the Astrup analysis. Astrup showed that there is virtually a linear line relationship between pH and log $PaCO_2$. If two points are known the line is defined and from a pH measurement of the blood, the $PaCO_2$ may be read off.

In order to assess the metabolic component of acid-base status Andersen and Engel (1960) introduced two additional scales, namely base excess and buffer base. BB is the sum of bicarbonate and buffering protein. BE expresses in mmol/1 the amount of acid which when added to one litre of blood (at N temperature and N $PaCO_2$) would bring it to its normal pH. In order to treat the patient it is essential to decide whether the primary abnormality is respiratory or metabolic, since compensatory mechanisms may confuse the acid-base picture.

Table 2.5. *Hydrogen ion metabolism*

$$C_6H_{12}O_6 + 6\,O_2 \longrightarrow 6\,CO_2 + 6\,H_2O$$

Intracellular carbohydrate breakdown

$$CO_2 + H_2O \rightleftharpoons H_2CO_3 \rightleftharpoons H^+ + HCO_3^-$$

Carbon dioxide combines with water to form carbonic acid which dissociates into one hydrogen ion and bicarbonate ion.

Primary acidosis

This can be due to deficient carbon dioxide elimination (respiratory acidosis) or be metabolic in origin. The metabolic causes are:

1. Increased intake of hydrogen ions.
2. Increased formation of hydrogen ions.
3. Retention of hydrogen ions.
4. Increased loss of hydroxyl ions.

In primary respiratory acidosis carbon dioxide production depends upon the metabolic rate and the quantity eliminated by the lungs. Acute cessation of ventilation leads to a rise in $PaCO_2$ and a fall in pH. When ventilation is insufficient for carbon dioxide elimination there is an associated decreased oxygen uptake. When the oxygen supply to the tissues falls below requirements, a hypoxic metabolic acidosis ensues. This clinical picture is designated as a primary respiratory acidosis with a secondary metabolic acidosis. A primary respiratory acidosis of long standing may be associated with renal compensation and a secondary metabolic alkalosis.

The management of respiratory failure is discussed in Chapter 8.

The management of a primary metabolic acidosis depends upon the initiating factors.

Increased formation of hydrogen ions

This may occur in tissue hypoxia and is treated by improving tissue perfusion and oxygenation. The management of diabetic ketosis is discussed on p. 341.

When acidosis follows acute stress or complicates chronic malnutrition energy is obtained from non-carbohydrate sources and enhanced lipolysis results in a marked rise in keto-acids and ketone bodies. When starvation is the cause the prime object is to correct the electrolyte and fluid imbalance and then to commence feeding as soon as possible. This should be preferably by intragastric tube but if this is not possible i v feeding will be necessary. Wretlind (1972) gives excellent advice about i v feeding.

Retention of hydrogen ions

This occurs in renal failure and generally requires dialysis for its correction. Renal tubular acidosis is characterised by a hyperchloraemic acidosis, a normal or slightly impaired creatinine clearance and a low urinary excretion of ammonia and hydrogen ions. Treatment consists in the administration of alkalies, correction of calcium deficiency with calcuim lactate and calciferol and potassium deficiency with potassium citrate. It may be necessary to give as much as 200 mmol potassium as potassium citrate daily and during this period the administration of sodium bicarbonate is decreased. Later the dose of potassium can generally be decreased and that of sodium bicarbonate increased.

Increased loss of hydroxyl ions

This may follow severe diarrhoea or result from losses via a recent ileostomy or a pancreatic or biliary fistula. Management consists in careful observation of the acid-base and electrolyte status. Some of the sodium ions replaced during the day should be as sodium bicarbonate in order to correct for the metabolic acidosis reflected in a base deficit on the Astrup analysis.

Primary alkalosis

This results from:
1. Excessive carbon dioxide elimination.

2. Increased intake of hydroxyl ions.

3. Increased loss of hydrogen ions.

4. Loss of potassium ions.

Primary metabolic alkalosis results from an increased intake of hydroxyl ions as in excessive intake of bicarbonate or citrate. Increased loss of hydrogen ions usually follows vomiting or gastric aspiration. Potassium deficiency leads to a shift of potassium ions from the cells to the extracellular fluid. The potassium exchanges with sodium and hydrogen ions which move into the cells. The resultant effect is an extracellular metabolic alkalosis and an intracellular metabolic acidosis. A metabolic alkalosis is therefore generally associated with a depletion of total body potassium. The serum potassium may be normal.

The correct treatment of a severe metabolic alkalosis is essential since these patients do not tolerate stress and may succumb to respiratory paresis or cardiac arrest from hypokalaemia. Tetany (p. 368) may also be a manifestation. Metabolic alkalosis can rarely be treated by mouth because of vomiting. The quantity of chloride ions required for the ensuing 6 to 12 hours can be estimated by electrolyte analysis of the gastric aspirate and assessment of its volume. The quantity of chloride ions already lost can be assessed by a careful history and observation of the fluid balance charts. An attempt should be made to correct over the first 24 hours half the total loss of chloride ions and then to keep up with the present chloride loss.

A severe metabolic alkalosis combined with dehydration and potassium deficiency may result in renal insufficiency. Hence renal function should be carefully observed.

Replacement of potassium is essential and it generally has to be given i v as potassium chloride. The number of potassium ions required over the next six hours should be assessed and replaced i v under ECG control. The serum potassium should be initially checked 6-hourly. One third to one half of the estimated potassium deficit should be given over the first 24 hours. Potassium chloride should be infused in isosmotic sodium chloride solution or glucose saline in a concentration of not greater than 1 litre every 4 hours, but occasionally in the presence of continuing losses the rate and concentration have to be increased. Tetany requires treatment with i v saline and calcium chloride (p. 369). On rare occasions the serum calcium is low and in such instances calcium gluconate will also be required (10-20 ml of calcium gluconate 10 g/dl given i v over three minutes).

GUIDE LINES ON WHEN TO ABANDON RESUSCITATION

Advice has already been given regarding cessation of resuscitation after cardiac arrest (see p. 724).

When to switch off a ventilator if resuscitation attempts fail to induce spontaneous breathing is difficult to decide. Each patient has to be assessed individually and the problem should be discussed with the nursing and medical staff. The patient's grave condition should be explained to the relatives. To avoid any appearance of self interest the doctors should not be those involved in any subsequent transplant procedure.

1. A decision should be reached as soon as possible for delay is unfair to the relatives (who hope for survival) and to the nursing staff (whose morale is likely to deteriorate).

2. Patients who are subjected to long-term ventilation associated with tranquillisation and sedation, accumulate the drugs and normal consciousness may not be achieved for many days. Under such circumstances, all drugs should be withdrawn and ventilation continued for 2-7 days (depending on the patient) before IPPV is stopped.

3. An EEG may help but should never be taken as the sole criterion for stopping IPPV. The EEG is an ancillary aid to clinical assessment and is of particular value following head injury where no sedation has been given.

4. In certain cases (hypothermia, severe barbiturate overdosage, drowning and electrocution) IPPV should go on longer than the clinical state alone would suggest.

5. Reflex iridoplegia may develop in certain comatose conditions where cerebral function may return to normal (e.g. methyl alcohol poisoning, atropine poisoning and following electrocution or lightning shock).

GILLIAN C. HANSON

REFERENCES

ASTRUP, P. (1961). A new approach to acid base metabolism. *Clinical Chemistry,* **7,** (1), 1.

EDITORIAL (1968). Consumptive coagulopathy in septicaemic shock. *New England Journal of Medicine,* **279,** 884.

GRUBER, U. F. (1970). Recent developments in the investigation and treatment of hypovolaemic shock. *British Journal of Hospital Medicine,* **4,** (No. 5), 631.

HARDAWAY, R. M., JAMES, P. M. Jr., & ANDERSON, R. W. (1967). Intensive therapy and treatment of shock in Man. *Journal of American Medical Association,* **199,** 779.

HERMRECK, A. S. & THAL, A. P. (1968). The adrenergic drugs and their use in shock therapy. *Current Problems in Surgery 1.* (July 1968.)

JOLY, H. R. & WEIL, M. H. (1969). Temperature of the great toe as an indication of the severity of shock. *Circulation, 39,* 131.

MERSKEY, C., *et al.* (1967). The defibrination syndrome: Clinical features and laboratory diagnosis. *British Journal of Haematology,* 13, 528.

MOTSAY, G. J., *et al.* (1970). Effects of costicosteroids on the circulation in shock. Experimental and clinical results. *Federation Proceedings,* 29, 1861.

NUNN, J. F. *Applied Respiratory Physiology.* London: Butterworth, 1971.

ROSS, B. A., LORD BROCK & AYNSLEY-GREEN, A. (1969). Observation on central and peripheral temperature in the understanding and management of shock. *British Journal of Surgery,* 56, 877.

SAMBLIN, M. P., WEIL, M. H. & VELHOJI, V. N. (1965). Acute pharmaco-dynamic effects of glucocorticoids. *Circulation,* 31, 523.

SIGGAARD-ANDERSEN, O. & ENGEL, K. (1960). A new acid-base nomogram. An improved method for the calculation of the relevant blood acid-base data. *Scandinavian Journal of clinical and laboratory Investigation,* 12, 177-186.

WRETLIND, A. (1972). Complete intravenous nutrition. *Nutrition & Metabolism,* 14, Suppl. 1.

CHAPTER 3

Acute Poisoning and Drug Dependence

(For Occupational Poisoning see p. 464)

(For Acute Food Poisoning see p. 133)

(For Poisons Information Service see p. 813)

ACUTE poisoning is a common clinical emergency. In 1971 there were 99 800 cases in England and Wales and of the 4 011 deaths more than 3 000 occurred before the patients even reached hospital. Roughly 10 per cent of the deaths are accidental, 10 per cent are suicidal, i.e. with death as the objective, and the remainder are the result of 'self-poisoning'—a *crie de cœur* with rescue as the objective.

While the circumstantial evidence of poisoning may be decisive this is not always so and hence it is important, when confronted with an obscure sudden illness, e.g. coma without lateralising signs or evidence of diabetes, that the possibility of poisoning should cross one's mind before valuable time is lost. Poisons sometimes enter the body by unusual routes, e.g. the skin. Venepuncture marks suggest drug addiction though some addicts now seek to avoid detection by using the vagina or rectum. Blood, albumin and sugar in the urine, and even extensor plantar responses and unequal pupils do not necessarily mean that the illness is 'natural'. Disease and poisoning may occur together and are not mutually exclusive. In 30 per cent of cases more than one drug has been taken and often alcohol too.

If foul play is suspected and the patient knows he is about to die a dying declaration might be made if the circumstances warranted this (p. 662). If the police have a suspect and the victim does not know he is dying a deposition may be taken (p. 662). Attempted suicide is no longer an indictable offence (p. 672) so there is no legal obligation upon the doctor or anyone else to report the matter to the police. In all cases he should do what is best for the patient. The Hill report (1968) advised that all cases of poisoning should be referred to a designated poisoning treatment centre regardless of seriousness. The size of the overdose bears no relation to the severity of the psychiatric upset and so all cases should receive psychiatric evaluation. If the patient refuses treatment and is deemed to be in need of it for the protection of himself and others, the procedure for compulsion is set out on p. 674. Children present special problems since for them the contents of the kitchen cupboard may be as hazardous as those of the unlocked medicine cabinet. Advice on the treatment of 'household' poisonings (as well as drug poisonings) can be obtained from the Poisons Information Service (see Appendix 12, p. 813).

Antidotes

True antidotes are available for only a few poisons: naloxone (morphine); oxygen (carbon monoxide); desferrioxamine (iron); BAL, dimercaprol and D penicillamine (mercury); CaEDTA (lead); atropine and pralidoxime, P_2S (organophosphorus insecticides); cobalt EDTA (cyanides). Even with these, general supportive measures are needed as well. The old idea of treating every poisoning by an antidote has given place to modern treatment based on two principles: (1) to keep the patient alive and (2) to remove or neutralise the poison. Treatment should begin as soon as the patient is seen. Pre-hospital life support is important and particularly maintenance of ventilation.

Identification of the poison

Time should not be lost in trying to identify the poison in the gastric aspirate, urine or blood at the onset for cardio-respiratory resuscitation (pp. 724 and 732) takes precedence over all other measures. The nature of the poison can usually be learned by ordinary policeman-like, not to say Sherlock Holmes-like, methods and circumstantial evidence. Specimens of tablets which may have been taken can be identified (p. 693). To the experienced doctor the clinical picture may be diagnosed as in poisoning by trifluoroperazine (Stelazine) which can be suggestive of meningitis. Other possibly poisonous material can be tested for by the Government Chemist Drug Test Scheme which can rapidly exclude such common poisons as cannabis, cocaine, LSD, amphetamines and barbiturates. The kit is available from BDH Chemicals Ltd., Poole, Dorset BH12 4NN. Tel. Parkstone 745520 (STD 0202) Ext. 256.

REMOVAL OR NEUTRALISATION OF POISONS

Inhaled poisons

Artificial respiration (p. 732) and hyperbaric oxygen (p. 814) may be needed.

Swallowed poisons

If seen early, vomiting may be induced as a first-aid measure before removal to hospital. There is a vogue for Syrup USP Ipecac 20 ml but this may not be at hand. A drink of salty water (for risks see p. 72) and putting the patient's fingers deep down the throat is simpler. If seen within four hours it is better to pass a large (30 gauge Jacques) tube and to draw off the stomach contents with a Senorans's evacuator (p. 722). If the patient is unconscious a cuffed endotracheal tube must be in place to safeguard the lungs. Gastric lavage is never too late in salicylate poisoning. Lavage is not necessarily contraindicated in corrosive poisoning for the risks from absorption may be more than those of passing a tube. A non-toxic binding agent (coconut shell activated carbon, ' carbon 315 '*) can be left in the stomach. The amount to use is five times the estimated weight of poison taken or ten times when there is food in the stomach. It is effective in poisoning by salicylates and tricyclic antidepressants.

Tap water is the best lavage fluid to use in most cases but other substances are used in special poisonings, e.g. 50 per cent castor oil in water for glutethimide (Doriden) poisoning; desferrioxamine in iron poisoning (p. 36); and weak (violet coloured) potassium permanganate in opiate poisoning.

DIALYSIS. Removal of poisons from the blood by dialysis, haemo (p. 805) or peritoneal (p. 716) is now a practical proposition and should be considered in poisoning by the following drugs: Aspirin (if blood level is above 55 mg/100 ml); barbiturates (phenobarbitone if above 10 mg/100 ml (431 μmol/l); amylobarbitone if above 3·5 mg/100 ml (155 μmol/l); bromides; ethylene glycol (p. 37), glutethimide (Doriden); isoniazid; methanol (methylated spirit); meprobamate (Miltown, Equanil, Mepavlon); phenelzine (Nardil).

Dialysis need only be used if it can clear the poison more quickly than the patient's own organs; if the blood level is dangerously high, or if renal failure supervenes. In all cases where dialysis is considered, the advice of the Haemo-Dialysis Unit (p. 805) should be sought.

FORCED DIURESIS. Acid diuresis is used in poisoning by amphetamines, pethidine and quinine; alkaline diuresis is used in barbiturate and salicylate poisoning. Many common poisons, being largely protein-bound, are only excreted in small amounts by the kidneys. Some are mainly fixed in the tissues with only traces in the blood.

* Sutcliffe Speakman & Co. Ltd., Leigh, Greater Manchester. WN7 2HE. Tel. Leigh 72101 (STD 052 35). See also Norit, p. 28.

KEEPING THE PATIENT ALIVE

Supportive measures may be needed to deal with:

1. Respiratory failure. Artificial respiration (p. 732) either mouth-to-mouth or by machine. This is necessary if the minute volume measured by a Wright flow meter is less than 4 litres a minute. Bronchial suction.
   Transfer to hospital for monitoring if arterial pH and $PaCO_2$ are necessary.
2. Shock (see pp. 238 and 618).
3. Dehydration and electrolyte loss (p. 602).
4. Convulsions. These may occur after a period of hypoxia and severe hypotension. Special measures may be needed to end a series of convulsions (p. 310).
5. Hypothermia, especially in poisonings by phenothiazines. A special low-reading thermometer must be used (pp. 362 and 694).

Except in the case of salicylate poisoning (where blood levels are necessary) it is satisfactory to assess the severity of poisoning according to the response to a painful stimulus (rubbing the sternum with the knuckles) as follows:

Grade I. Drowsy but responsive to verbal commands.

Grade II. Stuporose but responsive to minimal stimulation.

Grade III. Unconscious but responsive to maximal stimulation.

Grade IV. Comatose and unresponsive.

Most cases of poisoning can be managed successfully by the intelligent application of these principles. As well as the depth of coma the amount of respiratory depression and the presence or absence of shock and hypothermia should be taken into account. More detailed accounts of several of the commoner poisonings follow.

OUTMODED TREATMENTS

These are mentioned early so that time will not be wasted on them.

Analeptics. These do not shorten the period of unconsciousness or increase the clearance rate of drugs. Improvement in ventilation which they seek to provide is better attained by artificial respiration.

Lumbar puncture (p. 708). This is of little value because only low concentrations of poisons are found in the CSF.

Heat cage. This is inadvisable as it diverts blood from the vital centres to the vasodilated skin. Internal rewarming using a respirator with heated humidified air is better.

Antibiotics. These should not be used prophylactically but reserved for infection should it occur. Earlier use might mean that any infection would be by a resistant organism.

Catheterisation (p. 720). This can cause dangerous infection and should only be used when the bladder is not emptied by incontinence or pressure. It may be needed to measure the response to forced diuresis.

'Universal antidote'. The ingredients of this powder (charcoal, magnesia and tannic acid) react on each other and make it ineffective. But specially prepared activated charcoal of small particle size will absorb many poisons (Shell carbon 315 and Norit* powder). It is of value when made into a slurry with water and given early, especially in aspirin poisoning.

Corrosive Poisoning

1. Safeguard respiration. Call in the help of an anaesthetist. Tracheostomy (p. 737), oxygen (p. 740) and artificial respiration (p. 732) may be needed.

2. Try to find out what was taken. If it was Lysol or carbolic acid within the previous 15 minutes, induce vomiting or aspirate the stomach via a tube (p. 722). If acid give a thick paste of magnesia. Soapsuds, toothpaste or washing soda may be used instead. Bicarbonate is dangerous because of effervescence. If alkali was swallowed give vinegar diluted 1 in 3. If in doubt as to what was swallowed give white of egg.

3. Give morphine 15 mg to an adult. If respiration is depressed and morphine is needed naloxone (Narcan) 1 mg might be added.

4. Preserve any vomit for examination.

5. Contact a laryngologist or thoracic surgeon at once since by the prompt passage of a tube and the use of steroids a stricture may be avoided.

Carbon Monoxide Poisoning

CO poisoning is becoming rarer as North Sea gas (methane) replaces 'town gas' which contains up to 20 per cent CO. But it will still occur for CO is produced whenever there is incomplete combustion, as when a flame touches a surface cooler than the ignition temperature of the gaseous part of the flame such as in a water heater. Car exhaust fumes contain up to 7 per cent CO. ('Camping gas' consists of propane or butane and contains no

---

* Norit-Clydesdale Ltd., 105 Millerston Street, Glasgow, G31 1TG (041-554 8671).

CO). Victims of burns who have inhaled black smoke may have CO poisoning.

A proper understanding of the effects of CO will bring a better appreciation of what can be expected from treatment of poisoning by it. Haemoglobin combines with the same amount of CO as oxygen and produces HbCO. But CO has 200 times the affinity of oxygen for haemoglobin. Hence a partial pressure of CO only 1/200th that of oxygen (1 volume of CO in 1 000) will result in equal proportions of HbO_2 and HbCO in the blood. CO causes chemical tissue hypoxia of greater degree than would result from anaemia alone. This is because by shifting the disassociation curve of Hb to the left it impedes the release of oxygen from HbO_2 (p. 499).

The amount of CO in the blood depends on the concentration in the air, the length of exposure and the volume breathed per minute. Hence gassing is more severe in a person at work than in one at rest. Adults are less affected than children because a given mass of Hb is converted into HbCO whether in a child or an adult. As an adult has more haemoglobin the concentration is less. But the effects of CO poisoning are not simply due to the level of HbCO. After the initial hypoxic phase capillary damage leads to tissue and especially brain oedema with local hypoxia. The effects of this persist after the HbCO has fallen to a low level. The result may be irreversible brain damage and this can occur very quickly.

Another important point is that while about 50 per cent HbCO may be necessary to cause coma in non-anaemic healthy subjects, lower levels can be fatal in the decrepit, the diseased, the drugged and the drunk (the four D's of CO poisoning). Permanent nervous sequelae of CO poisoning include personality changes, Parkinsonism and other effects of cerebral atrophy. Myocardial ischaemia is usual. The classical pink colour due to HbCO is only seen in severe poisoning and then after death. More often there is simple pallor. Blisters occur as in barbiturate poisoning but are non-specific being trophoneurotic in nature from cerebral damage.

DIAGNOSIS. This is obvious when a suicidal person is found in a gas-filled room but accidental poisoning may be unsuspected. It is wise to test for barbiturates and salicylates in the urine lest more than one poison is acting. For estimation of CO 3 ml of heparinised blood covered with liquid paraffin should be sent. When coma persists after the CO level falls a cerebrovascular complication is likely.

RESCUE. Is it safe to enter? This question may not arise when the patient can be rescued quickly as from a gas oven but the rescuer should always go into the room crouching after taking a few deep breaths (coal gas, but not CO, is lighter than air). He should be 'roped' so that he can be dragged out if overcome and does not come out after an agreed time, say one minute. The gas should be turned off and the patient dragged out by the heels.

Rescue from a difficult position, e.g. a man-hole or bedroom, should make one pause to consider the best method, for it is foolish to rush in and become a casualty oneself particularly when it is unlikely that the patient can be rescued alive. The rescuer may lose the power in his legs while still conscious and so be unable to escape. There are various devices (chemical and electronic) for detecting and measuring the concentration of CO. While a man can work indefinitely in a concentration of up to 10 in 100 000 (0·01 per cent) a concentration of 200 parts per 100 000 (0·2 per cent) is dangerous for exposures of more than one hour. A fatal concentration for exposure of less than one hour is 400 per 100 000 (0·4 per cent). It must not be forgotten that the atmosphere may be low in oxygen and that other poisonous gases may be present also. For difficult and prolonged rescue attempts a fresh air respirator or a self-contained oxygen apparatus (p. 730) should be worn.

TREATMENT AFTER RESCUE. Clear the airway by pulling forward the tongue and using a swab. Avoid the crushing type of tongue forceps as they make the tongue swell rapidly. Breathing is usually normal but if it is depressed artificial respiration (p. 732) should be used. The mouth-to-mouth method provides roughly 16 per cent oxygen and 4 per cent CO_2. A specially made mixture of oxygen and CO_2 from a cylinder is not now recommended. The position of the limbs should be carefully watched, for the combination of hypoxia and vascular obstruction may quickly lead to gangrene. If it is thought that cerebral oedema is at all possible or if there is already papilloedema 500 ml of mannitol 20 g/dl should be given i v and followed by 500 ml of dextrose 5 g/dl over four hours (see p. 728).

Hyperbaric oxygen (p. 814) at 2 atmospheres pressure dissolves in the plasma and has been recommended with enthusiasm because it will greatly increase elimination of CO, though the levels in the animals used to establish this fact were much higher than those usually found in poisoned patients. As, however, it takes about 20 minutes for a hyperbaric oxygen chamber to reach 2 atmospheres pressure, and the HbCO will have fallen below a dangerous level from simply breathing fresh air for that time, the use of hyperbaric oxygen seems unnecessary in the stage of primary hypoxia. But it will greatly alleviate tissue hypoxia and cerebral oedema from capillary damage and so has a place in treatment especially in an atherosclerotic subject.

Exchange transfusion is sometimes suggested and while theoretically of some value it is a slow and inefficient method of getting rid of CO compared with breathing oxygen. Also it might push a hypoxic myocardium into failure.

ACUTE SALICYLATE POISONING

Aspirin tablets have become a domestic panacea and are the usual cause of salicylate poisoning. Methyl salicylate (oil of wintergreen) has a pleasant smell attractive to children. As little as one teaspoonful (5 ml) has proved fatal since this is equivalent to 4 g of aspirin.

DIAGNOSIS. There is a latent period of several hours after taking an overdose of aspirin (longer if enteric coated) in which the patient appears well and this is a trap for the unwary doctor. Drowsiness if not due to another drug indicates acidaemia. Later overbreathing (' air hunger '), low blood pressure and a positive ferric chloride test in boiled urine presents a characteristic picture. Phenistix will detect salicylate in plasma if the level is 20 mg/100 ml or more (below this level it is all protein bound and unreactive). (Colour changes with other drugs are too unreliable to be of value.) As the patient is not drowsy or unconscious until moribund he will give a history, often exaggerated, of what he has taken. He will complain of deafness and roaring tinnitus. Clinical assessment of severity is fallacious and so the plasma level should always be estimated. 50 mg/100 ml is serious (30 in children) and calls for diuretic treatment. If the high blood level is unrelieved circulatory collapse and unconsciousness will follow. Haematemesis (p. 157) from gastric irritation and hypoprothrombinaemia may complicate the picture. As aspirin causes shedding of epithelial cells in the renal tubules blockage may precipitate renal failure. Asthma (p. 194) is an occasional complication.

Adults tend to get a persisting respiratory alkalosis from the stimulating effect of the salicyl radicle on breathing. Children soon get over this and show a metabolic acidosis. The onset of acidosis is later in adults than in children. There is a marked loss of potassium especially in adults.

Treatment. This should be aimed at eliminating salicylate from the body and so blood should be taken at once in order to determine the initial level. Take 5 ml of blood into a heparin bottle for estimation by Trinder's method (Trinder, 1954). While correction of the complex metabolic disturbances would seem theoretically advisable, this would need elaborate monitoring techniques not usually available.

Since salicylate is held in the stomach for long periods as relatively insoluble clumps of tablets, gastric emptying by Senorans's evacuator (p. 723) followed by gastric lavage (p. 721) should always be performed. Renal excretion of salicylate is enhanced in an alkaline urine but oral alkaline fluids are insufficient. Forced alkaline diuresis should be started if the plasma level is 50 mg/100 ml or more (30 in children) or without this estimation if the clinical state looks serious. The risk of causing serious hypokalaemia is avoided by the ' cocktail ' diuretic described by Lawson *et al.* (1959) which renders biochemical control unnecessary. Give the following solution i v at the rate of 2 litres per hour for three hours.

Saline 0·9 g/dl (154 mmol/l)	0·5 litre
Laevulose 5 g/dl (278 mmol/l)	1·0 litre
Sodium bicarbonate 1·26 g/dl (150 mmol/l)	0·5 litre
Potassium chloride 3 g (in 2 l) (40 mmol/l)	
i.e. 20 mmol in the final volume of 2 l.	

Further infusion should go on at the rate of one litre an hour until the plasma salicylate level is below 35 mg/100 ml.

Contraindication to diuresis would be congestive cardiac failure with pulmonary oedema and failure to achieve diuresis after two hours because of poor renal function. (i.e. secretion rate less than 0·5 ml per minute.) Vitamin K_1 should be given by injection.

Elimination could be achieved by haemodialysis but as this would only be available at special centres diuresis is preferable for most cases. In small children exchange transfusion would be effective.

When there is very profound stimulation of breathing physical exhaustion may threaten. Curarisation and machine assisted respiration should then be considered. The acidaemia should be corrected by giving 500 ml of sodium bicarbonate 5 g/dl over 30 minutes (see p. 727).

BARBITURATE POISONING

Overdosage by barbiturates accounts for about half the annual mortality from poisoning in Britain. Although better drugs are now available barbiturates have not yet been superseded as hypnotics and so most practitioners will encounter barbiturate poisoning. The patient usually presents in coma with flaccid limbs. Sometimes he appears to be dead. The plantar reflexes may be extensor. An empty labelled bottle or bottles may point to the diagnosis and be helpful in those cases in which more than one poison has been swallowed.

A recognition panel of boxes of the various sedative tablets shown to the relatives may help to identify the one taken (see also p. 693). The effects of two or more sedatives are at least additive and one may even potentiate the other. In doubtful cases vomited or aspirated gastric contents should be tested for barbiturates (a laboratory procedure). Urine tests, particularly if short-acting barbiturates have been taken, may be inconclusive. Senility, associated disease, hypothermia, shock and hypoxia from pulmonary oedema and suffocation all play their parts in determining the outcome.

Short-acting barbiturates, such as pentobarbitone (Nembutal), quinalbarbitone (Seconal), cyclobarbitone (Phanodorm) are more dangerous in toxic doses than long-acting ones since they quickly cause severe shock and respiratory failure. Long-acting barbiturates such as phenobarbitone (Luminal) and sodium barbitone (Medinal) keep patients at a safer level of unconsciousness for longer periods.

The severity of poisoning will depend also on how habituated the victim was to barbiturates.

Treatment. Clinical evaluation of the severity of poisoning (p. 27) is important in deciding on treatment but there is no rule of thumb method. Reliance cannot be placed on any one sign. Absence of bowel sounds, however, indicates severe poisoning but their return may herald a period of further absorption and a worsening condition. Hypothermia (p. 361) is a bad sign.

Treatment begins as soon as the patient is seen and so, although he should be sent to hospital at once, he must be in the charge of someone capable of performing effective artificial respiration if need be. The effect of a period of apnoea in the ambulance may show itself disappointingly in convulsions later when the barbiturate blood level falls.

Gastric emptying and perhaps lavage (p. 721) should be carried out unless more than four hours have elapsed since the tablets were swallowed. For most cases no special measures are needed and supportive therapy is enough. The basic indications are as follows.

1. *To maintain respiration.* Most deeply unconscious patients are hypoxic and so oxygen should be given by a mask, at 10 litres per minute. Artificial respiration may be needed (p. 732). Sputum and inhaled material may have to be removed by bronchoscopic suction. Crusting of bronchial secretions becomes important if coma is prolonged. Inhalation of water vapour will discourage it but tracheostomy (p. 737) may be necessary. When the gag reflex is absent endotracheal intubation is indicated to avoid the risk of inhaled secretions.

2. *To combat shock.* Most poisoned patients show postural hypotension and this can be remedied by a head-down tilt. If there is also peripheral circulatory failure as shown by a fast pulse, low blood pressure and cold, cyanosed hands and feet other measures are needed. Give metaraminol (Aramine) 2 to 10 mg i v in repeated doses or 15 to 100 mg in a 500 ml i v drip.

3. *To give fluid.* Give 1 litre of dextrose 5 g/dl in 24 hours by i v or intragastric drip.

It is an advantage, particularly in phenobarbitone poisoning, to make the urine alkaline. Barbiturates exist in ionised and un-ionised forms and ionisation is increased when the urinary pH is increased i.e. when it is alkaline. Cell membranes are relatively impermeable to ionised forms. Hence bicarbonate will tend to lower tissue concentration and prevent renal tubular reabsorption. Sufficient bicarbonate should be given to keep the urine alkaline to phenol red indicator, i.e. to give a definite red colour (=pH 8·4). A first dose of 230 mg/kg is advised and can be given as Injection of Sodium Bicarbonate BP 5 g/dl.

Dialysis (haemo- or peritoneal) can be life-saving in exceptionally severe poisoning with long acting barbiturates but it is not indicated in most cases and has its own risks. Failing dialysis forced diuresis as described for salicylate poisoning can be used but only a little barbiturate is got rid of by this so called ' blood lavage '.

METHYL ALCOHOL (METHANOL) POISONING

This usually results from drinking methylated spirit which is 90 per cent ethyl alcohol and 9·5 per cent wood naphtha (mainly methyl alcohol). It may follow its use on the skin. Methyl alcohol is more toxic than ethyl alcohol because it is oxidised in the liver to formic acid and formaldehyde with resulting metabolic acidosis. It persists in the body for several days and much of it is excreted through the lungs. Individual tolerance varies greatly and depends partly on whether food and ethyl alcohol were also taken. Methanol poisoning is rare and only about 2 per cent of Britain's 350 000 alcoholics are meths drinkers.

Methanol is distributed largely in proportion to the water content of tissues. Hence intra-ocular fluids are greatly involved. Mild cases resemble ordinary alcoholism and may be mistaken for the common ' hang over '. Many conditions may be mimicked because of epigastric pain, persistent vomiting, blindness and delirium going on to coma.

Treatment. Only if the patient is seen within four hours need the stomach be washed out. Two or three tablespoonfuls of pectin (or Certo used for jam making) in water should then be given to delay absorption. The low intelligence of drinkers of 'red biddy' militates against early treatment. Ethanol competes successfully with methanol for oxidative enzymes and is preferred by them in a ratio of 9:1. It is preferentially oxidised to innocuous products while methanol is excreted as such. Even though the ethanol content of methylated spirit is 90 per cent it is fairly quickly oxidised and so it is advisable to give more in the form of brandy (40 per cent ethanol), say 30 ml per hour to keep the blood alcohol level above 150 mg per 100 ml. It should be continued for 3 or 4 days to avoid the late effects of methanol. The amount of ethanol which can be metabolised by an average adult is about 10 ml per hour. It is not advisable to try fructose in methanol poisoning as is done in ethanol intoxication as it would increase the acidosis from formic acid. A more effective treatment is haemo-dialysis (p. 805) and this should be considered if vision is impaired. Other measures are mainly symptomatic. Dextrose 5 g/dl should be given by i v drip and the blood electrolytes maintained at normal levels (p. 602). Bicarbonate is needed for metabolic acidosis if this is shown by a lower arterial blood pH (normally 7·35 to 7·45). As more than one person may have drunk methanol the police should be asked to look for possible victims.

SPECIAL FEATURES OF OTHER POISONINGS

If the poison is known and there is a good antidote, this may be used *when the general measures to eliminate the poison and to keep the patient alive have been started.*

'Home perm' solution

Outfits for hair waving at home contain a powder (potassium bromate) from which to make a neutralising solution to apply after the first one. It looks like water and is almost tasteless and so may be drunk in error. Should this happen, sodium thiosulphate (photographic 'hypo') 1 teaspoonful in a little water should be given by mouth and 10 to 50 ml of a 10 g/dl solution injected i v.

Arsenic (weed killer)

While preparing to wash out the stomach give a mixture containing 30 ml of Solution of Ferric Chloride BP (15 g/dl) and 30 g of sodium bicarbonate in 120 ml of water. (Add the bicarbonate bit by bit and allow each effervescence to subside. The mud-like resulting mixture contains ferric hydrate which with the arsenical stomach contents forms almost insoluble ferric arsenite.) BAL

(Dimercaprol) should be given i v in a dose of 4 mg/kg every four hours for 48 hours and then 3 mg/kg twice daily for eight days.

Paraffin oil (kerosene) and petrol

These substances are soluble in liquid paraffin and this should be given to prevent absorption. If it cannot be swallowed a tube may be used with full precautions against inhalation. Even small amounts which reach the lungs will disrupt lung surfactant and cause widespread pneumonitis. Hydrocortisone may be used to block any pulmonary reaction. After absorption kerosene will cause respiratory depression and convulsions. Occasionally addiction to petrol by inhalation is seen and then there is peripheral neuritis caused by the added cresyl phosphate.

Cyanide (p. 461)

Give amyl nitrite to inhale and use cobalt EDTA (Kelocyanor, Rona) promptly and even though the patient appears well for the action of cyanide is sometimes delayed.

Ferrous sulphate

Proprietary tablets containing ferrous sulphate are often brightly coloured and sugar coated and so they attract toddlers. When swallowed they dissolve fairly quickly and by corroding the stomach mucosa cause vomiting of black material, circulatory collapse and sometimes perforation. A prompt X-ray picture of the abdomen may reveal the number swallowed. If not fatal at this stage evidence appears after some hours or days of liver damage with jaundice, fever and metabolic acidosis, all attributable to the effects of absorbed iron. A serum iron of over 1000 μg/100 ml indicates dangerous poisoning. There may be encephalopathy with convulsions and coma. Iron poisoning is a serious emergency and energetic treatment is required. The drug of choice is Desferal (Ciba). This is desferrioxamine B mesylate, an iron-free derivative of ferrioxamine produced by *Streptococcus pilosus*. It combines with iron to form a complex which is rapidly excreted in the urine.

1. Inject 2 000 mg Desferal in 8 ml of water i m.

2. Wash out the stomach with sodium bicarbonate 1 g/dl and then give 5 000 mg of Desferal in 50 to 100 ml of water by mouth to chelate any free iron in the stomach.

3. Give Desferal in isosmotic sodium chloride solution by i v drip at not more than 15 mg/kg per hour; maximum dose 80 mg/kg in 24 hours.

Ethylene glycol ('Anti-freeze')

This is oxidised to oxalic acid which leads to death from acute renal failure caused by deposition in the renal tubules of calcium oxalate crystals. Calcium gluconate 10 ml of a 10 per cent solution should be given slowly by i v injection to convert oxalic acid to the relatively inert calcium oxalate.

Carbon tetrachloride

This is a popular household dry cleaner with a low boiling point and a highly toxic vapour. Whereas another dry cleaner, trichloro-ethylene, gives warning symptoms (giddiness and nausea), CCl_4 does not. The early symptoms of poisoning may resemble an acute abdominal emergency (p. 121) but acute renal failure is the main risk and it is increased by taking alcohol. Treatment is as on p. 374. When CCl_4 from fire extinguishers (and also methylene chloride, a paint stripper) comes into contact with a hot surface several toxic gases including phosgene (p. 463) are formed.

Phenol. Lysol. Cresol (For phenol burns see pp. 473 and 559)

These household antiseptics may cause poisoning quickly when swallowed and also when spilled on the skin (pp. 465, 473 and 530). If swallowed give white of egg and then empty the stomach and wash it out with water plus castor oil. Cleanse the skin with soap and water and other liquids as described on p. 530. Treatment for renal failure may be needed (see p. 374).

Morphine. Pethidine. Physeptone

The most powerful antidote is naloxone (Narcan) (p. 570) 0·4 to 1·2 mg i v in divided doses over three minutes. It does not depress the CNS except in the absence of opiates but even then artificial respiration would meet the emergency. With methadone (Physeptone) which has a long half life there is often a relapse and so the patient should not be discharged on recovering consciousness despite protests. Severe withdrawal symptoms may be precipitated.

DDT (Dicophane BP) poisoning

The minute quantities consumed in food are innocuous but if a very large amount of DDT is ingested it affects the nervous system and causes excitation, tremors, convulsions and paralysis. Treatment is by gastric lavage and purgation. The poison is soluble in fats and so these should be avoided until it is all excreted in about two weeks or until the urine is free from poison.

Fluoroacetate (1080; Tenate)

This very toxic substance contains a C-F bond and occurs naturally in a South African plant *Dichapetolum cymosum* which causes cattle poisoning. It is used as a rat poison mostly by Pest Control Officers. Not all substances with the C-F bond are toxic but those that are undergo ' lethal synthesis ' in the body to the very toxic fluorocitrate. This may be ingested, inhaled or absorbed from the skin and causes poisoning by halting oxidative processes. Acetamide, a protective substance, not strictly an antidote, 0·25 ml/kg BW should be given i m and repeated hourly for four doses (obtainable from Sigma, see p. 464). Failing this 1 litre of 5 per cent ethyl alcohol should be given i v.

Paraquat (see also p. 468)

Ingestion of a concentrated solution of Paraquat calls for immediate admission to hospital. Vomiting and diarrhoea are followed by painful ulceration of the mouth and oesophagus and then, after a misleading interval of 48 hours by hepatic and renal failure. Survivors may die later from progressive fibroblastic proliferation in the lungs causing respiratory failure. Induce vomiting (p. 26). Wash out the stomach (p. 721). Give 1 litre of a 30 per cent suspension of fuller's earth (Surrey finest grade. Laporte Chemical Industries) by stomach tube followed by Epsom salts. Repeat these measures at frequent intervals. If possible test for absorption (Goulding, 1976). If positive special measures are needed: diuresis and dialysis or charcoal haemoperfusion. Ask an Information Centre (p. 813). Check electrolytes every day. Send stomach wash, blood and urine and the Paraquat container to the laboratory (McGeown, 1975).

Mercurial salts

Give several raw eggs in milk to precipitate any mercury salts in the stomach and then wash it out preferably with 5 or 10 per cent sodium formaldehyde sulphoxylate (British Drug Houses).

Give BAL (Dimercaprol. Boots) as for arsenic poisoning. Treat for acute renal failure (p. 374).

Insecticide poisoning (p. 467)

Amphetamines (see also p. 43)

Excretion of amphetamines is enhanced by an acid urine and so addicts take bicarbonate to prolong its effect. Because of tolerance due to addiction the toxic dose is very variable and assessment has to be clinical. Restlessness, insomnia, delirium and panic attacks are common and give place to exhaustion. Sedation by barbiturates may be needed. Forced acid diuresis is likely to help. The following fluids are given in rotation in doses of 1 litre in the first hour and 500 ml hourly thereafter:

500 ml 5 g/dl fructose + 1·5 g ammonium chloride
500 ml 5 g/dl fructose
500 ml 0·9 g/dl sodium chloride

It is necessary to measure the serum electrolytes every hour.

Digoxin

The effect of massive overdosage of digoxin depends on whether the heart is normal as in children or damaged as it may be in adults. In children the more prominent symptoms are drowsiness and vomiting, the heart showing bradycardia with exaggeration of the normal sinus arrhythmia. Heart block is rare. Bradycardia calls for atropine 0·6 mg i m and repeated as necessary. Gastric lavage and activated carbon (p. 26) are indicated. In the elderly with damaged hearts the picture is that of ventricular ectopic beats, coupled rhythm and tachycardia (see p. 250). When there is doubt about the diagnosis a digoxin assay is helpful. Two or more ng per ml indicates probable toxicity. Normally the ' membrane pump ' maintains a high level of intracellular potassium but when it is poisoned by digoxin potassium leaks out and high serum levels result. This occurs with massive overdosage. With lower doses vomiting may cause hypokalaemia. Hence serum potassium estimations are mandatory. Digoxin is excreted by the kidneys and so a good urinary output must be maintained. In severe poisoning the insertion of a pacemaker is a wise precaution. For treatment of hypo- and hyperkalaemia see pp. 602 *et seq.* and for treatment of dysrhythmias see p. 249.

Non-barbiturate hypnotics

Glutethimide (Doriden) is fat soluble and so gastric lavage with Intralipid (Paines and Byrne) or a castor oil and water mixture is advised. Some oil should be left in the stomach. Variation in the depth of coma and periods of apnoea are probably caused by raised intracranial pressure. To prevent this treatment should be given as for cerebral oedema (pp. 301 and 728). Haemodialysis may be needed using oil with the dialysing fluid. Forced dialysis and peritoneal lavage are ineffective.

Methaqualone (Melsedin. Mandrax)

This drug causes deep coma with marked signs of damage to the pyramidal tracts. Haemodialysis may be needed but forced diuresis is not advised.

Lomotil

These tablets containing diphenoxylate and atropine are widely used for ' traveller's diarrhoea '. They may be taken by children and cause drowsiness, small pupils and hypotonia with depressed breathing. Gastric lavage and the use of naloxone (see morphine, p. 37) will rescue the victim.

Paracetamol (Acetaminophen) (see also p. 153)

This drug is issued in 500 mg tablets and is a common constituent of many compound analgesic preparations. As little as 10 g can cause severe poisoning. The main effect is on the liver and is potentiated by alcohol and barbiturates. If the patient reaches hospital within 12 hours gastric lavage should be performed and 20 g of activated carbon (p. 26) or the ion exchange resin cholestyramine (Questran Bristol 9 g sachets) introduced into the stomach. Attempts to prevent liver damage by forced diuresis will fail and haemodialysis is of doubtful benefit. The systemic use of cysteamine,* which may protect the liver by reducing covalent binding of paracetamol, is currently under evaluation. Should cysteamine be unobtainable, dimercaprol (BAL) 4 mg/kg should be given four hourly for the first 24 hours and 3 mg/kg four hourly for the second 24 hours. Side effects are abdominal pain and cramps. Plasma levels of paracetamol are easy to measure and, if greater than 200 μg/ml four hours after ingestion, are usually associated with clinically significant liver damage. Classically this appears 36-48 hours later, the most reliable parameters of severity being the prothrombin time and the plasma bilirubin level. The SGOT correlates poorly with the degree of liver damage. Fulminant hepatic failure with coma may supervene and treatment should then be as indicated on p. 155. The less severely affected may be discharged as soon as the prothrombin time has returned to normal and the plasma bilirubin is falling.

---

* Obtainable as a laboratory chemical under the name 2-Aminoethanethiol hydrochloride (Catalogue No. 12292-0) from Aldrich Chemical Co. Ltd., 264 Water Road, Wembley, Middx HAD IPY (01-998 4414); and as Mercaptoethylamine hydrochloride (Catalogue No. M 6500) from Sigma London Ltd. (see footnote p. 464).

Tranquillisers. Phenothiazines

Examples of drugs in this group are Largactil (chlorpromazine), Fentazin (perphenazine) and Stemetil (prochlorperazine). Severe hypotension, hypothermia and convulsions are liable to occur from overdosage. The biological half-life is very long (several months) and it is not possible to increase their excretion by dialysis. Poisoning by Librium (chlordiazepoxide), Valium (diazepam) and Mogadon (nitrazepam) resembles drunkenness but respiration is depressed also. General supportive measures usually bring recovery. As most of the drug is rapidly metabolised in the tissues methods to increase excretion are not needed.

Tricyclic antidepressants

After a brief period of excitement these drugs cause depression of consciousness and breathing together with convulsions and cardiac dysrhythmias. The pupils are dilated and the plantar responses extensor. Unless vomiting can be quickly achieved while the patient is conscious it should not be attempted lest it should happen when coma supervenes. The risk of inhaled vomit is too great. The nervous symptoms can be abolished by physostigmine (eserine) salicylate (Sigma, see footnote p. 464) giving 1 to 3 mg i v over 2 minutes and repeating in 10 minutes. Atropine Sulphate Injection BP should be available for eserine side effects. For convulsions Valium (diazepam) 5 mg should be given i v. For dysrhythmias Practolol or phenytoin should be used as described on p. 252. Cardiac arrest is a late event. Dialysis and forced diuresis are ineffective as the drugs are largely protein bound.

C. ALLAN BIRCH

FOR FURTHER READING

MATTHEW, H. & LAWSON, A. A. H. *Treatment of Common Acute Poisonings*, 3rd ed. Edinburgh: Livingstone, 1975.

REFERENCES

GOULDING, R., *et al.* (1976). Paraquat poisoning. *British Medical Journal*, **i,** 42.

LAWSON, A. A. H., *et al.* (1969). Forced diuresis in the treatment of acute salicylate poisoning in adults. *Quarterly Journal of Medicine,* **N.S. 38,** 31-48.

McGEOWN, MARY G. (1975). *Proceedings of the International Meeting on Clinical Aspects of Paraquat Poisoning.* Birmingham: Kynoch Press.

TRINDER, P. (1954). Rapid determination of salicylate in biological fluids. *Biochemical Journal,* **57,** 301.

DRUG DEPENDENCE

(For Drugs Branch of the Home Office see Appendix 21, p. 829)

Three types of emergency may be encountered among patients dependent on drugs:

1. Overdosage.
2. Drug psychoses:
   short-lived mental illnesses when such drugs as amphetamines and lysergic acid diethylamide (LSD 25) are taken in excessive amounts.
3. Abstinence syndromes from withdrawal of drugs causing physical dependence.

OVERDOSAGE

Although the treatment of narcotic overdosage should be straightforward there may be special problems when an overdose of an opiate is taken by someone who is physically dependent on it. If a morphine antagonist nalorphine (Lethidrone) or naloxone (Narcan) is used as an antidote the patient may have severe abstinence symptoms when he recovers consciousness and a further dose of the opiate may be needed to counteract them. This is clearly undesirable when treating overdosage, and narcotic antagonists are in general best avoided in these cases.

DRUG INDUCED PSYCHOSIS

Lysergic acid diethylamide

Short-lived psychoses may be seen in people who have taken LSD 25. This is a potent drug to which tolerance often develops rapidly without psychological or physical dependence. Its effects are uncertain and can sometimes be exceedingly unpleasant. Nevertheless, it is now widely used (or misused) in the United States, and to a lesser extent in Britain. The common complications are anxiety which can amount to severe panic, depression, confusional episodes with disorientation and psychotic reactions with hallucinations. These may occur at the time the drug is taken and may sometimes recur (particularly under stress) for several weeks afterwards (' return trip '). In most cases of a ' bad trip ' support and reassurance from friends is sufficient, and most ' bad trips ' settle down without specific treatment. In a severe case with marked panic or gross disorientation more active treatment may be required and a patient with an acute adverse reaction may need i m chlorpromazine, and immediate emergency admission to a psychiatric unit (p. 672).

Amphetamines

Amphetamines and amphetamine barbiturate mixtures may be taken at weekends by adolescents to produce euphoria and wakefulness and to increase energy and talkativeness. Occasional week-end use has been described as ' benign ' compared with ' malignant ' use when psychological dependence on amphetamines has developed. Those in this latter group use more amphetamines and are inclined to take a variety of forms in a reckless manner. They may have started taking amphetamine during the week as well as at the weekend and their physical health and work may have suffered. At this stage they may have short-lived mental illnesses with agitation, restlessness and a schizophrenic-like psychosis, frequently with persecutory ideas. They may develop depressive reactions ('coming down') when they stop the drug. These are sometimes described as ' the horrors ' (this term is also used for the acute psychotic illness). Amphetamines may be taken i v sometimes by opiate addicts (as an alternative to cocaine) and sometimes by amphetamine addicts who take larger amounts this way. The mental reactions are those of an acute amphetamine psychosis and urgent admission to hospital is sometimes necessary (p. 674). When the amphetamine is withdrawn the symptoms subside in two or three days. Chlorpromazine i m may occasionally be needed to control restlessness or an acute psychosis.

ABSTINENCE SYNDROMES

Two groups of drugs which when used regularly lead to physical dependence are important since if they are suddenly stopped at this stage, withdrawal symptoms may appear. Although the abstinence syndrome from withdrawal of opiates is better known, that from withdrawal of barbiturates is more severe and more dangerous.

Opiate withdrawal

The signs are craving for the drug, anxiety, restlessness and running of the nose. These and more serious abstinence signs are shown in Table 3.1. The symptoms are unpleasant but not usually dangerous and their onset is gradual. Heroin withdrawal symptoms can be treated equally well with morphine or methadone (Physeptone). The best way is to use oral methadone preferably in liquid form so that the patient does not know the amount he is given. (The amount of other opiates equivalent to methadone 1 mg are: heroin 1 mg, morphine 3 mg, pethidine 20 mg, codeine 30 mg.) Methadone itself is a drug of addiction and physical dependence to it develops but withdrawal symptoms are milder. In a doubtful case methadone 10 mg can be given and 20 mg an hour later if there is no improvement. This could be repeated after a further two hours but 50 mg should be adequate to cover the next 12 hours while other arrangements for treatment are made.

Only medical practitioners who hold a special licence issued by the Secretary of State may prescribe heroin or cocaine to addicts; other practitioners must refer any addict who requires these drugs to a treatment centre. All doctors may still prescribe heroin and cocaine for the relief of pain due to organic disease. The Misuse of Drugs (Notification of and Supply to Addicts) Regulations 1973 require all medical practitioners to notify particulars of addicts to the Chief Medical Officer, Home Office, *within seven days* from the attendance (when the doctor has confirmed his suspicion that the

Table 3.1. *Times of appearance of abstinence signs in physically-dependent opiate addicts* (*Modified from a table by P. H. Blachly, 1966*)

GRADE OF ABSTINENCE	SIGNS	HOURS AFTER LAST DOSE		
		HEROIN	MORPHINE	METHADONE
0	Craving for drugs, anxiety	4	6	12
1	Yawning, perspiration, running nose, lacrimation	8	14	34-48
2	Increase in above signs plus mydriasis, gooseflesh (piloerection), tremors, (muscle twitches), hot and cold flushes, aching bones and muscles, anorexia	12	16	48-72
3	Increased intensity of above plus insomnia, increased blood pressure, increased temperature, increased respiratory rate and depth, increased pulse rate, restlessness, nausea	18-24	24-36	
4	Increased intensity of above, plus febrile facies, position (curled up on hard surface), vomiting, diarrhoea, weight loss, spontaneous ejaculation or orgasm, haemoconcentration, leucocytosis, eosinopenia, increased blood sugar	24-36	36-48	

patient is an addict). A person is to be regarded as addicted if, and only if, as a result of repeated administration he has become so dependent on a drug listed in the Schedule to the Regulations* that he has an overpowering desire for its administration to be continued. (If an addict requires the drug concerned for the treatment of organic disease or injury, notification by the doctor is not necessary.) The particulars to be notified are name, address, sex, date of birth, National Health Service number, date of attendance, and the name of the drug or drugs to which the patient is addicted. Notification should be made in writing to the Drugs Branch, Home Office, Romney House, Marsham Street, London SW1P 3DY (see p. 829). If there is any doubt whether an addict has already been notified telephone the Home Office (01-212 0335).

Barbiturate withdrawal

Physical dependence (on barbiturates and other sedatives) may be found in persons dependent on barbiturates alone, also in alcoholics who have used barbiturates and have become dependent on them, and also in opiate and other addicts, who may simultaneously have physical dependence on barbiturates. The effects of large doses of barbiturates include ataxia, slurred speech, impairment of mental function, confusion, loss of emotional control, poor judgment and occasionally coma and death. Table 3.2 shows progressive signs of barbiturate-sedative intoxication.

When physical dependence on barbiturates has developed and they are suddenly stopped the withdrawal symptoms include in approximate order of appearance anxiety, involuntary twitching of the muscles, tremor of hands and fingers, progressive weakness, dizziness, distortion of visual perception, nausea, vomiting, insomnia, loss of weight, a precipitate drop in blood pressure on standing, convulsions of a grand mal type and a delirium resembling alcoholic delirium tremens. Where a major psychotic episode develops convulsions and delirium do not usually occur at the same time.

* Cocaine
  dextromoramide (Palfium)
  diamorphine (Heroin)
  dipipanone (Pipadone)
  hydrocodone (Dihydrocodeinone)
  hydromorphone (Dilaudid)
  phenazocine (Narphen)
  levorphanol (Levorphan)
  methadone (Physeptone)
  morphine
  piritramide (Dipidolor)
  opium
  oxycodone (Proladone)
  pethidine

3

Generally a patient may have one or two convulsions during the first 48 hours of withdrawal and then become psychotic during the second or third night. Table 3.3 shows progressive signs of barbiturate sedative drug withdrawal.

The barbiturate-withdrawal syndrome is best treated in hospital with barbiturates alone. The degree of tolerance should first be determined by systematically adjusting dosage until intoxication develops, to prevent the development of convulsions from premature withdrawal. Next the physical dependence must gradually be decreased. Physical dependence on barbiturates and other sedative hypnotics is more severe and dangerous than opiate dependence and more easily overlooked.

BARBITURATE WITHDRAWAL PROCEDURE

Withdrawal from physical dependence upon most sedatives, barbiturates and alcohol can be performed by substitution with the correct dose of pentobarbitone followed by daily reduction in its dosage. The withdrawal can be divided into four stages: (1) achievement of a 'normative' state (i.e. showing neither abstinence nor intoxication), (2) objective determination of the usual 24 hour dosage used, (3) withdrawal procedure, (4) post-withdrawal phase. Withdrawal should preferably be conducted on a closed ward prior

Table 3.2. *Progressive signs of barbiturate-sedative intoxication*

---

1. Depression of superficial skin reflexes
2. Fine lateral gaze nystagmus (see below)
3. Slight decrease in alertness with coarser rapid nystagmus
4. Diminished deep tendon reflexes
5. Minimal ataxia
6. Slurred speech
7. Pseudo-ptosis
8. Positive Romberg's sign
9. Thick speech
10. Moderate ataxia
11. Nystagmus on forward gaze
12. Somnolence
13. Marked ataxia with falling
14. Confusion
15. Sleep with difficulty in arousing
16. Semi-comatose with small pupils
17. Respiratory depression
18. Shock with dilated pupils
19. Death

Nystagmus should be sought by having the patient fix his gaze on the forefinger held at least 40 cm in front of the eyes. The finger is slowly moved laterally, then stopped abruptly. If horizontal nystagmus is present, the eyes will then begin a series of jerking movements. Vertical nystagmus is elicited by moving the finger up or down in the same manner. Nystagmus may be very fine and transient with early intoxication but becomes sustained, coarser and more rapid as intoxication deepens.

---

to objective determination of drug use. The patient must be in a 'normative' state. He should be observed closely from the time of admission till the following morning. During this period if he demonstrates a tremor, tachycardia, extreme irritability or a pulse rise on standing of more than 15 per minute this is interpreted as probable barbiturate/sedative (or alcohol) abstinence and he should be given 200 mg of pentobarbitone i m or orally. If at any time during the night these abstinence symptoms recur, the 200 mg of pentobarbitone should be repeated. Great attention should be directed to these early symptoms of abstinence. If they are not treated with doses of barbiturate, seizures or delirium tremens may follow within a few hours.

Objective determination of usual 24 hour dosage used

The patient (regardless of medication received during the night) is given a 200 mg of pentobarbitone (Nembutal) orally. He is then evaluated for signs of intoxication one hour later at which time examination is directed towards eliciting signs of intoxication:

Table 3.3. *Progressive signs of barbiturate-sedative drug withdrawal*

1. Weakness
2. Restlessness, tremulousness, irritability
3. Insomnia
4. Rising or elevated temperature
5. Increased pulse rate (over 100 per minute) and pulse rate increase of more than 15 minutes on standing (b.p.: the systolic pressure falls and the diastolic rises)
6. Increased muscle tone, fasciculations, twitching
7. Brisker deep tendon reflexes, coarse tremors of face and hands, ankle clonus
8. Fibrillary twitchings of the upper eyelids on loose closure
9. Distorted perception (e.g., walls appear curved)
10. Anorexia, nausea, vomiting, abdominal cramps
11. Dilated pupils
12. Convulsions and possible status epilepticus (see below)
13. Psychosis with visual and less frequently auditory hallucinations, confusion, paranoid ideation, formication, delirium. This is often preceded by 24 to 48 hours of insomnia. The delirium occurs especially at night with disorientation to time and place

The patient may be slightly confused for one to two hours but prolonged stupor as seen after a grand mal convulsion is seldom seen. Usually less than four major convulsions occur, whereas there may be many minor episodes, e.g. clonic twitching or athetoid movement may occur. Barbiturates will stop the convulsions but they may not halt the psychosis. Phenytoin (Dilantin) and phenothiazines will neither prevent nor control withdrawal convulsions, and are not indicated in the management of barbiturate, sedative or alcohol withdrawal.

nystagmus on vertical gaze, ataxia, pseudo-ptosis (inability to open the eyes widely on command) and slurred speech. If the patient is intoxicated on the examination he has no significant physical dependence upon barbiturates sedatives or alcohol. If the patient shows only minimal or no signs of intoxication he is given a 200 mg dose of pentobarbitone at two-hourly intervals until he does show significant intoxication, e.g. one or more of the symptoms of intoxication mentioned previously. The total intoxicating dose is recorded and the patient is given no further doses of pentobarbitone until the next morning. The total dose of pentobarbitone required to achieve intoxication when given in doses of 200 mg at two-hourly intervals is roughly equivalent (plus or minus 200 mg) to the patient's usual 24 hour intake of sedatives.

Withdrawal procedure

Generally the patient is given a 24 hour dose which is 100 mg less than his usual 24 hour intake and this is then dropped at the rate of 100 mg daily until abstinence is achieved.

THOMAS H. BEWLEY.

REFERENCE

BLACHLY, P. H. (1966). The management of the opiate abstinence syndrome. *American Journal of Psychiatry,* **122,** ii, 742-744.

CHAPTER 4

The Hazards of Medical Procedures

***Even the most simple procedures can sometimes be hazardous. It is
a good habit therefore to remind oneself before starting of what
might go wrong and to know what one would do if it did.***

ACCIDENTS WITH NEEDLES

Broken needles

SHORT needles usually break at the junction of the shaft and the
butt. Long needles may rust internally and break anywhere, especially if they have been in contact with iodine. Eccentric nozzles
reduce the strain on needles and so lessen the chance of breakage.
Nickel needles bend rather than break and may be used for lumbar
puncture if sudden jerks are expected. All needles should be tested
before use and a needle should never be inserted as far as it will go.
A guard may be placed on a needle to prevent too deep insertion
as in liver biopsy. Should a needle break in the tissues and project
sufficiently, it may be removed by forceps, but more often no part
remains visible though pressure on each side of the puncture may
reveal the end. Beware of making a small incision and poking
about. Prevent the patient from moving the part; tell him what has
happened but do not admit negligence or offer compensation. After
careful X ray localisation have the needle removed at a planned
operation, preferably by a surgeon who uses a metal locator.* If the
patient is too ill, say nothing and leave him alone. He may die. If he
recovers always X ray the part just before exploring. Small
portions of the needle have been left in the body and even in
the pleural cavity without causing untoward effects, and pieces of
dental needles in the pterygoid fossa are usually best left there. In
all cases the doctor would be wise to report the circumstances to
his medical protection society and to send them the pieces of the
needle.

Venepuncture

This may cause fainting which can be avoided by attention
to detail. Let the patient be seated and his arm comfortably
supported on a cushion. Don't use the word ' blood ' or let the
patient see the needle. Don't pinch the skin with the tourniquet.

* Metal Detection Ltd., Barnfield Industrial Estate, Tipton, West Midlands.
021-557 2104.

Don't let antiseptic trickle on the arm—he will think it is blood. Use a sharp needle but don't probe for the vein. It is there if you feel for it. Some find red fluoroscopic goggles a great help in seeing the vein. If, in spite of all this, the patient faints, lower his head quickly. Extravasation of blood is lessened if the arm is raised vertically to collapse the vein before removal of the needle. After this the site should be pressed with a swab for a brief period.

Needling of 'special' veins carries its own hazards. Infra-clavicular subclavian venepuncture (p. 747) may be complicated by pneumothorax but this is less likely in the supra-clavicular approach. With both routes haematomas may form and the vein may thrombose. If the needle is left 'open' too long and the patient is not flat air may enter the veins. The smallness of the groin vessels in infants makes damage to the femoral artery a real risk of femoral venepuncture. Serious arterial thrombosis has resulted.

Extra-venous injections (see also p. 85)

Many substances commonly given i v, such as calcium chloride, are highly irritant. Leakage of noradrenaline infusion (Levophed) may cause extensive necrosis (p. 85). Hypaque (Bayer) and Urografin (Schering) have the advantage of being relatively non-irritant if they leak into the subcutaneous tissues. Triosil (Nyegaard) and Conray (May & Baker) are even less irritant. For excretory pyelography under the age of 5 years it is possible to inject 10 to 20 ml of 45 per cent Hypaque i v (wrist, hand, scalp or external jugular vein) (p. 746). Useful results can be obtained by injecting half the volume into each subscapular region with hyaluronidase 1 500 units.

Although relatively non-irritant promazine (Sparine) can cause arterial spasm by inadvertent intra-arterial or peri-arterial injection. It should always be diluted first with at least an equal volume of isosmotic sodium chloride solution.

Prevention. When i v injection is likely to be difficult because of poor veins, measures should be adopted to ensure that they will be dilated. Flicking the vein with the finger will often make it dilate. Failing this the whole arm should be wrapped in a warm, moist towel and hot water bottles applied. Venous spasm is more likely in peripheral (especially leg) veins than in central ones because the muscle in their walls increases the further they are from the heart. As cold and pain may cause venous spasm, ether on the skin should be avoided and the subcutaneous tissues down to the vein should be infiltrated with 1 per cent procaine. A glass adaptor between the syringe and the needle (Fig. 4.1) makes it easy to see the blood on withdrawing the piston and thus indicates that the vein has been entered. This is otherwise impossible when using dark-coloured fluids. The eye must be fixed on the region of the needle point so that commencing extravasation ('tissuing') is seen at once. The risk of extra-venous injection or leakage of blood is said to be less if the needle is inserted in the bevel-down position. Unless the needle is very sharp, however, insertion is more difficult in this position. If a needle with a short bevel is used it can be inserted in either position without risk (see Fig. 4.2).

Treatment. If the injected fluid is dark in colour so that the extent of the leakage can be seen, it is good practice to incise the area, irrigate with isosmotic sodium chloride solution and stitch it up. In the case of small leaks of pale solutions an attempt to aspirate may be made. Infiltration with 1 per cent procaine with hyaluronidase may prevent damage from thiopentone. The limb should be immobilised and warmth applied.

Entry of an artery instead of a vein

This rare accident may happen when a tight tourniquet has obliterated pulsation in an aberrant artery lying between the fascia and the skin so that it looks and feels like a vein. It may also happen when, in exploring a plump ante-cubital fossa, a vein is transfixed and a deeper artery entered. In 18 per cent of people one or more arteries in the ante-cubital fossae are superficial. Most often it is the radial artery. Sometimes they appear as satellite arteries of ante-cubital veins and if parallel vessels are seen this should raise suspicion that one of them is an artery.

The outer rather than the inner aspect of the ante-cubital fossa should be used whenever possible so as to avoid the brachial artery but it would be safer to abandon the use of elbow veins in favour of hand veins. In right handed patients the left side should always be used. (As subcutaneous extravasation is more likely from small hand veins these should be avoided if a noradrenaline drip is

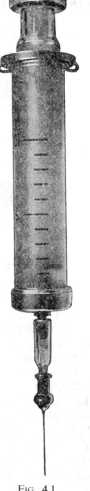

Fig. 4.1
Glass adaptor between syringe and needle.

being given (p. 85). In resuscitating the newborn it is thought
that nikethamide solution intended for the umbilical vein (which is
collapsed in asphyxia) might be injected into one of the umbilical
arteries. It could then reach the sciatic branch of the internal iliac
artery—the main supply to the leg in the fetus—and would account

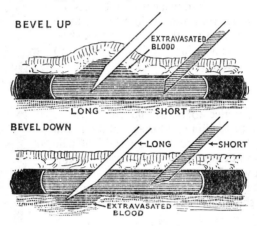

FIG. 4.2

To show the disadvantages of the long bevel
needle for venepuncture.

for cases of sciatic paralysis and gangrene of the buttock in the newborn. This accident can be avoided by isolating a stretch of cord
between clamps before blood drains from it and if necessary milking
the blood along to distend the vein. After injection the proximal
clamp is removed.

Two simple precautions should distinguish an artery from a vein.
Palpation *before applying a tourniquet* will reveal pulsation (though
this may be feeble in shock) and the blood withdrawn will generally
be bright red. Although thiopentone may cause venous blood to
darken a little in the syringe it will not make arterial blood look
like venous blood. Another point which should suggest in the case
of thiopentone that the injection is intra-arterial is that the onset of
narcosis will be delayed. It is always wise to wait a few seconds
after commencing a supposed i v injection and to proceed only if
no untoward effects appear.

The intima of arteries is specially sensitive to alkaline solutions
which if injected intra-arterially generally cause intense burning
pain. This may be absent, however, and then the only immediate
signs are coldness and blanching of the hand followed by urticaria.

Subsequent spasm, thrombosis and oedema may lead to gangrene. Blockage of vessels after injecting thiopentone seems to be due to its crystals which form when solutions (particularly strong ones) mix with blood. Such sequelae are infrequent, but not unknown, when weak solutions (2·5 g/dl) are used. Hexobarbitone soluble seems free from this risk and is almost as effective as thiopentone.

Treatment. Since the accident may have such serious consequences prompt treatment is indicated. The objects are to cause full vasodilation, to prevent thrombosis and to relieve pain.

1. If you have sufficient presence of mind don't remove the needle but inject into the artery at once (before blood clots in it) 5 ml of 2 g/dl procaine. This is likely to be at hand but tolazoline (Priscol, Ciba) 10 to 20 mg (25 mg in 1 ml) is better. Follow this with the first dose of heparin preferably into the artery so that it may act on blood trapped there.

2. Inject morphine 15 mg or pethidine 100 mg subcutaneously into the other arm.

3. Ask the anaesthetist (he is probably there already and the patient unconscious) to perform brachial plexus or stellate ganglion block (p. 711). Since the patient (because of thiopentone) will be unable to co-operate at least 20 ml of analgesic solution with 1 500 international units of hyaluronidase should be used. When the block is completed the subclavian artery should be punctured isosmotic sodium chloride solution injected into it. These procedures may be repeated several times if necessary though it may be wise to limit sympathetic block to two or three times while anticoagulants are used lest serious haematomas complicate the picture. Animal experiments have cast doubt on the efficacy of this procedure. Arterial neurectomy is an alternative.

4. Arrange for anticoagulant therapy to continue for at least a week.

5. Ensure warmth as advised for peripheral embolism (p. 244) but do not overheat.

Should oedema occur fasciotomy may be necessary. If operation is not urgent it should be postponed till heparin has had time to improve the arm and, if possible, until after a week's anticoagulant therapy. If operation becomes imperative protamine should be used to neutralise heparin (see p. 88).

Intravenous infusions

THROMBOPHLEBITIS. The risk of thrombophlebitis is ever present but it has lessened since plastic tubing has replaced rubber. It increases after eight hours and is greater in the leg than in arm veins and after giving crystalloid solutions rather than blood, particularly if the pH is on the acid side. Hydrocortisone 10 mg per litre of infusion lessens the risk. No infusion should run for longer than eight hours at a time. The vein used should be the largest convenient one, preferably in the arm just distal to a junction. For larger infusions a polythene catheter inserted into a large vein, such as the cephalic vein in the deltopectoral groove or even into the vena cava, is advised.

INFECTION. Careless preparation or faulty suturing after a cut down may lead to infection of the site of insertion. The skin should be prepared by applying iodine 1 g/dl in 70 per cent v/v alcohol or Betadine (povidone iodine); the cannula outside the vein should be cleaned daily with an antiseptic solution and the arm and cannula should be immobilised.

Intravenous plastic catheters

If the catheter is left attached to a needle a restless patient may cause the bevel to sever it and allow it to slip into the vein (' catheter embolism '). To prevent this the catheter should be attached to a wooden tongue depressor rather than just to the skin. There is also a risk of severance if the catheter is withdrawn through a metal cannula. Both should be removed at the same time. It is safer to use a catheter which is introduced *over* the needle (p. 748). Infection is an ever-present risk. Septicaemia makes CUP measurement inadvisable.

Intramuscular injections

Not infrequently the radial nerve in the upper arm and the sciatic nerve in the buttock are damaged by misplaced i m injections. It is safer to roll the shirt sleeve up high and inject into the deltoid or to use the outer side of the thigh. If the buttock is used there is danger especially for the nurse who regards the buttock as simply the ' cheek ' the upper and outer part of which is over the sciatic nerve. For the doctor the buttock is a larger area and its upper and outer quadrant is safe. A better surface marking, however, is (for a right-handed operator injecting the right buttock) to place the tip of the left index finger on the anterior superior iliac spine and the tip of the middle finger (abducted as in Sir Winston Churchill's V for victory sign) just below the iliac crest (Fig. 4.3). The injection site is then within the triangle formed by the fingers and the iliac crest. For the left buttock the position of the two fingers will be reversed.

An injection into relaxed muscles is less painful than into contracted ones and some of it is less likely to be forced back into the subcutaneous tissues. So lying is better than standing and the prone position better than the supine as the patient cannot then watch the injection. If the patient stands he should bear his weight on the opposite leg. To use a short fine needle as a gesture of kindness is mistaken for it will result in a painful subcutaneous injection. A sharp 5 cm needle of outside diameter 0·90 mm is best.

Refinements in i m technique are to draw the skin and subcutaneous tissues aside before inserting the needle so that when they slide back the needle track is broken; to aspirate for a few seconds after insertion to make sure that the blood vessel has not been entered; to inject a little 1 per cent lignocaine before the medicament to diminish pain; to inject a bubble of air or a little isosmotic sodium chloride solution to clear the needle and to leave it in place for a few seconds before withdrawal and then to press the site.

A haematoma may develop at the site of an i m injection in a patient receiving heparin (p. 88).

Intra-arterial transfusion

This is thought to have advantages in severe shock for the blood pressure is quickly raised, and circulatory overloading is less likely than with i v transfusion. But it carries the risk of ischaemic damage to the fingers, particularly if fluids other than blood are given. For this reason it is wiser in a right

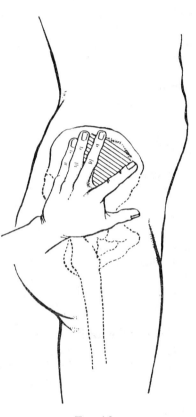

Fig. 4.3
Showing where to give an intramuscular injection into the buttock. (*Department of Photography and Illustration, Westminster Medical School*).

handed person to use the left radial artery, or better a femoral artery. Pressure must be applied and is safest if given manually from an aneroid sphygmomanometer as this ensures constant watching. Air embolism may be prevented by putting in circuit a safety drip chamber with a float which blocks the exit should the chamber run dry.

Cannulation of the radial artery

This procedure which is used for direct blood pressure monitoring and arterial blood sampling may be followed by necrosis of fingers and forearm skin. Total occlusion will follow cannulation at the level of the styloid process of the radius in 50 per cent of cases though the pulse may remain through retrograde filling from the ulnar artery if the palmar arch is complete. Otherwise finger ischaemia results. Radial artery obstruction in the forearm can cause skin necrosis because the superficial branches are without anastamoses. Whether distal or proximal cannulation is best is undecided but it is wise to allow flow around the catheter by using one of small gauge and preferably parallel-walled for as short a time as possible.

Intravenous injections

Anginal pain may be precipitated in patients with coronary insufficiency when too rapid injection particularly of iron and calcium preparations causes a fall of blood pressure. Even normal subjects may experience substernal discomfort. All therapeutic i v injections should be given slowly. Excessive i v dosage of hypertonic dextrose and saline solutions may so increase extra-cellular osmolality that the resulting intra-cellular dehydration causes neurological symptoms and coma. A similar picture can occur naturally (p. 345) and after peritoneal dialysis (p. 716).

Puncture of the trachea

The trachea may be damaged in an attempt to take blood from the internal jugular vein of an infant. Subcutaneous and mediastinal emphysema and pneumothorax may result and cause death.

Acupuncture

When a needle is inserted in the lower cervical region to treat painful conditions of the neck and shoulder the apical pleura may be punctured and a pneumothorax will result. Stellate ganglion block may be similarly complicated.

Pericardial haemorrhage

This is one of the remote risks of the now rarely used procedure of intracardiac injection of drugs (p. 714). It may also occur, but is less likely, when tapping a pericardial effusion by the epigastric route. The fact that the needle is in contact with the heart may be shown by connecting it to the precordial lead of the electrocardiograph. If blood is obtained when performing paracentesis there may be a doubt as to whether a ventricle has been entered. It is possible to make sure by leaving the needle in position and injecting saccharine (2·4 mg in 4 ml saline). If the patient tastes this (almost immediately from the left ventricle or in 17 or more seconds from the right ventricle) it means that the needle has entered a ventricle. Pressure of blood in the pericardial sac rather than its total amount is responsible for ' cardiac tamponade ' and as little as 200 ml has caused death. Haemopericardium from puncture is more likely to occur when the thin walled right atrium rather than the thick walled left ventricle is injured.

Pericardial tamponade (p. 248) from blood may be spontaneous in a patient overdosed with anticoagulants. It is indicated by a rising venous pressure, a small thready pulse, a narrow pulse pressure with increased cardiac dullness and distant sounds. Treatment is to remove liquid blood from the pericardium by tapping (p. 714) and to give vitamin K_1 (p. 755).

Lumbar puncture (For technique see p. 708)

Too much preliminary prodding of the back may precipitate hysterical phenomena in susceptible patients as may also the painful periosteal injury of clumsy manipulation.

When meningitis is thought to have resulted from lumbar puncture the organism should be carefully sought and its sensitivities tested as it may be a resistant one which has escaped sterilisation. Headache follows lumbar puncture when CSF leaks through the hole in the dura faster than it is formed by the choroid plexus. Prevention is achieved by adequate hydration and lying prone for a couple of hours so that by extending the spine the hole is closed.

Permanent paralysis has followed lumbar puncture in a few cases. It may have been caused by intrathecal bleeding, though this is usually harmless or causes only transient root irritation. A more probable cause is progression of a pre-existing lesion. Hence it is important to record carefully the physical signs present before puncture. Lumbar puncture should be avoided if possible during anti-coagulant therapy.

Insertion of the needle too far may damage or infect an intervertebral disc. This may be avoided by tilting the needle towards the patient's head. In this position it will encounter the next vertebral body above and not the disc. Lumbar puncture higher than the space between the third and fourth lumbar vertebrae should be avoided as a spinal cord extending lower than normal is not unusual.

Removal of CSF may, by vascular dilatation, initiate intra-cerebral or meningeal haemorrhage from diseased vessels. External rectus palsy may result from stretching of the sixth nerve from sudden alteration in intracranial dynamics.

Lumbar puncture should be avoided or only performed in a neurosurgical unit if papilloedema points to high pressure because of the risk of ' foraminal crowding ' in cases of subtentorial tumour. A supra-tentorial tumour may cause herniation of the uncus of the hippocampal gyrus into the tentorial hiatus. The risk is there also in the absence of papilloedema if the pressure rise has been too quick for it to develop. Those who claim that ' foraminal crowding ' is only a clinical ghost have probably been lucky. Prevention of the accident lies in avoiding lumbar puncture if there is papilloedema or if the picture suggests high pressure. If the puncture must be done as little fluid as possible should be removed though there is no guarantee that this will avoid trouble as leakage through the meningeal puncture may continue for hours. A very fine needle should be used. A refinement is to pass an introducer or cannula down as far as the ligament and then to pass the needle down it to complete the puncture. A Dattner double needle has the same object. Another precaution is to pierce the dura with the bevel of the needle in the spinal axis so that fibres are separated rather than cut across. The puncture will then close more easily. A ' pencil point ' needle with a hole at the side has the same effect.

Warning signals of collapse are sudden cessation of flow, neck stiffness, dysphagia. Respiratory failure can quickly follow. In this situation or if very high pressure (over 25 cm H_2O) is confirmed raise the foot of the bed, give 500 ml of sucrose 50 g/dl i v (see p. 298) and call the neurosurgeon. Record pupil sizes, pulse and blood pressure.

Cisternal puncture (For technique see p. 710)

An emergency may follow cisternal puncture if the needle is inserted more than 2 cm after the occipito-atlantal ligament is pierced. In this case the medulla is injured—usually with fatal results. Deviation of more than 18° from the mid-line may result in damage to a vertebral artery, with resulting subarachnoid haemor-rhage. This may also be due to damage to abnormal vessels inside the foramen magnum. As these are not uncommon, cisternal punc-ture is best avoided unless clearly indicated. In either of these emergencies little can be done, beyond the giving of analeptics.

Accidental intrathecal injections

During epidural and paravertebral block the analgesic solution may enter the subarachnoid space and produce the effect of a spinal anaesthetic. An aspiration test for CSF should prevent this accident. If it occurs the head should be lowered and a pressor drug given (metaraminol (Aramine) 2 to 10 mg i v). Artificial respiration may be needed.

Marrow biopsy

Marrow biopsy by sternal puncture presents few risks, but some accidents have occurred. A very ill patient might die from a cardiac inhibitory reflex caused by the puncture and to avoid this it is wise to give a sedative (Valium (diazepam)) first. Perforation of the sternum particularly if the inner plate is softened by some neoplastic disease has caused the syndrome of cardiac tamponade (quiet heart, hypotension and venous congestion) (p. 248) and death. Removal of blood from the pericardium is indicated (p. 714). Puncture as high on the sternum as possible and angulation of the needle into the manubrium is advised. A trephine instrument is safer than a needle. Haemorrhage might also occur if the patient is suffering from a haemorrhagic disease or is receiving anticoagulants. Blood transfusion and vitamin K therapy (p. 755) would be wise in such cases. The iliac crest or a lumbar vertebral spine is sometimes preferable to the sternum.

Liver biopsy

Needle biopsy of the liver may be complicated by haemorrhage and necessitate blood transfusion. It should be avoided if pro-thrombin activity is 50 per cent of normal or less or if the platelet count is less than 100 $10^9/l$. A preliminary course of vitamin K_1 (p. 755) is advised. Occasionally a hepatic friction rub can be heard during inspiration over the needling site for a short period. It is of no serious significance. If a large artery is impaled as well as a bile duct, bleeding may be into the duodenum. A rare complication is an arterio-venous fistula. Unless the patient controls his breathing by practice, the needle, fixed between the ribs, may tear the capsule as the liver moves. This is less likely when the puncture is made from behind. Puncture through the abdominal wall may avoid this risk but should not be made unless the liver is palpable. If the gall bladder is accidentally entered as shown by aspiration of bile or mucus have the presence of mind to leave the needle in situ and gently inject some air. This has on occasion shown up gall stones. It is best to limit the depth of liver puncture to 5 cm since beyond this a large branch of the portal vein may be entered. Incidentally, aspiration of much blood makes search for the bit of liver difficult. Needle biopsy should be avoided in obstructive jaundice because of the risk of puncturing a dilated biliary duct with resulting bile peritonitis or even bile embolism of the lungs. It is, of course, contraindicated when there is infection in the pathway of the needle. A transient episode of ' neurogenic hepatic hypotension ' may occur, the suggested mechanism being similar to that of a blow in the solar plexus. The mortality rate in 20 000 punctures was 0·17 per cent.

Renal biopsy

The chief risk of percutaneous needle biopsy is bleeding shown as haematuria or a perirenal haematoma, especially in hypertensive patients with small kidneys. The procedure should be avoided if there is severe hypertension or a bleeding tendency and if neoplasm, cystic disease or perirenal abscess is suspected. It is unwise if there is a single kidney or if renal calcification is present. It is best to reduce the diastolic pressure to under 100 by giving diazoxide 300 mg (Eudemine) i v immediately after the biopsy. This lessens the risk of haemorrhage. Intra-renal arterio-venous aneurysm formation has been recorded after needle biopsy.

Percutaneous lung and pleural biopsy

These procedures may be done by an aspirating needle, punch or air drill. All should be avoided in haemorrhagic disorders and pulmonary hypertension and if there are bullae. It is well to avoid them also if the FEV_1 (p. 195) is less than 1 litre. If any possible neoplasm looks operable biopsy should be avoided because of the risk of implantation of malignant cells in the needle track. Twenty five per cent of patients have a small, asymptomatic, pneumothorax afterwards but tension pneumothorax is a serious complication in an emphysematous patient. Reassure the patient by letting him see the drill and hearing its noise before using it. (Pleural biopsy using an Abrams' needle carries the same risk as other pleural punctures. The risks of ' brush biopsy ' are those of bronchoscopy (p. 75).

EMERGENCIES FOLLOWING LOCAL ANALGESIA
(For Emergencies in General Anaesthesia see Chapter 26.)

Toxic effects of local analgesics are very rarely due to sensitivity. Their commonest cause is overdosage or accidental i v injection.

Itching, sneezing and wheezing are the main symptoms. Sometimes fainting quickly follows an injection and is due to emotional causes. Occasionally the added adrenaline is responsible particularly if it enters a vein. The aspiration test should be repeatedly used during subcutaneous infiltration lest a small vein be entered.

Allergic and cerebral symptoms are less quick in onset. Occasionally unconsciousness is the first sign that anything is wrong. Slighter symptoms such as talkativeness, sweating and restlessness are common and may be overlooked or put down to ' hysteria.' They are due to cortical stimulation. Facial twitchings and dilated pupils follow and in severe cases go on to delirium, convulsions (p. 309) and respiratory failure. A local type of reaction may occur in the larynx when local analgesia is followed by intense spasm of the cords.

Prevention. Always read the label carefully. Never dismiss lightly a patient's statement that he had a reaction to a local analgesic previously. Give him a small amount (0·5 ml of a 1 g/dl solution) and wait. Avoid cocaine and adrenaline in any patient taking a monoamine oxidase inhibitor (p. 565). Cocaine should never be injected but faulty labelling has caused it to be used in error. When used in the nose, throat and eye the total dosage should not exceed 200 mg for a 70 kg adult. It has been largely replaced by procaine and lignocaine (for injection) and amethocaine, lignocaine or Butacaine Sulphate BPC for surface application.

The maximum safe dose of lignocaine injected or applied to a surface for a 70 kg man is 500 mg with adrenaline (7 mg/kg) or 200 mg without adrenaline (3 mg/kg).

The dose of a local analgesic varies with the patient's weight and general condition and also with the vascularity of the tissues injected, the concentration of the drug and the presence or absence of adrenaline. Toxicity increases in geometrical and not in arithmetical progression so that a 2 per cent solution is four times more toxic than a 1 per cent solution. Adrenaline should always be added except where contraindicated by ischaemic heart disease, a peripheral part (finger, toe, penis, ear or nose) or the subsequent use of chloroform, halothane or trichloroethylene. Table 4.1 shows how the maximum safe dose of lignocaine is calculated.

Prilocaine (Citanest) is as effective as lignocaine but is said to be less toxic—the maximum safe dose being 600 mg with adrenaline and 400 mg without it. Procaine is used as a 0·5 g/dl solution, the maximum safe dose being 200 ml. Amethocaine (Decicaine) is a good, long acting surface analgesic but rapid absorption facilitates overdosage. Not more than 80 mg should be applied and

Table 4.1. *Maximum safe volume of lignocaine to inject*

CONCENTRATION PER CENT	VOLUME OF SOLUTION IN ML
0·5 with adrenaline	100
1·0 with adrenaline	50
2·0 with adrenaline	25
0·5 without adrenaline	40
1·0 without adrenaline	20
2·0 without adrenaline	10

inflamed and vascular surfaces should be avoided. Butacaine Sulphate BPC 2 g/dl is probably the safest surface analgesic. All dosage figures refer to adults; children are less tolerant. Aged, shocked and myxoedematous patients need less. Concentration of solutions by evaporation or cracked ampoules (p. 80) should be borne in mind.

Too rapid absorption can be avoided by adding adrenaline to local analgesic solutions, the strength commonly employed being 1 in 250 000. Four drops of 1 in 1 000 adrenaline from a no. 12 needle added to 25 ml of analgesic solution gives this strength. Excess of adrenaline is harmful. The maximum safe adult dose is 0·5 mg (0·5 ml of 1 in 1 000 solution). Absorption is rapid from surfaces covered by other than stratified epithelium. Cocaine should preferably be avoided for surface analgesia except in the nose, throat and eyes. Urethral injection of it is specially dangerous and more so if a stricture is present or trauma has occurred. For pharyngeal analgesia by gargling it is better to tell the patient to ' gargle and spit ' rather than to ' gargle and swallow. '

Patients with myasthenia gravis are specially liable to collapse after injection of procaine or cocaine (p. 569).

A preliminary dose of Valium (diazepam) 2 mg is a wise precaution in nervous patients. When allergy is suspected a little of the drug may be appled intranasally to see if any reaction occurs.

Treatment. For a syncopal attack lowering the head will suffice (see also p. 228). Acute allergic symptoms should be treated with adrenaline injection 1 in 1 000 0·5 ml subcutaneously. Overdosage is best treated by lowering the head, giving oxygen and controlling convulsions by small doses of suxamethonium (30 to 50 mg) i v. Artificial ventilation will be needed. Alternatively thiopentone 2·5 per cent should be given slowly into a vein. When death from respiratory depression seems imminent, 100 mg of ephedrine hydrochloride should be injected i v. Treatment for circulatory arrest (p. 724) may be needed.

After recovery always tell the patient what happened so that he can warn the doctor on any future occasion. Advise him to wear a Medic-Alert bracelet (p. 822).

AIR EMBOLISM

Air embolism is of two clinical types—venous (or pulmonary) and arterial.

Venous (or pulmonary) air embolism

This accident is most likely to be fatal if a large quantity of air enters a large vein near the heart, as when a poorly filled vein is incised and held open by retraction of the edges of the wound. This mechanism is responsible for the very rapid death which sometimes follows a suicidal throat wound. To avoid its occurrence during neurosurgical operations in the posterior fossa, especially if the patient is upright, it is usual to insert a catheter into the right atrium or pulmonary artery before operation so as to allow removal of entrapped air. During neck and axillary operations, it is less likely to occur if the head is low, so that the veins are distended. It should be remembered also that damage to pelvic veins is more liable to be followed by embolism in the Trendelenburg position than when the patient is horizontal. Air embolism has complicated numerous other procedures such as operations on intracranial venous sinuses; forceful insufflation of air (e.g., with a Higginson's syringe) following an antral wash-out; irrigation of a submaxillary abscess; Eustachian tube insufflation; filling the bladder with air; aero-urethroscopy in the presence of urethral haemorrhage; peri-renal insufflation; intra-uterine injections; criminal abortions; vaginal insufflation; tubal patency tests; manual separation of the placenta; Caesarean section, and even normal delivery at term. (The marked solubility of CO_2 makes it a much safer gas than air for many of these procedures). Another cause is haemodialysis when air enters the heparin line or the blood pump insert.

Air embolism may complicate i v infusion:

1. If the tubing is loose or cracked, or incompletely emptied of air.

2. If the level of fluid in the bottle falls below the orifice of the exit tube. Probably only a little air would enter a vein if the bottle ran dry but it is bad practice to allow it to do so. The Barts-Enfield Drip Indicator gives visible or audible warning that the bottle is nearly empty, and so helps to avoid this risk. If the air inlet needle

is not pushed fully home it may allow air to enter the adjacent end of the outlet needle.

3. If positive pressure is created in the bottle by a Higginson's syringe or rotary pump when the level of the fluid has fallen below the top of the filter or when the filter is partly blocked. The use of a plastic bag for blood enables pressure to be applied by hand and obviates any risk of air embolism. A rapid inflow into the drip bulb may cause bubbles of air to be taken below the surface and when they are passed on by a pumped transfusion they can reach the coronary arteries via a patent foramen ovale and cause death. This risk can be avoided by keeping the drip bulb full of blood or by using a second drip chamber to act as a trap for air displaced from the first.

4. If cracks exist in the tubing. The common practice of injecting drugs into the tubing leaves small holes through which air can be drawn particularly if transfusion is being forced by a pump peripheral to the puncture holes. Such injections should be given as near the cannula as possible. The risk of causing invisible damage to tubing by injections into it can be avoided by using a small connector with a side diaphragm through which injections are given. The use of translucent tubing by enabling bubbles to be seen in it might obviate this accident.

Air embolism is less likely to happen if the clip on the tubing is near the vein rather than near the container, and it may be avoided by using a drip chamber containing a plastic float which blocks the exit should the chamber run dry. This should always be used if a drip is given under pressure. Such a drip chamber must be kept vertical. Arrangement of the tubing to form a loop below the level of the patient's vein is an additional precaution.

Air embolism may also complicate phlebotomy. When using a vacuum type of bottle to collect blood there is a risk of air embolism in the donor should the vacuum be lost and the tourniquet be released before clamping the tube or removing the needle from the donor's vein. This risk could be avoided by inverting the bottle during the collection of blood. Loss of vacuum can be detected by shaking the bottle. A loud clear splash is heard when the bottle contains air at normal pressure, whereas it is difficult to make a vacuum bottle emit even indistinct sounds. When blood is collected into an unevacuated bottle there must be an air vent. If this is a needle and it is not inserted far enough to penetrate the stopper blood flow will stop after some 100 ml of blood have entered. Release of the tourniquet before clamping the tube will then allow air from the bottle to enter the veins under pressure built up in the system. This is a combination of the pressure in the obstructed veins, the pressure of the tourniquet and the weight of blood in the tubing. Blockage of the air vent during a bleed as shown by slowing down the blood flow will cause the same chain of events. It is well always to see that the air vent is clear before releasing the tourniquet.

A small amount of air injected at the elbow is known to be harmless, and it is thought that not less than 480 ml must enter a vein to produce a fatal result though a much smaller amount will cause alarming symptoms and might kill an already gravely ill patient or one who has a (clinically undiagnosable) patent foramen ovale. The rate of injection is important. Large amounts of air have failed to kill animals if injected very slowly. Even so our aim should be not to allow any air to enter a vein.

In all serious cases the right heart is distended with foam and cannot empty itself. There is sudden failure of the pulses, and dilatation of the pupils. Auscultation over the heart reveals a characteristic ' water-wheel' splashing sound. The patient takes a few deep breaths and is dead within a minute from acute right-sided heart failure. Gas bubble formation in mesenteric vessels with subsequent gangrene can follow irrigation of the bowel of infants (as in meconium ileus) with hydrogen peroxide in concentrations greater than 7·5 parts per 1 000.

Treatment. Remove the needle from the vein and lower the head. In this position the air trap is less likely to be in the outflow tract of the right ventricle than when the patient is horizontal. Having done this watch for cardiac arrest. If this occurs (and an intra-atrial catheter is not already in place (see above)) open the chest, aspirate froth from the right ventricle through a large needle and then perform manual compression of the heart. To do this before aspiration of air from the right ventricle is dangerous for it will drive air into the pulmonary vessels. Artificial respiration will probably be needed. An oesophageal stethoscope can give early warning of air in the right heart. A catheter in the right heart, to measure venous pressure (p. 751) or deliberately placed before operation in cases where air embolism is a risk, can be used to aspirate gas. If nitrous oxide is being given it should be discontinued since it will diffuse into any gas bubbles and increase their size.

Arterial air embolism

The symptoms produced depend on the route taken by the air. Embolism of the coronary arteries can cause death quickly. Syncope, paralysis and paraesthesiae result from air reaching cerebral

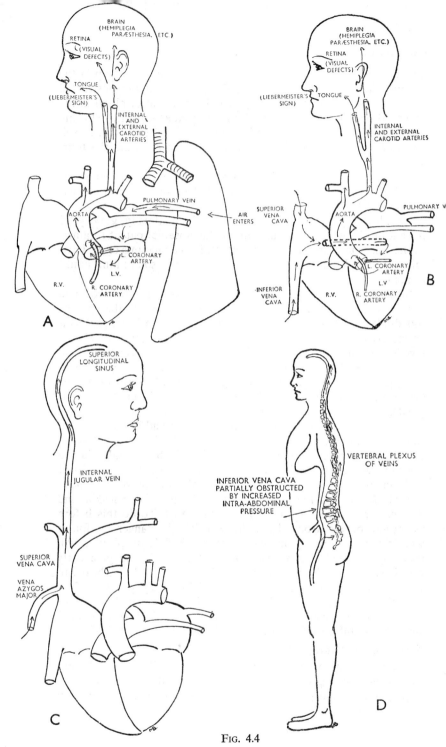

Fig. 4.4

Showing possible routes by which an air embolus may reach the
brain. (*The Practitioner.*)

Continued at foot of opposite page.

arteries. Retinal embolism causes visual defects and air entering peripheral arteries may cause areas of pallor in the skin and tongue (Liebermeister's sign).

Apart from intra-arterial transfusion and operations on the left ventricle itself the most obvious route is for air to enter a pulmonary vein, and go via the left heart to the systemic arteries (Fig. 4.4A). The accident was most often a sequel to the induction of artificial pneumothorax, but may complicate the opening of a lung abscess and irrigation of an empyema. It does not complicate haemoptysis. In the days of pneumothorax therapy it sometimes occurred when the needle entered an adhesion containing a radicle of the pulmonary vein. On inspiration the pressure in these veins is less than atmospheric, and so air was drawn into them. Death followed the injection of a small quantity of air since additional air reached the vein from the lung itself as well as from the needle. Arterial air embolism has complicated submarine escape training from ruptured lung capillaries caused by excessive intrapulmonary air pressure. (Air has also been found in the right heart in these cases, possibly getting there via pulmonary lymphatic vessels and the great veins of the neck). In cases where cerebral air embolism has followed puncture of a systemic vein, ' paradoxical ' embolism via a patent foramen ovale is the usual route (Fig. 4.4B). When a clot takes the paradoxical route there is usually a preceding pulmonary embolus. This raises the pressure in the right heart and makes incompetent a previously physiologically competent foramen ovale (present in a third of normal people). The stage is then set for a subsequent clot to pass through the foramen. In paradoxical air embolism, however, the position of the patient is probably the determining factor.

There are two other possible routes, both venous, by which air may reach the brain. Air may enter a tributary of the azygos vein or superior vena cava, and then rise in the jugular vein against the

---

Fig. 4.4—Contd.

A. Air enters a pulmonary venule when a needle punctures the lung and passes via the left auricle and the left ventricle to the aorta.

B. ' Crossed ' or ' paradoxical ' air embolism. Air enters a systemic venule in the chest wall or elsewhere and passes to the right auricle, and via a patent foramen ovale to the left auricle, left ventricle and the aorta.

C. Air enters a systemic venule and passes via the azygos vein to the superior vena cava where it rises against the blood stream (especially when the patient sits up) and passes up the internal jugular vein to the brain.

D. Air enters a systemic venule and passes via anastomoses with the vertebral venous plexus to the superior longitudinal sinus and so bypasses the heart.

blood stream to the cerebral sinuses (Fig. 4.4C). This route may explain those cases of cerebral air embolism in which symptoms do not follow quickly on the insertion of the needle, but come on later, particularly when the patient sits up.

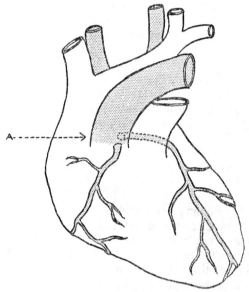

FIG. 4.5

The heart and great vessels showing the origin of the coronary arteries. It will be seen that a coronary artery does not arise from the part of the aorta marked A (right posterior aortic sinus) which will be uppermost when lying on the left side.

A further route is via anastomoses between systemic (or portal) venules and the paravertebral plexus of veins (Fig. 4.4D). Air is likely to take this route if for some reason such as coughing or high intra-abdominal pressure, the blood flow in the inferior vena cava is partially obstructed.

Treatment. In all cases cease pneumothorax induction, lower the head, and put the patient on his left sde. The reason for the left lateral position in arterial air embolism is that it lessens the chance of air entering a coronary artery (Fig. 4.5). Even though the patient quickly recovers, it is unwise to resume the operation. Pure oxygen should be inhaled since it lowers the partial pressure of nitrogen in the blood and so causes air bubbles in the circulation to shrink. Morphine should not be given lest depression of the respiratory centre be aggravated.

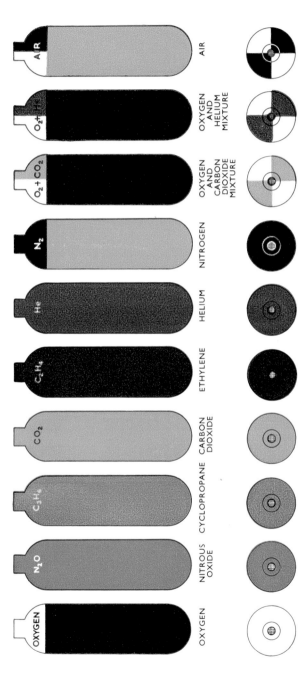

BRITISH STANDARD COLOURS FOR MEDICAL GAS CYLINDERS

OXYGEN

NITROUS OXIDE

CYCLOPROPANE

CARBON DIOXIDE

ETHYLENE

HELIUM

NITROGEN

OXYGEN AND CARBON DIOXIDE MIXTURE

OXYGEN AND HELIUM MIXTURE

AIR

Cylinders of British Oxygen Company's ENTONOX (pre-mixed 50 per cent nitrous oxide and 50 per cent oxygen) are blue with blue and white quartering at the valve end.

FIG. 4.6

British Standard colours for Medical Gas Cylinders.

MISCELLANEOUS MEDICAL ACCIDENTS

Taking the temperature

This can introduce a hazard in that hypothermia may be missed if the thermometer is not used properly. A notch at the base of the mercury column prevents the mercury from falling when the thermometer is removed. So it is essential to shake the mercury down *below the temperature scale*. If it does not rise to the scale the temperature is below 35°C and should be taken again with a special low-reading thermometer (see p. 362). It is the ' core ' rather than the skin or mouth temperature which is important. Taking the rectal temperature is a procedure not always acceptable to the patient. An alternative is the Uritemp bottle (Portex Ltd.) which records the temperature of the urine as it is passed.

Ice bags

Never put ' dry ice ' (solid CO_2) in ice bags. Its temperature is minus 75°C and it will cause tissue necrosis.

Bronchography

If the crico-thyroid route for bronchography is used it is possible to scratch the laryngeal mucosa and for the iodised oil to set up oedema. Tracheostomy may be required. Propyliodone (aqueous Dionosil) lessens this risk. In some cases tomography may yield the information and will avoid the risks of bronchography with iodised oil.

If a laryngeal catheter is used and the bronchi have not been previously emptied by tipping the patient, the retained sputum plus iodised oil may be enough to cause respiratory obstruction necessitating abandonment of the operation. Iodism (p. 86) is a further hazard. Intubation methods under anaesthesia have been complicated by heart stoppage from vagal stimulation.

The nasal catheter

This should never be passed beyond the pharynx. When it has entered the oesophagus and oxygen has been delivered other than through a reducing valve gross distension of the stomach and perforation has occurred.

Artificial respiration

The mouth-to-mouth method (p. 732) may transmit tuberculosis. The risk is lessened if a Brook airway (Fig. 32.18, p. 734) or Resusciade) (p. 733) is used.

Fractured ribs

Over-vigorous resuscitation measures in a frail patient may cause fractured ribs. Coughing may crack an apparently normal rib, though this mishap should raise the question of bone pathology (see p. 77).

Accidents with gas cylinders (see also pp. 578 and 743)

Explosion and fire can result from the careless use of gas cylinders. Grit, dust and even minute particles of cottonwool in the outlet of a cylinder may be blown into a regulator valve and cause fire. Cylinders should be turned on and off gently several times before use and turned on slightly before connecting to the regulator. Under no circumstances must oil, grease, or grease-containing substances be allowed to come in contact with cylinders or their valves. Oxygen, as well as mixtures containing ether and cyclopropane can, in the presence of friction, become highly explosive. Leaking reservoirs or rebreathing bags must be changed immediately.

Accidents have occurred because the wrong gas cylinder has been connected. The British Standard colours and labels for medical gas cylinders (Fig. 4.6) lessen this risk. The adoption of a non-interchangeable valve for cylinders of capacity not exceeding 682 litres (oxygen) or 1814 litres (nitrous oxide) makes it impossible to connect cylinders of these sizes wrongly to anaesthetic apparatus.

Telephoned instructions

These are easily mis-heard and disasters may result. So make sure that what you want is understood and so avoid a ' milk drip ' being given into a vein and ' formol saline ' being used when normal saline was intended. Be specially careful when mentioning ' sound alike ' drugs over the telephone.

Hyperbaric oxygen (p. 814)

The harmful effects to patients of breathing hyperbaric oxygen include oxygen toxicity (see below), pulmonary and aural atelectasis, pain in sinuses and teeth cavities and vomiting on decompression. Those who work in compressed air chambers may be affected by decompression sickness (p. 506), inert gas narcosis (p. 494) and avascular necrosis of bone. Various technical aspects of hyperbaric therapy present hazards. A hyperbaric environment affect flow meters, inflating cuffs and infusion bottles. The vaporisation of inhaled drugs is diminished. As in all procedures using oxygen the first risk must be guarded against.

Oxygen therapy (pp. 79 and 740)

Pure oxygen is irritant to the lungs and causes oedema and atelectasis with perhaps damage to surfactant. This only occurs at concentrations of over 70 per cent for more than 2 or 3 days. Such conditions would only apply to patients on IPPV and perhaps to air crew. (For risks in the new born see p. 397.) Oxygen therapy carries the risk of irritating the trachea from drying of secretions but only when the gas impinges on the mucosa from a nasal tube or when there is a tracheostomy or an endotracheal tube is used. In these conditions *all* the inspired gas should be humified preferably by an ultrasonic humidifier.

Draining of oedema fluid

Removal of large amounts of oedema fluid by Southey's tubes may, especially when the plasma proteins are low, be used to cause circulatory collapse, oliguria and acute potassium depletion with abdominal distension and mental confusion (p. 602). Apparently the mechanism was acute reduction in plasma volume which occurred despite the presence of oedema fluid because of poor circulation of blood in these cases.

Paracentesis abdominis

If ascites has to be tapped and a Southey's tube is used, omission of the guard makes it possible for the tube to slip into the abdomen at the time of insertion, or to part from the tubing and slip in later. It is always wise to search the bed clothes first and then to X ray the abdomen before calling a surgeon. The sudden relief of ascites may precipitate hepatic coma when liver function is greatly impaired.

Haemo-dialysis

Rapid dialysis removes relatively more water than sodium. The resulting hypernatraemia causes symptoms like those of hyperosmolar diabetic coma (p. 345). Glucose absorption plays a part also. Another complication of dialysis, especially haemo-dialysis, is headache with drowsiness and confusion coming on when the blood urea is very high. The gradient resulting from the time lag in removal of urea from the CSF as compared with blood, causes water to pass into the CSF with a rise of intracerebral pressure ('haemodialysis dysequilibrium syndrome'). More frequent and shorter periods of dialysis at lower levels of urea are preferable. Failure to stir the dialysing fluid has allowed concentrated solution to enter the circulation with resulting hypernatraemia and haemolysis. Sometimes a subdural haematoma forms because of shrinkage in brain volume with bleeding at a time when the blood is rendered incoagulable.

Peritoneal dialysis (for technique see p. 716)

If too much fluid is removed hypotension can result. Fluid which is not removed can cause circulatory overloading and cardiac failure. Glucose absorption from the dialysing fluid may lead to non-ketotic hyperglycaemic coma (p. 345). Insulin treatment may be necessary.

Gastric lavage and vomiting

The half-comatose patient may bite the doctor's finger (p. 636). Always, therefore, use a gag or boxwood wedge (p. 722). Emptying of the stomach may be very hazardous to the unconscious patient. Upper oesophageal spasm may cause a small tube to enter the larynx or, in the absence of the cough reflex, regurgitated fluid may enter the lungs. An asthma-like reaction with pulmonary oedema then occurs (p. 601). Gastric lavage, even in a comatose patient, should only be performed after full consideration of the indications. Whether prone or supine (see p. 722) the head must be low. We can prove that the tube is in the stomach by showing that fluid aspirated from it turns blue litmus paper red or by hearing injected air enter the stomach. The use of cuffed endotracheal and oesophageal tubes are the best safeguards (p. 572).

Barium placed in the drinks of old and ill patients has been shown later in the lungs even when there has been no vomiting. This emphasises the care that must be taken in feeding all such patients. They should only drink in the sitting position and should avoid going to bed with a full stomach. When dysphagia occurs in an elderly patient as after a cerebral vascular accident tube feeding is advisable. The finding of gastric contents in the lungs at necropsy does not necessarily mean that they were aspirated for they can reach the lungs by post-mortem gravitation.

The comatose patient is liable to accidents from vomiting and should always be watched until consciousness returns. The anaesthetised patient is similarly at risk and often more so as his oesophageal sphincters may be paralysed by relaxants. Vomiting is common after road accidents. Turning the patient on to his side is an important first aid measure (p. 318). After this it is wise to have an electric suction machine at hand to clear the pharynx if need be. Should inhalation of stomach contents occur, immediate broncho-scopic aspiration is desirable. It is of little use once pulmonary oedema has developed (p. 601). In an infant, an attempt may be made to aspirate milk from the bronchi by a large rubber catheter introduced through a laryngoscope. Failing these measures, postural drainage should be adopted. It would be wise to start penicillin treatment at once.

Saline emetics

As well as the mechanical hazards of vomiting saline emetics carry a risk of gross overdosage with salt resulting in metabolic acidosis and cerebral symptoms. This is particularly so if the poison taken has depressed the vomiting reflex.

Ingested mercury

The swallowing of mercury from a ruptured bougie creates a feeling of emergency but the situation is not immediately dangerous. A single bolus of metallic mercury is probably innocuous when surrounded by intact epithelium but if retained tissue damage and absorption may occur. A thermometer bulb has been bitten off and inhaled. Coughing (induced if need be by prethcamide (Micoren) i v (p. 76)) and up-ending may dislodge it. Failing this removal via a bronchoscope or by thoracotomy would be necessary. Spilled mercury is a risk in cardio-pulmonary laboratories for it breaks up into elusive globules from which it slowly evaporates at room temperatures. Treatment of the spill with a solution of zinc in $0·1$ N ($0·1$ mmol/l) hydrochloric acid will enable it to be swept up.

Mercury spillage in aircraft

Leakage of mercury from a doctor's sphygmomanometer may cause corrosion of the alloys used in aircraft construction. Aneroid instruments do not carry this risk. Mercury is a restricted article in air transport and if it has to be carried it must be specially packed.

Ingested plaster of Paris

When taking a dental impression some plaster may be swallowed. Pyloric or intestinal obstruction may follow. Glycerine followed by copious drinks of water may obviate surgical removal.

Swallowed Ryle's tube

When a Ryle's tube is completely swallowed by accident don't convert the situation to an emergency by letting the surgeon operate too soon. If there are no ill effects the patient can wait a long time (several weeks). Always use X rays *immediately before* operation for the tube may have passed on.

' Enema collapse '

A water enema in a patient already overloaded with fluid or who cannot excrete water freely may be followed by dangerous retention and ' water intoxication ' (weakness, drowsiness going on to coma, sometimes with convulsions and even focal signs (hemiplegia)) is the rare result of reduced osmolality of the blood from this cause. The risk is great in mega-colon for a water enema may not be returned. It is safer to use isosmotic sodium chloride solution. The amount given and returned should be noted. Any retained fluid should be siphoned back and not left to be absorbed.

Hydrogen peroxide when used for bowel lavage is readily absorbed and gives off oxygen in the blood. This may be enough to cause collapse possibly due in part to bacteraemia from alteration in the normal mucosal barrier against organisms (see also p. 65).

Rarely collapse has followed a barium enema when, because of a build-up of pressure below a stricture of the colon, some barium has entered a vein and reached the lungs. A misplaced nozzle has caused similar trouble from a vaginal tear.

Pacemaker hazards

A pacemaker is very unlikely to fail suddenly. If it does and there is time the patient should be taken immediately to hospital (preferably to the one which fitted it) and in an ambulance carrying a doctor with an external pacemaker. The patient should carry the address on the equipment. A patient will be in danger if a high level of electromagnetic radiation, e.g. from a diathermy apparatus or even from a combustion engine ignition system, is sufficiently close because the pacemaker output is affected. Pacemakers are unaffected by weapons detectors at present used at airports for the screening of passengers (see p. 702).

Electric convulsion therapy (ECT) (Electroplexy)

Temporary slowing of the heart and cyanosis are commonly encountered after electrically induced convulsions. Occasionally the heart may stop and then measures for circulatory arrest (p. 724) must be taken promptly. Artificial respiration may be necessary to restart breathing after convulsions. Very rarely status epilepticus has occurred and thiopentone has had to be given i v. Surgical complications, namely fractures, may also be present but can be avoided by preliminary use of a muscle relaxant. Death from ECT is rare (1 in 14 000 treatments) and is generally associated with coronary disease, a diseased heart being unable to survive the excessive demands put on it by a convulsion.

Gastroscopy

The risk of bruising or tearing the upper oesophagus during gastroscopy is slight with a fibreoptic instrument but is increased if the patient is an elderly vitamin-starved woman who has cervical osteoarthrosis.

Lower oesophageal perforation is generally associated with carcinoma of the oesophagus. X-ray after swallowing lipiodol will establish the diagnosis. Immediate resection offers the only hope of cure.

Gastroscopic perforation of the stomach is a rare accident. As the stomach is empty of food it can be treated expectantly.

Oesophageal tamponade

The chief danger is upward displacement of the Sengstaken-Blakemore tube causing laryngeal obstruction. A nurse must be in constant attendance. If respiration becomes laboured the oesophageal balloon must be deflated at once and if there is any doubt the tube must be cut across. Should the patient pull up the tube the gastric balloon may be forced away from its filling tube when it will be impossible to deflate it or remove it other than by gastrotomy. To ensure adequate tamponade the correct relative positions of the gastric and oesophageal balloons should be checked by a radio-opaque marker.

Bronchoscopy

The hazards of bronchoscopy include the following.

1. *Those due to the anaesthetic.* Local anaesthetics produce their own emergencies (p. 60). Thiopentone (Pentothal), if employed without a relaxant, is especially dangerous because any stimulus to the larynx may set up intense spasm. This is a very serious emergency since it prevents the passage of the bronchoscope through which oxygen might be given. Relaxation of the cords may occur even when death seems imminent but it should not be awaited since it can be produced by the prompt i v injection of 20 mg of succinylcholine. When relaxation occurs, the bronchoscope should be slipped through and oxygen blown in at 8 litres a minute. Failing all else tracheostomy (p. 737) should be performed and will give instant relief.

2. *Trauma.* Damage to the teeth and hyoid bone and perforation of the wall of the respiratory tract, are all possible but very unlikely. Bronchial perforation would lead to mediastinal emphysema. Passage of the bronchoscope through a tuberculous larynx may set up acute oedema and for this reason bronchoscopy should be avoided in patients with laryngeal tuberculosis. If it must be done, a tracheotomy set should also be at hand. Similar trouble may complicate the removal of tuberculous granulation tissue from the larynx.

Many of these hazards have been eliminated by the recently introduced fibreoptic instrument introduced transnasally under topical lignocaine anaesthesia.

3. *Bleeding*. Taking a specimen for biopsy, particularly in the case of an adenoma, may lead to profuse bleeding necessitating aspiration of blood through the bronchoscope and the application of an adrenaline-soaked pack. In one case of multiple bronchial papillomata, bleeding was stopped by inducing artificial pneumothorax. In another the placing of a cuffed endobronchial tube into the non-bleeding side was helpful in enabling a clear airway to be maintained. A blood transfusion may be needed.

Retained blood may lead to massive collapse. To prevent blood from passing into the lung, drainage should be promoted by lowering the head. To aid its expectoration prethcamide (Micoren) 225 to 450 mg i m may be used to make the cough reflex more sensitive.

Tuberculous patients should not be bronchoscoped until their sputum is negative and preferably absent. If there is any doubt the healthy side should be examined first to avoid the risk of carrying over tuberculous sputum.

Bronchoscopy in babies is easily complicated by spasm and oedema. It should only take a very short time and must be done by an experienced bronchoscopist.

Cardiac catheterisation

Catheterisation of the right heart carries a risk of death of 1 in 1 000. It is five times greater in the left heart.

The main hazards are cardiac arrhythmias and thrombosis of the vein at the site of insertion of the catheter. Air embolism is unusual. Blood in the pericardial sac resulting in tamponade is a rare complication. Less serious mishaps are venospasm and syncope. If a chemically sterilised catheter is introduced as far as a branch of the pulmonary artery infarction may follow. It would be safer to use an autoclaved catheter. If mercury is used as an anaerobic seal for the syringe used for blood sampling it is possible for some to enter the circulation. The resulting embolus can be shown in the lungs by X-rays. Chronic mercurialism has resulted (see also p. 73). The accident can be avoided by taking blood into a heparinised syringe and then transferring it via a 3-way tap to a syringe containing mercury.

Contraindications are ventricular tachycardia, recent pulmonary or cardiac infarction and bacterial endocarditis. The incidence rate of complications is 3·6 per cent and the mortality rate in a series of over 12 000 cases was 0·45 per cent. Cardiac catheterisation should only be done by those with special experience in the method. Any unusual feeling in the patient or persisting abnormality of rhythm should lead to termination of the examination.

Cardiac ' massage ' (p. 725)

Ribs are fractured in about a third of patients who are given cardiac ' massage ' by amateur first aiders. Injury to abdominal viscera is less common but liver bleeding can be fatal. The doctor usually knows that ribs have been broken and if there is an eventual necropsy the pathologist should be told. In the severely hypothermic patient cardiac ' massage ' may precipitate ventricular fibrillation (p. 254). Massage should wait until the patient has been warned.

Artificial ventilation

Pseudomonas lung infection is a risk for any patient on a ventilator. Antibiotics are not the answer. All filters and hoses must be changed before apparatus is used on a new patient and each day for the same patient. Models which allow for completely auto-clavable patient circuits are preferable.

Central venous pressure (p. 751)

Infection is the best recognised complication. All catheter tips should be cultured on removal. Mechanical risks are detachment of the tip or severance of the catheter ('catheter embolism'); pneumothorax, hydrothorax and perforation of the great veins. Deterioration of the patient's condition and respiratory embarrass-ment are warnings that the catheter is wrongly placed. Blood must be easily withdrawn from a catheter if it is in the lumen of a vein.

Angiocardiography

The chief hazard is syncope from sensitivity to diodone and the speed of giving it especially in patients with congenital heart disease. It cannot be predicted by preliminary testing or prevented by pre-medication.

Aortography and angiography

Aortography may be performed by injecting 30 ml of 70 per cent diodone into the aorta at the level of the twelfth thoracic vertebra by the percutaneous translumbar route. Should the bevel of the needle be partly in the aortic wall and partly in the lumen dissection may easily occur. (The position of the needle point should be checked by taking an X-ray film after 5 ml of diodone have been injected). Dissection may do no more than cause pain or confuse the diagnosis but it may damage the renal arteries by dissection or

4

thrombosis. This and also flooding of the renal arteries with diodone can cause serious anuria (p. 374). Aortography by femoral
catheterisation is less risky particularly if the patient can't keep
quite still. Multiple punctures and movements of the patient have
caused leakage of blood. Damage to lumbar arteries has caused
paraplegia.

Local haemorrhage, thrombosis, subintimal dissection and
aneurysm formation are all risks of arterial punctures. An arterial
catheter is damaging if too large and retained too long, particularly
if the cardiac output is low. Upper limb arteries are more liable to
spasm than are those of the legs. Most arterial puncture mishaps
are best treated surgically. A 'wait and see' policy can be
disastrous. An unusual result of carotid artery angiography is a
vertebral arterio-venous fistula which can occur if one vertebral
artery is abnormally large. The result is a continuous waterfall
sound which may be sufficiently disturbing to justify tying of the
vessels. For a threatened stroke during cerebral angiography give
5 per cent CO_2 in oxygen (p. 303) or let the patient rebreathe from
a paper bag.

Hysterosalpingography

Iodised oil injected into the uterus may enter the uterine venous
sinuses by 'venous intravasation' particularly if used under pressure
in the early post-menstrual period or after curettage. In most cases
a little lipiodol in the lungs is innocuous but there may be early
collapse with dyspnoea, cyanosis and cough. Sometimes symptoms
are delayed. X-rays show fine dense opacities throughout the lung
fields. Iodised oil has now been superseded by water-soluble
contrast medium (76 g/dl Urografin) which does not carry these
risks.

RADIOLOGICAL HAZARDS IN CHILDREN

The contrast medium Gastrografin (76 g/dl Urografin plus
flavouring) can seriously worsen a dehydrated child since it will
absorb 3 or 4 times its volume of water. For a small child, only
small amounts (5 ml) should be used.

When X-raying a child with Hirschprung's disease, the amount of
contrast medium should be limited to the minimum amount possible. It is better to use isosmotic sodium chloride solution than
water to suspend the barium (see Enema Collapse, p. 73).

When the oesophagus of an infant is flooded with contrast
medium, to demonstrate a tracheo-oesophageal fistula, there is a

risk of inhalation. An anaesthetist should be at hand, ready to treat this emergency by bronchoscopic suction.

SPECIAL HAZARDS IN THE NEWBORN

Artificial respiration in the newborn

Over-enthusiastic mouth-to-mouth insufflation (p. 732) and of intratracheal oxygen under pressure has caused alveolar rupture and mediastinal emphysema (p. 599). The resulting ' air block ' causes cyanosis and irregular breathing with the chest fully expanded. Diagnosis is confirmed if subcutaneous emphysema appears. After laryngoscopy and gentle tracheal suction treatment should be on the lines suggested on p. 392.

Oxygen therapy in premature infants

Prolonged administration of high concentrations of oxygen plays a part in causing retrolental fibroplasia in premature infants. Oxygen should not be given to premature babies unless ordered by a doctor. Its use should not be continued any longer than is necessary and the concentration should be kept at the lowest level necessary to relieve symptoms (preferably under 40 per cent).

Peroxide bowel lavage (p. 74)

Inhaled milk feeds

Inhalation of a large vomit may kill an infant. Smaller quantities of inhaled milk cause bronchopneumonia. Small vomits and unskilled and too early feeding of premature babies may lead to fatal post-feeding asphyxia from inhaled milk. These accidents can be avoided by abandoning two common practices, namely, leaving infants to feed themselves from a bottle while lying down and swaddling tightly after a feed so that movement is prevented.

Similar trouble may follow if a nasal feeding tube enters the larynx. Before giving a nasal feed therefore the position of the tube should be checked. The mouth and nostrils should be gently closed and the proximal end of the tube held under water or close to the doctor's conjunctiva. If the distal end of the tube is in the trachea a current of air will be detected. An alternative test is to blow down the tube while someone listens with a stethoscope over the stomach. Polythene tubing, particularly of large diameter (over 0·7 mm) may perforate the oesophagus in premature infants when used for nasal feeding. Vinyl tubing is more pliable. It would be wise to round the tip or to seal it by heat or wax and make lateral holes in it.

Another risk of careless feeding of infants, and particularly of those with cleft palates, is passage of infected milk up the Eustachian tubes with resulting otitis media.

Incubator hazards

Faulty insulation in an electrically heated incubator may easily cause fire in the oxygen-enriched atmosphere. Drops of oil and methylated spirit increase the risk. Ether should be avoided for cleaning since it gives rise to formaldehyde in contact with plastic material.

Drugs

Because of temporary enzyme deficiencies the newborn baby may respond abnormally to drugs which older children tolerate. Chloramphenicol is only slowly metabolised in the newborn and doses of 100 mg/kg/day (or 25 mg/kg in prematures) may cause a ' gray syndrome' with hypothermia, pallor and vasomotor collapse. Dosage should not exceed 25 mg/kg/day in prematures and 50 mg/kg/day in full term infants under one month.

Similar considerations apply to barbiturates, aspirin, ephedrine and probably many other drugs. Vitamin K analogues increase the risk of kernicterus in premature babies. The prophylactic dose should not exceed 1 mg. Preferably the mother should be given 10 mg not later than four hours before delivery. The treatment dose for haemorrhagic disease of the newborn should not exceed 10 mg.

EMERGENCIES FOLLOWING INJECTIONS

Cracks in ampoules

Invisible cracks in ampoules may lead to contamination of their contents with the antiseptic fluid in which they are stored. This should, therefore, have a distinctive colour. Ampoules should preferably be stored dry to avoid all risk of contamination. Even so water may be selectively lost from such an ampoule and lead to concentration of its contents. Plastic ampoules eliminate these troubles and also the risk of small particles of glass entering the contents when the ampoule is opened. The practice of inverting a ruber-capped bottle in antiseptic should be similarly condemned as negative pressure may allow antiseptic to enter.

Accidental i v injection

The plunger should always be withdrawn a little after inserting a needle subcutaneously or i m and before injecting fluid to make sure that a vein has not been entered. In the case of a thick suspension like procaine penicillin traction on the plunger must be prolonged. If one has to use the bad practice of mass vaccination where only the needle is sterilised gross contamination of the syringe with blood may be avoided by inserting the needle into a pinched-up fold of skin which is very unlikely to contain a vein. (Even so after several insertions enough tissue juice may enter the syringe to make the risk of transmitting hepatitis virus a real one.) In deeper injections if the needle can be turned through a right angle it is unlikely to be in a vein.

Accidental injection of a toxic dose

It may happen that an overdose of morphine or other drug is injected inadvertently. If this is subcutaneous or i m prompt action may obviate ill effects. If practical a tourniquet should be applied at once to prevent absorption and released at suitable intervals, so that a toxic dose is not absorbed and gangrene is avoided. Should the dose be very large, it might be advisable to incise the part and irrigate it with saline. If application of a tourniquet is impracticable, absorption can be delayed by application of ice or subcutaneous injection of adrenaline. In the case of **morphine** the antidote naloxone (Narcan) should be given. **Adrenaline** overdosage (minimum lethal dose 4 mg = 4 ml of 1 in 1 000 solution; maximum tolerated dose 8 mg) causes a reaction similar to, but more serious than, that seen in a phaeochromocytoma crisis (p. 356). The circulatory volume is depleted by intense vasoconstriction so that paradoxical hypotension occurs later. Overdosage calls for the use of an adrenergic blocking agent (pp. 232 and 357). A smaller dose of adrenaline may cause trouble if a patient's myocardium has been made more sensitive to sympathetic stimulation by isoprenaline (p. 89) taken by mouth or by excessive use of an inhaler.

Anaphylactic shock and allergic reactions

An alarming reaction may follow the sudden release into the circulation of histamine which results from an allergic insult such as injection of foreign protein or an insect sting. It can follow a dose of aspirin or penicillin. It is liable to occur when the patient has had an injection of serum of similar origin more than 10 days previously. The longer the interval between the injection and the onset of symptoms the milder the reaction. Non-protein substances may be responsible and it can follow skin tests in allergic subjects. Virus vaccines prepared from chick embryos may upset those allergic to egg protein. Anaesthetic agents may be responsible, the anaesthetist noticing severe resistance to ventilation caused by intense bronchospasm.

The reaction may be simply local swelling and urticaria and marked itching. Sometimes there is asthma. When more severe the patient experiences constriction of the chest and abdominal pain. He may vomit. Circulatory failure, coma and death may follow. Secondary complications such as coronary thrombosis precipitated by low blood pressure can complicate the picture.

Prevention. Forethought is important. A Medic-Alert bracelet may point to the diagnosis (p. 822). Use serum of human origin if available (see Humotet, p. 638). Avoid skin testing in children who have a history of being allergic especially to animal hair. Always read the label carefully. Put a sphygmomanometer cuff in position proximal to the site of an i m into the arm before you start. Ensure by pulling back the piston when giving an i m injection that a vein has not been entered. When giving serum take the precaution of using cautious diluted doses (p. 745). Lastly, have ready all the necessary drugs for use if need be (see anaphylaxis tray, p. 745).

Treatment. Lower the head and use any or all of the following measures.

1. Tighten the cuff if an i m injection has been given. Use Adrenaline Injection BP 0·3 ml around the site. These are measures to diminish absorption.

2. Give Adrenaline Injection 0·5 ml i m into the opposite arm and massage the place. Repeat if need be at 15 minute intervals. A 1 in 10 dilution can be given i v.

3. Set up an i v dextrose saline drip and add noradrenaline (Levophed) if the blood pressure is low.

4. If there is bronchospasm use aminophylline 0·5 g by very slow i v injection until relief is achieved, and other measures for asthma (p. 196).

5. Give oxygen by any convenient method (p. 740).

6. Give hydrocortisone hemisuccinate 100 mg i v.

Poliomyelitis following injections

Thirteen per cent of paralytic cases of poliomyelitis in children from 6 months to 2 years have been found to be causally related to vaccinations. The risk is greatest with alum-precipitated diphtheria-pertussis prophylactics but does not extend beyond a period of one month after injection. It would be wise not to inject prophylactics during a poliomyelitis epidemic. This advice does not apply in the case of very young infants (under 6 months) in whom the risk of poliomyelitis is less than that of the diseases against which they are routinely immunised. Two weeks should elapse after poliomyelitis vaccination before any other immunising injections or vaccinations are given. BCG vaccination should be separated from poliomyelitis vaccination by at least four weeks.

Tooth extraction and poliomyelitis

Extraction of teeth during a poliomyelitis epidemic is undesirable. If it has to be done human normal immunoglobulin (p. 794) should be given first. Similar considerations apply to tonsillectomy.

Neurological sequelae of prophylactic vaccinations

Complications at all levels of the nervous system may follow the injection of sera and various prophylactics. They are quite rare and not usually of an urgent nature. As they probably result from anaphylactic hypersensitivity treatment by antihistamine drugs would seem wise. As there is an appreciable risk of encephalitis from yellow fever vaccination in infants the requirement for international travel is generally waived for children under one year (p. 706).

Blood products and risks of hepatitis

See p. 95.

Smallpox vaccination (p. 757)

In sufferers from chronic eczema smallpox vaccination may cause severe generalised vaccinia with a mortality as great as that of smallpox (p. 757). It must not be forgotten that an eczematous child may catch vaccinia from close contact with a recently vaccinated sibling. If vaccination is imperative it should be accompanied by immunoglobulin and prednisolone as described below. Steroids inhibit antibody response to an antigen if given two days or less before vaccination but as all their metabolites are eliminated within 48 hours steroids given before then would have no adverse effect. However since vaccinia virus is live steroids can enhance its pathogenicity and cause vaccinia to be generalised. For this reason vaccination should be postponed for at least a month after steroid therapy ceases.

It is best not to vaccinate a pregnant woman and certainly to avoid doing it during the first three months of pregnancy.

Post-vaccinial encephalomyelitis (p. 441) is a rare complication. It is mostly confined to primary vaccination of adults and would be minimised if primary vaccination was done in infancy. The incidence is independent of the strain of virus used and seems to be related to different susceptibility of patients in different areas, e.g. its incidence is high in the Netherlands. An adult who feared the risk of it and yet had to be vaccinated in order to go abroad urgently (p. 702) could be given 5 ml of human specific immunoglobulin (p. 794) i m at the same time as vaccination. The value of steroids to prevent post-vaccinal encephalitis is very doubtful and their use is contrary to current belief. Revaccination should be avoided, and some countries will excuse it, if previous vaccination caused encephalitis. Even so it has been done without untoward results and it might have to be considered perhaps with human specific immunoglobulin as described on p. 794 if the risk of smallpox was great.

Although there is no evidence that smallpox vaccination has initiated poliomyelitis it is possible that it has increased the severity of an attack which the patient was incubating when vaccinated. In view of this and also of the difficulty of diagnosing bulbar poliomyelitis from vaccinal encephalomyelitis it would be wise to postpone routine vaccination during a poliomyelitis epidemic.

Loss of an eye has resulted from accidental inoculation of the conjunctiva from the tube of lymph or from scratching the arm and then rubbing the eye. Prompt irrigation may prevent trouble. Specific immunoglobulin from a recently vaccinated person (p. 794) should be given and also cortisone.

EMERGENCIES FOLLOWING THE USE OF CERTAIN DRUGS

The Jarisch-Herxheimer reaction

Mild forms of this ' therapeutic shock ' occur in over half the patients with early syphilis and show as an influenza-like illness with pyrexia, headache and a rigor within 12 hours of the first injection of penicillin. It rarely occurs when treating neurosyphilis and cardiovascular syphilis. The theory is that symptoms may be accentuated because of massive destruction of spirochaetes and liberation of toxin in a vital organ, such as the brain or the heart. The rapid softening of the wall of an aneurysm, acute oedema in a gummatous larynx, convulsions and coma in general paralysis of the insane and paraplegia in syphilitic lesions of the cord may all result. The reaction may also occur in leptospirosis.

When headaches and malaise follow the injections of penicillin for gonorrhoea, the coexistence of syphilis should be suspected. Sometimes a syphilitic rash is brought out or accentuated. Pyrexia to 37°C is very common following penicillin for neurosyphilis.

The reaction is ' all or none ' and cannot be prevented or diminished by starting with small doses of penicillin.

If a reaction occurs the treatment should be symptomatic. Antihistamine drugs have not been found helpful but prednisone will lessen the reaction.

Excretion urography

The dose of contrast medium should contain up to 600 mg iodine / kg BW. The incidence of major reactions is low (0·1 per cent). Death directly due to IVP is very rare (estimates vary from 1 in 40 000 to 1 in 116 000). Many patients have trivial reactions and about 8 per cent experience nausea (Davies, 1975). Pre-testing is unhelpful and there is no medical or medicolegal indication for its use. Prophylactic antihistamines are not advised. Patients with myelomatosis may suffer anuria but underhydration is probably a more important factor than alleged deposition of myeloma protein in the tubules.

Retrograde pyelography

Entry of the catheter into a vein in the renal pelvis has been followed by rigors. Contrast medium may be absorbed rapidly by an inflamed mucosa. The bladder should therefore be emptied at the end of the examination. Extravasation into the retroperitoneal tissues is not followed by any ill effects.

Intravenous cholecystography

This is more likely to cause a reaction if an oral cholecystographic medium has been given in the previous 24 hours. There should be a five day interval. I v cholecystography should be avoided in macroglobulinaemia.

l-noradrenaline (Levophed) drip

Extravasation (' tissuing ') of l-noradrenaline can cause extensive skin necrosis from ischaemia (p. 50). Multiple subcutaneous injections into the affected area of Piperoxan Hydrochloride BPC or phentolamine (Rogitine), using about 5 mg in 20 ml, will prevent this. When i v therapy is difficult and extravasation likely 5 mg of phentolamine may be added to each litre of l-noradrenaline given. This does not interfere with pressor effects but it obviates tissue necrosis if there is any leakage.

Paraldehyde (p. 755)

This has caused serious inflammation when given by rectum or by mouth because it has been slowly converted in the bottle into

acetic acid. Paraldehyde bottles should be of coloured glass and
kept in a dark, cool place. It is well to check them periodically.
Paraldehyde dissolves plastics and so must not be put into plastic
bottles or syringes. It could be given i v (p. 311) but it causes violent
coughing and has precipitated fatal pulmonary oedema.

Anti-thyroid drugs

On rare occasions, these cause agranulocytosis. Routine white
cell counts are, however, useless in its early detection, since the
typical disappearance of polymorphs may be very rapid in onset. If
a patient taking these drugs develops pyrexia and a sore throat, he
should be given penicillin 500 000 units at once and a white cell
count made. Should agranulocytosis be found, continue with penicillin and also give pyridoxine 50 mg daily.

Slow release tablets

Enteric coated tablets of potassium chloride can cause intestinal
ulceration and perforation. The wax-cored slow release tablets (Slow
K) do not appear to carry this risk.

Eye-drops

Watery fluorescein eye drops have been found to be easily contaminated with *Pseudomonas pyocyanea* which will cause serious
damage when there is a corneal abrasion. Only drops freshly made
up with Solution for Eye-Drops BPC and BNF or those dispensed
in individual dose containers are safe. Alternatively lamellae of
fluorescein 0·26 mg or fluorescein impregnated filter paper (p. 524)
should be used.

Eye drops containing mydriatics (atropine, hyoscine and cyclo-
pentolate) may be absorbed from the nose and cause toxic symptoms especially in children. It is well to press on the inner canthus
to prevent them from entering the lachrymal duct.

Iodism

Very rarely acute iodism follows injection of iodised oil into
the bronchial tree. Tests for iodine sensitivity are not very reliable
but at any rate will show that 'reasonable care' was taken. Weak
Solution of Iodine BP 0·3 ml in a little milk should be taken on the
previous day and the patient watched for a rash or coryza. Propyliodone (Aqueous Dionosil) is less likely to cause trouble. Acute
anaphylaxis may follow the injection of contrast medium for cholecystography.

If iodism occurs it is only rarely dangerous though it may cause alarm. Treatment depends on facilitating the excretion of iodine compounds in the urine. Simply stopping administration of the drug and insisting that the patient drinks freely—about eight pints of fluid a day—usually suffices. Calamine lotion should be applied to the eruption; bullae should be snipped with sterile scissors and penicillin given. In an iodine-sensitive patient brominized oil (May & Baker) could be used for any subsequent examinations.

Penicillin sensitivity

Penicillin sensitivity is the most common cause of acute anaphylaxis in clinical practice. It shows as an immediate collapse with bronchospasm, possibly fatal, or as delayed pyrexia, urticaria (especially round the site of injection), joint effusions and lymph gland enlargement. Contact dermatitis also occurs. The incidence varies from 1 per cent in the general population to 10 per cent in those who have had penicillin before. The risk of a reaction is greatest when penicillin is injected, especially i v, and least when it is given by mouth. The fact that sensitivity to one kind of penicillin normally implies sensitivity to all types, suggests that a common metabolite is responsible. Not every rash after penicillin is due to it and, since a diagnosis of sensitivity precludes further use of penicillin, the diagnosis should only be made after careful thought: this is especially true in children, in whom rashes are common but penicillin sensitivity is rare. There is no reliable test for sensitivity, and so all patients should be asked about it and a history of it should never be viewed casually. A sensitive patient's notes should be marked and he should carry a warning card or a Medic-Alert bracelet (p. 822). When giving penicillin, a tray should be at hand, as when giving serum (p. 745).

Insulin

Patients stabilised on insulin of predominantly bovine origin very occasionally develop hypoglycaemia if given the same dose of insulin derived from pigs. This is because bovine insulin produces antibodies which may partially neutralise its effect but which have little effect on porcine insulin. Little antibody to porcine insulin is produced as it is not a strong antigen. A change from porcine to bovine insulin does not appear to be hazardous. It is probably best for patients not to change brands of insulin without good reason.

Anticoagulants

Haemorrhage is the only hazard of uncontrolled dosage but it rarely occurs until the prothrombin concentration falls below 10 per cent. Haematuria is the first sign but more serious haemorrhage can occur spontaneously into the brain, pericardium and adrenals. Haemorrhage can be countered, though not immediately, by repeated small transfusions of fresh blood and by vitamin K therapy (p. 755). Contraindications to phenindione, nicoumalone and warfarin are liver and kidney disease, blood disease and bleeding tendencies, gross oedematous states and non-specific pericarditis. Prothrombin activity should not be depressed until 48 hours have elapsed since an operation, particularly on the brain and spinal cord. Anticoagulants should be used cautiously if the patient is known to have a peptic ulcer.

A patient receiving heparin is similarly liable to haemorrhage. I m injections of heparin should be avoided since they may cause haematomas.

Heparin overdosage is quickly countered by protamine sulphate by slow i v injection. 1 mg neutralises 100 units of heparin.

The effects of Arvin (Ancrod) (pp. 145 and 243) can be reversed by the slow i v injection of 1 ml of specific antidote (goat globulin). This plus 3 to 5 g of fibrinogen will bring back the clotting time to normal within an hour.

Transplacental iatrogenic neonatal disease (see pp. 355 and 413)

Dangerous combinations of drugs

Sometimes drugs innocuous in themselves prove dangerous in combination. Parenteral injection of soluble calcium salts potentiates the action of digitalis glucosides and increases the irritability of heart muscle. Occasionally, a digitalised patient has died from ventricular fibrillation induced by calcium. It is recommended that digitalis should be stopped for four days before calcium is given i v. A patient suffering from the ' milk alkali ' syndrome is similarly sensitive to digitalis and more so because his serum potassium is low also from alkalosis. Digitalis sensitivity may also result from potassium loss caused by chlorothiazide. In all cases i v injections of calcium, and particularly of calcium chloride, should be made very slowly (p. 56). Calcium is, therefore, not as suitable as other substances such as saccharin for determination of the circulation time. Many drugs like amphetamines and adrenaline and even trivial cough remedies containing phenylpropanolamine as well as tyramine-rich foods (beer, Bovril, broad beans, cheese, Cola drinks, figs, herrings, liver, yeast extract) will precipitate a hypertensive crisis (p. 356) in a patient taking a monoamine oxidase inhibitor (p. 565) for depression. Pethidine will render such a patient deeply comatose. (For details of treatment of these emergencies see p. 566). Another dangerous combination is adrenaline during anaesthesia with chloroform, cyclopropane, halothane and trichloroethylene. Adrenaline is also dangerous if injected within two hours of taking isoprenaline because the sensitivity of the myocardium to sympathetic stimulation is increased and ventricular fibrillation may result. The effects of morphine, barbiturates, bromides and alcohol are at least additive and may be synergistic.

OTHER REACTIONS FOLLOWING INJECTIONS

The wrong drug

Numerous examples could be found of emergencies due to injection of the wrong drug. The label should always be read carefully because some drugs such as carbachol are put up in various strengths of which only the weaker ones are suitable for injection. If the label is missing or illegible the drug should never be used. Even a substance as apparently innocuous as distilled water has caused trouble from haemolysis when given i v. Complicated techniques for preparing solutions for i v use such as I^{131}-labelled human albumin may in a mysterious way lead to reactions. Penicillin for injection has been dissolved in the fluid from a 2 ml ampoule which contained morphine. Diluents should be taken from larger ampoules to lessen this risk. Sudden death has followed the use of 10 ml ampoules of drugs, mistaken for water or saline, to dilute drugs for i v use of to flush i v cannulas. The risk is avoided by never omitting to read the label though something can be said for colouring certain solutions, e.g. potassium, as an extra safeguard.

The wrong route

Emergencies may also arise from the injection of the right drug by the wrong route. Adrenaline, unless very dilute and given very slowly, may cause death from ventricular fibrillation if injected i v particularly if given within two hours of a dose of isoprenaline. Less serious results are severe blanching, headache, palpitation, vertigo, and occasionally hemiplegia from vascular spasm. As adrenaline is rapidly oxidised in the tissues, useful therapeutic intervention is impracticable, but should adrenaline 1 in 100, which is meant for aerosol use, be injected it would be wise to counteract its effect by inhalation of amyl nitrite (see also p. 81). Adrenaline should not be injected i m, particularly into the buttock, because it lowers local oxygen tension by vasoconstriction and so may lead to gas gangrene infection. Carbachol given i v may cause collapse. The clinical picture of fat embolism (p. 653) may result if oily solutions are injected into veins. Aspiration should therefore always be tried before giving an i m injection particularly of an oily solution. A 'milk drip' has been given i v. It is safer to call it an intragastric drip. Too rapid i v injection of many solutions, especially cold ones, will cause chest pain and rigors. Ampoules of cold solutions should be warmed in hot water (43°C.) before use, or the syringe containing the drug should be ' sealed ' with a hypodermic needle and placed in hot water. Inadvertent injection of a vaccine into a small vein may quickly produce an alarming result. Material contaminated with bacteria or their products will cause sharp febrile reactions if given i v. If symptoms do not abate in a few hours, blood should be taken for culture and penicillin therapy started. If a patient complains of a queer taste in the mouth after a subcutaneous or i m injection one should suspect that the material has entered a vein and particularly if there is some bleeding at the puncture site.

Soluble sulphonamides cause disastrous results if used intrathecally and should never be given by this route. Care must be taken not to use intrathecally penicillin to which phenol has been added as a preservative since, though innocuous elsewhere, it may cause a severe and even fatal reaction. Procaine Benzylpenicillin is not simply a mixture of penicillin and procaine but a new compound which can cause severe reactions if injected i v or even i m. The anaphylaxis tray (p. 745) should always be at hand when procaine penicillin preparations are used.

CIRCULATORY ARREST

In about a quarter of the cases of sudden arrest of the heart beat the heart is diseased and the condition is ventricular fibrillation. Sudden stoppage may complicate many, even minor, procedures in patients with healthy hearts. The mechanism is vagal inhibition and hypoxia—a combination which may exist in a patient under an anaesthetic. A more direct mechanical cause is venous air embolism (p. 63). While the doctor should always be prepared for this emergency he should keep his sense of proportion and not by resuscitation simply prolong the act of dying in patients with serious heart or other disease. He should respect the dignity of death and avoid unnecessary procedures. His immediate problem is not to try to distinguish between ventricular fibrillation and simple asystole for it is impossible clinically but to keep oxygenated blood going to the brain. When this has been achieved the immediate emergency is over. A full account of what to do is given on p. 724.

Cardioversion

There is a risk of causing cardiac arrest if a DC shock is used in an over-digitalised patient. If a serious dysrhythmia resistant to drugs must be stopped by using a low energy (5 Joules) shock ventricular bigeminy will indicate when to desist.

LABORATORY HAZARDS

Special risks of contracting hepatitis face laboratory technicians in the handling of body fluids, particularly blood. Patients who present a higher risk than usual of transmitting serum hepatitis B to laboratory staff are: those who have had viral hepatitis; those on haemodialysis or immunosuppressive therapy; those attending haemophilia centres or clinics for drug addicts and mentally subnormal children in institutions (see p. 797). Specimens from such patients and their request forms should be marked ' Hepatitis risk '. Special care is needed at all stages: in taking the specimen: in transferring it to the container; in transporting it to the laboratory; in handling it by the office and laboratory staff and in its ultimate disposal. The technician should use special care in handling such specimens and wear goves and a mask. The hands should be washed with 1 per cent hypochlorite and the bench top washed down with it. Some tests such as sedimentation rates and platelet counts should be avoided in patients who are hepatitis risks. For specific immunoglobulin for prevention of serum hepatitis after accidental inoculation with hepatitis B associated antigen see p. 800.

DRUG-INDUCED SYMPTOMS

As well as accidents caused by the procedures already mentioned symptoms, sometimes urgent, can often be iatrogenic and due to the drugs prescribed. If these are unfamiliar because new or rare always check the information sheet supplied with them or phone the pharmacist before use. Symptoms may be dose-related (due to accumulation of a drug and so predictable) or non-dose-related (due to hypersensitivity and non-predictable). The mechanisms of dose-related effects can be altered rates of metabolism due to enzyme induction or inhibition as well as altered bioavailability (absorption). For example, when the enzyme-inducing effect of barbiturates is removed the dose of normally metabolised anticoagulant becomes excessive and serious haematuria can occur. Patients on long-term anticoagulant therapy should not be given other drugs without considering this question of enzyme induction. An example of enzyme inhibition is the removal of phenylbutazone which was inhibiting chlorpropamide causing the dose to be excessive with resulting hypoglycaemia. Plasma protein binding is another mechanism concerned in causing drug-induced symptoms. Many drugs after absorption are bound to plasma proteins and only the part remaining free is active. Some drugs such as phenylbutazone compete for binding sites with others such as warfarin and render a dose of the latter excessive which would be satisfactory if given alone. Adrenergic blocking drugs (clonidine, bethanidine, guanethidine and debrisoquine) are concentrated in adrenergic nerve endings as are catecholamines. Antidepressant drugs are similarly concentrated and will inhibit the effect of antihypertensive drugs with possibly disastrous results. Methyldopa is a safer drug for patients also needing antidepressants but as its side effects are similar to those of antidepressants a betablocker would be preferable for hypertensive patients who are depressed.

The doctor should familiarise himself with the side effects of all the drugs in his repertoire and be aware of the interactions between them. Possible side effects are: amphetamine (confusion and apprehension); chloramphenicol (aplastic anaemia); aspirin (asthma and gastro-intestinal bleeding); atropine or belladonna (confusion and excitement); chlorothiazide (gout and potassium depletion); chlorpromazine (jaundice); ephedrine (tremor, palpitation and difficulty in micturition); hypotensive drugs (coronary and retinal thrombosis and renal failure); steroids (potassium depletion, peptic ulcer complications and depression); imipramine (tremor, diplopia and hypomania); phenothiazines and haloperidol (Serenace) (Parkinsonism).

Drugs normally safe can be dangerous when past their shelf life. Deteriorated tetracycline, for example, causes renal damage but the tetracycline Vibramycin (doxycycline) is not known to deteriorate and in any case is not excreted by the kidneys and so is safe in renal failure.

Many drugs can cause trouble if added to i v infusions even though they cause no visible change. None should be put in a drip which is likely to run for over 6 hours. No drugs should ever be added to transfused blood (except perhaps chlorpheniramine, see p. 102) or blood products, lipid mixtures, aminoacids or mannitol. Gentamicin should not be added to an i v drip or given in a drip at all. This is because the serum levels thus attained are too low. It is best given as an i v bolus but should not be repeated unless blood levels can be estimated (see p. 388). Only isosmotic sodium chloride should be used for a penicillin infusion and this should be only made up just before use. When potassium chloride is added not more should be infused than 80 mmol (6 g KCl) in 24 hours. Heparin, antibiotics and hydrocortisone are incompatible if given in an infusion.

The following are incompatible with all other drugs if given by i v infusion: ampicillin, amphoteracin B, diazepam, frusemide, iron dextran, phenytoin sodium and compound vitamin preparations. Unless its compatibility is known the pharmacist should be consulted before adding any drugs to a drip. A 'Drug Added' label should be attached when appropriate.

Even when clear and cloudy (delayed) insulins are injected with the same syringe mixing should be avoided lest soluble insulin be partly converted to the delayed kind. Contamination of the clear bottle with cloudy insulin is avoided by putting air into the cloudy bottle first, then taking up the clear insulin and then the cloudy.

Not all supposedly inert substances added unnamed to drug formulations are without effects. Wheat flour as a tablet excipient may by its gluten content upset some patients. Lactose is another example and there are many others. The reader is referred to an article 'Problems presented by components of drug vehicles' by M. L. Rogers and C. W. Barrett in Adverse Drug Reaction Bulletin No. 47, August 1974.

It should not be forgotten that almost all the procedures we use in our daily work and even the most trivial of them may, under certain circumstances, cause emergency situations. This applies not only to the technical procedures already discussed but also to the routine methods of examination. We should not alarm our patient, for example, by raising our eyebrows on the unexpected discovery of serious disease or by thinking aloud. Careless use of words has frequently caused collapse of patient and relatives. 'Watch your word' is a good maxim for the doctor faced with an emergency, for his word is a therapeutic instrument no less powerful to avert and no less dangerous to produce an emergency than a surgeon's scalpel.

C. ALLAN BIRCH

FOR FURTHER READING

DAVIES, P., ROBERTS, M. B. & ROYLANCE, J. (1975). Acute reactions to urographic contrast media. *Lancet*, **1**, 434-437.

D'ARCY, P. F. & GRIFFIN, J. P. *Iatrogenic Diseases*. Oxford University Press, 1972.

HARVEY, R. F. & READ, A. E. *The Medical Annual*. Special article on Iatrogenic Disease, page 9. Bristol: Wright, 1973.

THE HAZARDS OF BLOOD TRANSFUSIONS

PROTECTION OF THE DONOR

In a properly organised service where only healthy volunteers are selected the hazard to the donor is negligible. Each donor's haemoglobin level should not be below 13·5 g/dl for males and 12·5 g/dl for females. Donors bled more than two or three times a year may show a reduction of serum iron concentration and a consequent increase in total iron binding capacity. Regular donors should be encouraged to take 0·4 g of ferrous sulphate daily for about a month after each donation. There is a small risk of a cerebral vascular accident if a hypertensive donor is suddenly depleted of 400 ml of blood. Hypertensives (BP 200/100) should only be bled as part of their treatment and then only under medical supervision. The risks of venesection are directly proportional to the experience of the doctor. A bruise will occasionally follow a difficult venepuncutre and if this is anticipated the donor should be warned lest he should worry unduly. All donors should be encouraged to rest for 20 minutes and have a drink of tea or fruit juice after each donation. This reduces the risk of an immediate faint. Delayed faints are more serious because the donor will have left the premises and may be at risk on the road or at work. Those known to be prone to fainting attacks are best advised not to be regular blood donors. It is a wise precaution to obtain signed statements from donors stating that they do not suffer from conditions such as heart disease, tuberculosis or epilepsy lest they blame a relapse on the doctor taking their blood. Those in hazardous occupations should not give blood within 12 hours of returning to work. When a glass bottle is used to collect blood there is a risk of air embolism if the air vent becomes blocked during donation (p. 63). This danger is avoided by using collapsible plastic bags for the collection of blood.

PROTECTION OF THE RECIPIENT

Donor blood should, whenever possible, be obtained from a recognised blood transfusion service. This ensures that carriers of disease will probably be excluded. But if in an emergency the clinician is forced to find his own donors he should only accept persons in good health and avoid any who have recently returned from tropical countries. A history of malaria, hepatitis or brucellosis or of contact should exclude a donor. Transfusion malaria is a risk in developing countries. It lessens with storage but prophylaxis is advisable. It is known that a permanent carrier state can arise following even a mild attack of infective hepatitis and it is assumed that in some carriers the original infection was subclinical. Homologous serum jaundice is clinically indistinguishable from infective hepatitis and occurs 40 to 150 days after transfusion. It is a great tragedy when a patient dies as a result of this after receiving a single unit transfusion and there appears to be little or no justification for such small transfusions in the adult patient in view of the risks involved. A well established blood donor panel is constantly cleared of assumed carriers, as and when the Regional Transfusion Director is informed of cases of post-transfusion homologous serum jaundice. The recent discovery that some carriers of viral hepatitis have an antigen (Australia antigen or HB_sAg) in their blood has led to the almost universal inclusion of a test for the antigen in all units of donor blood. About 1 in 1 000 donations are found positive and are discarded and the donor is advised never to offer his blood for transfusion in future. This precaution is also applied when the antibody to the antibody HB_sAg is found in the donor's blood.

An attack of brucellosis debars a donor as it can cause a life-long carrier state and is transmissible to the recipient. Transmission of syphilis is minimised by doing a Wassermann test or its equivalent on every donation of blood. Persons taking drugs should not give blood because they could transfer small amounts to the recipient. The risk is greatest when a single unit of blood is enough to replace the whole of the recipient's blood as in exchange transfusion in infants. In practice the condition for which drugs are being taken will often preclude the donation of blood.

Grouping and cross-matching

Blood grouping of donors and recipients, together with compatibility tests, are best left to the pathologist or technician properly trained in this work. The improved standard of safety in transfusion practice is largely due to the quality of methods, reagents and trained laboratory staff. The clinician should not unnecessarily hurry the laboratory to produce compatible blood. He should ensure that the sample is of adequate volume and that it comes from the right patient. The person taking the blood should sign the bottle label to this effect. The pathologist will want to know about any previous transfusions, pregnancies, miscarriages or injections of blood to help him decide the extent of the investigations required for the particular case. Suitable forms are supplied by the laboratory but it is a common failing on the part of clinicians not to complete them properly. Deaths have occurred through failure to give adequate details for identification and patients have suffered dangerous delays in receiving blood because insufficient information was available at the outset of laboratory tests.

In all non-urgent cases, blood grouping and cross-matching should be done a full day in advance. In urgent cases blood can be issued by the pathologist after a rapid test procedure or with no tests at all, but only on the responsibility and direct instruction of the clinician in charge who accepts the grave responsibility. In many cases of rapid haemorrhage low blood volume is the main difficulty. The value of plasma or a plasma substitute should be considered to allow time for laboratory tests to proceed. Blood samples to be used for grouping and cross-matching should be taken before plasma substitutes such as dextran are given as these substances in the blood make the laboratory tests difficult to interpret.

Cross-matching for babies

If a newborn baby needs a transfusion, whether for haemolytic disease or for any other cause, cross-matching should be done against the mother's and not the baby's blood. This is because any antibody in the baby's blood will have arrived there by transfer across the placenta. The baby does not develop isoagglutinins until some four to six months after birth. For purposes of cross-matching therefore, any antibody in the baby's serum is likely to be found in higher concentration in the mother's blood. Where ABO differences between mother and child prevent the use of blood of the baby's group in the cross-match, then group O blood of low antibody titre may be used and cross-matched against the mother's blood. In these circumstances the residual concentration of anti-A or anti-B in the infant's circulation is minimised by removing 150 ml or so of the supernatant citrate-plasma from the donor's blood. Such partially packed red cells are easily transfused. The need to reconstitute with fresh AB plasma is debatable and certainly exposes the patient to the risk of possible infection from two donors rather than one.

Auto-antibodies

Patients with acquired haemolytic anaemia present particularly difficult problems in finding compatible blood as the auto-antibodies they produce in their serum often react with every donor sample tested. Occasionally such patients have a specific auto-antibody, often with Rh specificity (e.g. anti-e). This finding is not uncommon after prolonged treatment with certain drugs such as methyldopa (Aldomet). Whenever a patient on this hypotensive drug needs a blood transfusion the drug history must be given to the pathologist who would then be certain to include the antiglobulin technique in the compatibility tests.

'Universal' and 'dangerous' donors

The aim of every blood transfusion should be to give the patient blood of his or her own ABO and Rh type. Failure to do this may result in the most severe reaction with shock, renal failure and possibly death. This is because naturally occurring isoantibodies are present in all persons other than those of group AB. Such antibodies in the patient's blood stream will rapidly destroy any donor red cells of dissimilar ABO group. It is commonly assumed that group O donors are 'universal donors' in that their red cells (lacking the A or B antigens) will survive happily in the circulation of any patient. What is very often forgotten is that group O donors have naturally-occurring anti-A and anti-B antibodies which are also being transfused and that if these antibodies happen to be very strong they will destroy a large number of the recipient's red cells if these are not group O. Reputable transfusion services either do not issue such 'dangerous donors' blood routinely, or label their containers with a warning such as: 'High Titre group O donor; blood not to be used for other than a group O recipient'. A group A patient who has received a *massive* transfusion of group O blood must be regarded as a group O recipient for the time it takes for most of the passively acquired anti-A to disappear from his circulation. He should not, therefore, receive a subsequent group A transfusion within the next two to three weeks.

Rh antibodies

With regard to the Rh system, we do not encounter naturally occurring Rh antibodies in either donors or recipients, but such antibodies (particularly anti-D) are not infrequently found in Rh negative patients who have been previously transfused or who have been pregnant. The existence of such 'irregular antibodies' will only become evident during cross-matching tests in the laboratory but then the patient's history will be most helpful to the pathologist who is anxious not to miss even a weak antibody.

Rh negative patients should be given Rh negative blood as they are more likely than not to produce anti-D if they receive the Rh positive antigen. The rule should never be broken where young girls or females below the age of menopause are concerned, since the stimulation of anti-Rh in their plasma could result in this antibody crossing the placenta during future pregnancies and destroying the red cells of any Rh positive fetus they may bear. Should a Rh negative female up to the age of the menopause be inadvertently transfused with Rh positive blood she should be given immediately an adequate amount of anti-D immunoglobulin provided she can be shown not to be already immunised to the Rh factor. (A usual dose is 20 μg for every ml of red cells transfused.) Once active immunisation to the Rh factor has occurred anti-D immunoglobulin is valueless. So the haematologist should be asked to have a closer look at the pretransfusion sample of the patient's blood for anti-D. Sometimes in patients previously sensitised a secondary response to D antigen may produce a rapid appearance of anti-D soon after the transfusion. In male patients (and nulliparous females past the menopause) who have never received previous transfusions or injections of blood, it is permissible, in emergencies, to transfuse them with Rh positive blood if Rh negative blood is not available.

Such patients should have their sera checked about two months following the transfusion to determine whether they have developed antibodies. If they have they should be told and should be given a suitable card bearing this information to carry as a safeguard in the event of a future transfusion. A Medic-Alert bracelet might be better (p. 822).

The overall risk of Rh immunisation following a first Rh positive pregnancy in Rh negative women is about 8 per cent. The risk is greatly enhanced following a ruptured tubal pregnancy as fetal cells are rapidly absorbed through the peritoneum (Katz and Marcus, 1972). Every effort should be made to remove all the blood from the peritoneum and on no account should this blood be collected and transfused back into the patient.

Other blood groups

Apart from ABO and Rh groups there are others such as Kell (10 per cent of the population are Kell positive) and Duffy (65 per cent of the population are Duffy positive). If a Kell negative recipent is transfused with blood from a Kell positive donor there is a chance of him suffering a haemolytic reaction if transfused again from the same donor or another Kell positive donor. Little can be done during the first transfusion to eliminate incompatibilities outside the ABO and Rh systems, but in subsequent transfusions careful cross-matching tests will reveal the existence of immune antibodies of any blood group system and allow an opportunity to select compatible blood. If the donor were a husband and the recipient his young wife, one transfusion could sensitise her to any blood group antigens he is carrying which she is not, so that her subsequent children (inheriting their father's antigens) may be injured. For this reason *a young wife should never be transfused with her husband's blood.*

For the situation where a clinician is faced with an imperative need to transfuse his patient and is unsupported by a laboratory service, guidance is given on the choice of donors, blood grouping, and cross-matching on p. 752.

Transport of blood

Having found compatible donors, proved by the most elaborate laboratory techniques, the patient is still not free from other immediate dangers. In the author's experience the greatest danger nowadays lies in the pathway from the blood bank refrigerator to the bedside. This is where the organisational errors occur and it behoves every hospital to study its blood transfusion procedure to ensure that every step is checked and double checked before the blood enters the vein. It is not unknown for the patient to point out to the nurse that the blood container label bears a different blood group from his own. Colour coding of blood container labels according to donor's blood group is standard practice in this country: group AB, white; group A, yellow; group B, pale red; group O, blue. If the blood is Rh negative the printing on the label is in red instead of black.

The administration of blood or its products should be considered in the same light as the administration of dangerous drugs. Only a responsible person should collect the cross-matched blood from the bank refrigerator and he should sign the blood bank register after ensuring he has the correct bottle. At the bedside two responsible people should carefully check the name, blood group, expiry date and number on the bottle label and compare with the patient's notes. Provision should be made on the bottle label for two signatures to signify that this procedure has been carried out. A careful watch should be kept on the patient during the whole transfusion and the doctor should personally observe the patient for the initial 15 minutes of the transfusion as any catastrophic reaction should be revealed during this time.

Warming blood (see also citrate poisoning p. 105)

It is unnecessary and unwise to warm blood routinely before transfusion. There is a great danger of overheating with consequent damage to the red cells and if, for any reason, the transfusion has to be delayed the once warmed blood may suffer from bacterial growth. Warmed, unused blood should never be returned to the blood bank but discarded. In special circumstances, such as the transfusion of newborn babies or in massive transfusions or adults, the consultant may want the blood to be warmed to 37°C. In these cases special methods should be used, such as passage through a disposable plastic coil immersed in a controlled water bath or by using a specially designed bottle heater and radiofrequency induction. Travenol Laboratories Ltd., Thetford, Norfolk, supply a dry heat warming device which overcomes the risk of infection when plastic containers are immersed in water. The apparatus makes use of a disposable plastic mattress which is compressed between heated plates. The system cannot be used in an environment of inflammable gases and this presumably precludes its use in operating theatres.

Bacterial contamination

Contamination of stored blood by bacteria is an ever present hazard. Some donor blood will be infected by skin contaminants at the time of withdrawal. Normally the organisms are destroyed by phagocytes and bacteriolysins in the freshly drawn blood and any surviving the early stages of storage will be prevented from multiplying by storing at 4°C.

Certain cold-growing organisms, usually coliforms or pseudomonas, may survive and even grow at this temperature and will be very likely to multiply rapidly if the blood is removed from the refrigerator and left at room temperature for any length of time. Hence it is a rule that the time during which blood is out of the refrigerator or other cold storage (such as insulated container) should not exceed 30 minutes on any one occasion. Similarly, bottles which have been opened or punctured for sampling and not used within 24 hours, although afterwards kept at 4°C should not be reserved for future use. Such containers should be suitably labelled and returned to the Regional Transfusion Centre. Containers of blood which have been partly used should never be reused even for the same patient. Concentrated red cells prepared by an open method should be used as soon as possible and certainly not more than 12 hours after preparation.

Some pathologists advocate the preparation of a stained smear of the donor blood as a routine investigation to eliminate the risk of issuing contaminated blood. For organisms to be seen in such a smear preparation the degree of contamination would have to be very gross. As stored blood contains so much debris the observer has difficulty in deciding whether he is looking at bacteria or not and is left in great doubt about its safety.

Haemolysis

Once the red cells in a unit of blood have settled it should not be issued unless there is a clear line of demarcation between the sedimented cells and the supernatant plasma, which should be straw coloured and free from visible signs of haemolysis. Haemolysis is shown by a reddish purple discoloration in the plasma immediately above the cell layer which gradually spreads upwards. Such haemolysis may be the only indication of infection but it is an equally valuable indication of haemolysis from other causes such as that following freezing and thawing of the blood. Absence of haemolysis, on the other hand, is no guarantee that the blood is not heavily infected. Blood should only be stored in a properly controlled refrigerator normally under the jurisdiction of the pathologist and his staff. It should never be placed near the cooling coils in case ice crystals form in the blood. General purpose ward refrigerators should be clearly labelled ' not for the storage of blood for transfusion '.

Preparation of apparatus

Extreme care must be taken in the preparaticn of solutions and apparatus for transfusions. If, for example, the anticoagulant solution becomes grossly infected before being autoclaved, although the final product may be sterile, large numbers of dead organisms will be present which, when transfused, can produce severe shock-like symptoms. Certain substances, known as pyrogens, when injected i v can cause an alarming rise in temperature. Pyrogens may be contaminants like methyl cellulose but most commonly they are the products of bacterial growth and a small number of bacteria can produce a very potent soluble pyrogen which, being heat-stable, resists autoclaving. All distilled water used for the preparation of i v fluids and for rinsing clean apparatus before sterilisation must be free of bacteria and pyrogens. The water must, therefore, come from a properly designed still and must be used within a few hours of preparation. Solutions made up from freshly prepared distilled water must be sterilised within four hours to avoid the possibility of bacterial growth. The water itself must be tested periodically for pyrogens. This can only be done bv carefully controlled injections into rabbits.

Pyrogens of non-bacterial origin can occur in the apparatus supplied for transfusion purposes. This was a serious problem in the days when blood taking and giving sets were manufactured from reusable red rubber tubing. Nowadays sets are made from plastics and are disposable. The incidence of pyrogenic reactions has, therefore, diminished greatly.

TRANSFUSION REACTIONS

Pyrexia

Patients vary considerably in the ease with which they show a mild pyrexia during transfusion. The complication is an irritating one both for the patient and the doctor who has to decide whether to stop the transfusion.

Provided the temperature does not rise above 38·3°C and is unaccompanied by other symptoms or signs, it is probably safe to continue cautiously. Sometimes a dose of aspirin settles the temperature but nothing else should be given lest it mask the onset of a more serious reaction.

A patient who becomes febrile during repeated transfusions must be fully investigated and the tests should include a search for platelet and especially leucocyte antibodies. The latter are likely to be found in those who have had multiple transfusions or pregnancies. When the cause of reactions is thought to be leucocyte incompatibility it may be necessary to give the patient leucocyte-poor blood, that is settled blood from which the buffy coat has been removed. In obstinate cases washed red cells can be provided.

If the cause of the reaction remains obscure it is worth prescribing 50 to 100 ml of platelet- and leucocyte-free plasma. Some patients develop antibodies to foreign protein in the donor plasma and this should be evident as a repeated pyrexia following the plasma alone. If this is the cause then washed red cells resuspended in isosmotic sodium chloride solution may have to be used. Requests for washed red cells must be limited to essential use only as their preparation is time-consuming and considerably increases the risk of infection.

Allergic reactions

These are rare but are most likely to arise during transfusions in patients with a history of allergy. They are reactions to transfused foreign protein and are just as likely to occur during plasma as whole blood transfusions. All grades of severity occur from urticaria to facial or laryngeal oedema and bronchial spasm. Obviously the transfusion may have to be stopped in the event of a sudden severe allergic attack but it may be possible after slowing the rate of transfusion to control the symptoms with an antihistamine drug such as chlorpheniramine maleate (Piriton). This is sometimes added to the blood before transfusion but as it may cause pain in the vein and increase the risk of infection it is best to give it by i m or i v injection. No other drugs should ever be added to the blood. They should always be given separately.

Allergy can be transmitted passively from donor to recipient. For example if a donor who is himself allergic to pollen is bled during the ' season ' his plasma will contain a high titre of antibody which will be transfused to a patient. Although the patient is not a sufferer from allergy, if he is now exposed to the pollen antigen he will react as if he were a hay fever subject. Even a mild attack of asthma in an otherwise dangerously ill patient is serious and for this reason donors must not be bled during the ' season ' if they have a history of allergy.

The incompatible transfusion reaction

This is the most serious reaction because it can easily prove fatal. It is almost always avoidable.

As pyrexia is often associated with this type of reaction it must be considered seriously and not dismissed as a simple febrile reaction. It is only possible to judge the significance of a transfusion pyrexia if the temperature has been recorded before the transfusion begins. The effect on the patient of transfusing incompatible blood will be governed by the dose of foreign antigen and the character of the antibody involved. If the patient complains of feeling ' flushed ' or has lumbar pain, faintness, nausea, throbbing headache, constriction of the chest, or if there is a rigor or a temperature rise above $38 \cdot 3\,^{\circ}$C the transfusion must be stopped at once. Circulatory collapse and the passage of free haemoglobin in the urine are alarming signs requiring prompt treatment to save the patient's life or prevent permanent renal damage.

Sometimes, depending on the blood group incompatibility, the immediate signs are less dramatic because the destruction of the donor's red cells does not occur in the patient's blood stream but extravascularly in the reticuloendothelial system. The amount of free haemoglobin liberated is minimal and the cell destruction is made apparent by a rise in serum bilirubin which, if sufficiently intense, will cause jaundice some hours later. Sometimes the first suspicion of incompatibility is a failure to maintain the expected rise in haemoglobin after transfusion.

During the massive destruction of red cells a substance is released which initiates the coagulation process with consequent utilisation of the patient's fibrinogen. This can lead to a haemorrhagic state with oozing of blood from operation sites and mucous membranes. Under anaesthesia or heavy sedation the obvious

clinical reaction is suppressed and unexpected generalised haemorrhage may be the first warning that incompatible blood is being
transfused. The patient will have a prolonged whole blood clotting
time and a diminished fibrinogen level.

Treatment. Having suspected an incompatible transfusion reaction, and having stopped the transfusion, the patient must receive
prompt treatment and the cause must be fully investigated. Circulatory collapse is dealt with as described on p. 238. Should anuria
prevail the patient is treated as described under renal failure (p. 374)
and the nearest haemo-dialysis unit should be alerted and the advice
of its experts sought as soon as possible. Generalised haemorrhage
complicating a transfusion reaction will require the transfusion of
fresh frozen plasma.

The full investigation of the reaction is the province of the haematologist and as he is to some extent involved in the whole transfusion procedure he should be notified immediately a severe
reaction occurs. For his investigation he will require :

1. A pretransfusion sample of the recipient's blood, which he
should already have in his laboratory if an adequate sample had
been provided originally.

2. Samples from the pilot bottles and residue of the donor blood.

3. A post-transfusion sample of the recipient's blood collected
into an anticoagulant such as citrate.

4. A clotted post-transfusion sample of the recipient's blood
(10 to 20 ml).

5. Any urine passed during or after the transfusion.

Every transfused patient should be put on a fluid output chart
for 48 hours. A low output of urine of specific gravity under 1 010
indicates renal damage.

As part of the treatment of oligaemic shock the haematologist
may be asked to provide *compatible* blood to continue the transfusion, so the less delay in providing him with the above samples,
the better.

Part of the immediate investigation rests with the clinician, who
should verify that all the precautions outlined earlier were in fact
taken, and satisfy himself that the blood obtained from the blood
bank was intended for his patient and that no organisational error
occurred. If a human error is revealed it would save considerable
time in providing compatible blood for the patient. The Regional
Transfusion Service which provided the blood may be involved in
a mistake and it is usual for the haematologist to notify the Director
of the Service immediately and sometimes enlist his help in the
investigation.

Out-dated blood

The transfusion of out-dated bank blood can lead to rapid destruction of the donor's red cells producing haemoglobinuria or marked jaundice which may at first be interpreted as due to an incompatible transfusion.

Infected blood

When blood containing a few virulent organisms is transfused the patient may develop a septicaemia some hours later. If the blood is heavily infected the patient becomes very ill very quickly after starting the transfusion. There is intense flushing of the face, headache, vomiting, diarrhoea, and profound hypotension. In spite of treatment with vasopressor drugs and broad spectrum antibiotics most patients fail to recover. Usually it is the intense toxaemia rather than the bacteraemia which causes the overwhelming collapse.

Once it is suspected that the blood is infected the transfusion must be stopped and the patient put on antibiotics and treated for circulatory collapse. The remains of the fluid being given should be sent to the laboratory without delay, with the giving set still in place in the bottle (or kept in the refrigerator if delay is unavoidable). A venous sample of blood should be taken for blood culture before antibiotics are given.

Citrate and potassium poisoning

During exchange transfusions in infants, or massive transfusions in adults, the toxic effects of citrate will be shown by tremors of skeletal muscles and electrocardiographic changes, usually marked prolongation of the ST segment. Citrate is rapidly metabolised by the liver and is only likely to reach toxic levels during transfusions if there is liver failure, or if the liver is premature as in babies. Massive transfusions can absorb much heat unless the blood is warmed and resultant cooling increases the hazard of acidosis and failure to metabolise citrate. Much of the citrate is removed with the plasma when concentrated red cells are used. Slow i v injections of 10 ml of 10 per cent calcium gluconate to an adult patient and proportionately less to an infant will control the effects of citrate. The dose may have to be repeated after every second container in long continued transfusions.

Potassium leaves the red cells during storage of blood and enters the plasma. When very fresh the plasma contains 4 to 5 mmol/litre of potassium. This rises to about 15 mmol/litre at 10 days storage, and to about 20 mmol/litre after 20 days. The massive transfusion of stored blood can, therefore, cause a rise in the recipient's circulating potassium level and if it reaches 8 mmol/litre ECG changes occur and at 10 mmol/litre sudden cardiac arrest following ventricular fibrillation. Blood for exchange transfusion of infants should be as fresh as possible and certainly not more than four to five days old.

Exchange transfusion

This carries a slight risk of causing peritonitis in the newborn. The mechanism is perforation of the bowel resulting from interference with its circulation, particularly if the catheter is inserted more than about 8 cm.

Intrauterine transfusion

When Rh isoimmunisation causes severe haemolytic disease an intrauterine transfusion may be given. Under radioisotope scanning control, a needle is introduced into the amniotic sac and then into the fetal peritoneal cavity. Thirty to 100 ml of Rh negative cells are injected. No serious mechanical damage results but infection is a serious risk. There is a chance of residual adhesions.

Circulatory overloading

Considerable judgment is required in assessing the volume of transfusion fluid necessary to correct blood loss and it is quite easy to over-transfuse. If the fluid being given to the patient can leave the circulation easily (such as saline) the danger is one of pulmonary oedema and virtual drowning. When blood is being transfused the danger is one of over-distension of the circulation.

Starling's work showed that a rise in venous pressure is associated with increased cardiac output; within certain limits the healthy heart adjusts itself to deal with as much blood as may be pumped into the right atrium. A stage may be reached, however, at which this physiological mechanism breaks down and it occurs earlier in chronically anaemic than in healthy subjects. It is apt to supervene with dramatic suddenness but sometimes the effects are delayed until after the transfusion. An early sign of overloading is distension of the neck veins from rising venous pressure. The first symptom is a persistent cough and this is a signal to stop the transfusion. Frothy sputum, sometimes blood stained, next appears and the patient becomes dyspnoeic and cyanosed. Auscultation of the chest reveals moist sounds. In a less acute form the water-logged lungs become the seat of pneumonia.

For exchange transfusion a nomogram to indicate how much blood should be exchanged is now little used by paediatricians. An exchange of 180 ml per kg body weight is usual. To lower the risk of cardiac failure it is wise to take out 40 ml more than one puts in. Most exchange transfusion outfits are satisfactory but disposable sets are to be preferred.

Apart from the ill effects of too great a volume the signs of circulatory overloading can occur because the rate of transfusion is too great. In the adult patient overloading is a likely occurrence if the rate of transfusion exceeds 2·2 ml/kg/hour, i.e. 140 ml/hour for a 65 kg man or half this rate if the initial haemoglobin is 4 g or less. The average drip bulb kept at 1 drop/second will deliver 3 ml/minute or 180 ml/hour since the size of the average drop is 1/20 ml. It varies with specific gravity and surface tension. The rate will fall during the transfusion due to the diminishing head of pressure and increasing viscosity of the blood and will be markedly slowed by any increase in venous pressure. In general the faster the drip rate the larger the drop. A useful rule for infants is that the normal requirement of 143 ml/kg/24 hours will be achieved if the number of drops per minute is half the weight in kg.

If transfusion is deemed necessary to save a chronically anaemic patient who is in serious cardiac failure (PCV less than 13 per cent) a slow (1 ml/kg/hour) infusion of packed cells may be given (the cells of 500 ml of blood will raise the PCV by 5 per cent). Exchange transfusion is an improvement on this, giving 1·0 to 1·5 litres of packed cells into an arm vein and removing 1·0 to 1·7 litres from a femoral vein. If a single vein is used a 10 second interval should be allowed between taking and giving blood, particularly if the catheter ends in a smallish vein.

Treatment. The immediate treatment of circulatory overload is as follows:

1. Stop the transfusion.
2. Give morphine 15 mg and atropine 1 mg subcutaneously.
3. Perform venesection or apply tourniquets to the limbs.
4. Give oxygen.

The risk of air embolism during i v infusion is dealt with on page 63.

W. J. JENKINS

CHAPTER 5

Acute (Non-surgical) Abdominal Catastrophes

THE clinical features of an abdominal emergency are pain, rigidity, vomiting and distension. All of these have well recognised 'surgical' causes, but each may be produced by a medical condition and mislead the surgeon into undertaking an unnecessary laparotomy.

A helpful way of dealing with the subject is to consider each symptom or sign in turn, noting what medical condition may cause it and how it may be distinguished from the same symptom or sign attributable to a 'surgical' cause. Each condition will have to be considered in some detail, since the physician's problem is not that of the surgeon, namely, whether to operate or not. While in most of the conditions which follow, acute abdominal pain is present, it is rarely persistent. *The old rule still holds that the majority of abdominal pains lasting longer than six hours are caused by conditions of surgical import* (Zachary Cope). Another old rule which has some foundation is that the patient with a surgical ' acute abdomen ' lies down and is disinclined to move whereas the one with a medical ' acute abdomen ' sits up. If there is real doubt it is best to operate for it is probable that more harm is done by remembering the medical snags than by forgetting them. It has been found that in 30 to 40 per cent of cases an incorrect diagnosis is made because the classic features are absent.

It is important to be on guard against the presence of an acute medical and surgical condition at the same time. Thus pyelonephritis and pneumonia may occur with appendicitis, and coronary occlusion with cholecystitis. Another source of trouble is the patient who is known to have had coronary thrombosis and who later has another somewhat similar attack which turns out to be a perforation. Ask the patient if he thinks the pain is the same.

Errors constantly occur because the surgeon neglects to use the stethoscope, or the physician the finger stall. No method of bedside examination is the prerogative of any one kind of doctor. Remember how Osler defined a consultant—' a man who makes the rectal examination after the other physicians passed it up.'

The medical ' acute abdomen ' is not a rarity, and has been found to account for 15 per cent of cases presenting abdominal symptoms. More than one of the cardinal signs are usually present but one is outstanding. In this account we shall be concerned largely with differential diagnosis.

PAIN

Abdominal pain causes most of our difficulties and is of two main types, visceral and peritoneal, according to its origin.

Visceral pain is caused by distension or spasm of a viscus. It is diffuse; it comes and goes and is unassociated with rigidity or pyrexia. Tenderness is marked and the patient lies still. Biliary ' colic' is a good example, while of the extra-abdominal causes, coronary thrombosis produces many of the features.

Peritoneal pain is caused by irritation of the peritoneum. It is localised, constant, and associated with rigidity and often with pyrexia. Tenderness is marked and the patient lies still. Perforated peptic ulcer causes this type of pain which also occurs as a reflex phenomenon in pleurisy. If raising the head off the pillow makes abdominal pain worse a peritoneal rather than a pleural cause is likely.

In addition to pain, of which the patient complains spontaneously, we must also mention tenderness, or pain elicited on palpation. A useful point in the differentiation of tenderness caused by some extra-abdominal condition is that in true peritonitis there is definite tenderness of the pelvic peritoneum on rectal or vaginal examination.

Tenderness is very important in small children and if a conscious child makes no attempt to remove the palpating hand, the condition is probabty not a local one such as appendicitis.

Hot water bottle burns are an index of a pain's severity but they do not point to its cause. Relief of pain after an injection of sterile water does not exclude organic disease for any pain may respond to suggestion. There is no easy rule and all depends on the doctor's assessment of the history and physical signs in the light of his knowledge and experience. Nowadays one must be alert to the possibility that a person dependent on drugs is simulating abdominal symptoms in order to get a further supply.

Coronary thrombosis

Coronary thrombosis with abdominal pain is a theoretical source of worry to the surgeon. A perforation with lower substernal pain is more likely to cause trouble than is coronary thrombosis with abdominal pain.

5

In practice confusion rarely occurs. Both conditions are commoner in men than in women A history suggestive of coronary disease is more helpful than one of indigestion, particularly if it can be established that there has been pain brought on by exertion, and if the present acute pain *began* behind the sternum rather than in the abdomen. A clear history is, however, often unobtainable and we are faced with a patient who has sudden, severe overwhelming epigastric and retrosternal pain. Usually by the time we see him, radiation has occurred. If this is up into the chest and down the arms it is in favour of coronary thrombosis, while radiation over the abdomen favours perforation. Shoulder and scapular pain especially on the right side is common after perforated duodenal ulcer with a subdiaphragmatic collection of fluid.

Other factors help us to decide. The pulse in perforation is slow at the onset, whereas it is rapid in coronary thrombosis. Respiration is grunting and thoracic in perforation, but abdominal in coronary thrombosis. Rigidity in perforation, other than into the lesser sac, is extreme and persistent, whereas the rigidity caused by cardiac infarction is not board-like and varies with respiration. Circulatory failure from the shock of perforation soon passes off, but in coronary occlusion it steadily dominates the picture. In perforation, escaped gas causes the liver dulness to disappear. As distended bowel may prove confusing by also obscuring the normal liver dulness, an X-ray film is often of great help by revealing an air bubble under both domes of the diaphragm. Leucocytosis, pericardial friction and signs of congestive failure appear later, and so are of no help at the onset of the emergency. Special consideration should be given to the following points:

1. The fall of blood pressure is greater and more sudden in coronary thrombosis than in the shock of an acute abdominal catastrophe but hypotension may not appear in the first few hours following the infarct. If the patient's previous blood pressure is known, this sign may be very significant.

2. Atherosclerosis of peripheral and retinal vessels is somewhat in favour of coronary thrombosis.

3. Dyspnoea, especially of Cheyne-Stokes type, suggests a cardiac cause.

4. In abdominal pain of cardiac origin the bowel sounds are normal whereas in perforation with peritonitis the abdomen is silent.

5 The response to morphine. Though morphine will relieve the pain of intra-abdominal disease, it acts best when the cause is extra-abdominal.

6. *The electrocardiogram.* Three standard leads, three unipolar leads and six chest leads should be taken. R-ST segment deviation is the characteristic feature of the muscle injury of cardiac infarction. In anterior cardiac infarction there is ST elevation and wide deep Q waves in lead I and the anterior chest leads. In posterior cardiac infarction there is ST elevation with wide deep Q waves in leads III and AVF. These changes may take several hours to appear. In pericarditis ST elevation occurs in all the standard leads and especially lead I but Q waves do not appear and the R waves remain. A snag is that abdominal distension causing a horizontal heart may result in Q waves with inverted T waves in leads III and AVF. There will be no RST changes, however, and another record in deep inspiration should resolve any doubts.

7. Serum glutamic oxaloacetic transaminase (SGOT) (aspartate aminotransferase. EC 2.6.1.1.) is raised in 80 per cent of cases of cardiac infarction within 12 hours of the onset and earlier in a smaller percentage of cases (normal levels 5 to 20 iu/l).

Dissecting aneurysm of the abdominal aorta (For dissection of thoracic aorta see p. 246)

Although radical surgical treatment is now possible this description is retained because of the resemblance to other painful catastrophes. Diagnosis during life has become possible in recent years. When it occurs in young adults it results from cystic medial necrosis of the aorta and there may be stigmata of other mesenchymal defects—tallness, high-arched palate and long fingers (Marfan's syndrome). An intra-mural haematoma forms which ruptures into the lumen. This is usually in the thorax but the dissection may spread to the abdominal aorta. In older people it is more often part of a generalised atherosclerosis and commonly starts close to the aortic cusps. It may be confined to the abdominal aorta. Very rarely the onset is painless and is simply associated with sudden loss of consciousness. More often pain is very severe and in the back. Occasionally it is associated with only part of the length of the dissected aortic wall. The picture following the pain of onset depends on which of the aortic branches is involved. When it is the coeliac axis an acute abdominal emergency is closely simulated. Haematuria may occur when one renal artery is occluded or anuria when both are blocked. Pain may radiate down both legs and be associated with evidence of poor blood supply to them. The picture may resemble that caused by a saddle embolus of the aortic bifurcation.

Pain is maximal at the onset and gradually improves with sometimes a distinct pause before it worsens. This is in contradistinction to the pain of coronary thrombosis which gets worse as time passes. Another distinguishing feature is that the blood pressure does not fall except when there is oligaemic shock from bleeding into the pleural space. The abdominal signs are never quite like those of perforation. X-rays do not show gas under the diaphragm. Calcification of the intima may enable the thickness of the aortic wall to be judged by X-rays and in this way a suspicion of dissecting aneurysm may be confirmed. Occasionally the dissection ruptures back into the aortic lumen and the patient may recover for a time. A similar result has been achieved by operation. Very rarely an old dissection may show as a calcified or 'double' aorta. When rupture occurs into the pleura, mediastinum or retroperitoneal tissues very confusing pictures may result. The patient who survives the onset should be transferred to a vascular surgical unit.

Ruptured abdominal aneurysm or aorta

Shock, abdominal pain and a pulsatile mass make the diagnosis of a ruptured aneurysm easy, especially if the doctor is forewarned of its presence. This is more likely if the anuerysm is syphilitic as syphilis usually affects the thoracic and upper abdominal aorta and the aneurysm causes symptoms from compression of the stomach and erosion of the vertebrae. An atherosclerotic aneurysm generally involves the aorta below the renal arteries and as often as not is long symptomless. When it starts to be painful rupture may be imminent. A lateral X-ray film of the abdomen may show the thin calcified wall of an aneurysm when an antero-posterior film would miss it.

After a period of retro-peritoneal leaking an aneurysm may suddenly burst into the peritoneal cavity and cause sudden severe abdominal pain and collapse. Early distension and rigidity may easily cause this catastrophe to be mistaken for perforation. Restlessness is a marked feature. The only effective treatment is surgical by clamping the aorta below the renal arteries and above the rupture and then to proceed to excision and grafting. Occasionally an aneurysm ruptures into the duodenum. Haematemesis is then a terminal event.

Intestinal or mesenteric angina

This rare extra-pectoral form of angina presents with otherwise unexplained attacks of dull aching pain around the umbilicus 15 to 30 minutes after meals and lasting up to three hours depending on the size of the meal. It may be provoked by exercise after a meal. Antacids bring no relief. There is usually some diarrhoea. The victim is usually elderly and atherosclerotic. Lack of tenderness is characteristic. A bruit over the upper abdomen may give a clue to the diagnosis. A barium meal is usually negative. A tablet of glyceryl trinitrate 0·6 mg under the tongue will often bring prompt relief. The more severe attacks probably result from minor infarctions of the bowel wall and eventually there may be a major mesenteric thrombosis. There is no effective medical treatment but surgery after arteriography in selected cases may bring relief.

Acute pancreatitis

This often misdiagnosed condition is described here because, if diagnosis from the other emergencies can be confidently made, as good results come from medical management as from operation. The patient is usually elderly and obese, with often a history of gall stones. Sometimes for some obscure reason accidental hypothermia (p. 361) is the predisposing cause. There is terrific epigastric and left upper abdominal pain passing through to the back. Tenderness is marked but there is not the abrupt onset or board-like rigidity of perforation. Shock is severe. Vomiting is profuse and diarrhoea may occur. Slight icterus and a tinge of cyanosis (from involuntary inactivity of the diaphragm) are often present. Discoloration in the loin (Grey Turner) and around the umbilicus (Cullen) are late and therefore unimportant signs. The fully developed picture is that of severe shock. About a third of cases the severe and there is necrotising pancreatitis. In the others the pathology is oedematous pancreatitis. Acute renal failure may be a complication (see p. 382).

A plain X-ray film of the abdomen will demonstrate the useful fact that there is no gas under the diaphragm. It may show gall stones. The plasma amylase AMS 3.2.1.1. level often shows a marked but short-lived rise to levels 10 to 30 times the normal of less than 300 iu/1 (60 to 160 Somogyi units per 100 ml). (The normal range for any particular laboratory should be known. The result can be given within an hour). The urinary amylase is raised but only after 24 hours and so it is not helpful in the early stages. It remains high when the blood level has fallen. Raised plasma levels may occur in perforation (from peritoneal absorption of pancreatic juice) and in intestinal obstruction. Morphine, renal failure and technical faults (contamination with saliva) may also cause raised amylase levels in the absence of pancreatitis but usually only two to five times the normal. Peritoneal exudate has a very high amylase content but needling to obtain it is dangerous and not recommended.

Confident differentiation from acute conditions which require operation is essential if medical measures only are to be used. The outstanding features of each of these conditions is: in perforation, rigidity and gas under the diaphragm; in acute cholecystitis, pyrexia (38·3°C) and tenderness under the right costal margin; in appendicitis tenderness in the right iliac fossa and sometimes per rectum; in small bowel obstruction, profuse vomiting, colicky pain and very active bowel sounds; in perforated diverticulitis exquisite tenderness in the left iliac fossa. In all of these the serum amylase is normal or only slightly raised. Pancreatitis mimics these conditions and the picture depends on the stage at which the patient is seen. Early it looks like acute cholecystitis, later it resembles a perforation and later still the picture is that of paralytic ileus. If there is doubt, the test for amylase should be repeated but when one is confident that a surgical emergency is present, operation must be undertaken regardless of laboratory tests. Hypocalcaemia may be a feature because calcium is fixed by fat ' necrosis '. It indicates a poor prognosis. The blood sugar may be raised. Some would disregard any diagnosis of acute pancreatitis not proved by laparotomy or necroscopy.

The immediate objectives of medical treatment are to relieve the intense pain and to treat shock (p. 8). Drugs should be given to suppress pancreatic activity. Pethidine is needed together with Pro-banthine (propantheline) (30 to 60 mg at once and then 30 mg six hourly) should be given and continuous gastric suction started to prevent acid gastric juice from stimulating the pancreas. Duodenal suction if it can be achieved is preferable. An alkaline mixture, if the patient can take it, has the same object. An antibiotic should be given. Claims have been made that corticotropin and corticosteroids are helpful. Trasylol (Bayer) (aprotinin), a non-toxic inhibitor of proteolytic enzymes, may help if given early enough. It is supplied in 5 000 ampoules, the recommended dose being 800 000 units by slow i v drip daily for five days or until serum amylase levels are normal (Trapnell et al., 1973; Editorial, 1974). Good results have been reported (Condon et al., 1973) from the use of glucagon (Lilly) 1 mg i v initially and then 1 mg by infusion over five hours but a controlled trial is awaited. If the patient fails to respond he must be given i v glucose.

Pyelonephritis (see also p. 383)

Acute pyelonephritis with pyrexia and pain in the right side of the abdomen may resemble appendicitis, but pyelitis usually causes a higher temperature and greater leucocytosis and is accompanied by

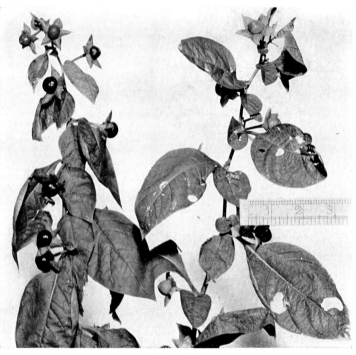

Fig. 6.3
Deadly Nightshade (*Atropa belladonna*). Yellow variety on right.
(*For each inch on scale read 2·5 cm.*)

Facing page 114

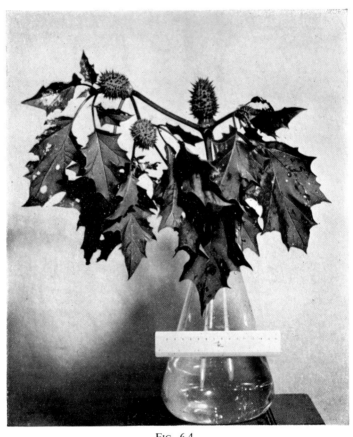

Fig. 6.4
The Thornapple (*Datura stramonium*). Scale divisions are 2·5 cm.

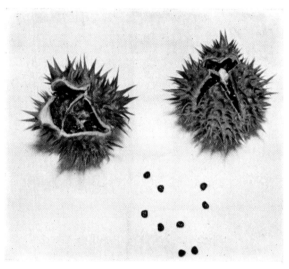

FIG. 6.5
Fruit and seeds of the Thornapple (*Datura stramonium*).
Scale divisions are 2·5 cm.

shivering. Examination of the urine reveals pus and organisms. Since these are almost normal findings in the 'ordinary' specimen of urine in many women, care should be taken in assessing their significance and a 'clean catch' specimen obtained. Occasionally urinary abnormalities may be absent because of blockage of a ureter. An emergency pyelogram may yield valuable information.

Great attention should be paid to the march of symptoms. Midline pain—vomiting—right-sided pain—fever—in this order are strongly suggestive of appendicitis. The absence of right-sided pain (of peritoneal origin) should not exclude appendicitis since the organ may be retro-caecal, pelvic or even right sided in situs inversus. Nor should dysuria necessarily be interpreted as a symptom of pyelitis since pelvic appendicitis may cause it.

Mesenteric vascular occlusion

This is mentioned briefly because although nowadays a surgical disorder it has medical aspects. The past history (of atrial fibrillation and aortic atherosclerosis) is important.

Superior mesenteric arterial obstruction causes intense continuous central abdominal pain with shock. Signs of peristalsis soon disappear but distension is not marked for many hours. There is no rigidity and little tenderness—the contrast between the severity of the symptoms and the paucity of signs being diagnostic. Melaena is rare since the infarction is ischaemic. Acute symptoms from inferior mesenteric arterial obstruction are rare but infarction at the splenic flexure can occur. Venous thrombosis is rarer than arterial in the mesentery. Its onset is more insidious without shock and the march of symptoms is slower.

Treatment. As soon as the medical state allows laparotomy should be undertaken in arterial occlusion for arterial surgery offers the only hope of cure. Venous mesenteric thrombosis may respond to streptokinase (Kabikinase 600 000 units i v and then 100 000 units per hour for several days. See literature supplied with the drug.)

Prednisolone 25 mg should be given first to control any febrile or anaphylactic reaction.

Congestive cardiac failure

Rapid distension of the liver in congestive cardiac failure quite commonly presents with right upper abdominal pain and vomiting, leading the inexperienced to suspect cholecystitis or a 'quiet' perforation. Careful examination should reveal other evidence of

cardiac failure. Sometimes there is a history of attacks of right hypo-
chondriac pain following exertion, and presumably caused by liver
distension. Occasionally the oliguria of cardiac failure is mistaken
for retention.

Acute idiopathic pericarditis

This uncommon condition may present as severe upper abdominal aching pain and the diagnosis may remain obscure until, after
two or three days, a pericardial rub is heard. It affects people of a
younger age group than coronary thrombosis and so a cardiac cause
of symptoms is apt to be forgotten. An ECG may clinch the diagnosis. Diagnosis in the early stages and before pericardial friction
is heard largely depends on one's clinical experience.

Pneumonia

This used to be notorious as a cause of right iliac fossa pain
resembling appendicitis (see Rigidity, p. 126) but seldom causes
confusion now that acute lobar pneumonia has become rare.

Biliary ' colic '

Biliary ' colic ' most commonly results from distension of the
biliary tract, due to spasm at the ampulla of Vater, caused by the
impaction there of a gallstone. It is one of the most severe pains
known. It is a visceral pain and so is felt centrally at first. When
cholecystitis follows cystic duct obstruction the pain radiates to the
right hypochondrium and right scapular region. It is not usually a
true colic in the sense that it waxes and wanes but is more often a
continuous pain.

The patient rolls about and is doubled up in agony and sweats
profusely. Vomiting may occur at the end of an attack, which may
last from a few minutes to several hours and leave the patient limp,
pale and sweating.

Examination during a paroxysm may reveal a tense painless
swelling, presumably the gall bladder, and resistance of the upper
right rectus muscle. Marked local tenderness and rigidity suggest
peritoneal pain from cholecystitis. Evidence of slight jaundice,
clinical or bio-chemical, helps to clinch the diagnosis. When colic
complicates acholuric jaundice pigmentation is obvious. When gallstones have formed, as they may do in long-standing cases of
acholuric jaundice, colic may be associated with true obstructive
jaundice should a stone block the common bile duct. Bile will then
appear in the urine.

Coronary thrombosis may be simulated (pp. 109 and 233). Acute pancreatitis (p. 113) may be an associated condition. Other abdominal colics are usually less severe and have their own charac· teristic distribution and accompaniments.

Treatment

Which of the several available remedies is used will depend on the circumstances. Mild attacks will respond to most analgesics.

1. Pethidine 100 mg with Buscopan (hyoscine N-butyl bromide) 20 mg i v is very effective. (Buscopan is inactive by mouth.)

Morphine is best avoided because it causes spasm of the sphincter of Oddi and so makes matters worse.

2. Glyceryl trinitrate 0·5 mg under the tongue. (Amyl nitrite should be avoided because of the unpleasant flushing and palpitation it causes.)

3. Aminophylline.

Very occasionally anaesthesia induced by i v thiopentone is necessary. Heat locally and a strong carminative mixture may help.

4. When cholecystitis is present antibiotics excreted in the bile should be used, such as ampicillin and rifamide (Rifocin-M) 150 mg i m every 8 hours.

Ascites

Sometimes attacks of severe upper abdominal pain occur mysteriously in cirrhosis and if there is some ascites an abdominal catastrophe may be suspected. In other instances ascites is mysteriosly fulminating and associated with diffuse abdominal pain. It is usually possible to demonstrate free fluid in the abdomen. Pyrexia and increased pulse rate are absent, so that observation rather than laparotomy and peritoneal aspiration to determine the nature of the fluid are justifiable. True peritonitis may complicate the now rarely-needed repeated tapping of ascites.

Tuberculous peritonitis is now a rarity in Britain but all manifestations of tuberculosis remain a problem in tropical and subtropical countries. A known case of tuberculous peritonitis may develop acute symptoms apart from those of an obstructive nature. The abdomen is tumid but there is no tenderness or rigidity. Presumably an increase in the number of tubercles is responsible and symptoms will settle down when treated with antituberculous drugs.

Benign paroxysmal peritonitis

This is a familial, life-long condition confined largely to Jews and beginning in childhood or youth. Because of its incidence in the Mediterranean area it is also called Familial Mediterranean Fever. There is sudden diffuse abdominal pain, vomiting and pyrexia lasting two or three days. Skin signs, erythema and purpura sometimes occur. Laparotomy is negative. Recovery is complete and health good between attacks. Amyloidosis has developed in later life in some cases.

The diabetic 'acute abdomen' (see also p. 340)

In a well controlled diabetic sudden abdominal pain is likely to have a surgical cause but occasionally diabetes will itself cause severe abdominal pain when the patient is in precoma (p. 337). The mechanism is obscure. If the patient is not a known diabetic the abdominal pain may make one suspect a surgical condition. The blood sugar should be estimated.

Drowsiness, anorexia, nausea, vomiting (often copious) and deep sighing respiration before the onset of pain are suggestive of diabetes. In acute surgical conditions vomiting follows pain. Ketosis does not include a surgical condition for this may coexist and if it be inflammatory it may have been the precipitating cause of coma. Nor will a leucocytosis help for this is usual in diabetic coma. The history is important. The diabetic acute abdomen occurs in someone who has been ill and dehydrated for several days. A surgical acute abdomen is a shorter illness and the patient has looked and felt well until the catastrophe.

A snag in children is that when they vomit they easily get ketosis and become dehydrated (p. 442). When dextrose-saline is then given i v some glycosuria may result and this finding may delay operation for the primary surgical condition.

The need for differentiation is not very urgent. We have to decide between ketosis only and ketosis plus perforation or other surgical conditions. Operations should not be undertaken until ketosis is yielding to treatment. If signs and symptoms are still present when ketosis has gone some cause other than diabetes is present (see also p. 340).

Faecal impaction

Sometimes elderly bed-ridden patients taking anticholinergic drugs accumulate inspissated faeces in the rectum and colon. Mild symptoms result or there may be none at all. Occasionally there is severe abdominal pain presumably from bowel spasm. Rectal examination reveals the diagnosis and a suppository or digital removal of faeces brings relief.

Acute non-specific mesenteric lymphadenitis

This condition occurs especially in children of the bright, alert type and causes recurrent attacks which are commoner than and often mistaken for appendicitis. There is often a history of previous attacks. While differentiation is often not sufficiently clear to justify expectant treatment certain points of difference should be noted. The child is restless and does not lie still or curled up as he does with appendicitis. In lymphadenitis the face is flushed but not ' toxic ' as in appendicitis and the tongue though red is hardly furred. The fauces are often inflamed and in many cases there is a history of a recent sore throat. As the condition is often associated with a respiratory infection its incidence is higher in the winter months. Pyrexia is not common and suggests a general cause (e.g. glandular fever). Vomiting occurs earlier but is rarer than in appendicitis. Diarrhoea practically never occurs. Pain is intermittent, severe and colicky and usually central. Tenderness is less local than in appendicitis and is more in the mid-line than in the right iliac fossa. Shifting of the point of maximum tenderness, from altered direction of the pull on the mesentery when the patient lies on the left side for a time, suggests adenitis but is difficult to elicit. Psoas spasm, rebound tenderness, rigidity and rectal tenderness all of which may occur in appendicitis are absent in adenitis. Glands may be felt by careful palpation in the left lateral position with the knees flexed.

If, as is often the case, differentiation from acute appendicitis cannot be made with confidence the abdomen must be opened for the penalty of a mistake in diagnosis is disaster. Otherwise expectant treatment should be adopted. Occasionally the appendix has already been removed.

Acute haemoperitoneum

Blood in the peritoneal cavity causes severe pain and most commonly comes from blunt or penetrating injuries of the abdomen. It may also arise from a ruptured ovarian cyst, a necrotic metastasis or a leaking aneurysm. Sometimes the small aneurysm is part of the picture of polyarteritis nodosa. Very rarely a ruptured Graafian follicle may produce severe intraperitoneal bleeding sufficient to require laparotomy (see ovulation pain, p. 172).

General infections and toxaemias

Abdominal symptoms may occur in the course of known infectious illnesses and suggest that some other condition is also present.

We should be chary, however, of diagnosing an acute abdominal condition when there are general symptoms especially if these over-shadow the local manifestations. It has been said that 'an acute abdomen with a headache is never an acute abdomen'. Tenderness and rigidity are usually absent.

Tonsillitis in children is often associated with abdominal pain and sometimes with true appendicitis. Appendicular pain and tender-ness over the appendix may occur in the prodromal stage of scarla-tina, measles and glandular fever, but true appendicitis is not part of the picture of these diseases. A white blood cell count and the finding of Koplik's spots in the mouth are useful aids in diag-nosis. Pancreatic mumps causes pain and vomiting but no rigidity. If abdominal symptoms follow parotid mumps diagnosis is easy. A history of contact is suggestive. The finding of raised serum amylase in mumps does not in itself indicate pancreatitis for it is of salivary origin.

When acute rheumatism was common severe, lancinating ab-dominal pain, worse on movement and associated with tenderness, used to occur. A history of acute rheumatism or chorea was usually obtainable. Polyarteritis nodosa may cause similar symptoms.

Vomiting is a common symptom of malaria and especially malig-nant tertian infections; in fulminating cases with visceral lesions there may be acute abdominal pain but there is no rigidity. The profuse sweating of malaria however may cause heat cramps of the abdominal wall so that an 'acute abdomen' is simulated.

In influenza there may be griping abdominal pain in addition to headache and pharyngitis. Rigidity is absent and the extra-abdominal symptoms suggest the diagnosis. (The risk of attributing a surgical condition to abdominal influenza during an epidemic must be remembered.)

'Food poisoning' (p. 133) is a well-known pitfall especially if only one person is involved. Not only may it be mistaken for an acute surgical condition but this, e.g. appendicitis, may be present and be attributed to food poisoning.

Acute alcoholism (p. 677) and particularly methyl alcohol poison-ing (p. 34) may be complicated by abdominal symptoms but there is usually a good response to gastric lavage and i v fluids. Hourly observation shows progressive improvement.

A spinal extra-dural abscess from osteomyelitis of a vertebra can cause severe root and abdominal pain in its early stages (before paraplegia) (see p. 314).

Acute diseases of the spinal cord (e.g. acute poliomyelitis) or nerve roots (e.g. zoster) may begin with abdominal pain. A period of watching will reveal typical signs (paralysis or a rash) of the true nature of the illness.

In rare cases when the small causal wound has been unrecognised, abdominal rigidity and pain have been the presenting signs of tetanus (p. 639). Toxins of industrial origin such as lead (p. 469) and carbon tetrachloride (pp. 37 and 464) must be remembered as causes of acute abdominal pain. It must not be forgotten that lead may be ingested in many unusual ways and that proprietary preparations containing carbon tetrachloride for cleaning clothes may cause poisoning at home. The bite of certain spiders (p. 628) in the southern states of the U.S.A. can cause severe abdominal pain and rigidity.

Abdominal pain and vomiting are occasional manifestations of idiosyncrasy to opium and morphine, usually in large doses and especially in women. The mechanism is probably intense spasm of involuntary muscle in the biliary tract or elsewhere.

Infective hepatitis can cause pain and tenderness in the right upper abdomen with vomiting and moderate pyrexia resembling appendicitis. Careful study of the march of events and a search for bile in the urine and slight jaundice of the skin and conjunctivae should point to the correct diagnosis.

Typhoid may be confused with appendicitis, particularly in sporadic cases in children. The immediate diagnosis in an isolated case presenting with acute pain in the right iliac fossa would be a matter for congratulation. Very few of these patients escape appendicectomy, but if a recent continental holiday or other feature brings the possibility of typhoid to mind the demonstration of a leucopenia may stay the surgeon's hand. A perforated typhoid ulcer may be very silent because the patient is so ill. It rarely presents as an emergency.

Acute gastroenteritis

The diarrhoea and vomiting of gastroenteritis may cause diffuse abdominal pain and tenderness. Care must be taken to exclude appendicitis, for it is too often forgotten that an inflamed appendix in the pelvis may itself cause diarrhoea. In a child the pain, tenderness and rigidity of appendicitis may be slight, and hence the need for great care in differentiating appendicitis from gastroenteritis. Special attention should be paid to tenderness since it is a much more important feature of appendicitis than pain.

Gastroenteritis in children resembles intussusception because in both conditions there is colicky pain with vomiting and in many cases, but not in all, bloody mucus may be passed. The important differential points are as follows. Passage of pure blood and clots does not occur in intussusception except in the rare case where an ulcerated Meckel's diverticulum (p. 160) forms the apex of the intussusception. Symptoms are less acute when the colon rather than the ileum forms the apex. Excoriation of the buttocks by evacuated succus entericus, and the peculiar smell which some can recognise, are indicative of gastroenteritis. Pyrexia may occur in both conditions but is more likely in gastroenteritis. Prolonged abdominal palpation, especially during a paroxysm, is important, and absence of the typical sausage-shaped tumour which contracts and relaxes is in favour of gastroenteritis. Microscopical examination of the faecal mucus shows numerous pus cells and a dysentery bacillus can often be grown on culture. The child with an intussusception is plump and healthy-looking by contrast with the usual case of gastroenteritis, and it is remarkable how well he may appear between the paroxysms. Indeed, after the first sudden severe bout of pain, the subsequent attacks may be relatively mild. Any sudden illness in an infant, however, with recurrent abdominal pain and vomiting especially if there is pallor and collapse should be regarded as intussusception until proved otherwise.

Now follow some rare conditions which can on occasion mimic an acute abdomen.

Henoch's (anaphylactoid) purpura (see also p. 229)

In this condition colicky pain is caused by spasm of the bowel and infiltration of its wall with blood and serum (' visceral hives '). Rigidity, vomiting, and distension are also present. Abdominal pain nearly always precedes the appearance of skin purpura, and until the latter appears the diagnosis may be in doubt. Joint pains and albuminuria are helpful differentiating points. The tourniquet test is almost invariably negative in anaphylactoid purpura. A past or family history of allergy should be sought. Even when skin lesions make the diagnosis certain it must not be forgotten that Henoch's purpura is not entirely a ' medical ' disease and that surgical complications such as necrosis and intussusception may arise. Abdominal colic may be a feature of hereditary (non-allergic) angio-oedema (p. 548).

Acute abdominal symptoms in blood diseases

Acute abdominal pain has been described in polycythaemia (p. 273) from rapid splenic enlargement and infarction. In 10 per cent of cases there is also duodenal ulceration. Pain also occurs in leukaemia (from perisplenitis and impending rupture) (p. 273) and haemophilia (p. 279) (from splenic haemorrhage). Acute haemolytic anaemias of various kinds may present with vomiting and abdominal pain. Sickle cell anaemia is a not very rare example sometimes met in the West Indies now in this country. Although surgical emergencies can occur in patients with blood diseases the chances are that bleeding is the cause of the pain.

Allergy as a cause of acute abdominal symptoms

Allergic abdominal symptoms are similar to those described under Henoch's purpura. Often there is a history that the attack began after eating some food such as strawberries or lobster to which the patient was known to be sensitive. If urticaria appears, the diagnosis is confirmed. The blood picture usually shows leucopenia with eosinophilia. Adrenaline Injection BP will alleviate the symptoms promptly. Cases have been reported of recurrent attacks of severe abdominal pain with pyrexia and signs suggesting appendicitis. Laparotomy in one such case revealed only great congestion of the subserous vessels.

Bornholm disease

This infection with Coxsackie virus B (also known as epidemic pleurodynia) presents with mild pyrexia and pain usually in the costo-diaphragmatic group of muscles. Children are specially susceptible. The disease is a great mimic and an acute abdominal emergency may be simulated. This should be excluded by other features of Bornholm disease such as myalgic pains elsewhere which shift about, tenderness of the costal margin, leucopenia and fever. There are remissions and exacerbations. Most patients have frontal headache and benign meningitis is an occasional complication. Cough and vomiting—the usual accompaniments of acute thoracic and abdominal disease—are almost invariably absent and there is no rash. When the disease is epidemic (usually in the hotter months) the diagnosis is easy.

Acute porphyria

Porphyrins are iron-free pigments formed during haemoglobin metabolism but they do not normally appear in the free state. In haemolytic diseases, lead poisoning, liver diseases and after barbiturates have been taken small amounts of porphyrins may be found in the urine or they may appear without known cause. This porphyrinuria is in itself symptomless. The term porphyria is used for the excretion of large amounts of porphyrins and the associated symptoms.

We are only concerned here with acute porphyria, a rare condition four times commoner in women than in men. Two distinct forms occur: (1) Acute intermittent porphyria. Here porphyrin precursors can be detected in the urine between attacks but the stool porphyrins are normal. It is prevalent in Sweden. (2) Variegate porphyria. Here bullous lesions occur on the sun-exposed skin. No porphyrin precursors are formed in the urine between attacks but stool coproporphyrin is always increased. It is prevalent in South Africa. Porphyria is a great simulator and may present as an abdominal or a neurological emergency. A family history of some manifestation of porphyria is often found. Acute attacks of severe abdominal colic occur, presumably from contraction of smooth muscle induced by the pigment. Many acute surgical conditions may be mimicked, and the vomiting and absence of diarrhoea suggest intestinal obstruction. The symptoms are marked, but are unsupported by signs and the belly is soft. There is usually a leucocytosis.

Associated findings—flaccid paralysis, mental change, fits and tachycardia—should suggest the diagnosis, but they are sometimes mistaken for hysteria. Confirmation depends on examination of the urine. This may be of normal colour when passed, but if allowed to stand in the light, and especially if acidified, a colourless precursor porphobilinogen is converted into deep reddish brown porphyrin pigment (' the window sill' test). The colour change is most marked near the surface where it is in contact with air. (Urines after blood transfusion may darken on standing.) Tests for blood are negative and the abnormal pigment may be identified spectroscopically. There is no regular relationship between symptoms and the amount of porphyrin in the urine. At room temperature even when the urine has darkened some porphobilinogen remains unchanged to pigment and so the following test for it may be helpful.

To one volume of urine add one volume Ehrlich's aldehyde reagent (sulphanilic acid and sodium nitrite), and allow it to stand for five minutes. Then add two or three volumes of a saturated solution of sodium citrate. Extract with 5 ml of chloroform. If the pink coloration remains in the upper aqueous layer it is due to porphobilinogen while if it is extracted into the lower chloroform layer urobilinogen is present. It is essential to neutralise all the HCl in the Ehrlich's reagent as otherwise false positive reactions may be obtained as when indole acetic acid is present, and is converted into pink coloured urosein by acid. Treatment is purely symptomatic and the mortality is high. Pethidine should be used for pain and a sedative to induce sleep. Barbiturates must be avoided. Griseofulvin upsets porphyrin metabolism and may precipitate an attack. The use of corticotrophin (ACTH) and also BAL (p. 35) and EDTA (p. 462) has sometimes been followed by improvement. Chlorpromazine (Largactil) 50 to 100 mg i m every six hours is reported to have relieved the abdominal symptoms. Some cases with paralytic ileus have responded to neostigmine (Prostigmine) 2·5 mg subcutaneously every six hours.

Paroxysmal myoglobinuria (rhabdomyolysis) (see also p. 323)

This is a rare cause of attacks of abdominal and generalised muscle pains which has led to an unnecessary laparotomy. The urine is very dark ' like stout '. It gives positive guaiacum and ' strip ' tests for blood but red cells (and porphobilinogen) are absent. Spontaneous recovery is usual (Berenbaum et al., 1955).

Essential hyperlipaemia

In this rare and rather ill-defined condition recurrent attacks of nausea, vomiting and abdominal pain occur. There is fever and a raised sedimentation rate. Hepato-splenomegaly, cutaneous xanthomata and lipaemia of the retina are diagnostic clues. In several reported cases it was discovered accidentally that the serum was very milky from lipaemia. If the condition is thought of this evidence should be deliberately sought. Adults have mild attacks with chronic low-grade pain but in children symptoms are more acute. It is thought that when lipaemia is sufficiently marked for the liver to be unable to remove it phagocytosis of fat by Kupffer cells begins and leads to painful distension of the liver. Starvation and i v heparin will improve symptoms by decreasing lipaemia.

Ferritin shock in haemochromatosis

Haemochromatosis, usually in elderly men, presents in about a quarter of cases with aching in the right hypochondrium, lower abdominal cramps and also attacks of generalised abdominal pain associated with shock and abdominal rigidity (MacSween, 1966). This pain is thought to be due to escape into the circulation of ferritin—the form in which iron is stored in the liver.

Abdominal epilepsy

Short recurring paroxysms of cramping abdominal pain from hypermotility of the bowel may occur rarely in epileptics and patients with focal brain lesions (injury or tumour). Epilepsy should not be considered as a cause until the commoner conditions have been reviewed. There may be some other epileptic feature such as somnolence or a disorder of behaviour to point to the diagnosis.

Hypercalcaemic crisis (see also p. 367)

The hypercalcaemia of hyperparathyroidism causes intestinal atony and constipation. When the serum calcium rises to about 3·75 mmol/l abdominal pain and vomiting may occur. The high calcium content of the urine causes polyuria and this in a drowsy, vomiting patient without glycosuria suggests the diagnosis. For treatment see p. 367.

Intestinal pain in aircraft (p. 504)

RIGIDITY

Abdominal rigidity of 'medical' origin is usually caused by disease of the lungs and pleura, particularly in children. It is more a stiffness of the abdominal wall than the board-like rigidity of perforation, and some prefer to call it resistance. When vomiting is an early symptom, as in a child, the resemblance to true abdominal disease is great. The only medical condition causing real board-like rigidity is the spasm of tetanus (p. 637) but in this case tenderness is slight or absent. Rigidity will be accompanied by pain whether the cause is in the chest or abdomen. If it is unilateral then pressure on the opposite side will cause pain if it is abdominal in origin. Pressure will be painless if the origin is in the chest.

Voluntary contraction of the abdominal muscles and abdominal rigidity of extra-abdominal origin can sometimes be made to relax by breath-holding and by pressure on the chest to restrict its movement. In this way any respiratory movement which the abdominal wall can make is brought out. The rigidity of extra-abdominal disease is a response to pain and, being central in origin, it diminishes after morphine. Rigidity in intra-abdominal disease persists after morphine.

Some unequivocal evidence of chest mischief such as a pleural rub or bronchial breathing often settles the matter. Slight cyanosis, inspiratory dilatation of the nostrils, raised respiratory rate, and the absence of rectal tenderness all point to the chest as the site of the trouble. Leucocytosis is higher in the initial stage of pneumonia than it is in appendicitis before perforation occurs.

Rigidity may be very marked in spontaneous pneumothorax and particularly haemo-pneumothorax. Typical signs of pneumothorax (resonance with silence or distant amphoric breathing) or of air and

fluid in the chest (splashing) are generally present. The chest should
be X-rayed.

Diaphragmatic pleurisy

This provides a special pitfall for the unwary for it causes referred
pain in the abdomen, and resistance. If the central portion of the
diaphragm be involved, pain may be referred to the shoulder tip.
Physical signs are disappointingly few, but lack of movement of one
side of the chest and dilatation of the nostrils on inspiration should
point to the chest as the seat of the trouble. A rare but helpful
symptom of pleurisy is persistent and painful hiccup. Other points in
favour of pleurisy are a flushed face with a tinge of cyanosis,
herpes of the lips, and a history of an initial rigor. Again, the march
of events should be carefully scrutinised for the patient with diaphragmatic pleurisy or pneumonia is 'too sick, too soon' to have
appendicitis. Rarely, however, are his symptoms sudden enough to
mimic a perforation. Sometimes an acute primary diaphragmitis
produces a similar picture but without evidence of pulmonary
disease.

Haematoma of the rectus muscle

Debilitating diseases, senility, arterial disease, coughing, pregnancy, a lower abdominal scar, injury by a retractor, peritoneal
dialysis and anticoagulant therapy are all factors which predispose
to bleeding from the inferior epigastric artery into the rectus sheath.
There may be premonitory soreness. Since the lower part of the rectus
abdominis muscle has no posterior sheath, bleeding there can form a
very large haematoma which may cause peritoneal irritation with
pain and rigidity. Sometimes the blood diffuses widely into the flanks
but such ecchymosis is a late sign. When a haematoma forms it can
be shown to be in the abdominal wall because it does not cross the
mid-line; it does not ascend or descend with respiration and it
remains palpable when the patient sits up or tenses his rectus
muscles. If the swelling increases in size, or the diagnosis is in doubt
(as it often is) operation should be undertaken to avoid the risks of
massive haemorrhage and infection.

VOMITING

When vomiting is the main symptom and pain is absent or
atypical a 'medical' cause is likely. Difficulty chiefly arises when
vomiting is associated with pain and distension, also of medical

origin. It must be emphasised that pain with vomiting is characteristic of small bowel obstruction, which should be diagnosed before the distension appears. Hence, very great care must be taken before deciding that there is no obstruction. (For bilious vomiting in the newborn see p. 410.)

Tabes dorsalis

Tabes is now rare but the gastric crisis can still prove a trap for the unwary by simulating an acute abdomen. It may also mask serious abdominal disease. True rigidity is not present and the finding of Argyll Robertson pupils with the absence of knee and ankle reflexes should stay the surgeon's hand. When an acute abdomen is thought to be present in a tabetic it is always wise to use X-rays to see if there is free gas under the diaphragm.

The periodic syndrome

This syndrome with ketosis has to be distinguished from surgical conditions and is fully discussed on p. 422.

Acute poisoning (see also p. 26).

Poisoning and ingested irritants may cause acute abdominal symptoms. Patients often try to attribute their symptoms to some dietary indiscretion. We must be on our guard against accepting their explanation too readily and missing a true appendicitis. ' Bolus colic ' may be suspected if a patient vomits a mass of obviously indigestible material.

Acholuric jaundice

Crises with abdominal pain and vomiting may occur in acholuric jaundice. The cause is biliary colic from ' bile mud ' produced by haemolysis. Sometimes tenderness is discovered and suggests intraperitoneal haemorrhage. The other features of the case should make the diagnosis clear.

Uraemia

Uraemia from chronic renal failure is a pitfall for the surgeon. The intense vomiting of sudden onset mimics high intestinal obstruction. The resemblance is greater if the patient is very thin, so that normal peristalsis is visible. The vomit is not faeculent as it may be in obstruction. Haematemesis from uraemic gastritis, or from bleeding gums may confuse the issue.

The general toxic appearance, the dry, furred tongue, and evidence incriminating the kidneys, such as a history of nephritis and hypertension or of excessive use of analgesics, together with the presence of urinary abnormalities, will indicate the correct diagnosis. In congenital cystic disease with uraemia, the kidneys are palpable. Peristaltic sounds are not increased in uraemic vomiting as they are in obstruction.

Sometimes the acute terminal pericarditis of uraemia causes upper abdominal pain, and the clinical picture closely resembles that of perforation.

Other medical causes of severe vomiting which may cause confusion are Menière's syndrome (p. 217), and the crisis of Addison's disease (p. 353). Should the eye condition be overlooked the vomiting of glaucoma may be misleading.

The vomiting of migraine may be severe but it usually follows the headache. Abdominal migraine without headache should be diagnosed with caution and only if there is a history of typical migraine attacks also and if other causes of vomiting can be excluded.

Local results of vomiting

Severe vomiting may cause lacerations across the gastro-oesophageal junction. Haematemesis follows. An attractive idea is that this Mallory-Weiss syndrome (p. 157) represents one end of the spectrum of lesions of which the other end is spontaneous rupture of the oesophagus (Boerhaave's syndrome). The victim of a rupture is nearly always a middle-aged man who has eaten well and is drunk. It is thought that the normal relaxation of the cricopharyngeus with vomiting fails to occur and so the gastric contents forced into an unyielding oesophagus cause it to rupture longitudinally where it is least supported, i.e. on the left side in its lower third. (In rare instances rupture has complicated status asthmatics, sea-sickness and an epileptic fit. It has also occurred very rarely without vomiting.) Severe retro-sternal pain followed by vomiting suggests the diagnosis. The patient feels worse (not better) after he has vomited. X-rays show a fluid level at the left base and sometimes in the mediastinum also. ' Crunching ' sounds synchronous with systole may be heard along the left sternal edge (Hamman's sign). When there is fluid as well as air in the mediastinum a peculiar sound may be heard. It is likened to a man sloshing through a marshy meadow with his galoshes awash (' sloshy galoshes ' sign). More definite confirmation is by showing leakage of swallowed gastrografin into the mediastinum and pleural space. There is no gas under the diaphragm. Surgical emphysema may be seen in the film of the neck and felt on palpation. The fluid on aspiration is acid and may clearly be the same as fluid, e.g. tea or milk, recently swallowed.

Without surgical intervention the condition is fatal within a few days.

DISTENSION

(See also p. 69)

Recent distension associated with vomiting indicates intestinal obstruction which, incidentally, should have been diagnosed at the stage of yellow-brown vomit before distension appeared. The hernial rings must not be forgotten. Abdominal distension and pain may be a marked feature of acute hydronephrosis. Other causes are myxoedema, hypokalaemia, ganglion blocking drugs and severe gastroenteritis. It can complicate operations on the vertebral spine.

Occasionally great distension complicates the picture of some other disease such as typhoid or ulcerative colitis, and make one wonder if a ' surgical ' cause is present. If the original diagnosis is firmly based, no difficulty should arise.

A rare condition, not very well known or understood, is that known as ' bloating ' or abdominal distension not due to gas. The distension is not present in the morning, but gradually appears as the day goes on, and may vanish suddenly without the passage of flatus. The intermittent nature of the swelling is emphasised in the picturesque name *ventre en accordéon*. Lying on the back and flexing the thighs will cause the swelling to disappear, as will a dose of morphine. It has the same mechanism as pseudocyesis namely pushing down the diaphragm, arching the back and cramp-like contraction of the abdominal muscles. It occurs in psycho-neurotic women and occasionally in men.

Tight distension or rigidity plus distension is a late picture and indicates intestinal obstruction with peritonitis. A rare cause of great abdominal distension in a young baby is an ano-rectal stricture. The distension is relieved by passing a catheter into the bowel, and cured by dilation with the finger.

' Toxic megalocolon '

The bowel wall cannot maintain its tone when the inflammatory process of ulcerative colitis involves its muscle. Enormous dilatation results; a very serious complication (mortality 25 per cent). It is usually preceded by increased pain and bloody diarrhoea but sometimes diarrhoea may cease and this is an ominous sign even when the general state remains fair. Often because of portal bacteraemia and liver damage there is rapid deterioration. Sometimes opiates, anticholinergic drugs and a barium enema appear to be precipitating causes. The essential clinical findings are abdominal distension and tenderness with absent bowel sounds. But the crucial sign is shown on a plain X-ray film of the abdomen. Bowel distension is seen with remnants of mucosa projecting into the lumen. These 'mucosal islands' are often called pseudopolyps. Treatment is by a short (48 hour) intensive course of transfusion of fresh blood, i v fluids and parenteral antibiotics (cephalothin and gentamicin) and naso-gastric suction. It is really preparation for surgery which is usually necessary. Indeed some (Brooke, 1968) regard the presence of 'mucosal islands' as an emergency situation and itself an indication for urgent surgery.

C. ALLAN BIRCH

REFERENCES

ANGELL, J. C. *The Acute Abdomen for the Man on the Spot*. London: Pitman, 1965.

BERENBAUM, M. C., BIRCH, C. A. & MORELAND, J. D. (1955). Paroxysmal myoglobinuria. *Lancet*, **1**, 892.

BROOKE, B. N. (1968). The indication for emergency colectomy in ulcerative colitis. *Diseases of the Colon and Rectum*, **2**, 85.

CONDON, J. R., KNIGHT, M. & DAY, J. L. (1973). Glucagon therapy in acute pancreatitis. *British Journal of Surgery*, **60**, 509.

COPE, SIR ZACHARY. *The Early Diagnosis of Acute Abdomen*. 14th ed. London: Oxford University Press, 1972.

EDITORIAL (1974). *British Medical Journal*, **2**, 133.

MACSWEEN, R. N. (1966). Acute abdominal crisis, circulatory collapse and sudden death in haemochromatosis. *Quarterly Journal of Medicine*, **35** (NS), 589.

TRAPNELL, J. E., RIGBY, C. C., TALBOT, C. H. & DUNCAN, E. H. L. (1973). Aprotinin in the treatment of Acute Pancreatitis. *Gut*, **14**, 828.

CHAPTER 6

Other (Non-surgical) Abdominal Emergencies

IN this chapter will be considered acute conditions affecting the abdominal organs which do not, as a rule, simulate acute surgical conditions, and which are not obstetrical or gynaecological.

VOMITING AS AN URGENT SYMPTOM

Vomiting is a common and sometimes a presenting symptom in many urgent illnesses. The following classification is therefore given as an aid in reviewing possible causes in an obscure case. Obvious causes such as anaesthetics and pregnancy (p. 177) are not included. Usually some associated symptom or sign such as headache or papilloedema will point to the diagnosis.

Causes of vomiting

In the stomach itself
> Poisons and unsuitable food. Alcohol.
> Morphine and other drugs.

In other viscera
> Intestinal obstruction. Appendicitis.
> Violent coughing.

Infective
> Onset of specific fevers.
> Epidemic vomiting.

Metabolic
> Addison's disease and other sodium deficiency states.
> Hyperparathyroidism.

Neurogenic
> The brain—increased intracranial tension.
> Meningitis. Migraine. Shock.
> The spinal cord. Gastric crisis of tabes.
> The special senses. Menière's disease.
> Motion sickness. Unpleasant sights and smells.

Psychogenic
> Cyclic vomiting. Air swallowing.
> Habit vomiting.

Treatment

This depends on the cause. Promazine (Sparine) 25 to 50 mg or metoclopramide (Maxolon) 10 mg by mouth or i m three or four times a day is recommended as symptomatic treatment or by using the proprietary combination Cyclimorph. Iced champagne is reputed to 'settle' the stomach. Gastric aspiration and lavage by the nasal route are temporary expedients in intractable cases (uraemia) or in those cases of unknown aetiology. Morphine-induced vomiting can be avoided by injecting cyclizine (Valoid. Burroughs Wellcome) 50 mg at the same time.

Acute complications of vomiting

Vomiting may cause urgent symptoms through its complications. These may be:
1. Mechanical
Inhalation of vomit:
  (a) In babies (p. 410).
  (b) During anaesthesia.
  (c) Causing peptic aspiration pneumonia (Mendelson's syndrome (p. 571) and 'food asphyxia' (p. 225).
Mallory-Weiss syndrome (pp. 157 and 129).
Rupture of the oesophagus (Boerhaave's syndrome) (p. 129).
2. Biochemical
Dehydration (p. 607).
Acute weight loss from dehydration.
Ketosis from carbohydrate starvation (p. 422).
Tetany (p. 368).
Hypochloraemic alkalosis from loss of chloride, with depression of renal function ('gastric uraemia').
Hypokalaemia (p. 602).
When vomiting complicates conditions like Addison's disease and renal failure, these effects follow more rapidly.

ACUTE FOOD POISONING

The modern trend is to abandon the term food poisoning when possible in favour of an aetiological diagnosis and the term should not be used when the cause is some condition notifiable in its own right, e.g. bacillary dysentery and typhoid. In some 35 per cent of sporadic cases no causal organism is found and for these the term food poisoning is retained as a working diagnosis. Since it may be a communal as well as an individual emergency it is important to realise its implications at the onset and to act before evidence is lost.
1. Make a note of food eaten before the attack.

2. Take charge of suspected food—not forgetting left-over scraps —and find out where it came from. Domestic pets and raw pet foods can harbour salmonella organisms.

3. Save specimens of vomit, urine and faeces for laboratory examination. A rectal swab may be used but faeces are more satisfactory.

4. Notification. Many doctors have long thought that food poisoning is not officially notifiable but this impression is not correct. It remains notifiable though this requirement has been poorly observed. Diagnosed or suspected food poisoning is notifiable forthwith to the doctor nominated by the Area Health Authority to receive such information. Early investigation in the hope of identifying the source of the poison and so preventing other cases depends on speedy communication by telephone or otherwise to the nominated doctor. The formal certificate of notification should follow by post in a sealed envelope. (Beware of giving a certificate of ' food poisoning ' to relatives until proved. It may be wanted simply to blackmail a restaurant.)

Chemical poisons

In all cases of chemical poisoning the interval between ingestion and the onset of nausea and abdominal pain is fairly short. Salts of lead, zinc, cadmium and antimony may contaminate acid fruit in metal containers. Home-made wine prepared in antique glazed earthenware may contain lead. Acidic beverages made in galvanised containers contain zinc which causes vomiting, diarrhoea and abdominal pain. Arsenic is rarely encountered and then only when added to food with malicious intent. Symptoms have followed the use of silverware cleaned with polish containing cyanide. Muscular paresis may follow abdominal symptoms if a kitchen insecticide containing sodium fluoride is taken in mistake for baking powder. Poisoning may occur if food is contaminated with DDT (p. 37) or organic phosphorus insecticides (p. 467). Permitted food additives can upset some people. Monosodium glutamate is used to enhance flavours and may cause a burning sensation in the face, arms and neck and palpitation—the Chinese restaurant syndrome or Kwok's quease. It does not herald a serious emergency and generally disappears within an hour or so.

Poisonous foods

These include fungi taken in mistake for mushrooms; belladonna leaves included in dry herbs; narcissus bulbs eaten as onions and rhubarb leaves used as spinach. Solanine is found in the potato

(*Solanum tuberosum*) especially just under the skin but not in toxic amounts except when the tubers are green and sprouting. It causes vomiting, diarrhoea and abdominal pain. Boiling diffuses the poison but baking conserves it. Mussels which have fed on red plankton may be poisonous. The flesh of many warm water fish contains ichthyosarcotoxin which can cause severe symptoms very soon after eating the fish, especially if it is raw.

Ackee poisoning, the vomiting sickness of Jamaica and other islands of the Caribbean, is caused by eating ackee (*Blighia sapida*). The unripe fruit contains a polypeptide which causes vomiting and marked hypoglycaemia. Most cases occur in children. Recovery is usual but drowsiness may call for gastric lavage and i v glucose. For other poisonous plants see p. 142.

Bacterial food infections

Here the illness is due to actual infection and not to preformed toxin. Hence the ingestion—onset interval is 12 to 24 hours or longer. The onset is sudden with diarrhoea, vomiting, abdominal pain and pyrexia. Salmonellosis is responsible for 63 per cent of sporadic cases.

Bacterial food poisons

Staphylococcal food poisoning is caused by preformed toxin in foods like cream cake and trifle. The food must have been at or above room temperature for several hours for toxin to be formed. The toxin is relatively heat stable and may withstand 30 minutes' boiling. The onset of salivation, nausea and vomiting is prompt— within 1 to 6 hours. On board ship it may be mistaken for sea-sickness (p. 479). *Cl. welchii* and many non-specific organisms when present in large numbers may cause similar symptoms. Strepto-coccal food poisoning is milder and less common. It has a longer incubation period probably because the organism as well as its toxin are both concerned.

Differential diagnosis

It must not be forgotten that patients with appendicitis may blame something they have eaten and lull one into accepting a diagnosis of food poisoning.

Bacterial food poisoning and infection have to be distinguished from the following:

Paratyphoid. The onset may be similar to Salmonella infection but the illness is prolonged.

Bacillary dysentery. Here there is marked diarrhoea and the passage of blood. Stool culture reveals the organisms.

Epidemic sore throat. Vomiting is a prominent symptom but group A streptococci can be found in the throat.

Epidemic nausea and vomiting ('Gastric flu'). Here nausea, vomiting and sometimes diarrhoea occur at intervals in a household. All bacteriological investigations are negative and the condition is presumably due to a virus of intestinal origin. Antibiotics should preferably be withheld until a bacteriological diagnosis is made. Even then they are not recommended for Salmonella food poisoning (other than by *S. typhi* and *S. paratyphi*).

Treatment

As vomiting has emptied the stomach it is unwise to wash it out but sometimes the simple procedure of putting two fingers into the throat after a copious drink of bicarbonate is advisable. A hot water bottle on the abdomen is comforting. In severe cases adequate hydration is very important and even when there is vomiting fluid should be given by mouth. Glucose accelerates the absorption of salt and water and so it or fruit juice should be added to isosmotic sodium chloride solution. Some prefer an effervescent drink. In collapsed patients 5 per cent glucose in isosmotic sodium chloride solution may be given i v. Modern practice is to use diphenoxylate with atropine (Lomotil) two 5 mg tablets (10 to 15 mg in 24 hours). Otherwise Kaolin and Morphine Mixture BNF 15 ml may be given four hourly but morphine by itself is best withheld until vomiting and diarrhoea abate.

Antibiotics should be avoided in uncomplicated gut-contained infections because they may convert patients into heavy faecal carriers. Co-trimoxazole (Bactrim. Septrin) is particularly bad in this respect. When there is blood stream invasion and toxaemia, however, chemotherapy with chloramphenicol is advised and failing this with ampicillin.

BOTULISM

This is a rare form of food poisoning by preformed toxin. The causal organism, *Clostridium botulinum*, is present in many soils, especially in California, but is rare in Britain. There is no special connection with sewage or farmyard material. The organism and its toxin are destroyed by moist heat at 121°C as in a pressure cooker but the spores can withstand 100°C for several hours. Ordinary domestic cooking does not eliminate them. (Nine instances of botulism following infection of a wound have been recorded.) Fresh food and recently made-up dishes are safe and so are canned foods made under factory conditions. At pH above 4·6 spores develop aerobically and toxin is produced. Home canned fruit being acid is safer than canned vegetables. The risk is greatest with root vegetables and those developed on the plant low down near the soil. Meat preserved in its own melted fat is also dangerous.

Cured meat has nitrite added to inhibit *C. botulinus* (botulus = sausage. Nitrite is not now used in British sausages.)

The characteristic symptoms which appear after a symptomless interval of 6 to 30 hours are diplopia, abdominal discomfort, peculiar speech and various paralyses caused by blockage of myoneural junctions similar to that caused by curare. Pyrexia is absent and the victim remains mentally alert. There may be initial nausea and vomiting caused by proteolytic products. When several members of a household have the same neurological symptoms this should alert us to the possibility of botulism. The mortality rate is at least 30 per cent.

Prevention

All home-bottled non-acid food, e.g. vegetables, should be boiled for 10 minutes. This destroys the toxin which has developed after bottling. Home bottling of non-acid foods is discouraged by women's organisations in the U.K.

Treatment. This may include artificial respiration and other general measures to keep the patient alive. Guanidine hydrochloride 10 to 30 mg/kg BW daily in divided doses in capsules may help. There is evidence that it enhances the release of acetylcholine at neuromuscular junctions. Antitoxin (p. 766) 50 000 units should be given i m. Expert help is advisable in its use and so the government health department (p. 764) should be consulted. It would be wise to give prophylactic antitoxin to all who had eaten the offending food even though still symptomless.

Any food suspected of being contaminated should be burned. If fed to animals they might develop botulism.

' MUSHROOM ' (TOADSTOOL) POISONING

Between 1920 and 1940 only 39 fatal cases of ' mushroom ' poisoning occurred in England and Wales. We know that in 12 of the subsequent years no deaths were recorded from ' noxious foodstuffs '. One death of a woman in 1970 was from ' mushroom ' poisoning. The hazard is rare and its serious consequences (mortality rate 30 per cent) easily forgotten. Fungus poisoning is commoner on the Continent.

Many non-poisonous fungi are avoided because of their peculiar shape or colour. Some members of the very poisonous *Amanita* genus and particularly the Death Cap (*Amanita phalloides*) are easily mistaken for the edible mushroom and have pleasant tastes.

Tests of edibility. Most of the often quoted tests are fallacious. The edible mushroom peels easily but so does the Death Cap. Some fungi change colour alarmingly when cut but this does not mean they are poisonous. Failure to blacken a silver spoon during cooking is no proof of edibility. The fact that fungi are eaten by rabbits does not mean they are safe for man since rabbits can eat the Death Cap with impunity. Hence the best test of non-edibility is to be able to distinguish the poisonous fungi on sight.

Distinguishing features. Serious poisoning is confined to two groups of the genus *Amanita.* Members of this genus are the only large ' mushrooms ' with both a ring and a volva though the volva will only be seen if the stalk at ground level is examined. The volva is the basal remnant of the membrane which covered the whole of the young fruiting body. The ring is what is left of the membrane which connected the edge of the gills to the stalk (Fig. 6.1). A very important distinguishing feature of *Amanita phalloides, verna* and *virosa* is that the gills are always white whereas those of the edible mushroom never are, but as this might not be appreciated when the fungus is small it is advisable to avoid the ' button ' stage of wild ' mushrooms '. The smell of the Death Cap is unpleasant. Other characteristics are shown in Table 6.1. Anyone collecting fungi to eat should avoid specimens growing near trees and should dig up the whole specimen so that it can be seen whether there is a volva or not. Any fungus with white gills must be avoided.

Poisoning by *Amanita muscaria* and *pantherina*

Vomiting, diarrhoea and abdominal pain come on between $\frac{1}{2}$ to 4 hours after eating the fungus. There is profuse sweating and salivation followed by wild excitement and delirium with visual hallucinations. The pupils are contracted. The muscarine-like alkaloid is present only in small amounts and is destroyed by cooking.

Poisoning by *Amanita phalloides, verna* and *virosa*

Symptoms come on after a latent period of 8 to 40 hours. There is sudden severe cramping abdominal pain and violent vomiting and diarrhoea with the passage of blood. Jaundice then appears and the patient dies of liver failure. Sometimes there is anuria.

Treatment

General measures (stomach washing and sedatives) will usually save the patient poisoned by *Amanita muscaria* and *pantherina*.

Atropine is not really necessary as muscarine for which it is the antidote is only present in minute quantities. The main toxin is

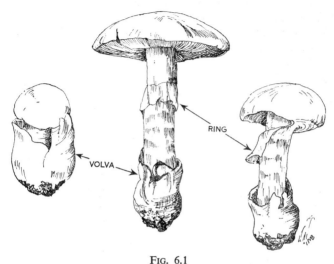

FIG. 6.1

The Death Cap (*Amanita phalloides*). Mature specimen in centre. (Height, 11·25 cm; width of cap, 8·75 cm; width of stem, 15·6 mm).

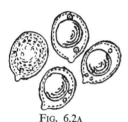

FIG. 6.2A
Spores of the Death Cap (*Amanita phalloides*). ×1 000.

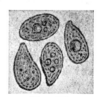

FIG. 6.2B
Spores of the Edible Mushroom (*Psalliota campestris*). ×1 000.

muscimol. Prompt measures are needed in Death Cap poisoning. Whether to treat for this or not can be decided by: (1) examining any uneaten fungi; (2) considering the time interval between ingestion and symptoms; (3) examining the vomit and stools for spores.

The spores of the Death Cap are sufficiently charcteristic to confirm a diagnosis. They are colourless sub-globoid bodies measuring 8 to 11 by 7 to 9 μ and contain a large oil drop (Figs. 6.2A and 6.2B).

If there is any doubt treat for the more serious condition as follows:

(1) Start treatment for liver failure and consider transfer to a liver unit for haemoperfusion through activated charcoal (p. 153).

(2) Give penicillin in large doses (1 g per Kg). This displaces the protein bound toxin α-amanitin which can then be excreted by the kidneys.

(3) Give the antidote cytochrome C 150 mg per Kg. It is obtainable from Fluorochem Ltd., Dinting Lane, Glossop, Derbyshire, SK13 9NU. Tel. Glossop 4917 (STD Code 04574) who hold a small stock for immediate dispatch. (Also from Sigma, p. 464).

(4) Treatment for oliguric renal failure may be necessary (p. 375) including the use of haemo- or peritoneal dialysis (p. 716).

Serious consideration should be given to offering emetics to or performing gastric lavage on all those who have shared the meal of fungi whether they have symptoms or not. Antiphallinic serum being useless and even dangerous is no longer available.

REFERENCE

FLOERSHEIM, G. L. (1972). Antidotes to Experimental α-Amanitin Poisoning. *Nature New Biology*, **236**, 115.

BELLADONNA POISONING

Every year at blackberry time, the country doctor is liable to meet belladonna poisoning. The patient is usually a child out for a day in the country. The berries eaten are usually those of the Deadly Nightshade (*Atropa belladonna*) (Fig. 6.3), like small black cherries three of which could kill a child. Those of Woody Nightshade or Bittersweet (*Solanum dulcamara*) like red currants, or of Black Nightshade (*Solanum nigrum*) like black currants, may also be responsible.

The Thornapple (*Datura stramonium*) (Figs 6.4 and 6.5) when ripe bursts open to reveal numerous small black seeds which are attractive to children. They contain 0·5 per cent of hyoscine and hyoscyamine and so cause symptoms similar to those of belladonna poisoning.

Some hours after eating these berries or seeds the child is found confused and excited and has a flushed face and dry mouth. He is ' hot as a hare, blind as a bat, dry as a bone, red as a beet and mad as a hen '. The widely dilated inactive pupils give him a startled appearance. The heart is rapid and the bladder distended, presumably from spasm of the external sphincter.

Table 6.1. *Poisonous Fungi*

	HABITAT	HEIGHT	WIDTH OF STEM	WIDTH OF CAP	COLOUR OF CAP AND OTHER FEATURES
Amanita phalloides	Woods and adjacent fields.	7·5 to 12·5 cm	15·6 mm	7·5 to 10 cm	Olive or yellowish green with brown centre (rarely white). Gills white.
Amanita verna	Beech woods especially.	7·5 to 12·5 cm	9·3 mm	6·25 to 7·5 cm	Usually white but sometimes as in *A. phalloides*. Gills white.
Amanita virosa	Damp woods.	10 to 18·75 cm	15·6 mm	7·15 to 12·5 cm	Usually white. Gills white.
Amanita muscaria	Near Silver Birch and conifers.	10 to 25 cm	25 mm	10 to 22·5 cm	The 'fairy toadstool'. Scarlet or orange with white or yellow warts.
Amanita pantherina	Woods, fields and moorland.	10 to 12·5 cm	12·5 mm	7·5 to 10 cm	Brownish with warts as in *A. muscaria*.

It is best to use an emetic of salty water rather than a stomach tube as the berries may block this. The specific antidote is neostigmine (Prostigmin) 0·5 to 1·0 mg i m. The excitement should not be treated with morphine since this might deepen the depression which will follow in any case. Sodium phenobarbitone 60 to 200 mg by i m injection is preferable. Similar symptoms more often result when atropine enters the body in excess from liniments, plasters, medicines and eyedrops (p. 86).

In a doubtful case a delicate test is to instil a few drops of the child's urine in a cat's eye. If belladonna (atropine) is present rapid dilatation of the pupil results.

POISONOUS PLANTS

Anxious parents may telephone the doctor urgently for advice when their children have eaten some odd berries. Knowledge of the plant concerned can often enable a reassuring message to be given, but the patient should preferably be seen.

About 200 British plants contain poisonous constituents but only a few cause serious illness. This, except for the special instances mentioned, will have to be treated on general lines. The seeds and berries of the following plants are harmless: cotoneaster, hawthorn, lily of the valley, nasturtium, pyracantha, sweet pea. Table 6.2 summarises the facts about common poisonous plants.

OESOPHAGEAL IMPACTION

Occasionally a too large piece of meat is swallowed and sticks in the oesophagus, usually at the lower end where there is narrowing from a Schatzki's ring. If X-ray examination confirms the obstruction and does not show any bone in it immediate oesophagoscopy is not always needed. This ' steak house syndrome ' can be relieved by enzymes. Give 50 ml of 5 per cent sodium bicarbonate and 400 000 units of chymotrypsin. Alternatively a vegetable enzyme, papain 500 mg, could be used. It attacks heat-coagulated protein rapidly but uncoagulated protein only slowly. Within a couple of hours the obstruction may have passed. This treatment should be used early. If delayed the impacted material may have damaged the oesophageal wall and this can then be digested itself.

TENESMUS

This means the urgent desire to empty the rectum, the act being accompanied by straining. It is a distressing symptom in some cases of diarrhoea. It may be caused by severe enteritis, impacted faeces,

Table 6.2. *Poisonous Plants, Shrubs and Trees*

(Modified after Matthew and Lawson, 1970).

A Comprehensive work such as British Poisonous Plants, H.M. Stationery Office 1954, should be consulted. The following summary is given for the species which are most commonly regarded as poisonous. Poisoning by deadly nightshade and thornapple is described on p. 140.

NAME	POISONOUS PART	CLINICAL FEATURES	TREATMENT
CONITE (Monkshood)	All parts but chiefly seeds and roots.	Tingling and burning of mouth and skin. Nausea, vomiting, diarrhoea, agitation, collapse, convulsions.	1. Symptomatic. 2. Atropine sulphate (2 mg) i m if severe.
RBERIS	Berries.	Purging.	Symptomatic.
ROOM	Poisonous only in very large amounts.	Similar to Laburnum but much less severe.	1. Gastric aspiration and lavage. 2. Symptomatic.
HERRY	Stones if chewed and broken.	As for cyanide poisoning.	P. 461.
AFFODIL	Bulb.	Nausea, vomiting, diarrhoea.	1. Gastric aspiration and lavage. 2. Symptomatic.
LDERBERRY	Leaves and bark.	As for cyanide poisoning.	P. 461.
EMLOCK	'Seeds'.	Paralysis. Slow pulse. Dilated pupils. Rapid breathing and then respiratory failure.	1. Symptomatic. 2. Artificial respiration. 3. Atropinisation (p. 468).
OLLY	Berries.	Nausea, vomiting, diarrhoea; mild sedation.	1. Gastric aspiration and lavage. 2. Symptomatic.
YDRANGEA	All parts.	As for cyanide poisoning.	P. 461.
ABURNUM	All parts, but when ripe, poison concentrated in seeds, pods and leaves. Next to the yew, is Britain's most poisonous tree.	Burning in mouth, nausea, intractable vomiting, diarrhoea, exhaustion, collapse. Delirium, convulsions and coma.	1. Gastric aspiration and lavage. 2. Symptomatic.
UPIN	Seeds, but other parts to lesser extent.	Depression of respiration, paralysis, convulsions, collapse.	1. Gastric aspiration and lavage. 2. Symptomatic.
ARIHUANA	Leaves.	Stimulation of senses. Hallucinations, ataxia, blurred vision, diminished consciousness.	1. Gastric aspiration and lavage if ingested. 2. Symptomatic.
ISTLETOE	Berries but also all parts.	Nausea, vomiting, diarrhoea. Slow pulse.	1. Gastric aspiration and lavage. 2. As for digoxin (p. 39).
ARCISSUS	Bulbs.	Nausea, vomiting, diarrhoea.	Symptomatic.
EW	All parts, but especially the red berries. Britain's most poisonous tree.	Vomiting, abdominal colic, diarrhoea, paralysis, circulatory failure. Convulsions. Death often within five minutes.	An acute emergency. 1. Wash out stomach. 2. Pentothal for convulsions. 3. Artificial respiration.

or even a foreign body. If rectal examination is negative, a starch
mucilage enema with opium, as a palliative measure, may be tried.
Fifteen grammes (a heaped tablespoonful) of starch are mixed with
30 ml of cold water to form a smooth paste. To this is added, while
stirring, 500 ml of boiling water. After allowing to cool, 120 to 180
ml, with 2 ml of tincture of opium are given slowly as an enema, at
body temperature.

RECTAL PAIN (PROCTALGIA FUGAX)

An urgent night call for the doctor may be occasioned by an
attack of boring unremitting cramp-like pain in the rectum just
above the anal sphincter. It begins as a slight pain and works up to
a maximum in 5 or 10 minutes but does not radiate. Sometimes in
men it is associated with sexual intercourse. There is no diarrhoea
but flatus may be passed in a severe attack. Abdominal cramps,
nausea and fainting, may complicate the picture. Local examination
is usually negative but sometimes reveals a tender band possibly the
result of spasm of the levator ani. It should always be made since
similar pain may result from impacted faeces. Sigmoidoscopy has
shown a swollen mucosa and prominent vessels and this has suggested vascular congestion analogous to that of migraine as a cause.

The taking of food and drink often brings prompt relief presumably because the gastro-colic reflex inhibits the painful spasm.
Other remedies are a small enema, a finger in the rectum and
pressure on the perineum (sitting astride the cold edge of the bath).
Sublingual glyceryl trinitrate 1·0 mg is said to bring prompt relief.
Pethidine 100 mg might be needed for a prolonged attack. The
attacks generally cease in later life.

THE HEPATORENAL SYNDROME

Various disorders may affect the liver and kidneys simultaneously
but in the present context the term means renal failure which
appears as a complication, often terminal, of failure of liver function.
While tubular necrosis may be precipitated in liver disease by
haemorrhage from oesophageal varices, loss of fluid volume from
the use of diuretics and the toxic effects of neomycin, it is thought
that in most cases the mechanism is renal circulatory failure. Some
degree of this is probable in most patients with progressive cirrhosis
especially when there is ascites. The pathogenesis is obscure. Treatment should be directed to preserving liver function on the lines
already suggested since only this offers some hope of recovery.

PRIAPISM

This rare tragic condition is a pathological persistent erection of the penis in the absence of libido. Erection persists because of multiple small thrombi in the corpora cavernosa or deep dorsal vein of the penis or at any rate impaired venous outflow. It differs from a physiological erection in that the glans and corpus spongiosum are not involved and remain flaccid. Retention of urine does not occur.

It is sometimes associated with a blood disease such as sickle cell anaemia and leukaemia and is a fairly common but mysterious complication of haemodialysis. The condition is serious for after recovery the penis is unlikely to erect again. Attempts to obtain relief by intercourse will fail. Success has followed forcible massage under anaesthesia probably from the dislodgement of clots. Two successes have followed therapeutic defibrination using Arvin (Ancrod) (Twyford Pharmaceutical Services Ltd., Rye Park House, London Road, High Wycombe, Buckinghamshire, HP11 1BN), a proteolytic enzyme fractionated from the crude venom of the Malayian pit viper. I unit per kg is infused i v over a 6 hours period. A second dose is given over 10 to 15 hours at the end of the first infusion and repeated every 12 hours. Failing Arvin, thrombolytic therapy with Kabikinase might be tried (p. 115).

Recurrent incomplete priapism is usually associated with diseases of the nervous system, e.g. disseminated sclerosis and then retention of urine is a common complication for the whole penis is involved. Suprapubic drainage is preferable to a catheter which might cause gangrene. Interruption of the nervi erigentes might have to be considered. Priapism is not uncommon in the newborn and is without signficance.

C. ALLAN BIRCH

HEPATIC COMA AND PRECOMA

It is essential to establish as early as possible whether hepatic coma or precoma has developed as a result of acute hepatic injury or is based on chronic liver disease. The latter is the more frequent clinical problem and, fortunately, its prognosis, at least for a single episode, is better.

HEPATIC COMA IN CIRRHOSIS

The usual sequence is that the cirrhotic patient, who may have been previously alert and well, becomes confused and drowsy (precoma) and may, if untreated, become progressively less aware, eventually reaching a deeply comatose state. The stages of hepatic coma have been conveniently graded (Table 6.3) for purposes of comparison. Often this progression is slow and occasionally bizarre psychiatric states including extreme somnolence, depression, paranoid delusions and violence are predominant. Convulsions are uncommon and usually only occur in the later stages.

Examination usually reveals the superficial stigmata of cirrhosis such as spider naevi, palmar erythema and leuconychia, although these may not be obvious, especially in the dark-skinned. Mild jaundice is often evident and ascites is common. Diagnostic difficulty may be experienced with patients in whom there is extensive portasystemic collateral circulation but well-preserved liver function, as such cases may show little external evidence of cirrhosis.

When coma develops the breath has a peculiar sweet sickly smell (fetor hepaticus). Neurological signs include a flapping tremor of the outstretched hands and the patient may experience difficulty in constructing simple diagrams (spatial apraxia) and with mental arithmetic. Useful tests include drawing or copying a five-pointed star or constructing one from match sticks. A daily specimen of handwriting should be obtained and the time taken to subtract serially from 100 measured repeatedly to follow the clinical progress. More sophisticated is the Reitan trail-making test in which the patient is asked to join scattered numbers together in sequence, the time taken to complete the test providing an index of abnormality.

Later on midbrain disturbances are dominant with symmetrical hyperflexia, ankle clonus and extensor plantar responses. Vasomotor instability and hyperventilation are pre-terminal and usually accompanied by decerebrate posturing. Eventually a flaccid paralysis with areflexia supervenes.

Essential investigations. A low serum albumin (3·0 g/dl) and a prolonged prothrombin time suggest severe impairment of hepatic synthetic function. An electroencephalogram may show a characteristic and symmetrical rhythm disturbance with slow triphasic waves (Fig. 6.6) but, like the blood ammonia, is only necessary when the diagnosis is in doubt. The ammonia level (normal arterial NH_3 <430 μmol/l) is usually but not invariably elevated, unless treatment with neomycin and a low protein diet has already been started. The blood sugar should be measured at once by dextrostix although hypoglycaemia is much rarer than in coma due to fulminant hepatic failure. In fact, the patient may be hyperglycaemic, as carbohydrate intolerance is common in cirrhosis, and occasionally the onset of clinical diabetes precipitates hepatic encephalopathy or is the cause of the coma.

Table 6.3. *Grading of hepatic coma*

STAGE	MENTAL STATE	FLAP	EEG CHANGE
I Prodroma, precoma	Euphoria, occasionally depression, fluctuant mood, confusion, slowness of mentation and affect. Untidy slurred speech, disorder of sleep rhythm.	Slight	Usually absent
II Impending coma	Accentuation of Stage I, inappropriate behaviour. Inability to maintain sphincter control.	Present (easily elicited)	Abnormal generalised slowing
III Stupor	Sleeps most of the time, rousable. Speech incoherent, confusion marked.	Present (if patient can cooperate)	Always abnormal
IV Coma	May or may not respond to painful stimuli.	Usually absent	Always abnormal

Investigation is principally aimed at discovering which of six common factors has precipitated coma:

Misuse of diuretics
Infection
Gastro-intestinal haemorrhage
Sedative or hypnotic drugs
Portacaval anastomosis
Progression of underlying disease.

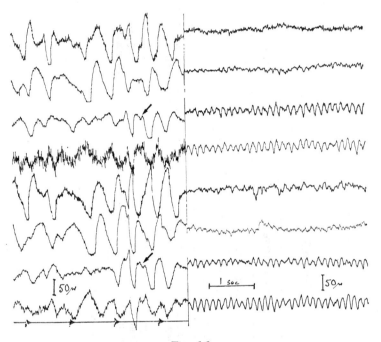

FIG. 6.6
Typical EEG abnormality in a patient with grade IV hepatic coma showing triphasic waves.

The misuse of diuretics may have precipitated hepatic coma in a variety of ways. **Hypokalaemia** is easily produced by potassium-losing diuretics (Frusemide, Ethacrynic acid, thiazides). For this reason potassium-sparing compounds such as spironolactone (Aldactone 100-400 mg daily), triamterene (Dytac) or amiloride (Midamor) are preferred in the initial drug treatment of ascites. **Uraemia** may be related to over-rapid diuresis, even when ascites is still present, and the daily weight loss whilst on diuretics should never be allowed to exceed 0·5 kg. Uraemia produced by diuretics must be distinguished from two other common causes—functional renal failure and acute tubular necrosis—on the basis of urinary volumes and urinalysis (Table 6.4). Functional renal failure, a common accompaniment of end-stage cirrhosis (see pp. 144 and 381) is probably related to a redistribution of blood flow within the kidney and is characterised by uraemia, oliguria and extreme sodium retention. This condition does not respond to diuretics. Acute tubular necrosis, as in other diseases, is often precipitated by hypotension (following haemorrhage) or septicaemia.

Table 6.4. *Urinalysis in the various uraemias seen in cirrhosis*

	ACUTE TUBULAR NECROSIS	FUNCTIONAL RENAL FAILURE	DIURETIC-INDUCED URAEMIA
Urinary sodium (mmol/l)	>20	< 5	>20*
Urine/plasma osmolality	< 1·1	> 1·1	> 1·1
Urinary sediment	Casts++	Casts±	Casts±
Glomerular filtration (ml/min)	< 5	<10	10-20

Life-threatening **infection** may be completely asymptomatic in the cirrhotic. Consequently, blood specimens (aerobic and anaerobic, 3 of each), a mid-stream urine, sputum, nose and throat swabs, and a sample of ascitic fluid must be cultured. The possibility of tuberculosis must always be considered, particularly in those on corticosteroids. Often antibiotic therapy has to be given before bacterial presence or sensitivities have been established. At the time of writing, the antibiotics of choice are gentamicin sulphate and cephalothin sodium. Gentamicin (Genticin) is given as a loading dose of 120 mg i v or i m, followed by 80 mg 8 hourly with subsequent dosage adjusted to give a peak level (15 minutes after i v injection or 1 hour after i m administration) between 6 and 8 μg of gentamicin/ml. Frequently, larger doses than those mentioned are necessary to obtain bactericidal concentrations. Gentamicin is highly active against *Pseudomonas, Staphylococcus aureus* (including penicillin-resistant strains) and the great majority of

* Whilst on diuretics; falling to <5mmol/l when diuretics discontinued.

coliform organisms. It is ototoxic and the recommended serum concentrations should not be exceeded. Cephalothin (Keflin) 1 g 8 hourly provides additional protection from *Staphylococcus aureus* and may be synergistic with gentamicin against coliforms. If the suspicion that this antibiotic combination may occasionally be nephrotoxic is confirmed, then cephalothin should be replaced by flucloxacillin (Floxapen) 500 mg 6 hourly if staphylococcal infection is suspected or by ampicillin (Penbritin) 500 mg 6 hourly.

Blood loss is usually self evident but occasionally the passage of a melaena stool may be delayed and haemorrhage suspected only because of hypotension, tachycardia and a low central venous pressure. The site of bleeding must be established by fibre-endoscopic examination when possible as in 30 per cent of cases peptic ulcer or acute gastric erosions rather than varices are responsible.

Control of haemorrhage from oesophageal varices (see also p. 166)

It is esssential both to restore the circulating blood volume and to arrest the haemorrhage. Vasopressin Injection BPC (Pitressin) 20 units (=1 ml) in 100 ml of dextrose 5 g/dl given i v over 10 minutes may be effective in stopping bleeding. It can be given more than once but becomes progressively less effective. It should not be used in the elderly or in those with known ischaemic heart disease. Haemorrhage from oesophageal varices may be effectively controlled by tamponade with the Sengstaken-Blakemore tube (see p. 724).

Control of haemorrhage from an erosion or ulcer

As in variceal haemorrhage the most important step is restoration and maintenance of normal blood volume with central venous pressure control. If coma of comparatively mild degree is present and the patient is considered fit on other grounds (mild jaundice only, little ascites, good general condition) then emergency surgery may be life-saving if haemorrhage persists. This is particularly so in the case of localised bleeding from a peptic ulcer.

Little is known about the cause of acute erosions and of the contribution of portal hypertension. Erosions are not confined to the alcoholic and enquiry into precipitating factors, including aspirin, is relevant though often negative. Conservative methods such as gastric lavage with ice-cold water and gastric cooling (p. 723) may be useful. Perfusion of the coeliac axis with vasopressin (0·02 u/min), although praised in the American literature (mainly for varices) has proved of little benefit in our experience.

Hepatic coma or precoma is an important complication following

portacaval anastomosis in cirrhosis, up to 30 per cent of patients being affected, though in varying degree. Coma is thought to develop because of an increase in the volume of portal blood by-passing the liver, and also because of an overall reduction in liver blood flow. In the presence of impaired liver function, hypoperfusion of the liver for any reason (myocardial infarction, shock, etc.) may precipitate hepatic coma.

Sedatives of all sorts are likely to precipitate hepatic coma in the patient with severe cirrhosis. Morphine derivatives are especially prone to do this and should never be given, particularly following gastrointestinal haemorrhage. The use of restraining binders and (if possible) extra nurses are a safer way of controlling the violent patient. Paraldehyde should not be used as its metabolism in the liver is impaired, coma and acidosis may develop and the breath may smell of it for days. If sedation is absolutely unavoidable, then small doses of phenobarbitone (60 mg i m), which is mainly excreted by the kidney, may be given. Some clinicians favour small doses of Phenergan (promethazine 25 mg i m). To control convulsions, diazepam (Valium) 5-10 mg by slow i v injection can be given but with considerable caution as respiratory arrest may ensue.

Treatment of hepatic coma in cirrhosis

Much of the standard treatment is designed to reduce the blood levels of compounds such as ammonia which have been formed as a result of protein breakdown in the gut but have failed to be metabolised by the damaged liver.

1. PROTEIN RESTRICTION AND PURGATION. When coma develops, protein must be withdrawn completely from the diet. With recovery, protein may be gradually reintroduced in increments of 20 g per day, but only rarely can the total daily intake exceed 60 g. Attempts must be made to purge the bowel, especially following gastro-intestinal haemorrhage (one pint of blood is equivalent to a meal of 60-130 g of protein). Magnesium Sulphate Mixture BPC 15 ml three times a day is given by mouth or through the Sengstaken tube and Magnesium Sulphate enemas (80 ml of a 50 per cent solution w / v, see p. 728) administered to ensure a daily bowel action. Constipation must also be avoided in cirrhotic patients verging on encephalopathy.

2. INTESTINAL ANTIBIOTICS. Neomycin sulphate (Neomin 1 g 4-6 hourly by mouth) is the usual choice, although some clinicians favour paramomycin (Humatin 4-6 g daily). Both antibiotics are assumed to act by reducing the numbers of colonic bacteria possessing urease activity (bacteroids, enterobacter, clostridia, Klebsiella),

but experimental verification is difficult to achieve. Small amounts of neomycin ($<$1 per cent) are absorbed from the gut and promptly excreted in the urine. In the presence of renal failure, the dose should be reduced because of the risks of nephro- or oto-toxicity.

3. LACTULOSE (DUPHALAC).* This synthetic disaccharide preparation contains per 100 ml lactulose 67 g, lactose 7·8 g and galactose 13·3 g. It is neither hydrolysed nor absorbed but is degraded by bacteria to lactic and acetic acids. It has a laxative action and may also produce a beneficial effect in chronic hepatic coma by affecting colonic pH and interfering with the degree of ionisation of ammonia and reducing its absorption. Lactulose may be substituted for neomycin for maintenance therapy and may occasionally provide an additive effect in resistant cases. The initial dose is 30 ml in the morning and 15 ml at lunch time, which is steadily increased until two or three soft bowel actions are obtained each day.

4. CARE OF THE UNCONSCIOUS PATIENT. When hepatic coma is prolonged, careful fluid and electrolyte balance, nutrition, physiotherapy and nursing care are of critical importance. A diet providing 2 500-3 000 calories per day should be the aim and this may be given via a Ryle's tube. If paralytic ileus (p. 609) develops then 10 per cent dextrose is given via a feeding catheter (Argyle feeding tube) advanced from the antecubital fossa into the superior vena cava. High concentrations of dextrose are to be avoided because the impaired glucose tolerance frequently present in cirrhosis may give rise to extremely high blood sugar levels. Intralipid 20 per cent may be used to boost the calorific value, provided that the patient is not too deeply jaundiced. Infusions of plasma or salt-poor albumin (if fluid retention is marked) may help to maintain the serum albumin level. Supplementary vitamins should be given in the form of Parentrovite Forte 2 (paired) ampoules i v daily, vitamin K_1 (10 mg i v daily), folic acid (5 mg twice a day) and vitamin B_{12} (1 000 μg weekly). Vitamin deficiencies are particularly common in the alcoholic cases especially with respect to thiamine, pyridoxine and folic acid, although vitamin B_{12} deficiency is rare.

Corticosteroid therapy is without benefit in hepatic coma or precoma complicating cirrhosis unless the underlying disease process is responsive to these drugs. One such disease is active chronic hepatitis for which prednisolone 20-30 mg daily should be given until the disease is brought under control and then 10-15 mg daily for maintenance therapy. Careful consideration of this diagnostic

---

*Duphar Laboratories Ltd., Gater's Hill, West End, Southampton, SO3 3JD. Tel. West End 2281 (STD 04218).

possibility must be given in each new case and blood sent for sero-logical examination and plasma protein electrophoresis. (Auto-antibody tests are available from Dr Deborah Doniach, Department of Immunology, The Middlesex Hospital Medical School, 40-50 Tottenham Street, London, W1P 9PG. 01-636 8333 Ext. 695. Send 5 ml of serum. Cost £2.10 per test.) Hypergammaglobulinaemia and increased aminotransferases (transaminases) are suggestive of this diagnosis and corticosteroids should be given without delay. Alco-holic hepatitis, usually but not always superimposed on alcoholic cirrhosis, is also often treated with corticosteroids, although the results of controlled trials to date are conflicting. This serious illness may precipitate coma and is suspected whenever a history of alcoholism is obtained and features including leucocytosis, fever, a raised aspartate aminotransferase (SGOT, EC 2.6.1.1.) of 100-500 iu/l and jaundice are present.

HEPATIC COMA IN ACUTE LIVER INJURY

This extremely serious complication of acute liver injury is for-tunately rare. The mortality rate among those reaching Grade IV coma is almost 90 per cent in most series. Early recognition of the condition is vital, as intensive care, rapidly instituted, may increase survival. (There is a special unit for the treatment of acute liver failure at King's College Hospital, Denmark Hill, London SE5 8RX. Tel. 01-274 6222 Ext. 2196. Between 1730 and 0900 hours dial 01-274 6222 and bleep the houseman.)

In this country hepatic coma is usually seen complicating one of the three types of acute liver injury: viral hepatitis; paracetamol (acetaminophen) self-poisoning and halothane hypersensitivity. Other less frequent causes include carbon tetrachloride poisoning, hypersensitivity to anti-tuberculous drugs (isoniazid, pyrazinamide) or monoamine oxidase inhibitors (Nardil, Marplan), tetracycline fatty liver, ' mushroom ' poisoning (*Amanita phalloides,* p. 137) and acute fatty liver of pregnancy.

Diagnosis

The tempo of the whole illness is usually quicker and more violent than in chronic liver disease. The cardinal signs of confusion and drowsiness may develop with alarming rapidity. Indeed, in this condition neuropsychiatric symptoms may precede clinical jaundice. With a paracetamol overdose (p. 40) there may be a delay of 24-48 hours before obvious signs of liver damage appear (usually severe damage is only seen in overdoses of 15 g or 30 tablets of 500 mg). Hypersensitivity to halothane, particularly if anaesthetics have been repeated for relatively minor procedures (cystoscopy, eye surgery) is usually manifest as fever followed by jaundice and then signs of encephalopathy, from five days to three weeks after the last exposure.

Physical examination reveals a confused and drowsy patient who may exhibit a flapping tremor and fetor hepaticus. Percussion shows liver size to be reduced. Ascites is a late manifestation. A haemorrhagic diathesis is almost always evident and bleeding is frequently severe. Neurological signs are as described in coma complicating cirrhosis, with emphasis on midbrain signs. The pupils are often dilated and slowly reactive to light. In fatal cases, progression to Grade IV coma is rapid and usually preceded by a violent phase in which the patient emits an inhuman and desolate cry and struggles against any restraint. Subsequently hyperventilation, hypotension and tachycardia predominate, leading to an areflexic, unresponsive coma with respiratory arrest and death. Oliguric renal failure, either of the functional variety or due to acute tubular necrosis, is usual in the late stages. Acute pancreatitis (p. 113) may accompany any form of acute hepatic necrosis.

Investigation

There is usually a polymorphonuclear leucocytosis, but fever is not prominent. Australia antigen should be looked for as soon as possible so that adequate precautions may be taken to protect staff. A latex fixation test provides a rapid and sensitive screen for the antigen, but as false positives are common with this technique each result must be checked without delay by counterimmunoelectrophoresis which is the standard technique used in regional transfusion centres.

The aspartate aminotransferase (serum glutamic oxaloacetic transaminase, SGOT, EC 2.6.1.1.) level is grossly elevated (>500 iu/l) when precoma first appears, but a rapid fall in the serum level is not necessarily associated with a good prognosis. Life-threatening hypoglycaemia may be an early phenomenon, sometimes associated with a severe lactic acidosis which requires urgent correction (50 ml of dextrose 50 g/dl i v and 100-400 ml of sodium bicarbonate 8·4 g/dl (1 mmol/l) (see p. 727). More frequently a respiratory alkalosis predominates, due to striking hyperpnoea so characteristic of the early stages. Attempts have been made to correct the arterial pCO_2 by elective ventilation, to augment cerebral blood flow, but no definite benefit has ensued. EEG abnormalities are similar to those described earlier.

The prothrombin time is the most useful single prognostic index.

When compared to the control sample the degree of prolongation may range from 30 seconds to 2 minutes, although occasionally more normal values occur despite severe necrosis. The prolongation is principally due to a synthetic defect in clotting factor production by the liver. In some cases, a major component of the haemorrhagic diathesis is provided by diffuse intravascular coagulation (DIC, see p. 283) possibly triggered by the release of tissue thromboplastins from the damaged liver cell. DIC produces a consumptive deficiency of clotting factors. Evidence of this is obtained by the development of purpura, a long thrombin clotting time (>40 seconds), a low fibrinogen level (<200 mg/dl), increased fibrin degradation products in blood and urine, and thrombocytopenia.

Table 6.5. *Physiological measurements and routine investigations in acute liver failure*

HOURLY	DIURNAL	DAILY
Blood pressure/pulse rate	Urea and electrolytes	Hb, WBC and platelets
Respiratory rate	Packed cell volume	Prothrombin time
Temperature	Blood sugar*	Blood culture
Central venous pressure		Bilirubin/AsT
Urine output		Arterial blood gases
Fluid balance		Chest X-ray

Clinical care

The patient should be transferred without delay to an intensive care unit. The general care is that of any other seriously ill individual. Regular recordings of pulse, blood pressure, central venous pressure and fluid balance are necessary, and a list of daily or diurnal investigations is given in Table 6.5. Careful and repeated physical examination is necessary to gauge the tempo of the illness and to anticipate respiratory arrest. Physiotherapy is essential and regular chest X-rays may reveal clinically unsuspected pulmonary oedema or consolidation. A cardiac monitor aids the rapid detection of arrhythmias.

The same general therapeutic measures apply in fulminant hepatic failure as in coma complicating cirrhosis, namely protein restriction, purgation and neomycin administration. In addition there are several special problems:

1. The haemorrhagic diathesis is corrected by infusions of fresh frozen plasma (one or two units, six hourly) aiming to keep the

* Check 2-4 hourly by Dextrostix.

prothrombin time below 25 seconds. When there is unequivocal evidence of DIC, controlled heparin therapy, using an *in vitro* protamine sulphate titration to check the heparin level, may be beneficial. Because haemorrhage is so frequent, blood should be ready crossmatched in the laboratory.

2. Fluid and electrolyte balance is complex, as in severe cases renal failure almost invariably develops. Once the intravascular fluid volume has been restored, frusemide (Lasix) 80-500 mg i v may be necessary to maintain urine output. Saline infusions are to be avoided as there is often avid reabsorption of sodium by the renal tubule and the salt content of the fresh frozen plasma is high. Hypokalaemia is common, and very large amounts of KCl (up to 12 g/day) are needed to maintain the serum K^+ level. Later on, hyperkalaemia may be seen. Once renal failure is established, the prognosis is extremely poor but if in other respects the patient's condition is not irreversible, the metabolic balance may be redressed by peritoneal dialysis.

3. Parenteral nutrition is best given by infusions of 10 per cent dextrose. Amino-acid preparations should be avoided as the plasma levels of most are already greatly elevated and some at least have been under suspicion of exacerbating hepatic coma. There is uncertainty as to whether fat emulsions can be utilised in the presence of gross liver function impairment and they are therefore best avoided. Vitamin replacement is as described on p. 152.

Despite the measures outlined above, the mortality of Grade IV coma remains depressingly high. This has led to various experimental techniques only practised in specialised centres. Exchange blood transfusion is no longer fashionable and may even be harmful to the patient. Pig or baboon liver perfusion has proved disappointing in the experience of most workers, and human cross-perfusion is difficult to justify ethically. Steroid therapy is unproven and at present is best reserved for the treatment of raised intracerebral pressure which develops late in the illness (Dexamethsone 8 mg at once and 4 mg eight hourly). Haemoperfusion through activated charcoal is currently being developed as the beginning of an artificial liver support system, the charcoal effectively adsorbing water-soluble toxins. Our first experience with this in patients with Grade IV coma from disparate causes has given nine survivors including cases of paracetamol poisoning, viral hepatitis, ' mushroom ' poisoning and halothane hypersensitivity.

Martin Smith
Roger Williams

HAEMATEMESIS AND MELAENA
(For intestinal bleeding in childhood see p. 421)

Haematemesis indicates an appreciable degree of blood loss, and so patients vomiting blood should be admitted to hospital. Symptomless melaena may result from quite a small haemorrhage—as little as 50 ml—and the patient may be initially observed at home. However, if there are already general symptoms of blood loss, admission should be arranged immediately. It is convenient to consider the management in relation to four clinical groups:—

(1) Patients with sudden, unheralded, life-threatening bleeding.
(2) Patients with steady, slow, continued bleeding.
(3) Patients with recurring separate crises of bleeding.
(4) Patients with known peptic ulcer.

(1) PATIENTS WITH SUDDEN, UNHERALDED, LIFE-THREATENING BLEEDING

These are patients in whom the severity of the haemorrhage may necessitate an early decision to operate, and, in spite of rapid transfusion, CVP (central venous pressure) measurements (p. 751) may indicate failure to restore or maintain blood volume. Most of these patients will in fact have acute or subacute painless peptic ulcers. Fibre-optic endoscopy is invaluable in demonstrating such acute gastric ulcers, which are commonly found high up on the posterior wall, often associated with varying degrees of gastric mucosal atrophy. They will be impalpable at operation from the outside of the stomach, but the bleeding vessel may be felt like a lead shot when the mucosa is palpated. Posterior wall duodenal ulcers may also be impalpable and their presence may not be appreciated until the duodenum is opened through a pyloroplasty incision. Sometimes a large, chronic ulcer may be found, in spite of the absence of any dyspeptic history. This can happen particularly in those patients who are relatively pain-insensitive to normal stimuli—a point which can be demonstrated clinically.

Mallory-Weiss syndrome

The important clue to the diagnosis in these patients is the fact that they vomited food first and then perhaps several hours later have had a haematemesis. The physical strain of vomiting has caused a laceration at the junction of the oesophagus and the cardia, especially if there is some degree of atrophic gastritis. If there is a sliding hiatus hernia as well, the pressure in the lower oesophagus builds up quickly and reaches a point at which the mucosa splits. The lesion can also result in patients who have had severe coughing bouts or status epilepticus. It can be demonstrated by endoscopy. The bleeding cannot be controlled by tamponage and if it persists, surgical underrunning may be needed. As it is a lesion easily overlooked at operation, it is one which must always be kept in mind.

Portal hypertension (see pp. 150 and 166)

A diagnosis of portal hypertension can fortunately be made clinically in the majority of patients, as hepatosplenomegaly may be found together with cutaneous stigmata of parenchymatous liver disease. Diagnosis of oesophageal varices can be difficult on barium swallow, but an increased diagnostic rate is achieved by using a small amount of thick barium paste with or without an i v injection of antispasmodic. However, even in the known presence of varices, endoscopy with a forward viewing instrument is essential since bleeding originates from other lesions in over half the cases, particularly from oesophagitis, acute gastric ulceration, or laceration of the gastro-oesophageal junction after vomiting. In cirrhotic patients whose venous obstruction is pre-sinusoidal as in splenic or portal vein block, congenital hepatic fibrosis and schistosomiasis elective surgery may be successful. Their prognosis is better than in those where obstruction is post-sinusoidal.

Leiomyoma

This tumour, arising from the smooth muscle of the stomach, characteristically causes sudden, entirely unheralded, severe haematemesis, but the diagnosis does not normally present much difficulty, as the smooth tumour can be easily seen gastroscopically or radiologically. Difficulty may occur, however, when a leiomyoma is present in the jejunum, as it may give rise to postprandial pain, and a diagnosis of duodenal ulcer may be readily accepted. However, at laparotomy the tumour should be felt in the region of the duodeno-jejunal flexure, where it had escaped palpation before operation.

A solitary, abnormally large submucosal artery

This congenital abnormality can cause sudden, very serious bleeding, due to the rupture of a single abnormal artery in the submucosa of the stomach. Such arteries may be otherwise quite normal and not showing any atherosclerotic change. Constant pulsation may have caused pressure necrosis of the mucosa and exposure of the artery to peptic digestion. The mucosal defect may be very small—only 2-5 mm in diameter. It is an important cause for the surgeon to be aware of, as such vessels may be quite difficult to palpate on opening the stomach. Bleeding from ruptured, normal-sized blood vessels may occur in patients with pseudo-xanthoma-elasticum and in the Ehlers-Danlos syndrome (cutis hyperelastica). In pseudo-xanthoma-elasticum there is alteration in the elastic tissue of the body and characteristic changes in the skin greatly facilitate the diagnosis. This skin is coarse, thicker than normal, looking like a crepe bandage, with elevations which are slightly yellow. There is loss of skin elasticity and a tendency to form folds easily. These changes are seen particularly in the neck, axillae, ante-cubital areas, inguinal folds and peri-umbilical region. Angioid streaking of the optic fundus may be seen. In the Ehlers-Danlos syndrome there is a generalised defect in the organisation of connective tissue, resulting in hypermotility of the joints, hyperelasticity of the skin, and wide thin scars which frequently overlie bony prominences.

Aneurysm

Atherosclerotic aneurysm of the aorta may cause pressure necrosis, and the third part of the duodenum is at particular risk. The diagnosis is now an important one to keep in mind, as successful excision of a bleeding aneurysm has been achieved. It is to be remembered that such aneurysms do not always pulsate, as they may contain laminated clots. There may be a history of episodes of quite intense pain associated with the phases of enlargement.

Biliary disease (haematobilia)

Massive, unheralded bleeding can occur into the biliary tree, as the result of gallstones, cholecystitis, aneurysm of the hepatic artery, and biliary tract tumours. Successful surgery for rupture of an aneurysm of the hepatic artery has been reported. Haematobilia is characteristically associated with upper abdominal pain and some degree of jaundice, both of which arise from blood clots in the common bile duct. Bleeding of the alimentary tract can occur from erosion of a large gallstone from the gallbladder into the duodenum, and bleeding can occur as well from within the pancreas, with pancreatic lithiasis associated with pancreatitis.

Carcinoma of the stomach

Brisk bleeding may be the very first symptom of carcinoma of the stomach, which may present without any previous digestive symptoms. The reason for this is the peptic digestion of a small malignant plaque in the stomach with exposure of submucosal blood vessels. Such patients may easily be thought to be bleeding from a simple gastric ulcer. Indeed, the ulcer may escape radiological detection, but should be found on endoscopy. Brisk bleeding also occurs in patients with advanced carcinoma, but the clinical picture does not offer any particular difficulties in diagnosis. The risk of these early cases being overlooked makes a follow-up for all X-ray-negative patients particularly important.

(2) PATIENTS WITH STEADY, SLOW, CONTINUED BLEEDING

These are patients who have a spongy, haemorrhagic mucosa, affecting part or all of the stomach or the region of a stoma. They tend to bleed at the rate of about 500 ml a day. This may persist for some days, necessitating repeated blood transfusions. These patients may be found to have achlorhydria and severe chronic atrophic gastritis, and there has presumably been a failure of the normal defence mechanisms of the stomach. The best policy is to persevere with medical management and not to operate.

(3) PATIENTS WITH RECURRING, SEPARATE EPISODES OF HAEMATEMESIS AND MELAENA

These patients have recurring episodes of acute bleeding, usually at intervals of months or several years. There are certain diagnoses which must be kept very much in mind, as special techniques may be needed for their diagnosis.

Post-bulbar duodenal ulcer

A very normal and indeed sometimes large duodenal bulb may dominate the radiological picture and conceal an ulcer just distal to it. This may be also missed at operation if the duodenum is not opened. However, it is likely that endoscopic duodenoscopy may help further in these patients, and furthermore present-day air-contrast techniques certainly help in the radiology.

Meckel's diverticulum

This remains a significant cause of recurring episodes of melaena. Such patients are liable to have a tender point in the right lower abdomen. X-ray visualisation is seldom possible, but a scanning technique has recently been introduced which may facilitate the identification of an acid-secreting Meckel's diverticulum (Jewett *et al.*, 1970).

Hiatal hernia

In a small group of patients with hiatal hernia who present with recurring episodes of haematemesis and melaena, the milder forms are due to erosive oesophagitis and the more severe examples have a fixed hiatal hernia and a gastric ulcer in relation to the ring constriction at the level of the diaphragm.

Leiomyoma

This can cause recurrent bleeding, but the diagnostic problems only arise when the tumour is in the upper part of the small intestine where it may have escaped detection, until laparotomy is performed at the time of bleeding.

Angioma

This constitutes a most difficult diagnostic group. Patients with capillary telangiectasia may have recurring epistaxis and cutaneous manifestations, but the cavernous group may present no clues. Angiography at the time of bleeding may pinpoint the bleeding site.

Post-surgical group

Patients who have had previous gastric surgery may have recurring episodes of bleeding, sometimes associated with unabsorbed catgut at the stoma.

Blood dyscrasias

The important one is von Willebrand's disease in which there is a deficiency of anti-haemophilic globulin (AHG or Factor VIII) (p. 281). Alimentary bleeding may be the only manifestation.

(4) PATIENTS WITH KNOWN PEPTIC ULCER

This is the most common cause of bleeding, the ulcers varying from small acute ones to large deep penetrating craters. Emergency endoscopy and emergency barium meal together now enable a very high proportion of acute ulcers causing bleeding to be identified. Nevertheless there remains a residual group with acute gastrostaxis, with rapid return to normal of the mucosa and which may defy detection.

GENERAL MANAGEMENT

The restoration of blood volume by transfusion is the first priority in the management of a patient with a serious degree of blood loss.

The second priority is the decision as to whether or not emergency surgery is required to deal with the bleeding point. Fortunately, in the great majority of patients bleeding ceases spontaneously. This will facilitate taking a simple clinical history and making a routine physical examination. After the restoration of blood volume there is a basic responsibility for trying to determine the cause of bleeding as quickly as possible. In practice, this may mean urgent fibre-optic oesophago-gastro-duodenoscopy, or an emergency barium meal. Each patient must be reviewed on individual merits. There is no doubt that urgent endoscopy can be a great help in identifying acute ulcers—which particularly in older age-groups may need surgical treatment, if bleeding recurs. It is a great help for the diagnosis of portal hypertension, although most can be diagnosed clinically by the bedside. Endoscopy may also provide the answer for bleeding from chronic ulceration or neoplasm, both simple and malignant, and may confirm a diagnosis of Mallory-Weiss syndrome. With the modern fibre-optic instrument and the use of iv diazepam (Valium), there is no doubt that patients can tolerate the examination very well, but every examination, however carefully done, carries some slight risk of mishap. Any such investigation should be made only when there will be therapeutic advantage to the patient commensurate with any discomfort or risk. An urgent barium meal is the simplest and safest investigation and can be given even when bleeding is continuing, but there are important pitfalls in diagnosis. Acute gastric ulcers and post-bulbar duodenal ulcers can very easily be overlooked. The basic points of management are:—

1. Reassure the patient by giving a simple explanation of the crisis.

2. Secure mental relaxation with diazepam (Valium) 10 mg by im injection, or alternatively sodium phenobarbitone 200 mg.

3. Order complete bed rest and make certain that bed blocks are available.

4. Request hourly initial blood pressure and pulse charts, changing to two-hourly or four-hourly as soon as is appropriate. (A diastolic blood pressure of 65 or less indicates serious blood loss and may provide a better indication initially than pulse rate or systolic blood pressure.)

5. Take about 14 ml of blood. Put 5 ml in an oxalate bottle for blood urea and haemoglobin estimation. 5 ml in a plain tube for serum for grouping. If liver disease is suspected, make up the special oxalate tube for prothrombin activity as directed.

The following points should be noted:—

(a) The haemoglobin may remain high for 6 to 18 hours after bleeding and so may be misleading.

(b) A blood urea of 70 to 100 mg per 100 ml (11·7 to 16·7 mmol/1 is common after a brisk haemorrhage. If over 25 mmol/1 consider the possibility of dehydration, chronic nephritis or alkalosis and give fluids i v.

6. Request soft diet with two-hourly feeds, with milk or other fluids on the locker, restricting intake only if the patient is nauseated.

The following diet would be suitable:—

6 a.m.	Cup of milky tea.
8 a.m.	Porridge and Bemax or lightly-boiled egg; thin bread and butter and jelly marmalade; cup of milky tea.
10 a.m.	Cup of milk and biscuit.
12 noon	Minced meat, chicken or steamed fish; mashed potato; puree carrot or cauliflower.
2 p.m.	Egg custard or cereal pudding or apple puree; orange juice.
4 p.m.	Cup of milky tea; three slices of thin bread and butter; bramble jelly; sponge cake.
6 p.m.	Cream of vegetable soup or minced chicken sandwich.
8 p.m.	Milk pudding or cup of milk.
10 p.m.	Cup of milk and biscuit.

7. Aluminium hydroxide gel 15 ml may be given as this has an anti-peptic as well as an acid-neutralizing action, and so may hinder the digestion of clot. Double doses at night may be given if the patient is awake. After three days reduce the dose to 15 ml four times a day.

8. Give effervescent ascorbic acid 1 g twice daily for five days. Ascorbic acid deficiency retards healing of the ulcer. This is particularly important in the early months of the year.

9. Review the need for blood transfusion or emergency surgery (see below).

10. Review the need for further diagnostic measures, including Hess test for capillary fragility, screening of blood for coagulation or bleeding defects, the bromsulphthalein test for liver dysfunction, emergency endoscopy and emergency barium meal.

11. The bowel is usually inactive for several days after haemorrhage. It is unwise to give aperients or early enemas. Reassure the patient and give a simple enema on the fourth day, using a plastic disposable bag.

SPECIAL INSTRUCTIONS CONCERNING THE SERIOUSLY ILL PATIENT

However seriously ill a patient may seem and however unpromising the prognosis, always persist with treatment unless there is clear evidence of advanced malignancy. Sometimes emptying the stomach, using Señorans's evacuator and washing out with water, may tip the scales in the patient's favour. Gastric cooling (p. 723) is best avoided as it may facilitate pneumonic complications. An oxygen tent or oxygen at 6 litres per minute through a mask may greatly assist a desperately ill patient. It is to be remembered that acute vitamin B deficiency (beriberi, p. 648) may be precipitated by giving dextrose i v to a malnourished patient. It can be prevented by giving vitamin B complex, Parentrovite—Bencard —i v or i m. This has the added advantage of augmenting vitamin C intake. If vitamin K deficiency is suspected or confirmed by estimation of prothrombin activity, vitamin K (phytomenadione, Konakion 10 mg) should be given i m.

There are four complications of gastroduodenal bleeding worth remembering:—

1. Temporary or even permanent blindness may follow recurrent bleeding in an already very anaemic subject, and this is a powerful argument in favour of adequate blood transfusion.

2. Coronary thrombosis and cerebral thrombosis may be precipitated by acute haemorrhage, and may cause diagnostic difficulties unless remembered.

3. Acute perforation occurs soon after bleeding in 1 per cent of cases. The diagnosis may be extremely difficult as the classical picture of perforation may be entirely lacking in a hypoxaemic patient. Unusual tachycardia or abdominal distension should prompt examination for absence of liver dulness and peristaltic sounds, and an X-ray film to seek air under the diaphragm may be needed.

4. A patient who has been kept flat on his back or with his head lowered, and when he has an indwelling naso-gastric tube, may have seepage of acid back into his oesophagus, and this may give rise to acute peptic oesophagitis with the risk of subsequent stricture,

BLOOD TRANSFUSION

Blood transfusion is an essential treatment for all patients who have a serious gastrointestinal bleed. The purpose of the transfusion is to help the patient to recover quickly from his oligaemic shock or to bring up the level of haemoglobin so that if further bleeding occurs the patient will be in a position to withstand it without the risk of passing into a state of prolonged shock or developing a serious degree of hypoxaemia. Clinical assessment of a serious bleed is not always easy, as the initial vasoconstriction reaction may give the patient a deathly pallor and which bears no relation to the severity of the bleed. Both the systolic blood pressure and the pulse may give quite misleading information, but a diastolic blood pressure of 65 or lower indicates a serious blood loss and is an indication for transfusion. The haemoglobin on admission is a notoriously misleading guide, as it will remain up until haemodilution has occurred, which may take 12 or 18 hours or sometimes several days. If the patient has had an initial phase of clinical shock, and if there has been vomiting of blood, or if the haemoglobin has already fallen to 8 g/dl, it is certainly advisable to transfuse to give the patient a greater margin of safety against further bleeding.

The management of patients with a serious degree of blood loss has been enormously improved by the use of the CVP line (p. 751) which enables the CVP to be recorded and rapid transfusions given sufficient to bring the CVP back to normal levels. It also enables a fairly accurate titration of blood loss to be undertaken. Furthermore, the CVP is an excellent indication of recurrent bleeding. It may enable emergency surgery to be undertaken without any undue delay. The supraclavicular subclavian vein technique, aiming to have the tip of the catheter in the superior vena cava, needs expertise (p. 747). It is essential that the patient be tipped head down to prevent any risk of air embolism (p. 63) during the introduction of the catheter, and it is very advisable for blood warmers (pp. 13 and 99) to be used so that cool blood in large volumes is not quickly introduced, as this may cause cardiac embarrassment. The patient needs quick restoration of blood volume, and this in fact is more important initially than restoration of the oxygen-carrying capacity. For this reason a plasma expander should be given while the blood is being cross-matched. Saline in practice is perfectly efficient in this respect, and unlike dextrans does not cause any subsequent complications with blood cross-matching, but there may be occasions when plasma is preferred. If haemodilution has already taken place and the CVP has returned to normal, it is necessary to give i v frusemide (Lasix) 80-120 mg to ensure adequate diuresis. In practice the increased potassium content of stored blood given fairly rapidly does not seem to constitute a problem (pp. 13 and 105), possibly because the blood is coming initially in contact with the endocardium and not initially affecting the coronary artery circulation. In practice also calcium injections are not necessary, although perhaps they might be kept in mind when really massive repeated transfusions have been required, for example in patients with portal hypertension. The serious complications of hypoxaemia remain a constant spur to prompt adequate replacement of blood loss so that if a patient should bleed again he is in a position to withstand further loss.

SURGERY

The mortality is concentrated in the older age-groups, but death can occur at any age. The initial objective is to establish whether the patient is in a high risk group, as this may indicate the likely need for emergency surgery. The clinical indications of a high risk are: age over 50; haematemesis; chronic gastric ulcer; severe haemorrhage; clinical shock; recurrence of bleeding after admission; the need for seven or more units of blood to restore central venous pressure; and associated diseases. Every patient is an individual problem needing individual assessment. The general policy should be towards operation at the earliest possible moment if the patient appears to be in an adverse situation prognostically. It is a better policy to be prepared to make up one's mind clinically in borderline cases rather than to delay too long on diagnostic procedures. These should certainly be made whenever possible but emergency treatment, both restoration of blood volume and surgical arrest of bleeding must have priority in appropriate circumstances. Recurrence of bleeding after admission is the most important single prognostic factor, and being 60 years of age or more at once brings the patient into the over 20 per cent mortality risk group, without surgery.

BLEEDING FROM PORTAL HYPERTENSION

Massive haemorrhage in portal hypertension usually comes from ruptured varices but lesser bleeding may arise from oesophagitis, acute gastric ulceration or laceration of the gastro-oesophageal junction after vomiting. In bleeding from varices the patient should be nursed with the foot of the bed raised to increase the rate of flow in the veins thus reducing the pressure on their walls. Gastric haemorrhage is particularly liable to precipitate hepatic coma if liver function is impaired for it provides a very large protein meal and consequent excessive production of ammonia (p. 146). Vaso-pressin Injection BPC may stop the bleeding (see p. 150). It acts by constricting the splanchnic arteriolar bed and so lowering portal venous pressure. These measures may have to be combined with oesophageal tamponade (p. 724). If bleeding recurs when the intra-oesophageal compression is released then emergency surgery may have to be considered. Tanner's operation of high gastric trans-section and resuture may be attempted but is not always successful and may result in a gastric fistula. An emergency porto-caval anas-tomosis may be made if liver function is good but it carries a high mortality. The recently described Boerema button appears to be effective in controlling the bleeding. It is a plastic device designed for facilitating oesophago-jejunal anastomosis after total gastrec-tomy. It controls bleeding from the oesophago-gastric junction by nipping the distended veins between the two parts of the button.

F. AVERY JONES

REFERENCES

JEWETT, T. C., DUSZYNSIK, D. O. & ALLEN, J. E. (1970). The visualization of Meckel's diverticulum with 99m Tc-pertechnetate. *Surgery* **68**, 567-570.

JOHNSTON, G. W. & KELLY, J. M. (1976). Early experience with the Boerema button for bleeding oesophageal varices. *British Journal of Surgery*, **63**, 117.

CHAPTER 7

Medical Emergencies in Obstetrics and Gynaecology

An emergency situation in this field generally presents in one of the following categories:
 1. Uterine haemorrhage, possibly associated with pregnancy.
 2. Abdominal pain, with or without uterine bleeding.
 3. Complications of pregnancy other than haemorrhage and pain.
 4. Emergencies of parturition.
In many cases accurate diagnosis and ideal treatment requires hospital facilities and specialised opinion but in an emergency much can be done to alleviate the situation and reduce risk pending further advice.

UTERINE BLEEDING—POSSIBLY ASSOCIATED WITH PREGNANCY

Diagnosis of pregnancy

The diagnosis of early pregnancy may be difficult and care should be exercised as in the presence of an absolute denial of the possibility a confident diagnosis of pregnancy may carry the risk of legal action. Amenorrhoea may be due to endocrine disturbance, or to systemic or local pelvic disease as well as being of psychological origin. Even in the nullipara breast secretion is not diagnostic of pregnancy and the condition of pseudo-cyesis (p. 130) may produce abdominal swelling and imaginary fetal movements. There are also many other causes of abdominal swelling.

The use of oral hormones such as Primodos as a test for pregnancy is not recommended as the positive and negative errors are too great and there is now considerable evidence that these substances are teratogenetic. Radiological methods are valueless before the sixteenth week and even then do not exclude pregnancy absolutely. They are best avoided until late pregnancy on account of the radiation hazards to the fetus.

Portable instruments utilising the Doppler effect and ultrasound can give positive evidence of the presence of a fetus by the twelfth week. The most satisfactory techniques for pregnancy testing are the immunological ones and in the absence of laboratory facilities the most convenient are the slide tests which take only two minutes to perform. They depend on the ability of human chorionic gonadotrophin (HCG) antiserum to agglutinate latex particles coated with purified HCG. The presence of HCG in the urine inhibits the agglutination. Pregnosticon Planotest (Organon) and Gravindex (Ortho) seem to offer the best compromise between sensitivity and an easily read end point.

Except in clearly menopausal women (and it is difficult to lay down an age limit for this) the possibility of pregnancy should always be suspected as the cause of uterine bleeding.

1. Examine vaginally. An intact pregnancy will never be disturbed by such an examination but an inevitable or incomplete abortion will readily be detected and removal of the placental tissue from the cervical canal often reduces the bleeding and shock sharply. Adnexal tenderness may be elicited (suggesting ectopic pregnancy) or a cervical lesion detected.

2. Give Syntometrine (Sandoz) 1 to 2 ml (ergometrine maleate 0·5 mg and syntocinon 5 oxytocic units per ml) i m and repeat if necessary in 30 minutes.

3. Ensure absolute bed rest and give morphine 15 mg i m.

4. If pregnancy seems an unlikely cause bleeding may be due to hormone imbalance or neoplasm. Rest in bed will do much to control the loss until expert opinion is obtained; ergometrine will do no harm and may be effective even in the absence of pregnancy. Bleeding from hormone imbalance will usually respond temporarily to Primolut N (norethisterone) 30 mg daily but a gestogen-oestrogen combination such as Enavid 5 mg a day may be necessary. The disadvantage of such hormone therapy is that it disturbs the endometrial picture and makes diagnosis by curettage less easy. It should not, however, be withheld if the loss is heavy and admission to hospital impossible. Vaginal bleeding due to neoplasm will respond temporarily to bed-rest, with perhaps the addition of morphine 15 mg. It must, however, be remembered that the neoplasm may be malignant and even though the bleeding ceases no time should be lost in obtaining expert opinion. This is particularly true of postmenopausal bleeding. Heavy periods occurring at or about the time of the menarche are usually self limiting but may require blood transfusion. A recurrence can usually be prevented by the administration of Primolut N (norethisterone) 10 mg daily by mouth during the second half of the cycle, or by controlling a few cycles with a low dosage oral contraceptive.

Hydatidiform mole

This should be suspected if recurrent bleeding occurs during the first half of pregnancy especially if it is associated with excessive vomiting or evidence of pre-eclampsia. The uterus is usually, though not invariably, large for the presumed duration of pregnancy and there is no evidence of the presence of a fetus.

Threatened and inevitable abortion

The distinction between these two conditions is usually easy on vaginal examination as the external os is closed in threatened and open in inevitable abortion. Even in the presence of a closed os, however, heavy and repeated bleeding in the first 10 weeks of pregnancy usually denotes an abnormal conceptus and evacuation may be indicated. In the presence of a threatened abortion bed rest is usually helpful and as an emergency measure Primolut Depot (hydroxyprogesterone caproate) 250 mg i m twice weekly may be useful and does not carry the risk of virilisation of the female fetus. The usefulness of such therapy is open to question and most certainly in non-urgent situations it is preferable to search for possible progesterone deficiency by having a lateral vaginal wall scraping examined by a competent cytologist.

Dilatation of the os in association with uterine bleeding is evidence of inevitable abortion, although if the membranes have not ruptured it is possible to salvage a small number of these pregnancies by inserting a stitch to encircle the cervical canal (Shirodkar operation).

Criminal abortion and septic abortion

Most, though not all, septic abortions are due to interference, and most criminal and all septic abortions are incomplete. Conservative treatment is only indicated until expert advice is available. The possibility of uterine perforation must be considered, and may require abdominal surgery. The administration of ergometrine as above, and also of oxytocin (Syntocinon, Sandoz) 1·0 ml will control bleeding, and a broad spectrum antibiotic (ampicillin 250 mg six hourly) should be given if there is significant pyrexia (38° C or more).

Transfusion of cross-matched blood, or in a great emergency, of Rhesus negative blood of the correct ABO group may be necessary but in shocked patients circulatory overloading (p. 106) must be avoided. Anuria (p. 374) may supervene in criminal and septic cases and medico-legal complications may arise (p. 476) with the possible need for a dying declaration (p. 662).

HAEMORRHAGE IN LATE PREGNANCY

Patients with vaginal bleeding after the twenty-eighth week should not be examined vaginally but should be admitted to hospital at once. After admission to hospital a gentle Sims' speculum examination is carried out in order to exclude lower genital tract bleeding as for example from a carcinoma of the cervix or a varicose vein. If there is no such lesion present the patient either has a placenta praevia or is suffering from ' accidental haemorrhage ' (abruptio). A significant number of patients show no obvious cause for the bleeding, and although these are grouped as ' antepartum haemorrhage of unknown aetiology ' it seems reasonably certain that most of them are ' accidental ' haemorrhages.

Placenta praevia

Unless it coincides with the onset of labour bleeding from placenta praevia is painless. The presenting part is usually high, although engagement does not exclude placenta praevia. Fetal heart sounds are usually present. Treatment is by bed-rest and sedation aided by blood transfusion when necessary. Preferably the pregnancy should be continued until the end of the thirty-eighth week when an examination under anaesthesia is carried out with all in readiness to perform an immediate Caesarean section. Occasionally heavy and repeated losses make earlier intervention mandatory.

Accidental haemorrhage (Abruptio placentae)

This implies premature separation of a normally situated placenta and it is associated in some 15 per cent of cases with hypertension. It occurs in all degrees from slight bleeding, which is none the less associated with a markedly elevated perinatal mortality, to the classical and serious concealed or mixed accidental haemorrhage. The more severe cases are associated with pain which usually precedes the bleeding and with early intrauterine death. Milder cases may simply show some tenderness over an area of the uterus and the fetus may survive for some time. Treatment is by immediate resuscitation, blood transfusion being of prime importance and then rupture of the membranes and the use of a Syntocinon drip. There is a small place for Caesarean section in the moderately severe cases in which the fetus is still alive, but the danger of operative bleeding necessitating a hysterectomy is real and in these circumstances Caesarean section should never be attempted by anyone other than the most experienced operator working in a fully equipped unit. Abruptio may be associated with or followed by defibrination (p. 283) and acute renal failure.

ABDOMINAL PAIN

If associated with uterine bleeding the likely causes are :
1. Abortion, threatened or incomplete.

2. Ectopic pregnancy.

3. Extrusion of an intrauterine fibroid. Rest and sedation will control the situation until diagnosis is clear and expert attention available.

4. Menstruation. This may occasionally be associated with more loss or pain than is customary for the patient, and may therefore present as an emergency, at least to the sufferer.

When unassociated with bleeding there is a wider range of causes but it must not be forgotten that the chance association of a normal menstrual loss may convert a case of abdominal pain alone into one with associated but irrelevant uterine bleeding.

The differential diagnosis of acute abdominal pain must include the following main causes:

1. APPENDICITIS (p. 173).

2. OVULATION PAIN (Mittelschmerz or middle pain). Pain at ovulation time is not infrequent. On its first occurrence it may cause difficulty in diagnosis for the symptoms may be quite acute, especially if accompanied by free bleeding into the peritoneal cavity. The attack usually occurs between the tenth and twelfth days of the menstrual cycle but since ovulation may be deferred from emotional or environmental reasons in a woman with previous regular cycles, it is possible for ovulation pain to occur three or four weeks after the previous menstrual period, the succeeding period being delayed correspondingly. There may be marked hyperaesthesia on moving the cervix from accumulation of blood in the pouch of Douglas. Treatment is conservative, with analgesics and rest in bed, but operation should never be deferred if the diagnosis is in doubt since in some rare cases quite severe intraperitoneal bleeding may arise from a ruptured Graafian follicle, in which case sutures will always control the bleeding. The ovary should *never* be removed.

3. OVARIAN CYSTS. Ovarian cysts may suffer torsion, haemorrhage or rupture. It will be usually possible to palpate a unilateral or bilateral pelvic mass. Unless there is shock or a rising pulse rate, conservative treatment is justifiable until the diagnosis is clear.

4. DYSMENORRHOEA. Dysmenorrhoea usually develops gradually, and rarely in the first few years of menstrual life, but the first attack may occasionally be so acute as to cause collapse and vomiting. As the pain may precede the menstrual loss by a few hours or even a day, the diagnosis may be difficult, but there is usually complete absence of abdominal rigidity. It must be remembered that during the postovulatory phase the temperature is usually elevated to 37·5°C.

5. PYELONEPHRITIS (especially in pregnancy). Urinary examination, together with a high temperature and back ache, will usually settle the diagnosis. Urinary frequency is not necessarily present.

Table 7.1. *Differentiation between salpingitis and appendicitis*

	SALPINGITIS	APPENDICITIS
Onset	Acute with steady improvement	Less acute with worsening
Appearance	Flushed and feverish	Not flushed. May be pale
Tongue	Clean and moist	Furred and dry
Vomiting	Not a feature	Usually an early feature
Backache	Usual. Low midline	Absent or negligible
Pain at onset	Low abdominal; bilateral	Mid-abdominal
Pain later	Unchanged but may be worse on one side	Right iliac fossa
Tenderness	Bilateral on deep suprapubic pressure	Right iliac fossa. Superficial. May be 'rebound'
Guarding	Ill defined and variable	Well marked and on right side
Vaginal examination	Bilateral tenderness and perhaps a mass	No tenderness (unless pelvic appendicitis and then only on right side and rarely a mass)

6. ACUTE SALPINGITIS. This is often confused with appendicitis but differentiation is important for the treatment differs, being expectant in salpingitis and active in appendicitis. During pregnancy salpingitis usually occurs after interference but appendicitis is not uncommon. The differential points may be set out as in Table 7.1, but it must be remembered that not only does the appendix move its site during pregnancy so that signs localised to McBurney's point are not to be expected but also that a white count of up to 15 000 is a normal finding in pregnancy.

7

Treatment. When there is doubt laparotomy is better than expectancy. If salpingitis is found the tubes should *never* be incised or removed.

The symptoms of acute salpingitis will usually respond to rest in bed in a semi-reclining position and the application of heat to the abdomen. Simple analgesics and sometimes pethidine should be used and the appropriate antibiotics given. Streptomycin should be avoided at first lest it makes the diagnosis of tuberculous salpingitis impossible.

The social and medico-legal implications of salpingitis must not be forgotten and if the endo-cervical and urethral swabs which should be mandatory in the management of this condition show gonococci the husband should be examined. In this case there is danger of infecting children and the patient must be isolated. When salpingitis complicates abortion the possibility of criminal interference must be considered (p. 170).

7. ECTOPIC PREGNANCY. Though uterine haemorrhage and pain usually coincide, in some cases severe pain precedes bleeding by 24 hours. Amenorrhoea is not always present. Referred pain in the shoulder tip, caused by free blood under the diaphragm, may be an important diagnostic point. A rapid pulse and shock denotes intraperitoneal bleeding, in the absence of pyrexia. There is abdominal guarding rather than rigidity but rebound tenderness may be marked. Vaginal examination may reveal exquisite tenderness in the pouch of Douglas. Movement of the cervix may provoke severe pain. The pregnancy test may be negative. Few cases present typical features and the condition is often misdiagnosed.

In the acute case with massive internal bleeding immediate laparotomy is essential. A transfusion may be commenced but *under no circumstances must operation be postponed* until the condition improves for no woman is ever too ill for this operation. Improvement begins as soon as the bleeding tube is clamped. Only light anaesthesia is required.

8. ANGULAR OR CORNUAL PREGNANCY. This condition is really half way between a uterine and an ectopic pregnancy and presents the symptoms of an intact ectopic pregnancy. The course is that of an intrauterine pregnancy. The uterus is asymmetrical and tender over one cornu rather than near the pelvic wall. Blood may leak along the tube and cause peritoneal irritation simulating bleeding from an ectopic pregnancy. With rest and analgesics most cases settle down.

Lower abdominal pain in women

A chronic condition may present as a new emergency if an exacerbation causes severe pain. Ill-defined lower abdominal pain may result from carcinoma of the ovary, chronic salpingitis, diverticulitis and even carcinoma of the colon, and any one of these conditions may cause a tender mass in the lateral fornix easily confused with an ovarian or tubal swelling. In general, lower abdominal pain due to pelvic disease is worse in the premenstrual phase and eased by the flow but these features are not always present. Depressed morale at the time of menstruation may make any chronic pain less tolerable, and therefore likely to present as an emergency.

Abdominal pain in pregnancy

Aches and pains are common in normal pregnancy and sometimes occasion an urgent call. Discomfort in the groins results from stretching of the round ligaments. Normal uterine contractions from the fifth month onwards may cause real discomfort but even when they are brought on by simple palpation of an irritable uterus they do not mean that labour is imminent. Red degeneration of fibromyomata occurs only during pregnancy and in women taking combined oestrogen-progestogen pills. It is related to haemolysis of blood extravasated into the fibromyomata but the precise reason for this haemorrhage is still unknown. What is certain is that surgical intervention is contraindicated. In a breech presentation there may be pain over the head relieved by external version. Acute hydramnios must be considered as a cause of pain even as early as the fourth month. Slipping of the tip of the twelfth rib over the eleventh may cause an acutely painful clicking sensation. Cough fractures of ribs may occur. Mediastinal emphysema (p. 599) and haematoma of the rectus sheath (p. 127) are rare but sometimes urgent complications of pregnancy.

Intercurrent unrelated conditions must not be forgotten. Pyrexia is rarely found in the complications of the pregnant state with the exception of pyelonephritis. A symptomless rise of temperature to 37·2°C is not uncommon in early pregnancy.

CHOLECYSTITIS AND PANCREATITIS. The symptoms of pre-existing gallstones and cholecystitis may worsen in pregnancy because of a rise in blood cholesterol. Acute pancreatitis (p. 113) is rare in young women but occurs in a severe haemorrhagic form in pregnancy.

ACUTE APPENDICITIS. This may be obscured by the pregnant uterus and after the fourth month the appendix itself is displaced upwards. The premonitory colic is unchanged but when peritonitis occurs the maximal tenderness is higher up and further out than the traditional McBurney's point. The mortality from incorrectly treated appendicitis during pregnancy is high. This is because spread of infection to the peritoneum is facilitated by uterine contractions and the fact that the uterus itself prevents omentum from reaching the site. Operation for possible appendicitis is indicated during pregnancy when in a non-pregnant patient a more expectant policy would be justified.

INTESTINAL OBSTRUCTION. The possibility of intestinal obstruction must be considered when there is vomiting with pain for the vomiting of uncomplicated pregnancy is painless.

COMPLICATIONS OF PREGNANCY OTHER THAN HAEMORRHAGE AND PAIN

It must be remembered that as pregnancy lasts nine months there is ample time for incidental disease to occur. We must distinguish between these incidental conditions unaffected by pregnancy; conditions directly related to the pregnant state and conditions which are made worse by pregnancy.

It is remarkably rare for pregnancy to be adversely affected by any intercurrent illness or disease. A severe infection with a high temperature may occasionally cause death of the fetus or abortion and severe trauma may very occasionally lead to separation of the placenta with accidental haemorrhage or abortion. Very rarely the management of illnesses late in pregnancy is complicated by the existence of the pregnancy, and after 34 to 36 weeks, it is justifiable to induce labour or even to terminate the pregnancy by Caesarean section in order more adequately to deal with the intercurrent illness. In general, however, treatment of intercurrent illness should continue regardless of the pregnancy since only in rare cases does treatment adversely affect the pregnancy (see below).

Rubella. If a pregnant woman contracts rubella in the first 14 weeks the fetus may be damaged. Her physical health is not affected, but anxiety may sometimes justify termination. Human normal immunoglobulin (p. 794), if possible from someone convalescing from rubella, offers protection in case of contact. Most obstetric units measure rubella antibody titres in early pregnancy. If high a suspect attack causes no concern but in a non-immune woman a rising titre means possible fetal damage. A woman whose baby at risk is born undamaged should be immunised soon after delivery.

Chorea gravidarum. This is a severe form of chorea with mental confusion, a rising pulse and pyrexia. If sedation fails, termination of pregnancy may be necessary.

Emergencies due to conditions directly related to pregnancy are vomiting, pyelonephritis and severe pre-eclampsia or eclampsia.

VOMITING IN PREGNANCY
(See p. 480)

It must not be assumed that vomiting in pregnancy is necessarily caused by it. Neglect of this fact has led to many tragedies. Vomiting persisting beyond three months must be regarded with suspicion and the possibility of urinary infection or cerebral tumour borne in mind. An incarcerated retroverted uterus is a rare cause and usually associated with urinary infection. A hydatidiform mole is frequently associated with excessive vomiting and in late pregnancy vomiting may occur in severe pre-eclampsia, chronic hydramnios and hiatus hernia.

Treatment. Hyperemesis is best managed by reassurance and frequent light dry meals. Recently the antiemetic compounds have been thought to cause fetal malformations but Ancoloxin BDH (meclozine 25 mg, pyridoxine 50 mg) has been cleared of suspicion and may be helpful in a dose of two tablets at night and repeated by day if necessary. Constipation is often present and should be relieved by senna (Senokot).

LIVER DISEASE IN PREGNANCY

Although it is rare in the United Kingdom there is a specific form of intrahepatic obstructive jaundice known variously as recurrent intrahepatic cholestatic jaundice, ' gestational hepatosis ' and ' the inspissated bile syndrome '. It is a benign condition and improves spontaneously after delivery.

In most cases jaundice in pregnancy is due to a co-existing condition such as infective hepatitis, or an impacted gallstone. Normal pregnancy does not damage the normal liver, but jaundice during hyperemesis in early pregnancy is a grave sign, and late in pregnancy a type of toxic vomiting occasionally occurs, progressing to acute yellow atrophy of the liver.

Attempts to abort an early pregnancy, especially if there is a dead fetus, may cause *Cl. welchii* septicaemia with haemolysis and jaundice (Jones, 1965). This infection may also occur when protracted labour is followed by death of the fetus. The diagnosis is confirmed by blood culture and vaginal swabs. Penicillin in massive dosage and anti-gas gangrene serum 100 000 units i v (p. 745) at once and 50 000 units six hourly afterwards may save the patient.

PYELONEPHRITIS IN PREGNANCY

Dilatation of the ureters and urinary stasis makes the pregnant woman especially liable to pyelonephritis (Kerr and Elliott, 1963). This presents as a rule between the third and sixth month with pyrexia, vomiting and backache (usually right sided). Frequency of micturition is not always present for cystitis is rare in pregnancy. Treatment is with fluids and sulphonamides although if severe vomiting is a feature parenteral ampicillin (Penbritin) may be required. It is difficult to sterilise the urine and recurrences are common. Ampicillin (Penbritin) throughout pregnancy is often advised in these cases, as it is harmless to the fetus although it may produce diarrhoea in the mother who may also develop monilial vulvo-vaginitis. Radiological investigations should be postponed for the enlarging uterus obscures the picture and there is also risk to the fetus. Anuria and oliguria in the obstetric patient should be dealt with on the lines described on p. 375. If all pregnant women were screened for the presence of significant bacteriuria and if treatment was given when necessary many cases of pyelonephritis during pregnancy could be avoided.

ECLAMPSIA
(See also p. 613)

This is a comparatively rare complication of pre-eclampsia, although it can arise dramatically after a very short and possibly overlooked episode. Usually the pre-eclampsia develops slowly over the preceding few weeks and eclampsia is thus usually avoidable. Convulsions arising more than 48 hours after delivery should never be ascribed to eclampsia.

Eclampsia consists of a short phase of headache, drowsiness and coma heralded by fits of epileptiform type. Other premonitory danger signs in the pregnant woman are epigastric pain, strangeness in manner and acute nasal congestion resembling a cold. Vomiting, a visual aura and oliguria are also dangerous signs in pre-eclampsia and call for heavy sedation and/or delivery.

Treatment. There are five main aspects of treatment in eclampsia :

1. Prevention of eclampsia is best achieved by treating mild pre-eclampsia before it becomes severe or, in the fulminating case of severe pre-eclampsia, by sedation and complete bed-rest in a dark quiet room. All urine should be tested for protein and the blood pressure recorded half hourly.

2. Sedation. Several regimes are in vogue but one which has stood the test of time is the initial injection, preferably i v, of morphine 15 to 20 mg. Watch must be kept for respiratory depression while bromethol (Avertin. Winthrop) is given rectally in doses of 0·075 to 0·1 ml per kg body weight as indicated. The dose should be dissolved in 250 ml of water at 37°C and a few drops of Congo red added. Any blueness of the solution, which should remain ' salmon pink ', indicates decomposition into toxic by-products and such a solution must not be given. An alternative

method of treating severe pre-eclampsia and eclampsia is the slow i v injection of 10 to 20 mg of diazepam (Valium. Roche) followed by 40 mg of diazepam in 500 ml of 5 per cent dextrose run in at about 40 drops per minute. If the hypertension does not respond to this sedative therapy 40 mg of hydrallazine hydrochloride (Apresoline. Ciba) may be added to the dextrose bottle. In circumstances where i v infusion is difficult a mixture of pethidine 50 mg, promethazine (Phenergan. M & B) 50 mg and promazine hydrochloride (Sparine. Wyeth) 50 mg may be given i m four to six hourly as indicated by the patient's condition.

3. The flying squad, when available, should be called to the patient's home to achieve sedation before moving her to hospital.

4. During a fit all attention must be as gentle as possible. Place the patient on her side with her head over the edge of the bed. If the mouth can be opened easily protect the tongue from being bitten by a gag or spoon. Don't let the mucus run back into the throat. Bromethol usually controls the fits but if necessary thiopentone 0·25 to 0·5 g i v may be needed. It is preferable to chloroform. Cyanosis calls for oxygen (p. 740) and perhaps artificial respiration (p. 732).

5. After the fit. Keep the patient in the quiet room between blankets with the foot of the bed raised and continue sedation. Change her position from side to side every two hours (p. 240). Leave a catheter in the bladder so that regular urine tests won't disturb her. Give fluids in small amounts, recording intake and output. Keep half hourly blood pressure, pulse and respiration charts. If expert help is not available labour should be induced 48 hours after fits have ceased. The specialist obstetrician may prefer to induce labour earlier or even to carry out Caesarean section. Such procedures are not to be embarked on lightly.

CONVULSIONS, COMA AND COLLAPSE IN PREGNANCY

Although eclampsia is generally the cause of convulsions in pregnancy, other conditions such as epilepsy and subarachnoid haemorrhage must not be overlooked. Important neurological complications of pregnancy and the puerperium are cerebral venous embolism via the paravertebral venous plexus (p. 68) and cerebral thrombosis.

CONDITIONS MADE WORSE BY PREGNANCY

HEART DISEASE. Ninety per cent of cases of heart disease in pregnancy are rheumatic in origin and the vast majority of these are mitral stenosis. Although hospital confinement is mandatory most patients do well during pregnancy, but the tight mitral stenosis may develop acute pulmonary oedema with alarming rapidity (p. 232). Any cardiac decompensation must be treated along general medical lines and no attempt made to interfere with the pregnancy. Decompensation is especially liable to occur in the presence of anaemia or an upper respiratory infection and these conditions should either not be allowed to develop or be treated energetically.

Congenital heart disease, especially of the cyanotic variety, can be an extremely dangerous complication of pregnancy. These patients must be under hospital supervision.

ANAEMIA. This can be avoided by the routine administration of supplementary iron together with 300 to 500 μg of folic acid throughout pregnancy, and the exclusion of any source of blood loss such as haemorrhoids or hookworm. Megaloblastic anaemia of pregnancy (confirmed by marrow biopsy) responds to folic acid 15 mg daily. Severe anaemia near term may indicate blood transfusion as even a moderate postpartum haemorrhage may cause collapse in anaemic patients.

POLIOMYELITIS IN PREGNANCY. Since severe poliomyelitis may develop rapidly during pregnancy removal to hospital should be prompt when it is suspected. An early sign is sometimes inability to pass urine with no history of previous urinary trouble. Labour during poliomyelitis may necessitate help from forceps. When respiratory muscles are paralysed Caesarean section with forced ventilation is necessary. Oral poliomyelitis vaccine should be given to pregnant women if they are not already immunised.

OTHER CONDITIONS CAUSING EMERGENCIES IN PREGNANCY

Diabetes

The mother. The unexpected development of diabetes or its neglect may cause it to present as an emergency. The chief risk is violent fluctuation in the insulin requirement and ketosis arises early. The lowering of the renal threshold makes control by urine testing impossible and frequent estimation of the blood sugar is essential. The demand for insulin increases as pregnancy advances. Pre-eclampsia and intrauterine death are particularly common in diabetes although much modern evidence goes to show that the incidence of these complications can be markedly reduced by strict control of the maternal diabetes.

Contrary to the common belief miscarriage is not very common in diabetes but there is an increased risk of it and of still births and large babies in latent diabetes.

The baby. The baby may be large and so is at risk from placental insufficiency and the trauma of labour. Hydramnios is a frequent complication and commonly associated with oesophageal atresia. There is little evidence for the common belief that neonatal death may occur from hypoglycaemia but it is certain that hyperglycaemia especially if associated with ketosis can lead to intra-uterine death.

Provided excellent control can be maintained Caesarean section or sometimes induction in the thirty-eighth week is the proper course, preferably in a department with full laboratory facilities. With the patient in labour the usual diet is best replaced by i v glucose and as the risk of hypoglycaemia increases with the exertion of labour it may be necessary to increase the amount of sugar given. The commonest complication of labour where antenatal control has been inadequate is impaction of the large shoulders. After delivery insulin requirements fall dramatically but if blood sugar estimations cannot be made it is usually safe to wait until glycosuria appears and then to give half the dose of insulin she was receiving before delivery.

Pulmonary tuberculosis in pregnancy

Pregnancy does not aggravate pulmonary tuberculosis or make chest emergencies more likely to occur. Rapid deterioration following parturition is rare except in patients with gross disease whose lives were already at risk. Chemotherapy should be continued as if the patient were not pregnant, although it may be necessary to suspend the administration of PAS if early pregnancy vomiting is troublesome. The risk of ototoxicity in the fetus is real but small and must be weighed against the hazards of withholding streptomycin from the patient with active tuberculosis. Surgical measures are not contraindicated. Termination of pregnancy for pulmonary tuberculosis is probably never justifiable on medical grounds. When it has been done the justification has been psychological.

Psychological emergencies in pregnancies and the puerperium

In early pregnancy neurotic manifestations are commoner than psychotic ones. An hysterical reaction to an unwanted pregnancy and worry about fetal abnormalities may prompt urgent demands for termination and threats of suicide. In countries with 'liberal' abortion laws it is as well to remember that the patient who shows the most severe hysterical reaction to pregnancy may also be the one who has the most severe reaction to having had it terminated. Although termination may be indicated on social grounds which may be inextricably linked with psychological disturbances it is nevertheless true that it is seldom indicated on pure psychological grounds although it may be necessary where there is a bad psychiatric history (Jeffcoate, 1960). In many cases a real emergency does not exist for not only do those psychiatric indications that justify termination also often justify sterilisation so that hysterectomy may be done but also mid-trimester abortion may be brought about by the use of prostaglandin (Midwinter, Bowen and Shepherd, 1972). There is, therefore, time for careful evaluation. Modern psychiatric treatment is compatible with continuation of pregnancy and does not affect the fetus. Termination, though improving the immediate situation, may not be beneficial in the long run because of feelings of guilt. Also the psychosis may continue and even worsen despite termination. Obstetrical stress and lactational difficulties may help to precipitate a psychosis. The warnings of sleeplessness, confusion and unusual behaviour should help the doctor to avert a catastrophe.

Syncope

Fainting may occur when an apprehensive patient has some obstetrical manipulation such as external version. It calls for a simple remedy (sal volatile, brandy or smelling salts) and lowering of the head. Postural hypotension may also occur when the woman near term lies on her back and is readily relieved by turning her on to her side. Postural hypotension may also be associated with manifestations of fetal distress.

Adrenal haemorrhage (p. 355)

Very rarely this may cause acute abdominal pain and collapse in the later weeks of pregnancy. There is usually some preceding complication such as pre-eclampsia.

Thrombocytopenic purpura (p. 276)

In pregnancy as at other times this may be secondary as well as idiopathic and so a causal factor must be sought. The idiopathic variety will usually respond to steroid therapy during pregnancy and splenectomy is rarely if ever indicated. While causing extensive bleeding and even accidental haemorrhage in late pregnancy thrombocytopenia often improves during labour and does not show any special tendency to cause post-partum haemorrhage unless laceration of the genital tract has occurred.

Hyperthyroidism

Pregnancy only occurs in mild cases of untreated hyperthyroidism but even in these may provoke a thyroid crisis (p. 358). Treatment with thiouracil throughout pregnancy may cause fetal goitre leading to dystocia but it seems possible to avoid this by the simultaneous administration of l-thyroxine 0·1 mg daily.

Addison's disease

Crises may occur early from vomiting and late from adrenal insufficiency (p. 353).

Dermatological emergencies

Most skin rashes during pregnancy are only urgent in the sense of their differentiation from the exanthemata. (For herpes gestationis and impetigo herpetiformis see p. 553.)

Air travel

For obstetric contra-indications see p. 517.

POST-MORTEM DELIVERY

When a pregnant woman dies suddenly the problem of delivery becomes urgent. The act of dying may precipitate labour and should the head be found on the perineum a forceps delivery may avoid the repugnant procedure of post-mortem section.

When death is not sudden the baby will usually predecease the mother. When the mother dies first the baby is not likely to survive long but may live for 20 minutes. If the fetal heart is beating a classical Caesarean section should be performed. Permission of the husband need not be awaited but incisions should be closed with care for a supposedly dead mother may revive. If a Roman Catholic mother dies in pregnancy the Code of Canon Law 1918 states that Caesarean section should be done in order that the fetus may be baptised. This applies whether uterine baptism was carried out or not but there is no obligation to carry out Caesarean section when both mother and fetus are known to be dead.

INCIDENTAL OPERATIONS DURING PREGNANCY

Pregnant women tolerate operations well but their diminished respiratory excursion increases the problems of anaesthesia as does the lessened gastric motility and misguided efforts to encourage oral fluids during labour. A small overlooked acid vomit may be inhaled during the induction of anaesthesia. All is well for a few hours and then the patient becomes very ill with cyanosis, dyspnoea and tachycardia. The lungs show extensive moist sounds—the picture of acute pulmonary oedema. The patient is unable when the stress of inhaled vomit occurs to meet the demand for adrenocortical hormones and the picture of acute adrenal insufficiency results (p. 353) (Mendelson's syndrome, p. 571). In addition to oxygen, antibiotics, bronchoscopy and general measures, hydrocortisone 100 mg should be given i v.

As anaesthetic complications are major causes of maternal deaths there is an increasing use of local anaesthesia for operations during pregnancy and labour. When general anaesthesia is required there is much to be said for attempting to neutralise the acid gastric contents with alkali by mouth. 15 ml of 0·3 molar sodium citrate flavoured with aniseed is effective (Lahiri *et al.*, 1973). (See also peptic aspiration pneumonia, p. 572).

EMERGENCIES OF PARTURITION

UNEXPECTED OR PREMATURE LABOUR. Some authorities feel that in many instances premature labour may be stopped by giving 10 per cent ethyl alcohol as an i v drip in dextrose saline. The results are not always convincing. Premature labour that cannot be arrested is usually short and easy. The birth is spontaneous and it is the baby that is the biggest problem. If a Paediatric Flying Squad is available it should be summoned but any baby born before 36 weeks or weighing less than 2·5 kg should be admitted to a special care baby unit. Pending such arrangements an emergency cot may be provided by a large box or clothes basket, well padded and supplied with hot bottles, care being taken to prevent burns to the baby. If possible a premature baby should be kept in a temperature of 26·6°C until skilled attention and advice is available.

PROBLEMS OF LABOUR. In the rare case of slow or obstructed labour under emergency conditions, without expert advice, the safest procedure both for mother and child is Caesarean section.

POST-PARTUM HAEMORRHAGE. This is the most serious and the commonest complication of an emergency labour. It may occur before or after the expulsion of the placenta when a multiparous woman has her baby unexpectedly or precipitately. Syntometrine 1·0 to 2·0 ml should be given i v. It will control the bleeding and if the placenta is not delivered will not prevent its removal. This, if performed before shock develops is a very safe operation. Transfusion with group O rhesus negative blood may be needed.

Reactionary post-partum haemorrhage from an atonic uterus may occur two or three hours after delivery especially in a multipara. Retention of a succenturiate lobe may be responsible and calls for exploration. Blood transfusion, ergometrine and bimanual compression will always control the bleeding (*British Medical Journal,* editorial, 1963).

ACQUIRED AFIBRINOGENAEMIA. Bleeding from a perineal laceration or the uterus may occur when afibrinogenaemia results from intravascular clotting or reduction by a fibrinolysin of the circulatory fibrinogen. Predisposing factors are antepartum haemorrhage, amniotic fluid embolism, prolonged retention of a dead fetus and sometimes incomplete abortion. Blood, saline or dextran should be transfused to maintain the patient until the diagnosis can be established by Wiener's test (dissolution of a deficient clot within an hour at 37°C). Simple observation of clotting of freshly drawn blood will help to confirm the diagnosis. A minimum of 100 mg of fibrinogen in 100 ml of blood is needed to ensure haemostasis. Four to six grams of human fibrinogen (p. 796) should be given but quadruple strength plasma i v is also helpful. Epsilon aminocaproic acid (Epsikapron) 0·1 kg body weight every four hours is helpful if given i v in isosmotic sodium chloride solution or 5 g/dl dextrose.

AMNIOTIC FLUID EMBOLISM (Aguillon 1962). This is a rare cause of collapse. After a short and ' stormy ' labour with rapid progress there is sudden cyanosis, dyspnoea and shock with widespread moist sounds in the lungs. Sometimes there is afibrinogenaemia. Many cases prove fatal but some will survive if treated for right heart failure with oxygen, morphine, aminophylline and digitalis. The danger is circulatory overloading (p. 106) and unless there is severe blood loss i v fluids should be restricted to those necessary for the administration of drugs and for correcting clotting defects. A quick acting diuretic such as frusemide (Lasix) 20 mg should be given i v. Corticosteroids are helpful in the more severe cases.

PUERPERAL INFECTION. Infection of the uterus is rare during pregnancy, except when caused by criminal interference. In the puerperium or following abortion, the staphylococcus has replaced the streptococcus as the most serious infecting organism. It is so often resistant to antibiotics, but the latest synthetic penicillins may be effective, and where other antibiotics fail, vancomycin (Vancocin, Lilly) may work. Steps to identify the responsible organism should always be taken before starting antibiotic treatment.

Elevation of temperature without much rise in pulse rate in an otherwise healthy patient may be treated expectantly. Breast infections may cause pyrexia before there is any flush or thickening. It must not be forgotten that carcinoma of the breast arising in the puerperium may closely resemble a breast abscess.

DRUGS HARMFUL DURING PREGNANCY

Implication of thalidomide (Distaval) as a cause of fetal defects has aroused the suspicion that many other drugs, helpful to the mother, may be harmful to the fetus especially in early pregnancy. In some instances drugs that are known to have or are suspected of having a teratogenic effect can easily be replaced by safe preparations. Chloramphenicol and tetracycline should be avoided during pregnancy and ampicillin used instead. Coumarin anticoagulants are a very real danger to the fetus in late pregnancy for they cross the placenta and are hepatotoxic. Apart from its other advantages in late pregnancy heparin does not cross the placenta and therefore carries no risk of fetal damage. Sulphonamides cross the placenta with ease and by causing haemolysis in the fetus can give rise to kernicterus. They should therefore not be used in late pregnancy.

The risk of fetal damage must be weighed against the risks to the mother (and therefore also to the fetus) of withholding treatment during pregnancy. Examples are the use of corticosteroids for the autoimmune diseases (although they are known to carry the risk of causing fetal abnormality) and streptomycin for active tuberculosis (despite the possibility that it may be ototoxic in the fetus). In these cases the decision to use the drug does not present difficulty for the indication is absolute. Apart from the known tendency of certain of the gestogen preparations to induce virilism in the female fetus (iatrogenic female pseudohermaphroditism), Herbst *et al.* (1971) reported that mothers of young women with adenocarcinoma of the vagina were found to have received stilboestrol during the relevant pregnancy. A high incidence of malformation and perinatal death in the babies of epileptics has been reported by Fedrick (1973) and both anti-convulsant drugs and phenobarbitone must be regarded with suspicion.

All the sedative and analgesic drugs given during labour may produce respiratory depression in the neonate and must be treated with great respect. A drug should be given to the pregnant woman only when a clear indication for its use exists and where the disadvantages of withholding it are thought to outweigh the possible risks of giving it. To some extent these considerations could be applied to all women who are at risk from pregnancy whether they are known to be pregnant or not as most drugs are likely to do most fetal damage at a stage when the patient may not realise that she is pregnant.

GEOFFREY DIXON

REFERENCES

AGUILLON, A., ANDJUS, T., GRAYSON, A. & RACE, G. J. (1962). Amniotic fluid embolism: a review. *Obstetrical and Gynaecological Survey,* **17,** 619.

BRITISH MEDICAL JOURNAL (1963). Editorial, **1,** 1359.

CHUKUDEBELU, W. O., MARSHALL, A. T. & CHALMERS, J. A. (1963). Use of 'syntometrine' in the third stage of labour. *British Medical Journal,* **1,** 1390.

EMBREY, M. P., BARBER, D. T. C. & SCUDAMORE, J. H. (1963). Use of 'syntometrine' in prevention of post-partum haemorrhage. *British Medical Journal,* **1,** 1387.

FEDRICK, Jean (1973). Epilepsy and pregnancy, a report from the Oxford Record Linkage Study. *British Medical Journal,* **2,** 442.

HERBST, A. L., ULFELDER, H. & POSKANZER, D. C. (1971). Adenocarcinoma of the vagina. Association of maternal stilboestrol therapy with tumour appearance in young women. *New England Journal of Medicine,* **284,** 878.

JEFFCOATE, T. N. A. (1960). Indications for therapeutic abortion. *British Medical Journal,* **1,** 581.

JONES, D. H. (1965). Gas gangrene complicating pregnancy. *Journal of Obstetrics and Gynaecology of the British Commonwealth,* **72,** 785.

KEMP, J. (1963). Clinical trial of 'syntometrine' in the third stage of labour. *British Medical Journal.* **1,** 1391.

KERR, D. S. & ELLIOTT, W. (1963). Renal disease in pregnancy. *Practitioner,* **4,** 59.

LAHIRI, S. K., THOMAS, T. A. & HODGSON, R. N. H. (1973). Single dose antacid therapy for prevention of Mendelson's Syndrome. *British Journal of Anaesthesia,* **45,** 1143.

LIEBSCHÜTZ, H. J. (1964). The effects of vaccination in pregnancy on the foetus. *Journal of Obstetrics and Gynaecology of the British Commonwealth,* **71,** 132.

MIDWINTER, A., BOWEN, M. & SHEPHERD, A. (1972). Continuous intrauterine infusion of Prostaglandin E for termination of pregnancy. *Journal of Obstetrics and Gynaecology of the British Commonwealth,* **79,** 807.

FOR FURTHER READING

BARNES, C. G. *Medical Disorders of Pregnancy,* 4th ed. Oxford: Blackwell, 1974.

BROWNE, J. C. M. & DIXON, G. *Antenatal Care* (Browne). 11th ed. London: Churchill, 1976.

DONALD, I. *Practical Obstetric Problems,* 4th ed. London: Lloyd Luke, 1969.

CHAPTER 8

Respiratory Emergencies

(For acute post-operative pulmonary complications, see p. 599)

HISTORY

WHEN there is doubt about the cause of a respiratory emergency the following information should be obtained, if possible, from a relative or other witness.

1. Mode of onset: presenting symptoms; sudden or gradual; whether in or out of doors; whether alone or in company; proximity to harmful physical agents.

2. Past history of respiratory, cardiac or neuro-muscular disorders.

3. Contact with certain infectious diseases, e.g. poliomyelitis, diphtheria, whooping cough, measles, influenza or other respiratory viruses.

4. Exposure to certain physical agents:
   (a) Inhaled: (i) Solid, e.g., foreign bodies (especially in children).
       (ii) Liquid, e.g., drowning; inhalation of vomit.
       (iii) Gaseous, e.g., domestic (CO, oxygen-deprived air); industrial (chlorine, nitrous fumes, toluene di-isocyanate).
   (b) Ingested or injected: Narcotic drugs; salicylates.
   (c) Electrocution.

5. History of trauma to throat or chest wall: accidental; surgical.

SYMPTOMS

Having elicited such history as may be available, the doctor should now consider those presenting symptoms which led to the emergency. These may include cough, stridor, dyspnoea, chest pain or haemoptysis.

Cough

The most important and urgent cause of violent coughing, especially in children, is the inhalation of a foreign body and this may also be associated with stridor. Severe bouts of coughing accompanied by cyanosis, jugular venous engorgement with congestion of the face, inspiratory stridor and even syncope also occur in whooping cough (p. 435) and in chronic bronchitis. These coughs are

188

usually dry. Cough in the early stages of pulmonary congestion is also dry but a sudden fit of moist coughing suggests acute pulmonary oedema if the sputum is thin, pink and frothy, and the rupture of an empyema or lung abscess if it is purulent. More rarely, a hydatid cyst can burst into the bronchial tree; this is sometimes accompanied by anaphylactoid features with circulatory collapse, and scolices or ' daughter ' cysts may be recognised in the clear thick expectorate.

Stridor

Stridor indicates obstruction to the pharynx, larynx, trachea or a main bronchus (p. 225). It is distinguished from asthmatic wheezing by the ' whooping ' character of the sound and by the fact that it is present and usually predominant during inspiration. Laryngeal causes are associated with dysphonia. Causes in the pharynx or larynx include a foreign body (e.g. inhaled food bolus) (p. 225), retropharyngeal abscess (p. 223); diphtheritic membrane; spasm or paralysis of the vocal cords as in tetanus or recurrent laryngeal palsy; glottic oedema as in certain acute infections, superior vena caval obstruction and angioneurotic states; haemorrhage into a superior mediastinal tumour (e.g. retrosternal goitre); trauma to the neck or throat; laryngeal tumours. A foreign body, carcinoma or tumours pressing from without are the main causes of stridor arising in the trachea and main bronchi.

Dyspnoea

Dyspnoea can be defined as an undue awareness of the need for increased breathing. Increased or irregular breathing alone, when due to cerebral or metabolic causes, does not necessarily result in dyspnoea. Nor does it usually constitute a respiratory emergency; the same holds true of periodic (Cheyne-Stokes) breathing. Indeed, the sensation of dyspnoea itself is mediated more by stretch and deflation receptors in the lungs and thoracic cage, operating through the Hering-Breuer reflexes, than by the central effects of hypoxia, hypercapnia or acidosis. True dyspnoea, therefore, should immediately direct attention to the thoracic organs themselves. It may result from obstruction to the airways, from restricted expansion of the lungs due either to a thoracic cage abnormality or to accumulation of air or fluid in the pleural cavity, or from an increased stiffness of the lung itself due to congestion, oedema, consolidation, infarction or fibrosis.

The sudden onset of dyspnoea in a previously symptomless person suggests bronchial asthma, spontaneous pneumothorax, pulmonary embolism or left heart failure. Sudden dyspnoea of cardiac origin is usually due to left ventricular failure (in hypertension, coronary occlusion and aortic valve disease), mitral valve disease or a ruptured valve cusp or papillary muscle. In these cases orthopnoea is usually prominent. Sometimes relatively minor complaints can precipitate extreme respiratory distress in patients with pre-existing disease of the thoracic organs. For example, cough fracture of one rib in a bronchitic subject, a small pneumothorax in a patient with emphysema or a segment of collapse or consolidation in a severe kyphoscoliotic can all provoke intense dyspnoea.

Chest pain

Pain in the chest of urgent significance is of two kinds. The first is sharp, related to inspiration, localised to one side and sometimes referred either to the abdomen or to the tip of the shoulder. This pain indicates inflammation of the parietal pleura but a similar pain can arise in the ribs or intercostal tissues from trauma or other causes. Pain originating in the chest wall may be made worse by certain movements of the thorax and upper limbs as well as by inspiration. In an emergency, this 'pleuritic' type of pain is important not only as a pointer to the diagnosis but also because it may interfere with efficient coughing and cause inadequate alveolar ventilation by limiting the depth of inspiration.

The second kind of pain is of sudden onset, gripping in character, central and retrosternal in site and is often associated with signs of circulatory collapse. Such a pain suggests myocardial infarction, massive pulmonary embolism or, less commonly, a dissecting aneurysm, ruptured oesophagus (p. 129) or tension pneumothorax.

Haemoptysis

Broncho-pulmonary haemorrhage must be distinguished from post-nasal epistaxis (in which blood may be seen flowing down behind the palate) and from haematemesis (in which the blood is dark red or brown in colour due to the action of gastric acid). Bright red frothy blood which is coughed up or simply 'wells up' into the mouth almost certainly arises from the respiratory tract. In certain respiratory emergencies the presence of blood in the sputum can be of diagnostic value. Examples of this include the pink frothy sputum of pulmonary oedema, the rusty sputum of pneumonia and the heavier blood-staining which occurs in pulmonary infarction. Massive haemorrhage creating an emergency in itself is more likely to result from bronchial carcinoma, bronchiectasis, cavitation due to tuberculosis and other causes, or mitral valve disease. The rupture of an aneurysm into the bronchial tree and the erosion of a major vessel by a malignant growth are causes of a rapidly fatal haemorrhage. Flooding of the airways rather than loss of circulating blood volume is the chief danger of broncho-pulmonary haemorrhage.

SIGNS

The physical examination of a patient presenting as a respiratory emergency must be comprehensive, but particular attention should be paid to the neck, throat and thoracic organs and to the extra-thoracic manifestations of impaired respiration.

In the neck, throat or thorax

The condition which demands the most immediate attention is major airway obstruction. This must be excluded first by careful examination of the neck, throat and, if indicated, the larynx (p. 225).

The examiner should then proceed to inspect the movements of the thoracic cage. The rate, depth and rhythm of breathing are noted, remembering that an abnormal pattern may be metabolic or cerebral in origin and not necessarily due to a primary fault of respiration. Certain movements indicate the degree of respiratory distress. These include activity of the alae nasi (especially in children), gasping movements of the mouth, contraction of the accessory muscles of respiration in the neck and indrawing of the intercostal spaces during inspiration. Inequality of expansion of the lungs and, especially in traumatic cases, paradoxical movements of the thorax should also be noted.

The position of the mediastinum (the trachea and apex beat) is of particular relevance to the respiratory emergency because any considerable deviation would suggest collapse, tension pneumo-thorax or a large effusion.

Percussion and auscultation will exclude these last three condi-tions as well as consolidation. Auscultation may also reveal the expiratory wheezing of asthma or the widespread crepitations of pulmonary oedema.

Finally, the cardiovascular system should be examined to exclude cardiac causes for respiratory distress. Hypertension, signs of aortic or mitral valve disease, and a triple rhythm over the left ventricle are signs of particular importance. Evidence of pulmonary heart disease may also be found, as in pulmonary embolism. This in-cludes the parasternal heave of right ventricular hypertrophy, ac-centuation of the pulmonary second sound, a triple rhythm over the right ventricle and jugular venous engorgement with pulsation.

Extra-thoracic signs

Signs of respiratory failure may be found outside the thoracic cage and these are mainly attributable either to oxygen lack (hypoxia) or to carbon dioxide retention (hypercapnia).

HYPOXIA. Hypoxia causes cyanosis, cerebral symptoms such as irritability, confusion and restlessness and also tachycardia. Cyanosis is an important but unreliable sign of respiratory failure. It is important because it may indicate a severe degree of hypoxia (i.e. an arterial oxygen saturation of less than 75 per cent and a PaO_2 of less than 50 mm Hg (6.65 kPa). It is unreliable because it may not be recognised in artificial light and also because it can be due to causes other than respiratory failure. If cyanosis is present, an attempt must be made to determine its cause.

Peripheral cyanosis. This is due to slowing of the circulation leading to excessive oxygen extraction by the tissues. The affected areas are cold as well as blue but regain their normal colour on warming; naturally warm parts, such as the tongue, are not involved. Peripheral cyanosis can occur in certain respiratory emergencies associated with circulatory failure and hypotension e.g. massive pulmonary embolism.

Central cyanosis. In central cyanosis the arterial blood is desaturated. The tongue as well as the skin is blue and warming the affected part does not abolish the cyanosis. Central cyanosis can be due to abnormalities in the quantity or quality of haemoglobin, or to diseases of the heart or lungs. An increase in the quantity of haemoglobin (polycythaemia) causes cyanosis because there is an absolute increase in the amount of desaturated haemoglobin. Abnormal haemoglobins (e.g. methaemoglobin and sulphaemoglobin) result from the ingestion of certain drugs and produce a form of cyanosis but do not interfere with respiration. There are four possible causes for central cyanosis of cardiac or pulmonary origin: (1) alveolar hypoventilation, (2) uneven distribution of air and blood to the alveoli, (3) impaired alveolar-capillary diffusion and (4) right-to-left shunts of blood, either in the heart or lungs, bypassing functioning alveoli. Shunt cyanosis is not abolished by giving 100 per cent oxygen for 10 minutes, thus distinguishing it from the other causes. It must be noted, however, that a significant shunt cyanosis can occur in any pulmonary disease associated with the continued perfusion of unventilated alveoli, e.g. collapse or consolidation.

Tachycardia. This is a valuable but neglected sign of hypoxia. Although less specific than cyanosis, it does sometimes provide a more reliable measure of the patient's progress.

HYPERCAPNIA. Hypercapnia is diagnostic of alveolar hypoventilation and is invariably accompanied by hypoxia unless oxygen is being administered. It rarely if ever results from an impairment of diffusion or from a right to left shunt.

Carbon dioxide is a potent vasodilator and the signs of hypercapnia are mainly those of cerebral and peripheral vasodilatation. The central signs include headache, mental confusion, drowsiness, flapping tremors, convulsions, papilloedema and ultimately coma. The peripheral signs include sweats, a warm moist skin, a full bounding pulse, injection of the conjunctivae and, later, circulatory failure with hypotension. Hypercapnia, however, can occur in the absence of these signs.

DIAGNOSIS AND MANAGEMENT

The diagnosis and management of respiratory emergencies not primarily due to disease of the lungs are dealt with in other chapters. These include neuromuscular disorders (p. 319), electrocution (p. 648), poisoning by narcotic drugs or carbon monoxide (p. 28), obstruction to the main airway (p. 567), drowning (p. 651) and pulmonary embolism (p. 241).

Respiratory failure

Respiratory failure is said to be present when the breathing mechanism permits the arterial tension of oxygen (PaO_2) to fall below 80 mm Hg (10·64 kPa) (normal level: 90 mm Hg $\pm$ 10; 11·97 kPa $\pm$ 1·33) or the arterial tension of carbon-dioxide ($PaCO_2$) to rise above 45 mm Hg; 5·99 kPa (normal level: 40 mm Hg $\pm$ 5; 5.32 kPa $\pm$ 0.665).

DIAGNOSIS. Hypoxia and hypercapnia, and the acidosis which may accompany these, can occur in any respiratory emergency and so it follows that measurement of blood gases and acid-base balance are essential to proper management. The PCO_2 of venous blood can be estimated by the rebreathing method, if the patient is cooperative, or measured in arterial blood (or arterialised capillary blood) by the Astrup technique which at the same time gives values for pH and plasma bicarbonate. Electrode methods are also available for the measurement of PaO_2 or, alternatively, spectrophotometry can be used to obtain oxygen saturation. If a spirometer is not available the Forced Expiratory Time provides a rough bedside assessment of impaired ventilatory capacity. The stethoscope is applied to the trachea after the patient has taken a maximal inspiration. He is then asked to blow out as fast and as fully as he can. The sound of the passage of air through the trachea should last for only two or three seconds in a healthy subject. A 5 second stop watch timing of a forced expiration as heard with a stethoscope over the trachea suggests significant airways obstruction. The degree is proportional to the duration of expiratory sounds. As the doctor may be shown the results of lung function tests these are summarised in Table 8.1.

MANAGEMENT. The management of respiratory failure clearly depends upon its cause but, in every case, hypoxia, hypercapnia and acidosis must be treated. *Hypoxia* may occur without hypercapnia and, if severe, can rapidly lead to a *metabolic acidosis* with low plasma bicarbonate due to the accumulation of lactic acid. Treatment includes the administration of oxygen and also of bicarbonate if there is an acidosis. *Hypercapnia* causes a *respiratory acidosis* (p. 19) and is invariably accompanied by hypoxia. The kidneys gradually compensate for the fall in blood pH by excreting a highly acid urine and by reabsorbing bicarbonate so that the plasma bicarbonate is raised. In chronic hypercapnia the respiratory centre may lose its sensitivity to changes in $PaCO_2$ so that breathing becomes dependent upon the stimulus of hypoxia. In these circumstances the administration of too much oxygen will suppress ventilation and aggravate the hypercapnia. Moreover, the administration of bicarbonate, while correcting any secondary metabolic acidosis, is ineffective against respiratory acidosis. Treatment, therefore, is to increase the output of carbon dioxide by improving alveolar ventilation and also to give oxygen so diluted that the hypoxic stimulus to breathing is preserved. The detailed management of respiratory failure is described in the next section which deals with its commonest and most important cause : airways obstruction.

The diseases characterised by airways obstruction include asthma, chronic bronchitis and emphysema. Each of these may occur in pure form or in association with one or both of the others.

ASTHMA

(For occupational asthma see p. 461)

An acute attack of bronchial asthma must always be regarded as an emergency especially if it is unrelieved by simple bronchodilator therapy. Attacks provoked by emotional causes are no less urgent than those brought on by allergens or infections, and the dangers of asthma are by no means confined to the elderly. Patients to whom narcotic drugs have been given or from whom steroid therapy has recently been withdrawn are at particular risk. A special hazard also arises from the self-administration of a sympathomimetic

Table 8.1. *Commonly used tests of lung function.*

TEST	DEFINITION	CONDITIONS IN WHICH IT IS MOST COMMONLY AFFECTED
SPIROMETRIC TESTS OF VENTILATION		
Vital Capacity (VC)	The volume of air which can be expelled after a maximal inspiration. Normal 3 to 5 litres.	Reduced in conditions restricting the expansion of the lungs, e.g. deformities of the thoracic cage, pleural thickening or effusion, lung fibrosis.
Maximum voluntary ventilation (MVV)	The amount of air which can be shifted in one minute by maximal respiration. Normal 120 to 160 litres per minute ($l \ min^{-1}$).	Reduced in diffuse airways obstruction, e.g. asthma, bronchitis, emphysema.
Forced expiratory volume in one second (FEV 1)	The amount of air which can be expelled in one second after a maximal inspiration. Normal 75 per cent of VC.	Reduced in diffuse airways obstruction, e.g. asthma, bronchitis, emphysema.
Minute and alveolar ventilation	*Minute ventilation.* The amount of air breathed in one minute during normal respiration, i.e. tidal volume × respiratory rate. Normal at rest 6 to 8 litres per minute ($l \ min^{-1}$). *Alveolar ventilation.* The amount of air ventilating the alveoli in one minute during normal respiration, i.e. tidal volume minus anatomical dead space† × respiratory rate. Normal at rest 4 to 6 litres per minute ($l \ min^{-1}$).	Increased in many lung diseases (e.g. pneumonia) and metabolic disorders (e.g. acidosis, thyrotoxicosis). Decreased in cerebral and neuromuscular diseases (e.g. by narcotic drugs, poliomyelitis).
TESTS OF GAS EXCHANGE		
Arterial oxygen saturation and tension (PaO)$_2$	*Saturation.* The oxygen content of arterial haemoglobin as a percentage of the content when blood is exposed to air. Normal 97 per cent. *Tension (PaO$_2$).* The partial pressure of oxygen in arterial blood. Normal 90 mm Hg ± 10 (11·97 kPa ± 1·33).	Hypoventilation e.g. cerebral and neuromuscular disorders. Continued perfusion of under ventilated parts of the lung, e.g. emphysema. Impaired diffusion, e.g. fibrosis due to dust diseases. Shunts of blood bypassing the lungs, e.g. Fallot's tetralogy.
Arterial CO$_2$ tension (PaCO$_2$)	The partial pressure of CO$_2$ in arterial blood. Normal 40 mm Hg ± 5 (5·32 kPa ± 0·665).	Increased in hypoventilation. Reduced in hyperventilation. Less affected by diffusion impairment or shunts because of the relatively high diffusibility of CO$_2$.

† Normal (approx.) 100 ml in women; 150 ml in men.

drug from an inhaler during an attack, for the dosage is not easily measured and excess can lead to cardiac arrhythmia and arrest (p. 724). The following treatment is recommended for the severe attack which has failed to respond to oral therapy.

Management

Steroids. Steroids are used at once for those patients from whom they have been withdrawn within the previous year or the amount is increased in those already receiving a maintenance dose. Hydrocortisone hemisuccinate 200 mg i v every two hours may be needed at first, reducing to 100 mg i v every six hours when a response is achieved.

Bronchodilator therapy. When steroids have not previously been used, aminophylline should be given. The optimum blood level of 10μg per ml can be attained by an i v loading dose of 5·6 mg/kg BW slowly over 30 minutes followed by a maintenance dose not exceeding 0·9 mg/kg BW per hour over a period of three hours. An alternative to aminophylline is salbutamol (Ventolin) given as a single dose of 200 μg i v over a period of 5 minutes or as an i v infusion at 5 μg per minute. (Add 5 mg salbutamol to 500 ml isosmotic sodium chloride solution and infuse 0·5 ml each minute for 1 hour.) If there is no improvement after this time hydrocortisone should be used. Bronchodilator drugs should not be administered solely by the oral, rectal or bronchial routes in an asthmatic emergency because the speed and amount of absorption cannot be predicted.

Oxygen. If the $PaCO_2$ is raised or not known humidified oxygen is given continuously by Venturi mask in a concentration of about 28 per cent or by nasal catheter at a flow rate of 2 to 4 litres/minute (1 min^{-1}). If the $PaCO_2$ is normal or low oxygen can be given freely but, in chronic asthma, especially if complicated by bronchitis, a close watch must be kept for signs of carbon dioxide narcosis.

Correction of acidosis. A severe and prolonged attack of asthma is usually accompanied by a metabolic acidosis which not only predisposes to cardiac arrhythmias but may also block the action of sympathomimetic drugs. This acidosis should be corrected by giving sodium bicarbonate i v (pp. 11 and 727).

Dehydration and any associated electrolyte imbalance are corrected by the i v infusion of the appropriate solution.

Antibiotics. If the attack has been precipitated or complicated by infection, amoxycillin 250 mg three times a day by mouth is prescribed, changing if necessary to the more appropriate antibiotic when the result of sputum culture is known.

Sedatives. Opiates, barbiturates and other drugs which suppress the respiratory and cough reflexes are contraindicated unless the patient is being ventilated mechanically. If sedation is needed either diazepam (Valium) 10 mg orally or i v or promethazine hydrochloride (Phenergan) 25 mg orally or i v should be used but even with these some respiratory depression may occur.

Removal of bronchial secretions. The retention of viscid bronchial secretions can lead to death from asphyxia, especially if the cough reflex has been suppressed by narcotic drugs. The following measures should be tried:

1. Physiotherapy to encourage and assist expectoration.

2. Water vapour delivered by nebuliser to the patient's mouth and nose. The ' hydrojet ' is a suitable apparatus for this purpose.

3. Mucolytic agents can be used but their effectiveness is as yet unproven. The preparations available include: Bisolvon 8 mg six-hourly orally, or acetylcysteine (Airbron) 5 ml of a 20 per cent solution by nebuliser. This treatment may result in an increased volume of liquid secretion and precautions must be taken to deal with this, by mechanical suction if necessary.

If these measures fail, per-bronchoscopic aspiration of secretions may be needed with or without saline lavage of the bronchial tree.

Tracheostomy and positive pressure respiration. In extreme cases, total ventilatory failure may supervene with cyanosis, diminished breathing effort, distant or absent breath sounds, carbon dioxide narcosis, hypotension and even cardiac arrest. These signs may develop quite suddenly but can sometimes be predicted from a rise in the $PaCO_2$, often from subnormal levels. This situation calls for tracheal intubation and assisted ventilation by intermittent positive pressure (p. 16). If prolonged assisted ventilation is needed the endotracheal tube must be withdrawn and a tracheostomy performed.

BRONCHITIS AND EMPHYSEMA

Chronic respiratory failure with hypoxia and hypercapnia is rare in pure emphysema but frequently complicates severe chronic bronchitis. In this situation not only is the respiratory centre relatively insensitive to changes in arterial CO_2 tension but the ventilatory mechanism itself is less able to respond to increased demand. Acute respiratory failure may thus result from anything which further depresses either central sensitivity (e.g. narcotic drugs or oxygen excess) or ventilatory performance (e.g. infection and trauma to the chest wall). Congestive cardiac failure, resulting mainly from hypoxic constriction of the pulmonary arterioles, may further aggravate the respiratory failure of chronic bronchitis.

Management

The principles of management are similar to those described for asthma except that, in the bronchitic patient, cardiac failure and carbon dioxide narcosis usually demand more attention than does bronchial constriction.

Oxygen, correction of acidosis and dehydration, antibiotics, sedatives, removal of secretions, tracheostomy and assisted ventilation—as under Asthma (p. 194).

Steroids and bronchodilator drugs. Unless there is a history of asthma, steroids are rarely effective in bronchitic respiratory failure and may only aggravate the infection and cardiac failure. Aminophylline is valuable not only as a bronchodilator but because it may promote a diuresis. It can be given i v (see under asthma) or as a suppository. Suitable oral bronchodilators include Orceprenaline (Alupent) 20 mg, terbutaline (Bricanyl) 5 mg or salbutamol (Ventolin) 4 mg given three or four times daily. Bronchodilators may also be given by inhalation (e.g. salbutamol (Ventolin)) but absorption is unreliable when the airways are obstructed by secretions. The delivery of a bronchodilator aerosol by positive pressure ventilation has also been advocated but the self-administration of an inhaler should never be permitted during a respiratory emergency.

Cardiac failure. If right heart failure is present with jugular venous engorgement and oedema, a diuretic is indicated. Lasix (frusemide) 40 mg may be given i v and then 80 mg orally each morning with Slow-K 2 g (potassium chloride) three times daily, but a close watch must be kept on the serum potassium level. Digoxin, although not always effective in cor pulmonale, may also be prescribed: 0·5 mg orally and repeated six hours later and then 0·25 mg two or three times daily so long as there are no signs of digitalis intoxication (see p. 250).

Carbon dioxide narcosis. The signs of carbon dioxide narcosis, including shallow respirations, suppression of the cough reflex and impairment of consciousness, may already be present when the patient is first seen and even small amounts of oxygen can then abolish respirations altogether and precipitate coma. In this situation every effort should be made to stimulate respiration and the cough reflex. Nikethamide (Coramine) 2 to 10 ml of a 25 per cent solution, or prethcamide (Micoren) 450 mg are given *slowly* i v. Cropropamide 225 mg can subsequently be given i m every hour. At the same time measures are taken to release the retained bronchial secretions (see p. 197). If there is no improvement within two or three hours, or if it is then still impossible to administer oxygen without worsening the narcosis, bronchoscopic aspiration of secretions, tracheal intubation and positive pressure ventilation are carried out.

The endotracheal tube must be removed after a few days to avoid laryngeal or tracheal ulceration and subsequent stenosis. If the patient is still unable to maintain an adequate level of ventilation as judged by clinical signs and blood gas levels than tracheostomy is needed. This is likely to be the case when the onset of respiratory failure was insidious and not obviously provoked by a transient and remedial cause such as an acute infection or narcotic drug. These patients are often suffering from advanced obstructive lung disease with emphysema and some will have been confined to their homes or even to their beds for many months. It is often said that the prospects for such patients and the quality of their lives are so poor that it is not justifiable to prolong life by a tracheostomy which may have to be permanent. In fact, response to tracheostomy is extremely difficult to predict, especially when the physician is dealing with a patient of whom he has no previous personal knowledge. Whereas the family doctor may properly decide not to refer such a patient for hospital treatment, the hospital physician himself can only rarely justify withholding life-saving treatment if the facilities for this are available.

PNEUMONIA

Pneumonia today more often creates an emergency in patients already ill from other causes than in previously healthy people. Urgency may arise either from the overwhelming nature of the infection itself or from interference with respiratory function. The response to infection in the lung depends upon the nature of the invading organism and the resistance of the patient. The *Streptococcus pneumoniae* causes a pneumonia of lobar distribution without tissue breakdown and may affect healthy subjects. The same is true of virus and mycoplasma infections but then the pneumonia is more patchy and rarely embarrasses lung function, although a dangerous toxaemia accompanies infection by viruses of the psittacosis group. Most of the other organisms causing pneumonia, including the staphylococcus, *Haemophilus influenzae* and *Klebsiella pneumoniae,* do so only when either the local bronchial defences or the general resistance of the patient has been lowered by previous disease. Prolonged treatment with broad-spectrum antibiotics may

clear the way for infection with Gram-negative bacilli (e.g. *E. coli,
B. proteus* and *Ps. pyocyanea*) and fungi (e.g. *Aspergillus fumigatus*
and *Candida albicans*). *Pseudomonas* infections are a special hazard
to the patient with a tracheostomy. The pneumonia in these cases
is usually of patchy peribronchial distribution and, especially in
staphylococcal and klebsiella infections, can lead to abscess formation. The nature of the resulting emergency is mainly determined
by the conditions predisposing to the pneumonia and may take the
form of a septicaemia in patients whose general resistance is lowered
or acute respiratory failure in those with previous chronic chest
disease.

Diagnosis

Classical lobar pneumonia presents with a rigor, pleuritic pain,
cough with ' rusty ' sputum, cyanosis, a pleural friction rub and the
signs of consolidation: impaired percussion note, bronchial breathing, bronchophony and fine inspiratory crepitations. In other types
of pneumonia the onset can be masked by pre-existing disease and
even by antibiotics used for the treatment of that disease. Pneumonia
should therefore be watched for whenever a patient, especially
an elderly one, is already ill with a chronic chest condition or
general debilitating disease, or confined to bed after an operation
or from any other cause. Evidence of pneumonia in these cases
may be limited to a sudden rise in temperature, pulse or respiratory
rate, cough with pleuritic pain, cyanosis and patches of crepitations,
often basal in site, without the typical signs of consolidation. In
elderly debilitated patients there may be a rise in pulse and respiratory rate without fever. A fall in blood pressure occurs with more
severe infections.

There are two conditions which can be confused with pneumonia
and which are especially liable to affect patients kept in bed for
any length of time: pulmonary collapse (p. 205) and embolism with
infarction (p. 241). The clinical features of these two conditions and
the special investigations which help to identify them are described
on pp. 205 and 241.

Management

Investigation. Immediate arrangements should be made, if facilities are available, for a chest radiograph, culture of the blood
and sputum and a white cell count.

Treatment of the infection. Typical lobar pneumonia in a previously healthy patient is probably due to *Streptococcus pneumoniae*
and should be treated with penicillin 1 mega unit six-hourly. Pneu-

monia arising in patients with chronic chest disease, especially those who have already had antibiotics in the past, is unlikely to respond to penicillin. The same is true of pneumonia complicating other diseases, particularly among hospital patients. In these circumstances a broad-spectrum antibiotic, either amoxycillin 500 mg eight-hourly or co-trimoxazole (Septrin) 2 tablets eight-hourly by mouth in patients allergic to penicillin, should be started pending the result of the sputum culture. If the patient is desperately ill or if the pneumonia is cavitating then a staphylococcal infection must be suspected and fusidic acid (Fucidin) 300 mg six-hourly by mouth with flucloxacillin (Floxapen) 250 mg six-hourly by mouth is given in addition to a broad-spectrum antibiotic. Bronchopneumonic infections by Gram-negative bacilli (e.g. *pseudomonas*) are becoming an increasing problem in intensive care wards among tracheostomy patients who may be already receiving a variety of antibiotics. In these circumstances a serious pneumonia should be treated with Gentamicin (Genticin) 80 mg eight-hourly i v, but the subsequent dosage should be adjusted according to serum levels of the drug and signs of renal damage must be looked for (see p. 388). Treatment is subsequently adjusted according to clinical response and the sensitivity of the organisms grown on culture.

Treatment of hypoxia. When pneumonia complicates chronic respiratory failure with hypercapnia, oxygen must be given by Venturi mask or nasal catheter and a careful watch kept for carbon dioxide narcosis (p. 198). Otherwise pneumonia itself usually causes hypoxia without significant hypercapnia and then oxygen may be given by the most effective available method. Either a well-fitting mask or oxygen tent is appropriate but, if these are not tolerated by the patient, oxygen can be delivered at a high flow rate (8 to 10 litres/minute (l min^{-1})) through a nasal catheter.

Relief of pleuritic pain. The rapid shallow respirations induced by pleuritic pain can aggravate hypoxia by diminishing effective alveolar ventilation. It is therefore important to relieve pain and, if simple analgesics fail, it is even justifiable to use drugs which depress the respiratory centre unless there is a previous history of chronic chest disease. In the first instance it is worth applying local heat in the form of a kaolin poultice with either aspirin or dihydrocodeine tartrate (DF 118) 60 mg by mouth. If these measures are ineffective then pethidine 50 mg i m or morphine 10 mg subcutaneously can be given and repeated in four hours if there have been no adverse effects. Certain preparations, such as Pethilorfan (pethidine and levallorphan tartrate), are supposed to cause less respiratory depression, but some degree of depression is inevitable with most potent analgesics so far available.

Treatment of cough. In the early stages of pneumonia a frequent dry cough can aggravate the pain and exhaust the patient. Linctus codeine (BNF) may be sufficient to alleviate it, or, failing this, pholcodine linctus BPC 4 ml or methadone linctus BPC 4 ml can be tried. Later in the course of the illness, especially in cavitating pneumonia, cough may be productive and should be encouraged; preferably with the help of the physiotherapist (see also p. 210).

Treatment of fulminating pneumonia. Certain forms of pneumonia can kill the patient in a matter of hours with widespread oedema of the lungs and peripheral circulatory failure. Staphylococcal infection complicating virus influenza is one of the commonest causes of fulminating pneumonia. Immediate treatment consists of continuous oxygen, amoxycillin 500 mg with hydrocortisone 200 mg, flucloxacillin 500 mg and gentamicin 80 mg i v. Digitalis 0·5 mg and frusemide (Lasix) 40 mg i v are also given to those patients with atrial fibrillation or congestive cardiac failure. Tracheal intubation with intermittent positive pressure respiration may be needed in the more severe cases.

SPONTANEOUS PNEUMOTHORAX

Spontaneous pneumothorax is common in relatively healthy young people but, like pneumonia, it more often creates an emergency among older patients with pre-existing lung disease such as emphysema. The causes include the rupture of a subpleural bleb, a cyst, an emphysematous bulla or, more rarely, a lung abscess. Pneumothorax (although not strictly spontaneous) may also complicate the intensive therapy of chronic lung disease: it may be provoked by corticosteroids and positive pressure ventilation or induced by attempts to insert a jugular central venous line (p. 751).

The raised intrathoracic pressure resulting from pneumothorax has two serious consequences: impaired ventilation due to lung collapse and a fall in cardiac output due to diminished venous return to the thorax. Sometimes the tear in the lung or the rupture of an adhesion produces a haemopneumothorax (p. 209).

The urgency of the situation depends upon the type of pneumothorax and the state of the underlying lung. Three types are recognised: closed, open and tension pneumothorax. In *closed pneumothorax* the leaking point quickly seals off as the lung collapses, the intrapleural pressure remains negative and the air is gradually reabsorbed. This type rarely causes anxiety. In *open pneumothorax*

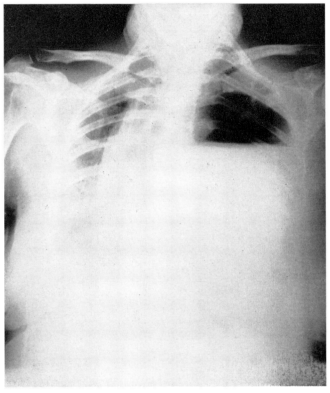

Fig. 8.1
Tension haemopneumothorax with displacement of the mediastinum.

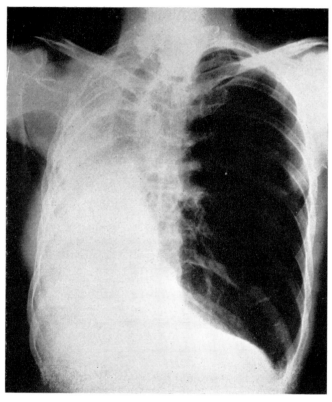

Fig. 8.2
Massive collapse of right lung.

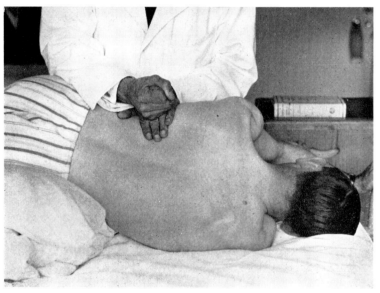

Fig. 8.3
Postural percussion drainage for massive collapse of the lung.

the hole in the lung surface is held open by rigidity around it or by an adhesion, the mean intrapleural pressure is atmospheric and the air is not absorbed. This is particularly likely to happen in patients with pre-existing lung disease and can lead to dangerous encroachment upon their respiratory reserve, but it rarely impedes cardiac output and more often creates the long-term problem of re-expanding the lung than an acute emergency. *Tension pneumothorax,* on the other hand, is invariably an urgent matter (Fig. 8.1). Here the tear in the lung closes during expiration but opens with inspiration, thus producing a valvular mechanism whereby air can enter but not leave the pleural space. Cough and airways obstruction will also force air out through the leak so that a tension pneumothorax is more common and also more dangerous in bronchitic subjects. The mean intrathoracic pressure rapidly becomes positive and, unlike the other two types, tension pneumothorax thus causes a fall in cardiac output due to diminished venous return.

Diagnosis

Pneumothorax most commonly presents as sudden unilateral pleuritic pain and dyspnoea in a young subject who may have had similar attacks before. The classical signs are found mainly in the tension variety and include cyanosis, tachycardia, diminished expansion of the hemithorax, mediastinal deviation toward the opposite side, a hyper-resonant percussion note, reduced or absent breath and voice sounds and a variety of auscultatory signs including distant amphoric breathing, ' tinkling ' crepitations, a clicking sound synchronous with the heart beat and the coin sign. When the pneumothorax is under extreme tension there may also be jugular venous engorgement, hypotension and visible distension of the affected hemithorax. In older patients, particularly those with chronic chest disease, the symptoms and general effects of a pneumothorax can be out of proportion to local signs which may also be masked by underlying emphysema. Pneumothorax must therefore be suspected whenever a patient with chronic airways obstruction has a sudden increase of dyspnoea or cyanosis or a chest pain which, particularly in the older patient, can be central and constricting in type rather than pleuritic. In this situation, and also when the pneumothorax is relatively small and not under tension, local signs may be limited to a relative reduction in breath sounds on the affected side.

Pneumothorax must be distinguished from other causes of sudden chest pain and dyspnoea, including pulmonary embolism (p. 241) and myocardial infarction (p. 233) and from conditions such as large

cysts or emphysematous bullae which can not only cause a pneumothorax but also mimic its physical signs.

Management

If the diagnosis is in doubt, it is safer to await the result of a
chest radiograph than to plunge a needle into the chest and thus
risk inducing a pneumothorax in a patient already seriously ill from
some other cause. Films taken during full expiration with lateral
and postero-anterior views are needed to exclude a small pneumothorax, and an electrocardiogram should also be done if there is
any suspicion of either pulmonary embolism or myocardial infarction.

Only very rarely does a pneumothorax present such an extreme
emergency in the home that the patient cannot safely be transferred
to hospital. When this does occur and there is no doubt about the
diagnosis, a large bore needle should be inserted into the second
intercostal space about two inches from the sternal edge. A length
of rubber tubing (stethoscope tubing can be used) is attached to the
needle and the other end is put into an open bottle of clean water.
Alternatively, the punctured finger of a rubber glove can be tied
around the end of the needle to form a non-return flutter valve.
The patient should then be moved to hospital.

In less urgent cases the diagnosis is confirmed by a radiograph
which will also indicate the optimum site for drainage. Providing
that the lung is not adherent at this level, the second intercostal
space 5·0 cm from the sternal edge is selected. After local anaesthesia with 15 to 20 ml of 1 per cent lignocaine, a small skin
incision is made with a tenotomy knife and a trocar and cannula
are inserted. The trocar is then withdrawn and replaced by a
catheter with 6 to 8 cm inside the pleural cavity and with a sufficient
length outside to permit the patient to move about freely in bed.
A Malecot catheter or the Trocath apparatus (see Peritoneal Dialysis,
(p. 716)) are suitable for this purpose. It is kept in position by
a suture which is passed through the skin and then lashed around
the tube without transfixing it. A mattress suture is also left
ready to close the wound when the tube is ultimately withdrawn.
The other end of the catheter is placed beneath the surface of water
in a bottle with a double-lumen stopper (the other lumen being left
open to the air) or is connected to an electric suction pump if
more rapid re-expansion of the lung is thought necessary. A
regular inspection must be carried out to ensure that the catheter is
not obstructed by pleural secretions, kinking or local re-expansion
of the lung. Obstruction may lead to clinical deterioration and can

be recognised by the cessation of bubbling through the water. Palpable surgical emphysema may also occur.

Other measures which may be needed include the relief of pleuritic pain and cough (p. 210), the aspiration of fluid, pus, or blood from the pleural cavity, antibiotics if there is an empyema, blood transfusion to replace a large haemothorax, bronchodilators to alleviate airways obstruction and bronchoscopy if the lung fails to re-expand because of absorption collapse due to bronchial occlusion.

Finally, before the lung has fully re-expanded, a decision must be made as to whether a sclerosing material should be injected into the pleural space to effect a pleurodesis. This may be considered advisable in those patients who have had a previous pneumothorax but, since it can cause a severe reaction, it should never be done when the pulmonary function or general condition of the patient are still causing concern. An elective surgical pleurodesis at a later date is often safer and usually more effective.

COLLAPSE OF THE LUNG

The urgency of pulmonary absorption collapse depends upon its extent, the speed with which it develops, and the function of the unaffected areas of lung. For example, gradual collapse of a lobe due to bronchial carcinoma may be quite symptomless, whereas the sudden occlusion of a major bronchus by viscid secretions in an asthmatic subject can create a dire emergency.

Causes

There are two main causes for collapse of an urgent nature:

1. *Bronchial obstruction.* Collapse due to bronchial obstruction may result from inhalation of foreign material, an increase in the quantity or tenacity of secretions, loss of the normal ciliary action or suppression of cough.

2. *Failure of alveolar inflation.* Even when the bronchi remain patent the alveoli may collapse because of adherence of their walls when respiration is unduly shallow. This is especially so if the surfactant lining, which normally ensures that surface tension falls during deflation, is destroyed.

It follows that pulmonary collapse is especially likely to arise in bronchitic subjects whose cough and respirations have been suppressed by narcotic drugs or by the pain which follows surgical or other trauma to the chest or upper abdomen. Other factors contributing to post-operative collapse include the inhalation of vomit, the increase in secretions provoked by tracheal intubation or

8

the anaesthetic agent itself, the greater tenacity of secretions due to dehydration or inadequate humidification of inspired gases, and the shallow breathing associated with delayed reversal of curarisation. Inactivation of surfactant may be responsible for alveolar atelectasis in the adult respiratory distress syndrome or 'shock lung' (p. 207).

Diagnosis

Collapse should be suspected when, in any of the circumstances already described, a patient develops dyspnoea, cyanosis, fever or an increase in the heart and respiratory rate. The classical local signs are found only when there is collapse of a lobe or lung. These include mediastinal deviation toward the affected side. reduced expansion, a dull percussion note, and absent or bronchial breath sounds. (Fig. 8.2). The lower lobes and right middle lobe are most often affected. Collapse may be associated with considerable hypoxia, usually without hypercapnia. This is due to a shunt caused by continued perfusion of the unventilated area of lung. However, as the collapse progresses, blood supply to the affected part is gradually shut off with relief of the hypoxia. The disappearance of cyanosis may therefore indicate increasing collapse rather than reaeration.

The differential diagnosis of collapse, especially during the post-operative period (p. 600), includes pulmonary embolism with infarction (p. 241), and pneumonia (p. 199). Collapse usually occurs within 48 hours of the operation whereas embolism is commoner after the end of the first week. The onset is often more dramatic in embolism and haemoptysis is more frequent. The chest radiograph (Fig. 8.2) and electrocardiogram help to distinguish these two conditions. In collapse the electrocardiograph is normal and the radiograph shows an opacity corresponding to a contracted anatomical lobe or segment of the lung with a line of demarcation which radiates towards the hilum. Post-operative pneumonia, especially when it affects the lower lobes, is so frequently associated with collapse that it is safer to assume for purposes of treatment that both conditions are present.

Management

Postero-anterior and lateral radiographs of the chest should first be taken.

Percussion postural drainage is carried out with the patient so placed that the collapsed lobe or segment drains towards the hilum of the lung (Fig. 8.3). The patient is encouraged to cough at regular intervals while the wound (if any) is supported by hand. Postural drainage may be more effective if a bronchodilator and a mucolytic agent or water aerosol (p. 197) is given beforehand.

Deep breathing exercises are then performed to help full re-aeration of the affected alveoli.

Bronchoscopy to aspirate retained secretions is necessary if re-expansion has not occurred within 24 hours, or sooner if pulmonary function is seriously impaired.

Other measures may be needed, including oxygen (p. 740), antibiotics and bronchodilator drugs (p. 196).

ACUTE PULMONARY OEDEMA AND 'SHOCK LUNG'

Pulmonary oedema of cardiac origin is described on page 229. Non-cardiac causes include fulminating pneumonia (p. 199), the inhalation of certain fumes (e.g. nitrogen dioxide, p. 463) and the ingestion of toxic substances (Paraquat, p. 38). Pulmonary oedema also occurs in the syndrome of 'shock lung' and in mountain climbers.

The onset of these forms of pulmonary oedema is characteristically delayed until hours or days after the initial insult; up to 36 hours in the case of nitrous fumes and for a week or more in Paraquat poisoning and 'shock lung'.

Damage to the alveolar lining cells with inactivation of surfactant causing increased surface tension may be an important factor in these non-cardiac forms of pulmonary oedema. The pathological findings include proliferation and desquamation of alveolar cells with hyaline exudate, haemorrhage and atelectasis as well as interstitial and alveolar oedema.

'SHOCK LUNG'

(Adult respiratory distress syndrome; Post-traumatic pulmonary insufficiency, Traumatic Wet Lung syndrome)

It has been recognised in recent years that progressive pulmonary insufficiency can follow an incident of 'shock' due to trauma, major surgery, burns, haemorrhage, infection, myocardial infarction or pulmonary embolism. The syndrome usually supervenes some days after a precarious resuscitation has been achieved with large infusions of blood or other fluids, prolonged oxygen therapy and a variety of drug regimes. Indeed, the syndrome has in some cases been attributed to excessive therapy of this kind. The earliest sign is hyperventilation with hypocapnia, respiratory alkalosis and a progressive hypoxia which cannot be corrected by giving oxygen.

Patchy crepitations are associated with radiographic signs of oedema and segmental atelectasis mainly in the dependent areas of the lungs. Secondary pneumonic infections are common. Spontaneous ventilation eventually fails, but adequate pulmonary inflation and oxygenation of the blood may prove impossible even with mechanical ventilation. In these more severe cases, hypercapnia and hypoxia lead to respiratory and metabolic acidosis and death from a cardiac dysrhythmia.

Management

No specific or consistently effective therapy is available for the various forms of non-cardiac pulmonary oedema. Digitalis and diuretics are rarely helpful but corticosteroids have been used with success in acute pulmonary oedema due to nitrous fumes. Tracheal intubation or tracheostomy with intermittent positive pressure ventilation will be needed in the more severe cases whatever the cause. The appropriate antibiotic should be given when there is secondary infection. Oxygen, the correction of acid-base imbalance and fluid replacement may also be required but, in some cases of 'shock lung' especially, these forms of treatment must be closely monitored by frequent blood gas, electrolyte and central venous pressure measurements.

HAEMORRHAGE

Spontaneous thoracic haemorrhage may present as haemoptysis or as intrapleural bleeding (haemothorax) complicating spontaneous pneumothorax (p. 202).

HAEMOPTYSIS

Although haemoptysis usually arises from serious bronchopulmonary disease it rarely constitutes an emergency and, when it does so, this more often relates to interference with ventilation than to actual loss of blood. Flooding of the airways and collapse due to bronchial obstruction by blood clot are particularly dangerous when the disease causing the haemoptysis has already encroached upon the respiratory reserve.

Management

An attempt is made to determine the cause and to locate the source of the bleeding so that appropriate surgical treatment can be undertaken at a later date if this proves necessary. A chest radiograph with lateral views will usually reveal the disease causing the haemoptysis but, where this is widespread or bilateral, the precise origin of the haemorrhage may remain uncertain. Bronchoscopy will demonstrate a source of bleeding in the proximal parts of the bronchial tree or, when the haemorrhage is of pulmonary origin, blood may be seen emerging from the bronchus supplying the affected segment of lung. If bronchoscopy is negative then a bronchogram should be carried out.

Reassurance plays an important part in treatment and, in most cases, this can be given with confidence. Anxiety can be allayed with chlorpromazine (Largactil) 25 mg by mouth or i m injection, but morphine and other drugs which suppress the cough reflex must be avoided. The patient should be encouraged to cough in order to clear clot from the bronchial tree, but vigorous postural drainage is inadvisable. He should be nursed in the semi-sitting position leaning towards the side of the haemorrhage to prevent blood from entering the other lung. Blood transfusion is rarely needed but surgical excision of the bleeding segment of lung may have to be undertaken in intractable cases.

HAEMOTHORAX

Haemothorax is an occasional complication of spontaneous pneumothorax (p. 202). It may be evident within hours of the lung rupture or not until several days later. There may be local signs of pleural effusion and systemic manifestations of haemorrhage. Haemothorax should therefore be suspected when a patient with spontaneous pneumothorax develops increasing dyspnoea, cyanosis, mediastinal displacement, dullness to percussion at the lung base, pallor, sweating, tachycardia or hypotension. The chest radiograph will show a basal opacity bounded above by a horizontal fluid level (Fig. 8.1).

Management

Management includes pleural aspiration and replacement of blood by transfusion. If the chest tap confirms a haemothorax, however small, the whole of the blood must be removed immediately, not only to alleviate dyspnoea but also to ensure full re-expansion of the lung before clotting occurs. In cases of massive haemorrhage or when bleeding recurs after aspiration, an intercostal catheter should be inserted and attached to an underwater seal. This facilitates accurate measurement and replacement of blood loss. Thoracotomy may eventually be needed either to secure the bleeding point or to re-expand the lung by the removal of blood clot or by decortication.

COUGH AS AN URGENT SYMPTOM

Prolonged irrepressible coughing may be the reason for an urgent call.

Management

The correct approach is to find the cause; it might, for example, be an unsuspected foreign body or high altitude as in mountaineers. The following purely symptomatic measures may be used:

1. Narcotic drugs which depress the cough centre:
   - (a) Codeine phosphate 15 to 60 mg six hourly. Syrup of codeine phosphate contains 15 mg in 5 ml.
   - (b) Dihydrocodeine (DF118) 30 mg tablets and 1 ml (50 mg) ampoules.
   - (c) Pholcodine linctus BPC 5 ml (about 5 mg) four hourly for an adult. It does not cause addiction.
   - (d) Methadone hydrochloride BP (Physeptone) in a linctus, e.g. methadone linctus BP 5 ml (2 mg methadone) every three or four hours for an adult.
   - (e) Heroin (diamorphine). The usual dose, 6 mg, is contained in 10 ml of linctus of diamorphine. As it is very liable to cause addiction it is best reserved for hopeless cases.

   Paraldehyde (p. 755) will enhance the effect of these drugs without further depression of the respiratory centre.

2. Non-narcotic drugs which depress the cough centre. Pipazethate (Selvigon) has an activity equal to or greater than codeine but without side effects. Adults should take two 5 ml doses of syrup or two tablets (40 mg) three times a day but a smaller dose may be effective. The dose for infants is 1 to 5 mg (3 to 20 drops of syrup).

HICCUP

Hiccup is a reflex activity mediated by afferent pathways in the phrenic and vagus nerves and the sympathetic chain from T6-12. The efferent route is now believed to include the intercostal as well as the phrenic nerves. It consists of spasmodic contractions of diaphragmatic and external (inspiratory) intercostal muscles with inhibition of expiratory intercostal activity. The resulting inspiration is cut short by closure of the glottis so that the spasm has very little effect on ventilation.

Hiccup may have central or peripheral causes. Central causes include arteriosclerotic and other forms of brain disease or general toxic states, such as uraemia, but psychological factors may also be important. The local causes are more often below than above the diaphragm, the commonest being a simple digestive disorder, but hiccup may also accompany serious conditions like peritonitis.

If frequent and persistent, hiccup may exhaust the patient and call for urgent treatment especially in those already ill from other causes. The following measures can be tried:

(1) MECHANICAL MANOEUVRES: These probably act by interrupting the reflex arc but are rarely lasting in their effect. They include breath-holding, rebreathing from a bag, drinking cold water, pulling the tongue forward, massaging the paraspinal areas of the neck and stimulating the pharynx with a nasal catheter or a teaspoonful of granulated sugar swallowed dry. The occasional efficacy of a sudden fright probably reflects the psychological rather than the reflex basis for some cases of hiccup.

(2) DRUG THERAPY: A variety of remedies have recently been recommended:

1. Metoclopramide (Maxolon) 10 mg i v followed by 10 mg orally or i m every six hours.

2. Chlorpromazine (Largactil) 25 mg three times a day (orally or i m) alone or with metoclopramide.

3. Orphenadrine citrate (Norflex) 2 ml (60 mg) i v and then 100 mg orally three times a day.

4. Haloperidol (Serenace) 3 mg i m three times a day.

5. Diphenylhydantoin (Epanutin) 200 mg i v over five minutes and then 100 mg four times a day by mouth. This is based on the theory that there is an irritable focus in the area of the respiratory centre in the medulla.

It remains to be seen whether these will prove any more effective than those remedies listed in the ninth edition of this book: inhalation of amyl nitrite, atropine 1 mg i v, methylamphetamine 4 mg and promazine 25 to 50 mg.

COLIN OGILVIE

FOR FURTHER READING

D'ABREU, A. L., TAYLOR, A. B. & CLARKE, D. B. *Intrathoracic Crises.* London: Butterworths, 1968.

COTES, J. E. *Lung function, Assessment and Application in Medicine.* 3rd ed. Oxford: Blackwell, 1974.

SYKES, M. K., MCNICOL, M. W. & CAMPBELL, E. J. M. *Respiratory Failure.* 2nd ed. Oxford: Blackwell, 1974.

CHAPTER 9

Emergencies in Ear, Nose and Throat Disease

ADEQUATE diagnosis and treatment in ENT emergencies are only possible when both light and sight can reach the depths of such narrow and inaccessible passages as the external auditory meatus and the nose. The head mirror reflecting a strong light and the reflecting mirror head-lamp are both satisfactory in permitting vision along the centre of the illuminating beam and thus eliminating difficulties caused by parallax (Fig. 9.1).

THE EAR

Any pus present should be taken on a swab for culture of organisms and determination of sensitivities to antibiotics. The meatus may be cleaned by syringing with tap water, the stream being directed against the posterior meatal wall. The water should be at body temperature (36·6°C) to avoid inducing caloric vertigo. A 100 ml plastic syringe (Medi-plast) is now available with detachable nozzle for easy filling and safe use. Besides pus and wax many foreign bodies may be removed by syringing. Alcohol may be used in the syringe instead of water to remove an hygroscopic foreign body such as a dried pea which would swell when wet. After syringing, the ear should be dried by mopping with cottonwool on a wire wool carrier. To prevent damage to the tympanic membrane care should be taken that the wool projects freely beyond the end of the wire.

Impacted wax

Wax may cause pain as well as deafness, when swollen from contact with water. Painful manipulation of the external auditory meatus must be avoided and the wax softened by the instillation of warm sodium bicarbonate ear drops (BPC and BNF) thrice daily for four days after which the softened wax can be syringed away painlessly.

Haematoma of auricle

This, the ' pugilist's ear ', is the result of trauma causing sub-perichondrial haemorrhage of the pinna. Organisation of the blood clot and subsequent fibrosis results in a thickened and distorted pinna. If seen early aspiration of the fluid blood through a wide-bore needle is possible. A firm pad and bandage will prevent recurrence of the haematoma. At a later stage incision and evacuation of the clotted blood is necessary.

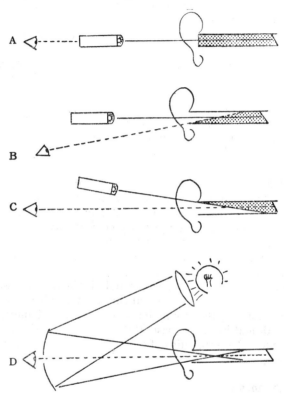

FIG. 9.1. The problem of parallax. Comparison of head-mirror and torch or head lamp.

    A. Head lamp or torch obscures view.
    B. Light adequate but vision obstructed.
    C. Eye can see deeply but shadow is cast.
    D. Light and vision unobstructed.

Foreign body in the ear

Most commonly the patient is a child who has inserted a stone, pea or bead into his ear. Shaking the head with the affected ear undermost may dislodge the foreign body, particularly if a little lubricant such as liquid paraffin is first instilled. A smooth-surfaced foreign body so lubricated may be attracted out of the meatus by a suction cannula (filed needle) gently advanced on to it without touching the tender meatal skin.

If this fails, removal should be attempted under anaesthesia as the procedure may be very painful and movements of the child's head uncontrollable by any other method. An adult may permit manipulation without anaesthesia. Forceps must never be used to remove a hard foreign body as closure of its jaws may impel a smooth foreign body further into the meatus or even through the tympanic membrane into the middle ear. The outline of the external auditory meatus being oval, a hook can be passed beyond the foreign body, turned, and on withdrawal the foreign body can be readily removed. Syringing the ear with water will suffice to remove many foreign bodies in older patients. Soft material like paper or sponge may be removed readily with angled forceps.

Furuncle

A boil in the ear may be extremely painful because the skin is tightly bound down. Pus should be obtained for culture and vaccine preparation. Antibiotics are of little value. Incision under anaesthesia to evacuate pus may be necessary but short-wave diathermy applied to the ear twice daily may abort the incipient furuncle. It is difficult to modify the course of a single furuncle and treatment is mainly directed to preventing recurrence by scrupulous attention to cleanliness of the hands and elimination of associated infections of teeth, nose, tonsils and sinuses. Immediate recurrence may be prevented by the prompt introduction of a wick impregnated with bismuth and iodoform paste ('BIPP'). An occasional patient is sensitive to it. External otitis of an infective type will also respond to the same care.

Acute otitis media

Most common in children, this condition is usually secondary to infection in the nose and throat. Any respiratory infection may precede it. Predisposing factors are the short freely patent Eustachian tube of the infant and the obstruction of it that accompanies adenoid hypertrophy in the older child. Sinusitis, unhealthy tonsils, and carious teeth, may play their part.

Severe otalgia, pyrexia and the observation of an inflamed tympanic membrane make the diagnosis comparatively simple. Antibiotics in large doses will bring rapid relief of pain and prompt resolution in most cases. Having ascertained by questioning that the patient is not allergic to penicillin a single dose of Procaine

Penicillin Injection BP should be given and followed by booster doses of phenoxymethylpenicillin (Penicillin V) 250 mg four times a day by mouth. Myringotomy is rarely called for. Early patency of the Eustachian tube is desirable and decongestant nose drops, e.g. Argotone (weak silver protein 1 per cent and ephedrine 0·9 per cent in isosmotic sodium chloride solution), are advisable for a short period. A swab should be taken of any pus which escapes through a perforated tympanic membrane. To secure an adequate view of the tympanic membrane it may be necessary to syringe the meatus clean with warm (36·6°C) tapwater.

Acute mastoiditis

Some mastoid tenderness may be found with otitis media and rarely a true mastoiditis may occur simultaneously when a debilitated patient is infected by virulent organisms. More often acute mastoiditis develops after the onset of otitis media, particularly if antibiotics have been omitted or their dosage inadequate. Antibiotics may mask the symptoms of acute mastoiditis and so enquiry about previous treatment is essential. Post-auricular abscess formation is now rare and calls for mastoidectomy as does persistent otorrhoea after otitis media.

Otorrhoea

Scrupulous cleanliness is essential where there is any discharge in the external auditory meatus whether from furuncle, external otitis, or otitis media. Frequent cleansing by cottonwool moistened with 1 per cent cetrimide should be followed by the instillation of auristillae consisting of mixtures of hydrocortisone acetate BP and neomycin sulphate BP (Neocortef).

Bell's palsy

For emergency aspects see p. 317.

For emergency aspects see p. 317.

DEAFNESS

Sudden deafness may occasion an emergency call. The type, conductive or perceptive, may be distinguished by simple tuning fork tests and by audiometry.

Conductive deafness

Here sound waves are prevented from gaining access to the intact nerve mechanism of the cochlea. Thus a vibrating tuning fork can be poorly heard at the meatal orifice but when pressed on the mastoid process the intact cochlea is adequately stimulated by bone conduction and appreciates the tuning fork note for a longer period than it can be heard by air (Rinne's test negative). Normally air conduction is appreciated longer than bone conduction and Rinne's test is positive.

Conditions giving rise to such conductive deafness acutely are swelling of impacted wax, a furuncle occluding the meatus, a foreign body, acute otitis media and exudate in the middle ear. Not uncommonly a child's scholastic progress is retarded by painless conduction deafness. Examination shows the tympanic membrane to appear yellow as a result of exudate ('glue') in the middle ear. Under anaesthetic aspiration of fluid through a myringotomy incision restores hearing dramatically and insertion of a plastic 'grommet' into the incision maintains tympanic ventilation indefinitely. Factors interfering with Eustachian tube drainage—enlarged adenoids and nasal sepsis—will require simultaneous attention.

Perceptive deafness

Here there is no interference with the conduction of sound waves through the external auditory meatus and the middle ear. The perceptive element, the cochlea, is diseased and unable to pick up stimuli adequately conducted to it. The tuning fork can be no better perceived by bone conduction than by air conduction and Rinne's test remains positive, but the tuning fork placed on the forehead is heard on one side—the normal one. (In conductive deafness it is heard best on the deaf side—Weber's test.)

The causes of sudden perceptive deafness are haemorrhage into the cochlea due to trauma or blood dyscrasia and virus infection which may produce complete sudden deafness without vertigo.

If treated promptly acute perceptive deafness due to failure of blood supply may respond to vasodilatation produced by stellate ganglion block (p. 711).

Spontaneous perilymph fistula

The onset of sudden unilateral deafness following un-noteworthy exercise was formerly attributed to vascular occlusion. It can result from spontaneous perforation of the round window membrane in the middle ear with consequent perilymph leak. Deafness may be profound. It should be treated by immediate surgical exploration of the middle ear (tympanotomy) and occlusion of the perilymph leak by a fat graft taken from the lobule of the ear. The risk of infection of the inner ear is not high but the perilymph fistula does provide direct access to the subarachnoid space for any infection in the middle ear.

Deafness due to malingering

A malingerer may complain of complete deafness in one or both ears. When deafness is said to be bilateral there may be difficulty in diagnosis but partial anaesthesia with i v thiopentone will enable a question and answer conversation to expose the deception. Unilateral feigned deafness may be discovered by placing the ear-pieces of a stethoscope into the subject's ears and speaking into the bell-end behind the patient, asking him to repeat numbers. Alternating compression of the tubing to the good and supposedly deaf ear will inevitably result in the patient being caught out repeating numbers which should not have been heard.

VERTIGO

DIAGNOSIS. Although the sense of position may be upset in many disorders severe vertigo results only from some disturbance of the labyrinth, cerebellum and the associated pathways. In most cases an otological cause is present and this should be looked for first. The following procedure is suggested.

1. *Take a detailed history.* Is it the first attack or one of a series? Recurrent attacks in a deaf middle aged person suggest Menière's disease. Migraine and epilepsy may have vertigo as the aura. Head injury may result in vertigo after months or years. A first attack suggests the possibility of non-otological causes such as disseminated sclerosis and posterior inferior cerebellar artery thrombosis.

Is there a history of previous ear infection or evidence of it now?

Is there a history of other periodic nervous upset?

Is the patient taking drugs (quinine, salicylates, streptomycin)?

Is there tinnitus? This suggests an otological cause.

2. *Examine the ears.* Vertigo is only rarely caused by disease of the external ear but caloric vertigo may be induced if very cold water enters the ear. Geniculate herpes is a rare cause of vertigo; vesicles are found in the external auditory meatus or throat and there is a seventh nerve palsy. Suppurative otitis media, particularly in the presence of a cholesteatoma, may lead to the formation of a fistula into the labyrinth with serous or suppurative labyrinthitis. A fistula can be demonstrated by raising the pressure in the external auditory meatus in cases of chronic suppurative otitis media. The pressure transmitted to the labyrinth causes vertigo and deviation of the eyes to the opposite side with nystagmus to the same side. Radical treatment is necessary.

3. *Carry out hearing tests.* If the patient is deaf to speech and watch tests, use a tuning fork (C 256) to distinguish nerve (perceptive) from middle ear (conductive) deafness (p. 215). Table 9.1

outlines the salient features of the four principal types of otological vertigo.

4. *Examine the nervous system.* Although raised intracranial pressure may cause vertigo this is rarely the primary symptom and from the emergency point of view the only likely cause under this heading is **posterior inferior cerebellar artery thrombosis.** Here a wedge-shaped infarct on the side of the medulla causes a characteristic syndrome with very severe vertigo and inco-ordination. There is Horner's syndrome (meiosis, ptosis and enophthalmos) and paralysis of the palate, pharyngeal muscles and vocal cord on the side of the lesion. The face on this side shows loss of pain and temperature sense and these are lost also in the limbs and trunk of the opposite side.

5. If the diagnosis is still in doubt hysteria should be considered.

Treatment. Specific treatment depends on diagnosis but the immediate problem is the relief of giddiness and the associated vomiting. The patient will have taken to bed or should be moved there.

In otological vertigo phenobarbitone sodium 200 mg should be given by i m injection if there is nausea. Hyoscine 0·3 mg may be added if vertigo is uncontrolled.

Migrainous vertigo should be treated by ergotamine tartrate 1 mg i m.

Infective conditions call for penicillin or other antibiotics.

For vascular causes papaverine 65 mg should be used. Anticoagulant therapy should be considered.

If an intracranial tumour is present phenobarbitone should be used. Morphine should be avoided for it causes respiratory depression.

THE NOSE

Epistaxis

Nose bleeding becomes an emergency when it is profuse or when the patient is already ill from some underlying disease. In its treatment it is important to recognise two important principles: (1) That intravascular clotting will arrest haemorrhage but that extravascular clotting is of little value. (2) That the identification of the bleeding point is essential for rational treatment.

When first seen the nose may be full of clot preserved carefully *in situ* under the mistaken impression that haemostasis is thereby encouraged. If the patient is lying back no blood may appear at the nares but inspection of the pharynx in a good light may reveal it trickling down the posterior wall of the pharynx.

Table 9.1. *Otological causes of vertigo*

	CHARACTER OF VERTIGO	COURSE OF VERTIGO	RELATIONSHIP OF VERTIGO TO HEAD POSITION	CALORIC RESPONSES	DEAFNESS	TINNITUS	CHARACTER OF DEAFNESS	PATHOLOGY
Ménière's disease	Paroxysmal with nausea and vomiting	Attacks often severe. Long periods of freedom	Absent	Abnormal responses occur in 95 per cent	Always present	Always present. Often severe	Variable. Sounds and voices distorted	Distension of endolymph system. Degenerative changes present in end organs. Nerve fibres and ganglion cells not affected
Tumours of cerebello-pontine angle	Paroxysms rare. Persistent imbalance usual	Slight in early stages, thereafter progressive	Rare	Abnormal responses occur in 100 per cent	Always present	Always present. Not often severe	Progressive	Degeneration of fibres of VIIIth nerve and associated ganglion cells. Degeneration of end organs not usual but may result from derangement of vascular supply
Vestibular neuronitis	Blackouts or drop seizures. Sometimes persistent imbalance	Attacks frequent during active stages. Recovery or long remissions usual	Absent	Abnormal responses occur in 100 per cent. Often bilateral	Cochlear symptoms and signs absent			Unknown. ? Toxic degeneration of vestibular neurones
Positional nystagmus of benign paroxysmal type	Paroxysmal	Attacks frequent during active stages. Recovery or long remissions usual	Always present	Often normal	Cochlear symptoms and signs present only when condition is associated with ear disease. Usually middle ear infection			Degeneration of maculae of otolith organs. Character of tissue changes suggestive of trauma, infection or vascular upset

The patient should sit up with his face over a large bowl and by forcible blowing expel all blood clot from each side of the nose. His comfort is improved immediately as nasal respiration is restored. Do not mix any swabs with the blood as the quantity lost into the bowl must be measured. If bleeding continues identify the side from which the blood is dripping and then inspect the nasal cavity. To facilitate examination a wool plug soaked in 4 per cent lignocaine (or Citanest, see p. 61) may be inserted into the nose for two minutes. Adrenaline is to be avoided since any temporary arrest of haemorrhage will prevent recognition of the bleeding point. A head-mirror and good source of light are essential and a nasal speculum must be used. If bleeding is so brisk as to flood the nose and obscure vision a nasal sucker facilitates the examination. Pledgets of cottonwool may be used to shut off areas from which the bleeding may be arising to ensure that the bleeding does not come from some other site.

In most cases the site of bleeding can be identified and the bleeding arrested by the insertion of a firm wool plug against the bleeding point. Used in this way under direct vision cottonwool makes a much firmer and more success-ful pack than ribbon gauze. Although applied dry the wool becomes moistened with the nasal secretions and readily slides out on traction 24 to 48 hours later. Plugs to be left *in situ* for any period should not be soaked in agents such as cocaine or adrenaline but lubrication with liquid paraffin may be used.

In many cases the shape of the nose allows a small wool plug to be inserted exactly where wanted and yet so firmly as to be secure. The patient is then able to breathe round the plug and does not suffer the inconvenience of a blocked nostril. Use of ribbon gauze, however, means that the nostril is completely blocked and is to be deplored unless all else fails. Great care must be taken to

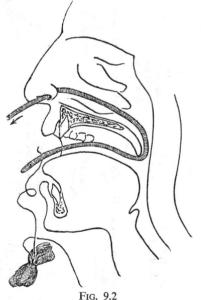

FIG. 9.2

Postnasal packing showing catheter inserted and tied to the pack.

ensure that all wool is removed in due course and for this purpose it is again essential to use the head-mirror and nasal speculum.

Recurrent epistaxis should be treated by sealing the bleeding point or surrounding vessels with the electric cautery at cherry-red heat or with a silver nitrate bead and this cauterisation is best done on removal of the wool plug when the dry area can be clearly seen. The nostrils should then be kept supple and crusting prevented by a bland ointment. The site of haemorrhage in the posterior part of the nose or from the posterior margin of the nasal septum can sometimes be seen by using a head-mirror with a good light and a post-nasal mirror. A post-nasal pack could then be introduced into the choana (Fig. 9.2). A pad of gauze or sponge 1·5 cm in diameter and about 3 cm long is tied securely to the middle of a 60 mm length of 1·25 cm tape. A lubricated catheter is passed through the nose, seized in the pharynx and withdrawn through the mouth. One end of the tape is tied securely to the catheter which is then withdrawn through the nose. The other end of the tape is similarly drawn through the other side of the nose. The gauze pad is then insinuated gently above the soft palate into the postnasal space and secured by tying the ends of the tape over the columella which can be protected by a small piece of gauze. The pack must not be too large and its size depends on the age and size of the patient. Such a pack will serve also to arrest haemorrhage after adenoidectomy. In rare cases of very profuse haemorrhage in the elderly, from ruptured athero-sclerotic vessels which cannot retract, it may be necessary to intro-duce a postnasal pack and then to pack ribbon gauze on to it from in front. More heroic measures may become necessary if this fails to control the bleeding and surgical intervention to tie off the internal maxillary artery or the anterior ethmoid artery may be necessary. It is to be stressed, however, that the most important single consideration in the arrest of epistaxis is to observe the actual site of bleeding and direct attention to it. Sedation and bed rest are essential adjuncts to treatment.

Epistaxis complicating haemorrhagic disorders. When a bleeding disease is known to exist the cautery should be avoided. Blood transfusion may be needed and a firm wool adrenaline pack at the site of bleeding.

Congenital occlusion of the posterior choanae

Failure of canalisation of the posterior choanae in the newborn results in complete nasal obstruction. The infant is unable to feed since his mouth must remain open for breathing. This emergency can be diagnosed as the nose will be seen to be full of mucus and a fine nasal catheter introduced along the floor of the nose fails to emerge along the posterior pharyngeal wall. Where one side is patent the child will be able to take his feed when the closed side of the nose is pressed against the mother's breast, nasal respiration still being possible. When the child is turned round and put to the other breast the free nostril becomes occluded against the mother and feeding becomes difficult. In such unilateral cases the child may be fed against each breast with the patent nostril unobstructed. The only permanent treatment is surgical and an early opinion should be sought.

Haemorrhage following removal of tonsils and adenoids

This calls for early recognition and prompt treatment for it can be fatal rapidly. The site of bleeding must be found and attention directed to it. Since the patient returns from the theatre lying on his side, haemorrhage may occur from the nose or the corner of the mouth. Blood in the throat will induce reflex swallowing and the up and down movement of the Adam's apple is a warning that must be heeded. An increase in the pulse rate, recorded every 15 minutes, will show that blood loss is going on. Inspection of the pharynx will confirm this and show its site of origin. A postnasal pack (p. 221, Fig. 9.2) will control adenoid bleeding and should be left in place for 24 hours. Occasionally an anaesthetic is needed for its insertion, but not for its removal.

Useless extravascular clot should be wiped out of a tonsillar fossa with gauze soaked in 4 per cent lignocaine. This minimises discomfort and by anaesthetising the exposed nerve endings facilitates further manoeuvres. Pressure on gauze applied to the fossa and kept up for 15 minutes may suffice to promote intravascular clotting. Should it fail, the patient should be returned to the operating theatre for control of haemorrhage under anaesthesia.

Foreign body in the nose

In the adult foreign bodies may enter the nose by accident and removal may be attempted with a hook, gravity being used to aid withdrawal. Most commonly the patient is a child who has inserted a pea or bead in his nose. Attempts to remove this without anaesthetic are painful and frightening and should be avoided. Forced expiration through the nose should not be used as a method of removal because the deep inspiration prior to forced expiration may cause the foreign body to be inhaled. The child should be anaesthetised and the nasal mucosa sprayed with a decongestant such as Solution of Adrenaline Hydrochloride BP. He should be placed on his back with a pillow under the shoulders (the tonsil position) so that should the foreign body inadvertently be pushed further in it will then come to lie in the postnasal space from which it can be recovered. If the patient were sitting up the foreign body might be pushed further into the nose and inhaled, a minor mishap becoming a major emergency. Forceps should not be used to remove the foreign body but a hook should be passed behind it, turned, and the object withdrawn. The light from the reflecting head-mirror facilitates this operation.

THE THROAT

Quinsy (peritonsillar abscess)

Although rare in children quinsy is not uncommon in adults and may occur even if only tonsillar remnants are present. The patient may or may not have had preceding tonsillitis. With progressive oedema of the soft palate talking and swallowing become increasingly difficult and the patient's condition is extremely uncomfortable. Examination shows the tonsil, or both tonsils to be pushed towards the mid-line and the soft palate near the upper pole inflamed and oedematous. Immediate emergency tonsillectomy with antibiotic cover is the most satisfactory form of treatment. Relief may be otherwise obtained by the insertion of a pointed scalpel into the soft palate at the upper pole of the affected tonsil and making a small cut. Local anaesthesia with a 4 per cent lignocaine spray is often used but the large amount of mucus present on the palate renders this of little value. If pus is not obtained after the knife blade has been inserted a distance of 6 mm sinus forceps may be introduced to open the abscess cavity, when a free gush of pus may be obtained. Intensive antibiotic therapy and frequent warm gargles suffice to secure resolution. The patient should be referred for tonsillectomy in due course.

Acute retro-pharyngeal abscess

The patient is a child and presents with dysphagia and inability to speak. Examination is difficult and the diagnosis best made by palpation for the swelling is not obvious and may be missed. The child should be well swaddled and placed on his back with the foot of the table raised and head down. A (protected) forefinger may be used as the only gag. The abscess should be opened without anaesthesia and care taken that no pus is inhaled. A sucker should be available. (In the adult a mid-line retropharyngeal absess is probably tuberculous and must not be opened into the pharynx.)

Swallowed foreign bodies

Sensation arising from foreign bodies impacted above the level of the crico-pharyngeus is usually referred to one side of the throat. Such foreign bodies are often visible on examination through the mouth, using a head-mirror with a powerful external source of light and laryngeal mirrors to examine the hypopharynx. Foreign bodies which the patient feels in the mid-line, however, are almost invariably impacted in the oesophagus for this is a mid-line structure. They require oesophagoscopy for their removal. The diagnosis of impacted foreign body can almost invariably be made from history and physical signs. X rays offer little additional help. It is no use X raying for swallowed fish bones for they are not radio-opaque. Meat bones and radio-opaque foreign bodies produce their clamant symptoms. X rays are not needed and indeed a barium swallow renders subsequent oesophagoscopy more difficult. The axiom is that *if the patient says he has swallowed a foreign body and can still feel it then that foreign body is present and the patient is to be believed.* A tired house officer who has been called to Casualty in the night by a patient kept awake by an impacted fish bone may say that the swallowed bone has scratched and gone on. This mistake must be avoided. If the patient says the fish bone is still there, then it is there.

Where the patient indicates that the foreign body is in the throat meticulous examination is required for which a head-mirror is indispensable. Sharp foreign bodies such as fish bones, even minute ones, often find their way into lymphoid follicles at the base of the tongue or in the tonsils. Much time should be spent examining carefully each part of the tonsils and the base of the tongue, using small pharyngeal mirrors to observe otherwise inaccessible parts. Local anaesthesia using a spray of 4 per cent lignocaine is often useful to facilitate this examination and manipulation of the tonsils to expose each surface. The patient wearing an upper denture is not uncommonly the one who swallows a sizeable piece of bone, for his dental plate prevents detection of the foreign body by contact with the hard palate at the early stage when rejection is possible. By the time the patient feels the bone against the soft palate the mechanism of deglutition has been initiated and it is too late to stop the bone being swallowed.

EMERGENCIES IN DISEASE OF THE LARYNX

No emergency can be more urgent than that caused by acute laryngeal obstruction. This may be associated with the following conditions:

Congenital laryngeal stridor.
Impacted foreign body.
Acute oedema of the larynx (from quinsy and trauma, or allergy).
Retro-pharyngeal abscess.
Diphtheritic and streptococcal laryngitis (pp. 418 and 433).
Acute on chronic obstruction.

Congenital laryngeal stridor

Congenital stridor occurs when a web persists across the anterior junction of the vocal cords. Where respiration is adequate no treatment is necessary as the enlargement of the larynx both actual and relative will result in eventual disappearance of the stridor. Diagnosis, however, is essential and can be made by direct laryngoscopy.

Impacted foreign body

When small a foreign body may cause complete laryngeal obstruction by superadded spasm of the larynx. In a child inversion and a sharp blow between the shoulder blades may dislodge it. A large impacted body such as a denture or the epiglottis (following explosion) may be disimpacted by the finger. A foreign body may be pushed into the oesophagus whence it can be recovered. Masseter spasm may prevent this. Prompt opening of the airway by laryngotomy ('mini-tracheostomy', p. 737) below the level of impaction will save life and will also permit removal of the foreign body. Alternatively, a classical tracheostomy (p. 737) may be performed with subsequent removal of the obstruction under direct laryngoscopy. Children are the common victims of inhaled foreign bodies and a history may be difficult to obtain. Where a child has been known to be playing with an object which has disappeared, radiological and if necessary bronchoscopic investigations are essential.

Impaction of a piece of meat in the larynx is a not uncommon cause of sudden death. There were 297 such cases in adults in Britain in 1972. The elderly victim in trying to swallow something solid suddenly becomes unable to breathe. The fact that he cannot groan or speak is significant. He pitches forward on to the table clutching his throat. This sudden collapse when eating is not due to a so-called 'café coronary' but to laryngeal obstruction ('food asphyxia'). Recognition of this has enabled some victims to be rescued either by removal of the piece of meat with the middle and index fingers or by the manoeuvre of Heimlich (1975) which depends on a quick upward thrust on the diaphragm by pressing inwards and upwards on the epigastrium. The sudden rise of intrathoracic pressure ejects the bolus. If these measures fail immediate tracheostomy must be performed.

Acute oedema of the larynx

Acute oedema of the larynx is particularly prone to occur in the infant or young child (p. 419) where the lax sub-mucosa connective tissue readily swells. Early tracheostomy has been superseded by prompt endotracheal intubation using a polythene catheter. The polythene is well tolerated unlike earlier rubber catheters and may be left *in situ* for several days. Tracheostomy is not without risk in the infant and infection and difficulties with detubation may arise. Systemic penicillin in large doses may have a profound and dramatic effect in reducing laryngeal oedema and preventing the need for intubation.

Acute epiglottitis

See p. 434.

Acute on chronic laryngeal obstruction

The commonest cause of chronic progressive laryngeal obstruction is carcinoma in the elderly male. Slowly progressive laryngeal obstruction can be compensated for to an astonishing degree, the patient learning to breathe through a progressively smaller hole. Sudden reduction of the lumen to a similar size would cause death from asphyxia. Similarly, bilateral recurrent nerve paralysis following thyroidectomy results in complete laryngeal obstruction on inspiration, the valve-like shape of the vocal cords results in inspired air forcing them together. In both these conditions tracheostomy (p. 737) is essential pending further planned treatment.

LEWIS CITRON

REFERENCE

HEIMLICH, H. J. (1975). A life-saving maneuver to prevent food-choking. *Journal of the American Medical Association,* **234,** 398.

CHAPTER 10

Cardiovascular Emergencies

(For Circulatory Arrest see p. 724)

SYNCOPE

(For Cough Syncope see p. 288)

(For Micturition and Prostatic Syncope see p. 289)

CARDIOVASCULAR syncope is ' loss of consciousness caused by an acute decrease of cerebral blood flow '. This flow depends on cardiac output and systemic vascular resistance. When peripheral blood vessels are dilated and the cardiac output is unchanged or reduced, syncope will result from diminished blood flow to the brain. An acute fall in cardiac output without peripheral vasodilatation may have the same effect. The commonest kind of syncope is the simple faint or vasovagal attack but there are many other causes, which may be listed as follows:

DISTURBANCES OF RHYTHM		Cardiac standstill
		(Ventricular fibrillation. Heart block)
		Extreme bradycardia
		(Heart block. Sinus node arrest)
		Extreme ventricular tachycardia
REFLEX		Vasovagal faint
		Micturition syncope
		Orthostatic hypotension
		Carotid sinus syndrome
OBSTRUCTIVE		
	Intracardiac	Aortic stenosis
		Hypertrophic obstructive cardiomyo-pathy
		Tumours
		Pulmonary embolism
		Obliterative pulmonary hypertension
	Extracardiac	Tamponade
		Constrictive pericarditis
		Cough syncope
CEREBROVASCULAR		Carotid or vertebral artery stenosis or kinking
		Cerebral embolism

The vasovagal attack (simple faint or vasomotor syncope)

The common faint, associated with bradycardia and a sudden fall of blood pressure is due to rapid vasodilatation in muscle. It may be initiated by an emotional upset which causes a powerful autonomic discharge, producing vagal stimulation accompanied by depression of the vasomotor centre, bradycardia, sweating, fall in blood pressure, dizziness and loss of consciousness. Although there is vasodilatation in muscle and the splanchnic bed, the skin vessels are intensely constricted so that there is pallor and sweating. Bradycardia from excessive vagal action contributes to the effect of the fall in blood pressure. The onset is always gradual and preceded by nausea and sometimes vomiting. In severe faints, cerebral blood flow may be so diminished as to induce an epileptiform convulsion (p. 308). The pulse is always slow, sometimes exceedingly so, but cardiac standstill does not occur.

Treatment. This is merely to lay the patient flat when consciousness will automatically return. Unconsciousness removes the trigger mechanism and acetylcholine produced by vagal stimulation is rapidly destroyed by cholinesterases and so the attack is self-limiting. The erect posture, during or after a faint, can be very dangerous since it may then be impossible to maintain a satisfactory cerebral blood flow. Any patient who threatens to faint should be promptly laid flat. Elevation of the legs may hasten the return of consciousness by increasing the venous return to the heart. Although atropine has a dramatic vagal-blocking action the patient usually recovers before it could have time to work.

Those who are predisposed to these attacks should avoid stuffy atmospheres and prolonged standing in crowds. While the characteristic prodromal symptoms, the cold, clammy skin, slow pulse and small pupils, with rapid recovery on lying down make the diagnosis clear, anyone who has a faint should be assessed for serious trouble such as gastrointestinal haemorrhage, coronary occlusion or a cerebral vascular accident.

Hypersensitivity of the carotid sinus

This may be tested for in persons subject to syncope by carotid sinus *massage* (p. 714). This triggers powerful vasodepressive reflexes, leading to a rapid fall in blood pressure and/or extreme bradycardia producing what is, to all intents, a vasovagal attack. In those who seem specially liable to vasovagal attacks it is wise to have the patient supine and to look for bradycardia and a fall of blood pressure rather than syncope. The hypersensitivity usually has no obvious cause but sometimes it occurs temporarily after cardiac infarction. Occasionally there is a carotid body tumour. Prevention may be achieved by a sympathomimetic agent such as ephedrine or isoprenaline. Digitalis may accentuate the symptoms.

Postural hypotension

Some people have deficient autonomic reflexes which fail to cause normal vasoconstriction on standing. When they stand up blood pools in the peripheral and splanchnic vascular beds and hypotension, leading to syncope, is the result. These autonomic abnormalities may be associated with anhidrosis and impotence (idiopathic postural hypotension). Secondary postural hypotension may result from deficient blood volume, Addison's disease or ganglion blocking drugs, as well as some neurological disorders affecting autonomic reflexes. Attacks are best prevented by a sympathomimetic drug, or, in severe cases, by compression of the abdomen and legs, as is done by an airman's suit, to counter vasodilatation on standing. 9-α fluorohydrocortisone may be effective.

ACUTE LEFT VENTRICULAR FAILURE
AND PULMONARY OEDEMA

This is precipitated by sudden insults to the left ventricle, notably cardiac infarction and hypertensive crises, including those due to a phaeochromocytoma (p. 356). The sudden increase in the left atrial and pulmonary venous pressure causes dyspnoea from acute pulmonary oedema. Other causes of acute pulmonary oedema are mitral stenosis, especially in pregnancy, cardiomyopathy, space-occupying lesions in the left side of the heart, aspiration of liquid vomit (Mendelson's syndrome, p. 571) and ingestion of some poisons (p. 463). (For cardiac failure in beriberi see p. 648.)

Whatever the cause the symptoms are the same. There may have been a period of exertion, especially when the attack occurs in a pregnant woman who has mitral stenosis. Often, the patient wakes after two to three hours sleep with an irritating dry cough, restlessness and a sense of uneasiness; then the attack develops, the patient becoming progressively more dyspnoeic so that he has to sit up or stand to get his breath. All his accessory muscles of respiration come into use. He is very distressed, sweating and pale from vasoconstriction, secondary to heart failure. The sputum is frothy and often blood stained.

Slipping down from the semi-recumbent position, depression of the respiratory centres by sleep and a pulmonary venous pressure in excess of the osmotic pressure of the plasma are all factors which favour accumulation of oedema fluid in the lungs. This fluid interferes with the normal stretch reflexes in the alveoli and so causes dyspnoea.

Early in the attack pronounced wheezing may give an erroneous impression of bronchial asthma (p. 194). Differentiation is usually possible from the history of a recent cardiac illness such as a cardiac infarction, the absence of a history of true asthma and the finding of evidence of cardiac disease such as a loud, early diastolic gallop rhythm or the signs of mitral stenosis.

In mitral stenosis, pulmonary oedema is not due to left ventricular failure but to sudden increase in pulmonary venous pressure, secondary to impairment of left atrial output as the result of obstruction at the mitral valve. Attacks are favoured by tachycardia, which, by reducing the filling time of the ventricle, tends to increase pulmonary venous pressure further. Other precipitating causes are an increase in circulating blood volume, high cardiac output and salt retention (as in pregnancy), chest infections, excessive exertion and the onset of rapid atrial fibrillation. A further cause is acute subvalvar mitral regurgitation due to chordal rupture or papillary muscle infarction. The sudden onset of acute pulmonary oedema with an ejection type of systolic murmur at the cardiac apex suggests the diagnosis. Left ventricular function may be adequate and pulmonary oedema is due to the transmission of high pressures directly into the left atrium and pulmonary veins (Goodwin 1968). Acute pulmonary oedema would be commoner in mitral stenosis than it is, were it not for the long-standing atrial hypertension, increased compliance of the atrium, lung lymphatic enlargement, chronic thickening of the alveolar-capillary membranes and regional vascular changes, all of which tend to be associated with chronic interstitial oedema, but which reduce the tendency to acute massive alveolar oedema.

Unacclimatised persons with normal hearts exercising at high altitude may suffer from pulmonary oedema ('the pulmonary oedema of mountains'). The mechanism is not fully understood but pulmonary hypertension is always present. Treatment is by oxygen and diuretics with descent to lower altitude.

Treatment

This is to use immediate measures to improve cardiac function and reduce pulmonary congestion. The patient should be propped up at once and given oxygen. The i v injection of 0·25 g of theophylline with ethylenediamine (Aminophylline), slowly, is of great value and may terminate the attack. A 'bloodless venesection' by placing sphygmomanometer cuffs on the thighs is also of value. A cuff should be pumped up to a pressure midway between the systolic and diastolic arterial pressures so that it produces venous congestion in the limb without impeding arterial inflow. Cuffs should be inflated and deflated alternately every 10 minutes. In this way an appreciable amount of blood can be trapped in the limbs, away from the lungs, so that the procedure acts in the same way as classical venesection. If rapid atrial fibrillation is present, and particularly if this has just developed, **digoxin** should be given i m or i v if necessary, provided that the patient has not been receiving any for three weeks before the attack. Half a mg may be given, well diluted, over a period of five minutes, and followed by a further 0·25 mg six to eight hours later. Morphine may be needed to allay restlessness but it can cause vomiting and is dangerous if there is obstructive airways disease (p. 197).

DIGITALIS. Digitalis therapy in acute pulmonary oedema is mainly indicated in patients who have mitral stenosis with rapid atrial fibrillation of recent onset. In patients in whom pulmonary oedema is due to left ventricular failure, the use of i v digoxin may further increase the load on the left ventricle by peripheral vasoconstriction. In left ventricular failure, following acute cardiac infarction, i v digitalis is often frowned upon because of the possible dangers of ventricular tachycardia or fibrillation. Except where there is also hypokalaemia, the risk has possibly been over emphasised and such arrhythmias are more likely to be due to a hypoxic myocardium than to the effects of digitalis. But vagal stimulation tends to occur in acute cardiac infarction and may be exceedingly disadvantageous. I v digitalis, which tends to increase vagal effects, should be avoided in the early stages of the disease. This in no way contraindicates the use of digitalis by mouth in patients with cardiac infarction, in many of whom it is clearly of great merit.

DIURETICS. With these measures, the average attack of acute left ventricular failure can usually be brought rapidly under control. It is wise to give also a diuretic, which will take effect during the ensuing 12 hours and tend to maintain improvement and prevent further attacks. **Frusemide** (Lasix) 20 to 60 mg i v, has a rapid and intense action and is highly suitable for this purpose. This will produce a diuresis which starts in 30 minutes and is complete within 90 minutes to two hours. An oral dose of frusemide, given at the same time as the injection, would ensure prolongation of the diuresis. Ethacrynic acid (Edecrin) may also be used in this way. Other treatment is by IPPR (intermittent positive pressure respiration) and anti-foaming agents such as alcohol vapour by a mask.

The patient should subsequently take a low sodium diet. Every effort should be made to investigate and treat the underlying cause in addition to any associated conditions such as severe anaemia, chest infection or bacterial endocarditis.

VALVOTOMY. Pulmonary oedema in severe mitral stenosis is due to mechanical obstruction rather than myocardial failure. If medical measures fail to end an acute attack valvotomy becomes essential, especially in early pregnancy when oedema may develop suddenly. Warning signs are persistent tachycardia, basal râles and wheezing, dyspnoea at rest, orthopnoea and haemoptysis in a patient with tight mitral stenosis.

HYPOTENSIVE DRUGS. Left ventricular failure is usually associated with some systemic hypertension but not when severe cardiac infarction is the cause. When a usually normotensive patient develops left ventricular failure, not due to cardiac infarction, the significance of any rise of pressure is doubtful. In hypertensive failure the pressure readings tend to be higher than when some other condition is causing the failure. There will be other evidence such as fundal changes of hypertensive disease and the attack will be relieved by reduction in blood pressure. This reduction must be achieved rapidly by giving a small dose of a ganglion blocking agent such as **hexamethonium** i v. Since these patients are often very sensitive to such drugs and have a high degree of sympathetic tone and peripheral vasoconstriction, very small doses may be effective and moderate doses may cause an unwelcome fall of blood pressure. The usual initial i m dose is 5 to 10 mg, or the drug may be injected i m at the rate of 1 mg a minute while the effect on blood pressure is noted. Alternatively, **pentolinium** (Ansolysen), which is more powerful weight for weight than hexamethonium, may be used but, since the dose for an equivalent effect is one tenth that of hexamethonium, only very small doses, in the order of 0·5 to 1 mg are required (see also p. 382).

Methyldopa (Aldomet) has been used i v for the treatment of acute hypertensive crises but it requires two to three hours to become fully effective and is not, therefore, likely to be of help in an emergency. The best drug for an immediate effect is probably Diazoxide (Eudemine) which can be given in a single i v dose of 300 mg (see also p. 382). This causes an immediate fall of blood pressure lasting 4 to 12 hours. Peripheral vascular resistance, systemic blood pressure and end-diastolic left ventricular pressure are reduced while renal plasma flow is maintained. Diazoxide tends to improve the response to the usual hypotensive drugs. (It also causes moderate hyperglycaemia.)

In severe heart failure glucagon may be considered (p. 347). **Phentolamine** (Rogitine), an alpha-adrenergic blocking agent, has been used successfully in severe heart failure due to ischaemic heart disease. Reduction in systemic vascular resistance due to excessive sympathetic tone leads to an increase in cardiac output. Initially administration is by i v infusion of 5 mg followed by 0·1 to 2·0 mg per minute as required. The systemic blood pressure in the supine position must be carefully watched; a reduction of 25 mm Hg (mean) has been advised.

Careful observation will be necessary to determine whether other methods of treatment for left ventricular failure will be required once the blood pressure has been reduced. Further oral hypotensive therapy will be needed in the ensuing days. Most patients with hypertensive left ventricular failure subsequently require digitalis and diuretics in addition to hypotensive therapy. For acute pulmonary oedema caused by a phaeochromocytoma see p. 356.

Left ventricular failure due to acute cardiac infarction is commonly accompanied by cardiac pain and often extreme hypotension and circulatory failure so that it may be necessary to nurse the patient flat. The relief of pain by morphine or pethidine is a paramount need, but, it should be remembered that large doses of morphine may produce undesirable vagal stimulation while pethidine may lower blood pressure and thus the smallest dose consistent with relieving pain and anxiety should be used.

The management of the crisis due to acute coronary occlusion is discussed later but in contrast to left ventricular failure due to hypertension, the blood pressure may have to be supported by pressor agents rather than reduced by hypotensive drugs.

ACUTE CORONARY OCCLUSION

Coronary occlusion most commonly results from thrombosis consequent upon atherosclerotic disease of the coronary arteries. Rarer causes are coronary embolism, dissecting aneurysm and coronary arteritis. (For ECG changes see pp. 111 and 236.)

The commonest presenting symptom is intense, crushing, praecordial pain often radiating up to the neck or jaw and down to the left or both arms, and coming on both at rest or on effort. It may go through to the back but rarely spreads down to the abdomen (p. 110). Rest does not relieve the pain which continues relentlessly and is accompanied by sweating, pallor, and great distress. There is often dyspnoea also from left ventricular insufficiency. Disturbance of consciousness may occur from a sudden fall in cardiac output and cerebral blood flow, while excessive vagal action, secondary to the infarction, may further reduce output. Conduction defects may cause Stokes-Adams attacks. Vomiting is common and may be preceded by flatulence so that the patient calls his trouble ' indigestion '. The pain has to be distinguished from that of acute pericarditis, pulmonary embolism, dissecting aneurysm and acute cholecystitis and sometimes from that of hiatus hernia.

Treatment

Early management in specially equipped coronary care units has reduced mortality to 15-20 per cent but many patients with severe infarction die in the first one or two hours before admission. Immediate treatment in the home and ready access to resuscitative facilities is of great importance.

Morphine, 10 mg subcutaneously or 3 mg i v, while of undoubted value in relieving pain and distress has a number of variable effects in coronary occlusion. A fall in blood pressure may occur, the heart rate may increase, and cardiac output may increase or remain unchanged.

In some patients, perhaps from vagal stimulation, morphine may exaggerate the bradycardia or heart block caused by the infarct and a distastrous fall in blood pressure may result (Shillingford, 1965). Morphine may also induce vomiting, which in turn, perpetuates the vagal stimulation. It also depresses the respiratory centre and may further compromise respiratory function. Careful observation is thus necessary after giving morphine. While the patient should be kept as flat as possible to maintain the blood pressure, the sitting position is best if there is left ventricular failure. This therapeutic paradox must be resolved by judging each case on its own merits. The recumbent position is the one usually employed. Acute left ventricular failure should be managed as described on p. 230. Morphine may be combined with promethazine 10 to 25 mg to reduce vomiting. Pethidine 50-100 mg i m or by mouth has little euphoriant effect and may cause hypotension. Pentazocine (Fortral) 50 mg by mouth or 30 mg i v tends to increase pulmonary arterial pressure and so may be undesirable also. Morphine remains the best drug when used with discretion. Its disadvantages may be partly avoided by using papaveretum (Omnopon) or diamorphine (heroin).

PRESSOR DRUGS. Severe hypotension formerly called for the use of pressor drugs. Originally noradrenaline in dextrose solution was used successfully but the necessarily slow infusion is difficult to give. Patients tend to become dependent on it, developing tachyphylaxis and requiring increasing doses to maintain their blood pressure. Local skin necrosis may occur at the site of infusion (p. 50 and 85). It may cause dangerous arrhythmias.

Metariminol (Aramine), like nor-adrenaline, has a positive ino-tropic action through stimulation of beta-adrenergic receptors in the heart. It has a vasoconstrictive action and does not cause dysrrhythmias. Metariminol is given in a dose of 1 to 10 mg i m, i v or in an i v infusion. Some feel that it does not cause sufficient peri-pheral vasoconstriction to maintain coronary blood flow and so prefer noradrenaline. Other pressor amines may act by releasing nor-adrenaline from tissue stores and prolonged use may lead to failure of response because of exhaustion of these stores. More knowledge of the haemodynamics in cardiac infarction is needed before the exact place of pressor agents becomes clear. They may even aggra-vate the situation by further reducing tissue perfusion through vaso-constriction and there is much to be said for using isoprenaline which causes peripheral vasodilatation. While pressor agents may be unavoidable every effort should be made to maintain good cardiac action and adequate blood pressure by correction of arrhythmias, adjustment of acid-base balance and effective oxygen therapy.

The clinical picture does not always follow the haemodynamic state. Sometimes cardiac output is high while blood pressure is low; peripheral resistance may be falling as cardiac output falls. A slow heart rate may be accompanied by hypotension, the pressure rising as the rate subsequently increases. Possibly reflexes from receptors on the surface of the left ventricle may be involved in causing bradycardia and hypotension.

It has been concluded that in the absence of clinical ' shock ' cardiac output is normal or low but blood pressure is maintained. Patients with cardiogenic shock have very low cardiac outputs, poor peripheral compensatory vasoconstriction and heart failure. Such patients also have arterial blood hypoxaemia, metabolic acidosis (p. 19), lactic acidaemia and hyperglycaemia. The place of intra-aortic balloon pumping is still under investigation.

OTHER CARDIAC DRUGS

DIGITALIS. Because of electrolyte disorder, tendency to ventricular arrhythmias, and lowered threshold for toxicity, digitalis is probably best avoided in the absence of congestive heart failure and/or supra-ventricular tachycardias (Pertroth and Harrison, 1973).

GLUCAGON. This has a transient effect in increasing cardiac output without increasing ectopic beats. It is not antagonised by beta-adrenergic blocking drugs. It must be given by i v infusion (1 to 2 mg/hour) but may cause vomiting. Close watch must be kept on the blood sugar which tends to rise. It may be of value in severe heart failure or shock.

OXYGEN. Although some doubt exists as to the effect of oxygen in cardiac infarction, for it can cause a fall in output and a rise in blood pressure, current practice is to give a concentration of 30 to 40 per cent at 10 litres per minute via a facial mask (p. 740).

HEPARIN. Some hold that heparin may diminish cardiac pain by causing coronary vasodilatation but its best use would seem to be for the prevention of subsequent venous thrombosis or embolism. A recent controlled trial (Medical Research Council, 1969) of short-term use of heparin followed by phenindione for 28 days showed a significant reduction in thromboembolic incidents though not in the total mortality from all causes. Hydrocortisone must not be included in a heparin drip (see p. 242).

STREPTOKINASE was shown in one trial to be superior to heparin for acute myocardial infarction. Heparin alone has not been shown to lessen mortality significantly so that streptokinase, although not new therapy, may find a place in the future. Details of its administration are on p. 243.

ARRHYTHMIAS. About 90 per cent of patients with acute myocardial infarction develop some disturbance of rhythm. The commonest form is the premature ventricular contraction. Ventricular ectopics are not always serious. They may be reduced in frequency by lignocaine i v (see p. 255).

Some form of atrioventricular block occurs in around 20 per cent of patients. Sinus bradycardia, 2 : 1 heart block or complete heart block may occur. A/V heart block is more common in patients with inferior or posterior rather than with anterior infarction. Fascicular block (p. 262) and bundle branch block may occur, the latter carrying a poor prognosis. Bradycardia should be treated with atropine 0·2 mg i v whatever the cause but care should be taken in the presence of Mobitz type 2 block (Fig. 10.11), for atropine may increase the degree of block. A temporary pacemaker should therefore be inserted. Pacing should be employed for any patient in complete heart block with a ventricular rate of less than 40/min. or if heart failure is present. The presence of bifascicular or trifascicular block (p. 264) indicates the need for pacing if conduction defects increase. Isoprenaline by infusion at the rate of 1

μg/min may be of value in bradycardia. The elevation of ventricular rate and blood pressure may also reduce the incidence of ventricular ectopics released by the slow rate.

Supraventricular arrhythmias, particularly atrial fibrillation, may be associated with pump failure and shock, when they carry a poor prognosis. Management is discussed on p. 252. Patients whose pain is of short duration and who have no evidence of circulatory disturbance or arrhythmias may sometimes be managed at home but frequent observation in the first five days is essential.

Prognosis

Recent work has shown that three main factors, arrhythmia, respiratory disorder and acidosis are important in prognosis. Arrhythmia, particularly if associated with bradycardia, may be followed by a catastrophic fall in cardiac output which may be masked clinically until cardiac arrest occurs. This complication may be prevented by careful monitoring of the ECG, by avoidance of vagotonic drugs and stimuli and the use of atropine if the heart slows to below 60 beats per minute.

Respiratory abnormalities cause patchy pulmonary oedema and this means that blood passes through vessels inaccessible to pulmonary gas for exchange. This predisposes to arterial desaturation and impaired pulmonary function.

Metabolic acidosis occurs when there is cardiogenic shock with low cardiac output and poor regional perfusion. This further lowers cardiac output and compromises ventricular function. It calls for treatment with sodium bicarbonate (p. 727). Tachycardia increases oxygen demand and may increase the size of the infarct and so its control is important. Factors which reduce oxygen demands and increase oxygen supply to the myocardium may reduce the size of the infarct as may glucose, insulin and potassium which enhance anaerobic metabolism and increase substrate transport (Braunwold & Makoro, 1974).

The management of patients with acute cardiac infarction is now under review and the general opinion favours special intensive care units for the first few days. During this period arrhythmias may occur in patients whose initial attack was not severe. They can be treated satisfactorily in a special unit equipped for instant resuscitation. The availability of mobile coronary care systems to bring early aid to patients is an important aspect of therapy. There is, therefore, an increasing argument in favour of treating any patient with acute cardiac infarction in hospital. After five to seven days many patients can be nursed at home.

9

UNSTABLE ANGINA. CRESCENDO ANGINA.
INTERMEDIATE SYNDROME

Unstable angina occurs irregularly with increasing frequency and often at rest. It responds poorly to nitrites. It probably represents unstable ischaemia but, contrary to previous belief, many patients do not develop myocardial infarction. Enzyme changes do not occur.

Patients should preferably be admitted to hospital for rest, monitoring, relief of pain and correction of arrhythmias. Pain may be relieved by simple analgesics but morphine may be needed. Beta-adrenergic blocking agents are of value in aiding resolution of the episode, in preventing arrhythmias and perhaps diminishing the area of ischaemia. Propanolol (Inderal) may be given starting with 10 mg eight-hourly and increasing gradually. A third heart sound indicates left ventricular insufficiency and is an indication for digitalis. This may help patients with nocturnal angina in which there is often an element of left ventricular failure. Propping the patient up in bed and the use of diuretics may also help. If, despite full medical measures, angina increases, emergency coronary arteriography may be needed with a view to coronary artery bypass grafting. The exact indications are not yet fully agreed.

Persistent pain may also occur in patients with severe aortic incompetence or stenosis.

PERIPHERAL CIRCULATORY FAILURE
' SHOCK '

A useful definition of shock is ' a state characterised by protracted hypotension, prostration, cold moist skin, pallor, collapse of visible veins, reduced urine formation and clouding of consciousness '. The symptoms reflect the basic underlying disturbance which is poor perfusion of tissue by blood to a point where physiological and metabolic abnormalities in tissue function appear.

The causes underlying shock are not fully understood but there is no doubt that they are multiple and so a unified concept is not possible. Shock may be divided into the following varieties: cardiogenic, hypovolaemic, neurogenic, anaphylactic, bacteraemic and haemo-obstructive.

Cardiogenic shock implies the characterisic circulatory state following a major cardiac insult such as a large cardiac infarction. Hypovolaemic shock occurs when fluid is suddenly withdrawn in large quantities from the circulation as in massive haemorrhage, extreme dehydration, or extensive burns. Neurogenic shock is related to vasodilatation and may occur after spinal anaesthesia or the use of ganglion-blocking drugs. Perforation of a peptic ulcer or acute pancreatitis may produce a ' shock-like state '. Anaphylactic shock may follow the administration of non-human serum which causes the release of histamine. This, in turn, causes profound peripheral vasodilatation and fall of blood pressure as well as bronchospasm and angioneurotic oedema. Bacteraemic shock denotes a profound failure of the circulation consequent upon overwhelming septicaemia or bacteraemia.

In many types of shock, and particularly the hypovolaemic type, there appears to be pooling of blood in certain circumscribed areas. Vasodilatation is probably the basis for this and the prototype is anaphylactic shock. It has been thought that there is a constriction of small hepatic veins and pooling of blood in the portal venous system with resulting diminution of venous return to the heart, reduced cardiac output and hypotension. Experimental injections of histamine and the absorption of toxic substances may cause similar changes.

Treatment

Cardiogenic shock demands maintenance of adequate cardiac output, blood pressure and regional perfusion, control of respiratory function and regulation of acid-base balance. Maintenance of peripheral vascular tone is also important and drugs which combine a central inotropic cardiac stimulant action with a peripheral vasoconstrictive one are theoretically ideal. But it may be difficult to decide whether peripheral vasoconstriction to maintain blood pressure will offset the possible deleterious effect of an increased afterload on a failing left ventricle. Noradrenaline, although of value in this respect, has certain disadvantages so that metaraminol (Aramine) may be more satisfactory. Treatment must also be given for any coexisting left ventricular failure. Hydrocortisone, in large doses, has been advocated to reduce peripheral vasodilatation and venous pooling but it is uncertain whether it is beneficial. Unfortunately, severe and persistent cardiogenic shock due to cardiac infarction often fails to respond to any known methods of treatment. Newer drugs which improve cardiac performance such as phentolamine (Rogitine, p. 357), glucagon (p. 347) and salbutamol may be tried. If shock is due to or complicated by perforation of the ventricular septum (severe heart failure, raised jugular venous pressure and pan-systolic murmur at the left sternal edge) or by mitral regurgitation (pulmonary oedema and systolic murmur at the apex) appropriate surgical correction can reverse it.

Hypovolaemic shock requires replacement of the necessary fluid, usually blood, dextrose or plasma. Needless to say, underlying diseases such as diabetes, massive septicaemia or adrenocortical failure must be recognised and treated. It is worth recalling that sudden circulatory collapse in old people may be due to massive concealed gastrointestinal haemorrhage or an overwhelming septicaemia. In the latter case it is wise to take blood cultures and to start massive antibiotic therapy.

In experimental haemorrhagic shock in animals, Mellander and Lewis (1963) have shown that there is impairment and even abolition of the responses both to the precapillary arterial sphincters (resistance vessels) and the postcapillary venous sphincters (capitance vessels) of skeletal muscles. These studies suggest that a pressor drug producing vasoconstriction might be useful in the early stages of haemorrhagic shock by aiding the maintenance of venous return and maintaining cardiac output. The ideal pressor drug should also possess inotropic properties to stimulate a failing myocardium in the later stages of shock. Where bacteraemic shock is suspected, cortisone in large doses should be given i v and combined with massive antibiotic therapy.

Adrenolytic and pressor agents have been shown to be effective in preventing tissue necrosis, possibly because imbalance between precapillary and postcapillary sphincter tone may be corrected by sympatholytic drugs with resultant improved capillary tissue perfusion. Many of the abnormalities in severe shock may result from inadequate and unequal tissue perfusion and it is possible that vasoconstrictor drugs may aggravate matters by reducing the blood flow to vital areas. Symmetrical limb gangrene, after perfusion for cardiac operations when pressor agents have been given, suggests that this explanation may be true. However, in the present state of knowledge, the use of pressor agents is still indicated in some states of shock and there is some evidence that their effect may be increased by large doses of glucocorticoids. Lillehei et al. (1965) (p. 565), in pointing out the importance of blood flow as well as blood pressure, have suggested that when blood pressure and volume have been restored, a vasodilator (phenoxybenzamine (Dibenyline)) should also be used. The i v dose is 1·0 mg/kg diluted well and infused slowly. Large doses of hydrocortisone (0·5 to 1·0 g daily) should also be given (see also p. 430). Severe shock may be followed by renal tubular necrosis and anuria for which dialysis will be needed. Careful watch should, therefore, be kept on urinary output, blood urea and blood potassium levels.

ACUTE PULMONARY EMBOLISM

Pulmonary embolism is apt to complicate operations and child-birth but may occur also in any patient in bed for a long time, especially if in heart failure. The clinical picture depends upon whether infarction occurs and, if so, its site. With infarction, there is acute pleural pain, fever, tachycardia, haemoptysis and perhaps a pleural rub. Without infarction, the main features are those of syncope caused by circulatory obstruction. There may be some insignificant praecordial discomfort but pleuritic pain does not occur. The blood pressure suddenly falls and consciousness is clouded. There are signs of acute right ventricular failure with increased jugular venous pressure and a loud gallop rhythm over the right ventricle at the left sternal edge. Pulmonary valve closure may be slightly accentuated by the acute pulmonary hypertension. True dyspnoea is uncommon but tachypnoea and hyperventilation occur. Death may follow

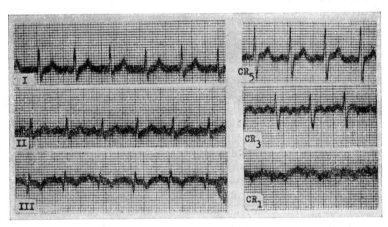

FIG. 10.1

ECG in acute pulmonary embolism showing S waves and upright T waves in lead I and Q waves and inverted T waves in lead III. There is an rsr pattern in CR_1 and T wave inversion in CR_1 and CR_3. CR_5 shows a deep S wave.
(Reproduced from *Clinical Disorders of the Pulmonary Circulation*. Ed. Daley, Goodwin and Steiner, by permission of J. & A. Churchill, London.)

rapidly but, in those who survive, the picture is one of hypotension with acute right ventricular failure.

If taken early in the attack, the electrocardiogram is extremely valuable in diagnosis, showing S waves in standard lead I and Q waves with inversion of the T waves in lead III, the ST segment remaining isoelectric (Fig. 10.1). The chest leads show evidence of acute right ventricular embarrassment with inversion of T waves in right and central precordial leads. The appearances may be mistaken for those diaphragmatic cardiac infarction but it should be remembered that, in pulmonary embolism, ST segment elevation in lead III does not occur and Q waves in VF are not usually present. The characteristic S1, Q3 pattern in the standard leads and T wave inversion in the central praecordial leads should permit further differentiation (Fig. 10.1) but sometimes the changes of true cardiac infarction may also occur.

Massive pulmonary embolism is seldom the first event in the thrombo-embolic story. If the patient has been under observation, a tell-tale increase in the pulse rate or slight fever, possibly associated with mild, dizzy attacks or unexplained ' dyspnoea ' which have been dismissed as unimportant, point to small previous emboli which have culminated in a larger one. The acute right ventricular failure which ensues is the result of organic obstruction to the pulmonary vessels by blood clot. Vasoconstriction plays little part.

Treatment

This is to give vasopressor drugs to increase systemic blood pressure, digoxin to support the right ventricle, and i v heparin to discourage further thrombosis and the spread of emboli from the original thrombus. Circulatory arrest may occur and call for external cardiac massage (see p. 725). Morphine is not always required, for pain may not be a prominent feature unless the infarction has involved the pleura. Respiratory stimulants will not be needed since the patient tends to hyperventilate. If the heart rate is slow, a satisfactory response may be obtained by the use of isoprenaline which has a powerful beta-adrenergic action and causes cardiac stimulation with an increase in pulse rate and cardiac output and a consequent increase in blood pressure. Although isoprenaline produces peripheral vasodilatation, this effect is always less than the effect on cardiac output so that blood pressure rises rather than falls. Isoprenaline may also be given i v in a dose of 0·05 to 0·1 mg which can be repeated. A smoother and longer action can be obtained by the use of suppositories of 2·5 to 5 mg given per rectum every three to six hours. **Heparin** must be given immediately to prevent further embolism. An initial i v dose of 10 000 units is given, followed by an infusion (preferably by a constant infusion pump (p. 342)) at a rate of 20 000 to 30 000 units in 24 hours and continued for two weeks. (If the use of hydrocortisone also is contemplated it should not be mixed in the heparin infusion as the two are incompatible.) (See p. 93.) Daily whole blood coagulation time should be estimated, aiming at a range of 15 to 25 minutes. Monitoring of coagulation time is essential since sensitivity to heparin is often reduced in the early stages of pulmonary embolism and an arbitrary dose may be too small. Following heparin oral anticoagulants should be given and continued for at least three and preferably six months.

Evidence is accumulating that **streptokinase** (Kabikinase, p. 115), which activates plasminogen, and, unlike heparin, lyses thrombi, is more effective than heparin. It may be given if the complex tests necessary for effective control are available. After 10 000 units of heparin 600 000 units of streptokinase should be given i v over a period of 30 minutes and followed by 100 000 units hourly for 72-100 hours. Control should be maintained by daily estimation of plasma thrombin time aiming at 20 to 30 seconds using a control level of 10. The initial streptokinase should be covered by chlorpheniramine (Piriton) 10 mg and hydrocortisone 100 mg to discourage allergic reactions. After 72 hours no anticoagulants or antithrombotic drugs should be given for four hours to allow the fibrinolytic system to recover and then heparin should be given by i v infusion for two weeks and followed by warfarin.

A recent multicentre trial of heparin and urokinase (which acts like streptokinase) in USA (Report 1973) showed an advantage to urokinase in terms of more rapid resolution of emboli and more complete return of haemodynamics to normal as compared with heparin but no significant difference in mortality. Urokinase is prohibitively expensive, but the use of streptokinase should be considered in massive pulmonary embolism where the need for rapid resolution is greatest and the risk of the emergency highest.

The use of **Arvin** (Ancrod, p. 145) a defibrinating agent as an alternative to heparin is under study but it must not be given unless the fibrinolytic system is intact as this is essential to remove the split products of fibrin produced by defibrination. Arvin is probably less effective than streptokinase in that it does not lyse thrombus.

Patients who do not rapidly improve on a medical regime should be considered for pulmonary embolectomy which may be combined with plication of the inferior vena cava or venous thrombectomy. Preliminary pulmonary arteriography and lung scanning will be required to localise the areas of embolisation in the lungs.

The most important aspect of pulmonary embolism is prevention. Leg vein thrombosis (p. 617) may occur during or immediately after an operation and may be present without any signs whatever. Early ambulation, elastic stockings worn in bed and frequent leg exercises are important preventive measures in any patient confined to bed. Heparin in low dosage (5 000 units 12 hourly) subcutaneously has 'been shown to reduce the incidence of venous thrombosis and possibly pulmonary embolism but monitoring of clotting time is advisable.

Venous thrombosis must not be forgotten, for appropriate anti-coagulant therapy is needed.

Repeated pulmonary emboli involving the medium sized or small pulmonary arterioles may occur silently and show themselves only by unexplained attacks of syncope. Thus, the possibility of recurrent pulmonary thrombo-embolic disease should be considered in any patient who develops unexplained syncopal attacks which are clearly not simple faints. Such syncopal attacks may be accompanied by unexplained dyspnoea for which there is no obvious clinical cause (Goodwin et al., 1963).

SYSTEMIC EMBOLISM

Systemic embolism occurs when a fragment of thrombus or tumour is discharged from the aorta, left ventricle, left atrium or pulmonary veins into the general circulation. In paradoxical embolism, a fragment from the right side of the heart or the systemic venous system crosses to the left side in patients who have a communication between the right and left sides of the heart, such as a patent foramen ovale or an atrial or ventricular septal defect. The commonest condition in which a systemic embolism arises from the right side of the circulation is the tetralogy of Fallot.

Conditions which particularly predispose to systemic embolism are obstruction to left ventricular inflow, as in mitral stenosis, atrial fibrillation or an intraventricular thrombus over a large cardiac infarct. Occasionally, atheromatous plaques or thrombi may be detached from the aorta and lodge in more peripheral arteries. Rarely, an embolus may arise from a thrombus in a pulmonary vein, while intracardiac tumours on the left side of the heart, such as left atrial myxoma, may give rise to thrombus or tumour emboli.

Atrial fibrillation predisposes to stasis in the left atrium and favours thrombosis in it. If, in addition, there is obstruction to the left ventricular inflow, as in mitral stenosis, the stage is set for systemic embolism.

The clinical picture depends on the site of the embolism. When the cerebral vessels are involved, acute hemiplegia, loss of consciousness or the results of brain stem damage may be the presenting symptoms. A renal embolus will cause acute loin pain and haematuria and an embolus to the mesenteric arterial system (p. 115) will cause the passing of blood per rectum followed by signs of intestinal obstruction. Probably the commonest systemic embolism is that which occurs in the lower limbs. In many cases, the bifurcation of the aorta is obstructed (saddle embolus). Quite often, however, the clot breaks up at the bifurcation, showering fragments into one or both femoral arteries. The attack starts suddenly with acute pain, loss of sensation and coldness of the limb involved, or both lower limbs, in the case of saddle embolus. The amount of ischaemia, and the severity of the symptoms, depend upon the size of the arteries blocked and the number of smaller arteries which receive secondary emboli. When severe obstruction is present, pain is usually intense but sensation may rapidly be lost. The limb is pale, mottled, cold and pulseless. Loss of sensation to objective testing is followed by loss of reflexes and, in severe cases, inability to move the limb. Usually the origin of the embolus will be apparent and is commonly a fibrillating atrium in association with mitral stenosis.

Treatment

Early treatment is essential if the limb is to be saved. Morphine or pethidine will be required. The limb should be exposed and on no account should any active source of heat, such as hot water bottles, be applied to it. Heating to the trunk, however, to induce reflex dilatation in the limb, may help. I v **heparin** is indicated immediately to prevent further emboli and to discourage spread of the clot. 10 000 units should be given i v and continued as for pulmonary embolism (p. 242). **Streptokinase** may prove to have a place in the treatment of systemic embolism but this has not been fully defined. Additional help can be provided by the use of **Rheomacrodex** (Powley, 1963). This high molecular weight dextran expands the circulation and discourages sludging of cells in small vessels, thus diminishing the risk of gangrene due to small vessel obstruction. One half to one litre of 10 per cent Rheomacrodex is given in 5 per cent dextrose solution by i v infusion, but it should be remembered that Rheomacrodex, in itself, has some anticoagulant properties and may potentiate the effect of heparin. The coagulation time, using the Lee and White method, should not exceed 30 minutes. Rheomacrodex must be used with care in patients with heart failure, for it expands the blood volume although subsequently acting as a diuretic. Renal tubular failure may occur if urine flow is reduced. The next step will be to control rapid atrial fibrillation, if present. by suitable doses of digoxin and to treat cardiac failure in the usual way.

The decision regarding embolectomy must on no account be left too late. Any patient who has peripheral embolism should be seen by a vascular surgeon unless satisfactory circulation returns to the limb within an hour, with increase of skin temperature, flushing and return of pulses. If ischaemia persists after three hours, despite Rheomacrodex and other measures, embolectomy should be undertaken. Undue delay may be disastrous with loss of limb or life. This is particularly true in the case of saddle embolism, where embolectomy is usually required and should be carried out as soon as the diagnosis is made. Without operation a complete persistent saddle embolus is usually fatal but a successful result can be obtained by early embolectomy.

Less severe degrees of peripheral systemic embolism may present merely with pain and a little coldness in the limb and may be mistaken for ' rheumatism ' or similar affections. Failure to recognise the true cause may delay anticoagulant or surgical treatment and lead to loss of function in the limb or even, ultimately, loss of the limb itself. Any sudden attack of pain should be considered as possible embolism and careful examination of the limb for temperature, colour and pulses should be made, especially in patients who have a predisposing cause.

DISSECTION OF THE THORACIC AORTA AND DISSECTING ANEURYSM

(For dissection of the abdominal aorta see p. 111)

Dissection of the aorta commonly occurs in persons, around the age of 60, with systemic hypertension and is due to cystic necrosis of the muscle of the media. Similar necrosis has been found in young subjects. Dissection may occur anywhere in the aorta, but it is commonest in one of three sites: immediately above the aortic valve, in the arch of the aorta and at the beginning of the descending aorta. The first and third of these sites are the most common. Although often associated with atherosclerosis, dissection is not due to this and occurs in an area free from atheroma. The attack starts with severe pain in the chest which often spreads down to the abdomen and through to the back. This may be accompanied by low blood pressure, peripheral circulatory failure, and collapse. If the dissection spreads rapidly to involve the descending aorta there may be paraplegia from interference with the intercostal and lumbar spinal arteries and anuria from dissection of the renal arteries. Intestinal infarction may also occur. The cardinal sign of dissection is disappearance, fluctuation, or inequality of the arm, neck or leg pulses. Hemiplegia may occur and consciousness may be lost if dissection involves the arteries to the brain. Sometimes the dissection spreads backwards to involve the aortic valve, causing acute aortic insufficiency and, sometimes, haemopericardium. There is often a bloodstained pleural effusion and X rays show dilatation or localised expansion in the region of the ascending aorta or arch. A double contour of the aortic wall may be seen (Fig. 10.2).

The condition must be distinguished from other causes of chest pain but the diagnosis can usually be made if the condition is thought of and the abnormality of the pulses, radiation of the pain and involvement of other organs detected. The electrocardiogram usually shows merely signs of left ventricular enlargement due to hypertension or pericarditis (if the dissection has involved the pericardium) and does not show the classical signs of major cardiac infarction unless the dissection has involved the orifice of one of the coronary arteries.

Treatment

This is aimed at relief of pain and the reduction of blood pressure. It is thought that continuing hypertension may tend to favour a further dissection and so blood pressure should be reduced to subnormal levels by one of the methods mentioned for acute left ventricular failure (p. 229). In the acute stages surgical treatment should be considered and, as soon as the diagnosis is entertained, the patient should be transferred to a centre where angiocardiography (Fig. 10.2) and appropriate surgical treatment can be carried out. The immediate medical mortality is high, about 80 per cent of patients dying within the first 24 hours. Of the small proportion who survive this period, a number may live for up to two or three years and, if the dissection appears to have re-entered the lumen of the aorta, and the patient's condition is satisfactory, there may be no indication for surgery. While acute dissection of the distal aorta may be treated conservatively acute dissection of the ascending aorta may call for urgent surgery and valve replacement because it often causes acute aortic regurgitation. Watch must be kept for the development, later, of an aneurysm, for progressive dissection is usually an indication for surgical treatment, as is continuing pain, involvement of branches of the aorta or increase in the size of the aneurysm. In those who survive the acute attack, and are treated medically, prolonged bed rest is important and anticoagulants should be avoided. Satisfactory blood pressure control should be maintained with hypotensive drugs. In addition the use of propanolol

(Inderal) is advisable to reduce the force of ventricular contraction and thus the impact of the pulse wave on the damaged aorta. Heart failure, if present, should be treated in the usual way. Aspiration of the haemothorax may be required in some cases.

CARDIAC TAMPONADE

Cardiac tamponade occurs in an acute form when fluid accumulates rapidly in the pericardium and compresses the heart by restricting diastolic filling. This seriously reduces cardiac output. The severity of the tamponade depends upon the rapidity with which fluid collects and upon the elasticity of the pericardium. Thus, in the normal, somewhat inelastic pericardium, the rapid accumulation of even a few hundred millilitres of blood may produce extreme tamponade. Conversely, the gradual accumulation of large amounts of fluid may by progressive stretching of the pericardium be accommodated without serious effects. Tamponade should be thought of in any patient in whom sudden circulatory failure develops with or without syncope, in association with a rapid, small volume pulse, low arterial systolic and pulse pressures and elevated venous pressure. The diagnosis becomes even more likely if a pericardial friction rub is present or if the patient is known to have had some recent involvement of the pericardium by trauma, infection or some other condition. The presence of a pericardial rub in no way denies the possibility of tamponade and, in fact, is an important clue to its presence. Typically, the venous pressure in the neck rises on inspiration and the arterial pressure diminishes (paradoxical pulse). This is due to the downward movement of the diaphragm on inspiration, tightening the pericardium on the already constricted heart and increasing the degree of compression on inspiration. The cardiac impulse is usually difficult or impossible to feel and heart sounds may be muffled. Differential diagnosis is from other causes of acute hypotension and circulatory failure with or without syncope. Myocardial failure, cardiac infarction and occult blood loss must all be considered. The raised venous pressure makes blood loss unlikely, while the characteristic signs of tamponade on respiration do not usually occur in acute myocardial failure. A third heart sound, heard in myocardial failure, is usually absent in tamponade unless there is associated myocardial disease. The electrocardiogram will show low voltage complexes with flat or slightly inverted T waves and a tachycardia. Electrical alternans is a valuable sign, the alternate QRS complexes varying either in direction or amplitude. X ray examination of the heart may show the characteristic globular heart shadow or pericardial effusion (Fig. 10.3), but the heart silhouette may be little enlarged if tamponade is due to rapid accumulation of a small amount of fluid or blood.

The diagnosis may be confirmed by ultra-sound scan or if circumstances are less urgent by angiocardiography, with injection of contrast medium into the right atrium. The collection of pericardial fluid can be seen as a clear space between the lateral cardiac shadow and the cavities of the right atrium and right ventricle (Fig. 10.3). The right ventricle appears to be ' lifted off ' the diaphragm.

Treatment

Immediate aspiration is needed for acute tamponade (p. 714). Subsequent management will depend upon the cause. It is always wise to suspect the possibility of acute tuberculous pericarditis and examination of the pericardial fluid, X ray examination of the lungs and Mantoux testing are important. When the patient is seriously ill, and the diagnosis of tuberculosis seems reasonably sure on clinical grounds, anti-tuberculous drugs should be started without delay, although, whenever possible, bacteriological or other confirmation should be obtained first.

DYSRRHYTHMIAS

The dysrrhythmias may broadly be divided into disorders of impulse formation (ectopic rhythms) and disorders of impulse conduction. The former usually produce tachycardia (tachydysrrhythmias) and the latter bradycardia (brachydysrrhythmias). Disorders of impulse conduction may be physiological (as when protective AV block develops in the presence of rapid supraventricular rhythms) or pathological as in the various forms of heart block.

TACHYDYSRRHYTHMIAS

Tachydysrrhythmias may arise in the atria, junctional tissues or ventricles. In paroxysmal atrial tachycardia, atrial fibrillation and flutter there are two main mechanisms: volleys of activity from an ectopic focus in the atria, or re-entry of excitation into an area previously refractory. It is thought that re-entry mechanisms play an important part in many dysrrhythmias. In the Wolff-Parkinson-White syndrome there is a tendency to re-entry or reciprocating tachycardia due to an anomalous pathway (bypass) which short circuits the AV node. Enhanced automaticity of conducting tissue due to electrolyte disorders, digitalis effects, hypoxia or local oedema favour the development of ectopic tachycardias. Attacks often start and stop suddenly. Atrial fibrillation and flutter are special forms of atrial tachycardia in which physiological AV block develops to protect the ventricles from the excessive rate of discharge from the ectopic focus.

Simple clinical points may help in the differential diagnosis of the type of dysrhythmia. Supraventricular tachycardias usually occur in younger people who often give a history of repeated attacks which start and stop suddenly. The function of the heart is usually not disturbed. The rhythm is quite regular and the first heart sound constant in intensity. Atrial flutter may be diagnosed by noting jugular vein pulsation at twice the ventricular rate at least. Atrial fibrillation produces a completely irregular arterial pulse. Paroxysmal ventricular tachycardia is usually associated with considerable circulatory disturbance. The rate is slower than in supraventricular tachycardia, the patients are often older and the first heart sound may vary in intensity.

SUPRAVENTRICULAR TACHYCARDIAS (see also pp. 408 and 409)

Paroxysmal atrial tachycardia. Here, the ectopic focus is in the atrium, outside the sino-atrial node. The resulting tachycardia is rapid (170) and absolutely regular. The ventricles respond to each atrial stimulus producing a regular rhythm, usually without any conduction defect, but sometimes with a 2 : 1 block (multiple atrial foci may cause irregular atrial tachycardia which clinically resembles fibrillation). Attacks may last from a few moments up to hours or, occasionally, days. They occur in patients without serious heart disease, the arrhythmia being important mainly for its unpleasant symptoms and accompanying anxiety. The cardiac output is maintained and the jugular venous pressure and the systemic blood pressure remain normal. The ECG shows normal QRS complexes at a rapid, completely regular rate with P waves (perhaps inverted) preceding each QRS complex (Fig. 10.4).

Due to digitalis. Digitalis overdosage may cause a characteristic paroxysmal tachycardia with an atrial rate of 200 to 250 per minute—i.e. slower than atrial flutter. Bidirectional tachycardia may be seen. The patient is usually seriously ill and often in severe heart failure with signs of a low cardiac output and evidence of digitalis intoxication, such as nausea and vomiting. The pulse is regular in contradistinction to that in atrial fibrillation. The ECG before the attack may or may not show signs of excessive digitalis effect as ST depression and coupled ventricular beats (Fig. 10.5). These are an important indication that digitalis should be temporarily withheld. The ECG may also show sagging ST segments and U waves of hypokalaemia. Carotid sinus massage fails to slow the atrial rate but may increase the degree of block (Oram *et al.*, 1960).

Digitalis intoxication is often precipitated by potassium depletion such as may occur after a brisk diuresis. It is more common in the elderly who have impaired renal function and a raised blood urea correlates particularly with the risk of digitalis intoxication. Digitalis blood levels are of some limited value in diagnosis: patients who are well controlled have levels of 0·5 to 2·5 ng/ml while toxic effects are usually found with levels over 2·0 ng/ml. Blood levels of digoxin may now be measured by a number of techniques, that of radio-immunoassay being employed by Chamberlain *et al.* (1970). Un-labelled digoxin of the unknown serum competes with titrated digoxin for binding sites of digoxin of digoxin-specific antibody.

The biological availability of Lanoxin brand of digoxin now (1973) being manufactured is approximately double that of earlier preparations, 80 per cent being absorbed as compared with 40 per cent. Patients who take the new preparation of Lanoxin at the old dose may run the risk of intoxication. Any patient taking digitalis and diuretics who becomes seriously ill, with increase of heart failure and a change from sinus rhythm or fibrillation to a rapid rhythm, should be suspected of having a digitalis ectopic tachycardia. There is also extreme muscular weakness from potassium deficiency. Failure to recognise the condition may lead to increased digitalis dosage with disastrous consequences (ventricular fibrillation and cardiac arrest). Other disturbances of rhythm due to digitalis include ventricular tachycardia, bidirectional tachycardia, heart block and slow idioventricular rhythm.

Atrial flutter. When the rate of discharge from the ectopic focus is faster (around 300) than that in atrial tachycardia, some degree of atrioventricular block develops. The flutter waves have an inverted ' saw tooth ' appearance with an isoelectric base line (Fig. 10.6). Occasionally the atrial rate can be counted in the jugular venous pulse at double the ventricular rate, but usually clinical differentiation from atrial tachycardia is extremely difficult. Atrial flutter is rather more common in patients with rheumatic heart disease than in those with otherwise normal hearts. It can occur in thyrotoxicosis.

Atrial fibrillation. Here the ectopic impulses are too rapid for normal atrial contraction and a writhing motion without any effective pulsation results. Atrial activity is totally irregular and some degree of atrioventricular block must occur. The totally irregular rhythm gives rise to a pulse deficit, the heart rate being faster than the pulse rate at the wrist. Atrial fibrillation usually starts suddenly and is first seen in an established form although repeated paroxysmal attacks are common. Rapid atrial fibrillation seriously compromises effective ventricular filling and output so that congestive heart failure or left ventricular failure often develop. The main causes are mitral valve disease, thyrotoxicosis in older persons, constrictive pericarditis, ischaemic heart disease, congestive cardiomyopathy and sometimes, acute myocarditis. It may occur in apparently normal hearts.

Unlike paroxysmal tachycardia with a regular ventricular rhythm, the irregularity of the ventricular rate in atrial fibrillation and the lack of effective contraction of the atria, predispose to systemic embolism which often occurs at or shortly after the onset of the paroxysm. The ECG shows total irregularity of the ventricular rhythm with normal QRS complexes and fine or coarse irregular oscillations (f waves) due to atrial fibrillation (Fig. 10.7).

Paroxysmal junctional tachycardia. This closely resembles atrial tachycardia, but the P waves are buried in the QRS complex.

Treatment of supraventricular tachycardias

The understanding of the action of drugs in controlling dysrrhythmias and the genesis of dysrrhythmias has been greatly improved by modern electrophysiological techniques. Details are beyond the scope of this chapter but reference is made to the work of Krikler (1974) and Vaughan-Williams (1973).

Supraventricular tachycardia may be terminated by simple manoeuvres such as carotid sinus massage (p. 714), eyeball pressure or a gentle thump on the chest, all of which depend on vagal stimulation. For carotid sinus massage, the patient should be lying down in case the blood pressure falls and only one artery should be compressed at the same time to lessen the risk of cardiac standstill (p. 714).

The principal drugs are digitalis,* phenylephrine (Neophryn) and propranolol (Inderal), practolol (Eraldin)* and Verapamil (Cordilox). Antazoline, reserpine and phenytoin may also be used. Procainamide and lignocaine are less effective for supraventricular tachycardia.

Digitalis is the best of these. It depends for its effect on its vagotonic action. The initial dose is 0·25 to 0·5 mg digoxin followed by 0·125 to 0·25 mg doses at six-hourly intervals (total 1·0 to 2·0 mg). The attack may cease after a single dose of 0·25 or 0·5 mg or the

_____

* Digoxin Tablets BP are now more potent than they were before 1 Oct. 1975. Eraldin tablets are issued for short term use to hospitals only because peritoneal lesions have followed their prolonged use. Injectable Eraldin is generally available.

ventricular rate may be well controlled, the patient remaining in fibrillation. It is rarely necessary to give it i v. Subsequent digitalisation is not usually required but occasionally a small maintenance dose appears to prevent further attacks.

Phenylephrine (Neophryn) is a peripheral vasoconstricting agent which increases blood pressure and reflexly causes bradycardia. A dose of 0·5 mg may be given i m or i v but it is contraindicated in hypertensive patients.

In very rapid atrial fibrillation, procainamide is unlikely to achieve conversion to sinus rhythm. In atrial flutter, it may convert the rhythm to a one to one atrioventricular response at a disastrously fast ventricular rate unless digitalis has been used first to block atrioventricular conduction and slow the ventricular rate. Long-acting quinidine (Kinidin Durules) is safe and useful in preventing supraventricular dysrrhythmias.

Propranolol (Inderal), a beta-adrenergic blocking agent, may be effective in inhibiting sympathetic inotropic effects on the heart. It is also of value for dysrrhythmias due to digitalis. Its use should be restricted to patients who do not have heart failure since interruption of the sympathetic drive may cause extreme bradycardia and a catastrophic fall in blood pressure. Despite a report to the contrary (Snow, 1965), propranolol can be dangerous after recent cardiac infarction and, even more so, following operations on the heart. For patients with normal hearts, or without heart failure, the dose must not exceed 10 mg i v given slowly, with careful note of its effect on heart rate and blood pressure.

Alternatively it can be given by mouth in a dose of 10 to 20 mg. If it is essential to use the drug in patients with heart failure or following recent cardiac infarction or cardiac surgery, very small doses, say 0·5 mg i v or 2·0 mg by mouth should be used. Care should be taken in patients with obstructive airway disease or asthma since it may cause bronchospasm. Practolol (Eraldin) has little or no membrane effect on the cardiac cell and thus does not depress the action potential as does quinidine. It has a cardioselective beta-adrenergic blocking action and is an alternative to propranolol, especially in patients with airways obstruction. The dose is 5 mg i v repeated up to a total of 25 mg. It is of particular value in supraventricular tachycardia after cardiac surgery but must be used in smaller doses (1 to 10 mg) and with great care. Oral use is not advised as serious side effects involving the eyes, skin and mucous membranes may occur. Verapamil (Cordilox) is a vasodilator with antidysrrhythmic properties due to calcium antagonism. It is often effective in atrial fibrillation and may restore sinus rhythm. It is less effective by mouth (40 mg) than by parenteral injection (5 mg). It must not be given to patients taking propranolol (Inderal) or practolol (Eraldin) since cardiac arrest may follow. Verapamil may be of especial value in reciprocating tachycardia of the Wolff-Parkinson-White type.

Antihistamine drugs have been used successfully; the one recommended being antazoline (Antistin) which is of low toxicity. The dose is 100 mg i v, repeated at five-minute intervals up to a total dosage of 10 mg per kg. It may be given in 5 g/dl glucose as an i v infusion or by mouth in a dose of 200 mg (Leon-Sotomayor, 1963).

Dysrrhythmia which proves resistant to drugs may be treated by direct current counter shock, using a synchronised capacitor discharge but description of this technique is beyond the scope of this chapter. Great care must be exercised in patients who have long been receiving digitalis, as heart block may ensue and conversion to normal is more difficult.

Atrial flutter is treated in the same way as atrial fibrillation. Slowing of the ventricular rate by digitalis will often convert flutter to fibrillation. When the drug cannot be taken by mouth, i m injection should be used.

Once the ventricular rate has been slowed the acute emergency is over and the subsequent management will depend on the underlying disease. In those with mitral disease it is advisable to give heparin because of the risk of embolism. If the ventricular rate cannot be slowed by digitalis, direct current counter shock should be tried, bearing in mind the danger of heart block and of pulmonary oedema in patients with tight mitral stenosis or myocardial disease.

Reserpine is occasionally valuable in paroxysmal tachycardia and the anticonvulsant drug sodium phenylhydantoinate (Dilantin) has also been shown to have antidysrrhythmic properties similar to quinidine. It is mainly of value in ventricular dysrrhythmia.

Quinidine has no place in the management of rapid atrial fibrillation or atrial tachycardia, but long-acting quinidine (Kinidin Durules) is safe and may be valuable in preventing recurrent supraventricular dysrrhythmias.

PAROXYSMAL VENTRICULAR TACHYCARDIA

Here the ectopic focus lies in the ventricle outside the atrioventricular node. It is extremely dangerous for, although the ventricular rate is often slower than in supraventicular tachycardia, the quality of the ventricular contraction is very poor. Attacks are commonly associated with severe impairment of cardiac action with low blood pressure, raised venous pressure and anginal pain due to inadequate coronary flow. The dysrrhythmia is most often the result of ischaemic heart disease and may occur after cardiac infarction when it is usually fatal unless quickly stopped. Local ischaemia, oedema and electrolyte imbalance increase automaticity by affecting the slope of diastolic repolarisation in conduction tissue. Varying degrees of exit and entrance block around the site of an ectopic pacemaker facilitate re-entry mechanisms. The ECG shows wide, bizarre splintered complexes resembling bundle branch block at a rapid and slightly irregular rate (Fig. 10.8). Independent P waves may be seen. Because the atria are acting independently, the PR intervals and thus, the intensity of the first heart sound vary, a point which may aid clinical detection.

Treatment

The most satisfactory treatment is usually by electroversion (for risks see p. 91). Failing this, procainamide 500 mg by mouth every three hours is indicated. I v procainamide can have serious effects for it is a myocardial depressant and tends to lower cardiac output and cause peripheral vasodilatation. High doses excite the spinal cord and cause muscular twitchings. Often more urgent treatment is needed and then lignocaine should be given i v because it causes less cardiac depression and hypotension than procainamide. Multiple ventricular ectopic beats can be suppressed by it. A bolus dose of 50 to 100 mg should be given. Conversion may occur quickly and so small increments only should be made preferably by an i v infusion of not more than 4 mg/min. A 200 mg dose i m can produce adequate plasma levels. Propranolol (Inderal) may be used with great caution (p. 253) but is more dangerous than electroversion.

Quinidine carries risks often equal to those of the dysrhythmia itself and should only be used if no other treatment is available. Quinidine gluconate 300 to 500 mg parenterally can be given i v, very slowly, monitoring the heart as with procainamide. Facilities for prompt cardiac resuscitation should always be available. Dilantin (with quinidine-like properties), 50 mg i v or 100 mg orally every eight hours, and bretylium (which reduces catecholamine action) have been used for ventricular tachycardia. Bretylium is sometimes effective when other drugs have failed and increases the threshold for ventricular fibrillation. Hypotension may be a problem. Mexiletene (Mexetil, Boehringer) 100 to 200 mg eight-hourly may be used by mouth. It has properties similar to lignocaine.

The possibility that ventricular tachycardia is associated with a low serum potassium (p. 602) and perhaps digitalis intoxication should always be considered. Potassium chloride, 24 to 50 m mol (2 to 4 g) should be infused slowly over a period of three to four hours in cases of ventricular tachycardia associated with potassium deficiency. Small single doses of 2 to 4 mmol may be surprisingly effective. It should not be used i v if renal function is impaired as it may cause cardiac standstill and it is best avoided altogether if correction of the dysrrhythmia is not urgent. It is important to correct electrolyte imbalance, heart failure, acidosis, and hypotension to prevent further attacks.

Treatment of dysrrhythmia due to digitalis intoxication

Once the diagnosis has been made, digitalis should be withdrawn and, if the situation is not urgent, potassium chloride, 15 mmol (1 g) should be given every three or four hours as wax cored tablets (Slow K, Ciba). These carry the risk of causing oesophageal ulceration if the left atrium is enlarged. When more urgent treatment is needed, procainamide or lignocaine can be used but it carries some risk and does nothing to abate the toxic effects of digitalis. Beta-adrenergic blockade by propranolol (Inderal) given cautiously has been useful in digitalis dysrrhythmias. Unfortunately, it is just those patients who need the most urgent treatment who are often most at risk from the use of propranolol as they can be particularly sensitive to the drug. As little as 0·5 mg should be given i v and then 10 mg three or four times daily by mouth. Larger doses may be used for patients not in heart failure. Practolol (Eraldin) may be safer though sometimes less effective than propranolol (Inderal). Chelating agents have been suggested to diminish digitalis effects in intoxication. The best treatment is probably with propranolol. Dilantin has been particularly recommended for digitalis-induced ventricular tachycardia. Three mg/kg body weight in dextrose 5 g/dl is given i v over a 20 minute period and may be repeated in one to two hours. The solution is irritant and liable to cause thrombosis.

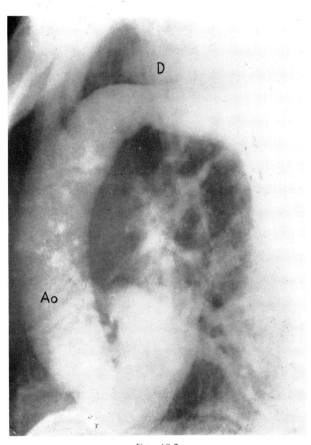

FIG. 10.2

Dissection of the aorta. Lateral projection of angiocardiogram
showing unfolded aorta (Ao) and a double lumen due to
dissection (D) in the arch.

Facing p. 256

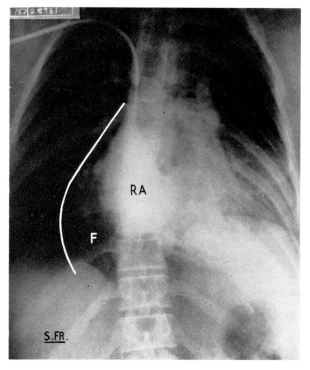

Fig. 10.3

Frontal projection of angiocardiogram in a patient with a large pericardial effusion. The right atrium (RA) is filled with contrast medium and the outer border of the heart shadow is shown by a white line. The space between this and the RA is occupied by pericardial fluid (F).

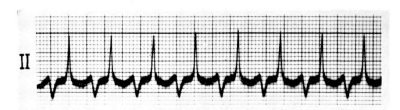

Fig. 10.4

Lead II of an ECG showing supraventricular tachycardia of the coronary sinus type due to an ectopic focus near the coronary sinus. The P waves are inverted; the PR interval is ·022 second and the atrial and ventricular rates 130 per minute.

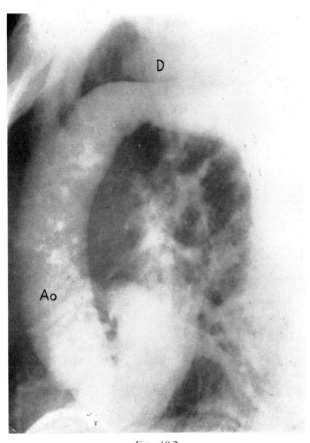

Fig. 10.2

Dissection of the aorta. Lateral projection of angiocardiogram showing unfolded aorta (Ao) and a double lumen due to dissection (D) in the arch.

Facing p. 256

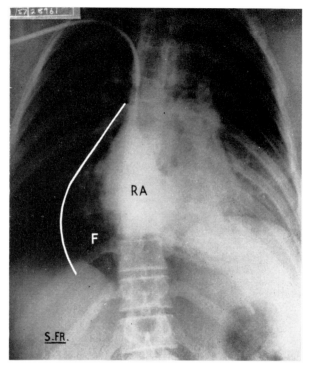

Fig. 10.3

Frontal projection of angiocardiogram in a patient with a
large pericardial effusion. The right atrium (RA) is filled
with contrast medium and the outer border of the heart
shadow is shown by a white line. The space between this
and the RA is occupied by pericardial fluid (F).

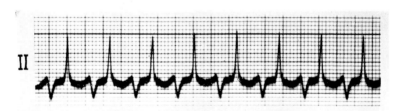

Fig. 10.4

Lead II of an ECG showing supraventricular tachycardia of the coronary
sinus type due to an ectopic focus near the coronary sinus. The P waves
are inverted; the PR interval is ·022 second and the atrial and ventricular
rates 130 per minute.

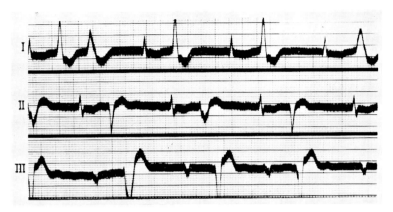

FIG. 10.5

ECG showing ST depression and coupled ventricular ectopic beats due to digitalis. The basic rhythm is atrial fibrillation.

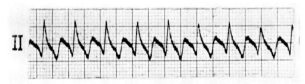

FIG. 10.6

Lead II of an ECG showing atrial flutter.

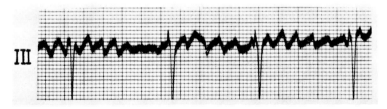

FIG. 10.7

Lead III of an ECG showing coarse atrial fibrillation.

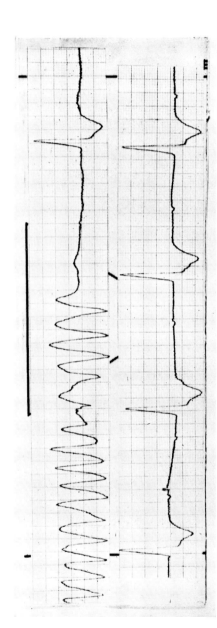

FIG. 10.8

Continuous strip of ECG (lead 1) showing (upper left) ventricular tachycardia followed by (upper and lower) complete heart block and idio-ventricular rhythm with wide QRS complexes. Ventricular rate 30 and atrial rate 70 per minute.

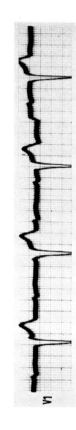

FIG. 10.9

Lead V of an ECG showing complete heart block. Ventricular rate 37 and atrial rate 110 per minute.

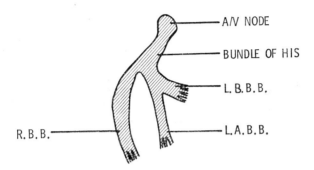

Fig. 10.10
The conducting system and fascicles.
RBB = right bundle branch.
LBBB = left posterior bundle branch (fascicle).
LABB = left anterior bundle branch (fascicle).

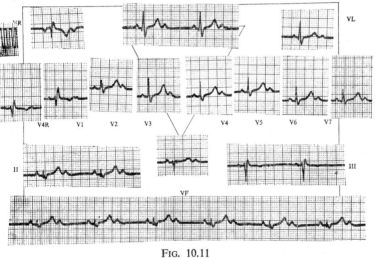

Fig. 10.11
Electrocardiograms showing right bundle branch block and 2 : 1 atrio-ventricular block, Mobitz type II with normal PR interval.

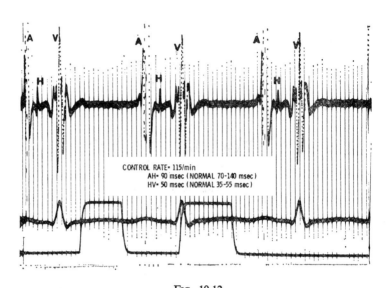

FIG. 10.12

a

His bundle electrograms.

a. Normal.

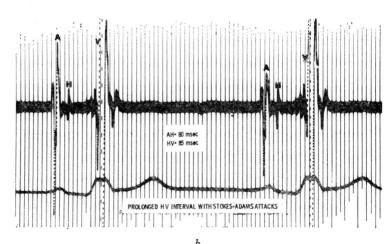

b

b. Prolonged HV interval indicating disease of the His-Purkinje system.

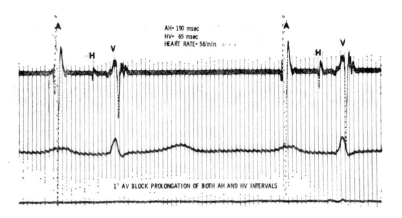

c

c. First degree heart block with prolongation of both AH and HV intervals suggesting disease of the His-Purkinje system.

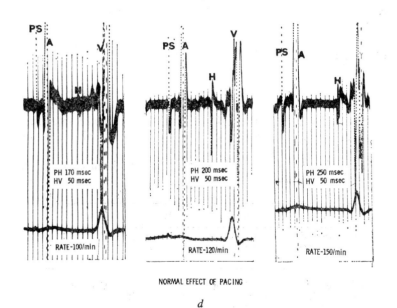

d

d. Normal effect of atrial pacing up to 150/min. No AV block produced.

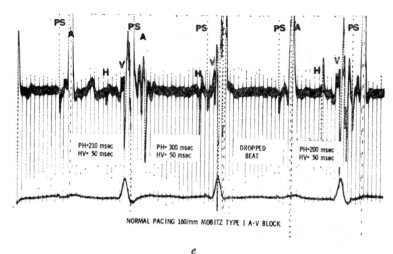

e

e. Normal effect of atrial pacing at 160/min producing Mobitz type I atrioventricular block.

General comment on the immediate management of ectopic paroxysmal tachycardia

Dangerous drugs should never be given parenterally for arrhythmias not of serious import. Thus, paroxysmal atrial tachycardia which is not disturbing the patient should be treated with safe drugs orally or even by simple sedation after methods of vagal stimulation have been tried.

The anti-dysrrhythmic actions of drugs have been classified as follows (Vaughan Williams, 1973):

CLASS I	CLASS II	CLASS III	CLASS IV
Slowing rate of rise of depolarisation	Anti-sympathetic	Prolongation of action potential	Calcium antagonism
Quinidine Procainamide Lignocaine Phenytoin	Beta-blocking agents Bretylium	Quinidine Procainamide	Verapamil

Whenever possible, ECG confirmation of the type of tachycardia should be obtained. This is most important before giving digitalis, for, in ventricular tachycardia, digitalis may cause ventricular fibrillation. In patients with atrial fibrillation aberrant conduction of supraventricular impulses may closely resemble ventricular ectopic beats. The difference can be readily appreciated by His bundle electrography. Quinidine should on no account be given without monitoring control. Enquiry should always be made about previous digitalis therapy. Tachydysrhythmias refractory to drugs may be suppressed by pacing to capture the impulse and terminate re-entry mechanisms. If AV conduction is normal pacing may be from the right atrium. But if atrial capture is difficult to maintain or if AV block develops, ventricular pacing may be indicated.

DISORDERS OF IMPULSE CONDUCTION. BRADYDYSRRHYTHMIAS

Extreme sinus bradycardia, first and second degree heart block and complete heart block all produce disturbance of consciousness or congestive cardiac failure. Sinus node disease causes alternating sinus bradycardia or sinus arrest and tachydysrrhythmias (Sick sinus syndrome. Bradycardia/Tachycardia syndrome). Subjects are usually elderly; embolism is not uncommon and death may occur (Rubenstein *et al.,* 1972).

Second degree heart block may be of the Mobitz type I variety (Wenckebach periods) with increasing PR interval until a sinus impulse is blocked after which the PR interval becomes shorter and the cycle begins again. Mobitz type II block occurs with a fixed PR interval (which may be prolonged but is constant) and regular 2 : 1 or greater degrees of AV block. Increase in heart rate tends to cause increase in the degree of block. Complete heart block commonly develops and this fault is much more serious than type I. When Mobitz type I block is associated with normal QRS width the site of the block is usually at AV junctional level. When the QRS is wide and bundle branch block is present the site of the block is less certain. His bundle electrography is necessary to delineate the site.

Complete heart block may occur at the AV junctional level with narrow QRS complex and moderate bradycardia from the nodal pacemaker, as in congenital complete heart block. More serious block results from distal and more extensive conduction disturbance with wide QRS complexes from idioventricular pacemakers with extreme bradycardia and irritability which may lead to ventricular fibrillation.

THE HEMIBLOCKS (Rosenbaum, 1970)

The intraventricular conduction system is divided into three main fascicles—the right bundle branch, the anterior and posterior divisions of the left bundle branch (Fig. 10.10). Block of the left anterior division produces left axis deviation with frontal plane QRS axis—60, QI, SIII patterns and normal QRS duration (left anterior hemiblock). Disease of the posterior division causes right axis deviation and is usually associated with right bundle branch block. The combination of left anterior hemiblock with right bundle branch block is called bifascicular block. If the PR interval is also prolonged trifascicular block is said to be present and complete heart block may readily occur. This is especially imminent if Mobitz type II block is present (Fig. 10.11).

BUNDLE OF HIS ELECTROGRAPHY (Fig. 10.12 a, b, c)

The AV node, bundle of His, bundle branches and Purkinje fibres form the specialised conducting tissue which transmits atrial impulses to the ventricles. The potentials from the bundle of His may be recorded by a special electrode placed in the region of the bundle by right heart catheterisation. The PR interval can be divided into three components. The two main ones are the AH interval from the onset of the right atrial electrogram to the first high frequency component of the H (His) potential (which measures AV nodal conduction time) and the HV interval from the H potential to the onset of ventricular activation (which measures conduction in the His-Purkinje systems). Normally right atrial pacing increases A-H, H-V remaining constant. At critical rates Mobitz type I block may develop proximal to the His bundle. The development of block distal to the His bundle at less than the normal critical rate indicates disease in the Purkinje system. His bundle electrography and programmed stimulation are of value in analysing the site and extent of conduction defects and can be helpful in determining the need for demand pacemaking in patients who may be likely to develop complete heart block or Stokes-Adams attacks (Fig. 10.12, a and b).

HEART BLOCK (STOKES-ADAMS ATTACKS)

Stokes-Adams attacks are episodes of syncope or near syncope associated with a conduction defect in the heart. They result from inadequate cerebral blood flow consequent upon too slow a heart rate. Any patient with a history of such attacks should be regarded as a potential emergency.

Attacks occur in established complete heart block (Fig. 10.9) and also when there is a change from partial to complete block. They begin when the heart rate suddenly drops to an unacceptable level (10 to 15 per minute). The patient rapidly loses consciousness, falls to the ground and is pulseless. Breathing continues and the pupils are not always widely dilated. When the heart rate speeds up consciousness is regained suddenly with an intense flush due to oxygenated blood in the left ventricle being suddenly expelled into dilated peripheral vessels. Severe attacks may be accompanied by convulsions and these simulate epilepsy (p. 308). Minor attacks may be no more than a transient giddiness but often they are associated with a distressing sensation of impending doom. A ventricular ectopic beat often heralds the return of effective cardiac action. Sometimes similar symptoms are due to repetitive short bursts of ventricular tachycardia or fibrillation (Fig. 10.8). The attacks occur at short intervals, the patient passing from consciousness to coma in rapid succession. Persistent attacks are usually of very bad prognostic significance.

The subjects of Stokes-Adams attacks are usually elderly. They do not usually have overt coronary or other disease (Zoob and Shirley Smith, 1963) but attacks can follow immediately after cardiac infarction, particularly of the infero-posterior variety (James, 1962) and they can be caused by digitalis and quinidine). Normal sinus rhythm between attacks in no way contraindicates the diagnosis of Stokes-Adams attacks in a patient with a suggestive history. There is a high incidence of right bundle branch block in patients with Stokes-Adams attacks. A history of syncopal attacks in a patient with sinus rhythm and right bundle branch block suggests that there are episodes of complete block, especially if there is also left anterior hemiblock. Attacks may occur when complete heart block comes on during or after an operation on the heart and when the surgeon has to work near to the conducting tissues in closing a ventricular septal defect.

A less sinister form of heart block, atrio-ventricular disassociation, may occur after cardiac surgery or from digitalis toxicity. The atrial rate is slower than the ventricular and both chambers beat independently.

PROPHYLAXIS

An understanding of the natural history of conduction defects is important in prevention of Stokes-Adams attacks. Bifascicular block with a history of syncope requires insertion of a demand pacemaker triggered to fire when the heart rate falls below a critical level, usually 70 per minute. Bifascicular block without symptoms may usually be left alone but cardiac depressant drugs should be avoided if possible and the patient kept under careful observation. Bundle branch block with prolonged HV interval is not an indication for pacing unless there is a history of syncope and block develops distal to the His bundle on atrial pacing. Trifascicular block or Mobitz type II block is an indication for pacing. Since the site of complete block cannot be defined with certainty by surface electrography second or third degree block with block in or distal to the His bundle is an indication for pacing. Congenital heart block with block proximal to the His bundle, narrow QRS complexes and adequate ventricular rate without symptoms does not usually require pacing.

In cardiac infarction heart block persists in only a minority of patients who survive the acute episode. Pacing is therefore usually a temporary measure. Conduction defects in inferior infarction are relatively benign and pacing is only needed if there is undue bradycardia with hypotension, heart failure or Stoke-Adams attacks. Heart block in anterior infarction usually denotes widespread myocardial damage and carries a poor prognosis even with pacing. The development of junctional block, bundle branch block or third degree AV block is an indication for insertion of a prophylactic pacing electrode wire in the demand mode.

Prevention of attacks of syncope due to the cardio-auditory syndrome (long QT interval and syncope or sudden death with or without deafness) is very unsatisfactory. Digitalis may be dangerous. Demand pacemaking is rational but may give rise to ventricular fibrillation because the impulse may fall in the vulnerable period due to the long QT interval. The cautious use of propranolol may be considered.

Drugs to prevent Stokes-Adams attacks are of doubtful benefit. Isoprenaline may be given i v or as suppositories or as a delayed action preparation by mouth (Saventrine, 30 mg four- to six-hourly). The effects are erratic, the protection uncertain and side effects such as multiple ectopic beats or ventricular tachycardia are not uncommon with Saventrine. An increase in rate may not be due to improved conduction but to ectopics. If Saventrine is to be used it should be preceded by a slow test infusion 1 μg per minute to see if ectopics occur. Long-acting drugs of the atropine series are really not practicable. Digitalis should only be given if a pacemaker is in position and functioning on demand.

Steroids are sometimes thought to be beneficial in the prevention and treatment of Stokes-Adams attacks, either by favourably influencing the intra- and extra-cellular potassium balance (in chronic cases) or from an anti-inflammatory effect in patients with recent cardiac infarction.

Oral prednisone 40 to 60 mg may be used following initial doses of 100 to 200 mg hydrocortisone i v. Too much importance should not be attached to steroids and they should not blind the physician to the need for electrical pacemaking.

Treatment

This should be as for circulatory arrest (p. 724) and when the circulation has returned the exact type of rhythm must be determined. In the event of asystole or a very slow heart rate, atropine may be tried but preferably isoprenaline should be given by intracardiac (p. 724) or i v injection. External pacing, followed by internal pacing, may be needed and, if ventricular fibrillation occurs, external defibrillation will be necessary.

Any drugs which have a cardiac depressant effect, particularly quinidine and procainamide are absolutely contraindicated in threatened or actual Stokes-Adams attacks. Digitalis is contraindicated in variable heart block unless this is the result of an ectopic tachycardia.

INTRACARDIAC OBSTRUCTION

Syncope may result from acute obstruction within the heart or great veins. Pulmonary embolism (p. 241) is the commonest example. Syncope may also occur in acute stenosis, hypertrophic obstructive cardiomyopathy and with intracardiac tumours.

Aortic stenosis

In aortic stenosis, syncope commonly occurs after effort. Vasodilatation in skeletal muscle absorbs much of the cardiac output which fails to rise adequately on effort. Inadequate filling of a grossly hypertrophied left ventricle may also be a factor. Cerebral blood flow is diminished and consciousness is lost. Death from ventricular fibrillation may occur. Coronary blood flow is inadequate and this explains angina on effort in severe aortic stenosis. Treatment is to keep the patient lying flat and, if the blood pressure remains low, to employ metaraminol (Aramine) which has a cardiac stimulant action. Nitrites should generally be avoided if angina occurs, since they merely increase the peripheral vasodilatation and may make matters worse. Oddly enough, the angina of aortic stenosis does sometimes improve with nitrites, probably because, during an attack of angina, some degree of left ventricular insufficiency occurs and nitrites act by diminishing venous return and reducing the work of the heart. Any patient who is suffering from syncopal attacks due to severe aortic stenosis should be considered for urgent surgical relief, since removal of the obstruction is the only measure likely to effect any substantial improvement and prevent intractable heart failure or sudden death.

Hypertrophic obstructive cardiomyopathy

In this condition digitalis, nitrites and inotropic drugs must be avoided. Phenylephrine or propranolol are indicated.

Intracardiac tumours

The commonest intracardiac tumour is a myxoma which usually arises in the left atrium. It is an amorphous, jelly-like mass, often pedunculated, although sometimes sessile, which grows from the fossa ovalis. The clinical effects of a myxoma depend upon three actions. First, obstruction to the left atrium which produces effects similar to mitral stenosis with pulmonary venous congestion, haemoptysis and pulmonary hypertension. If the tumour blocks the mitral orifice from time to time, syncope will occur, often when the patient changes position. Second, the tumour may give rise to multiple emboli which consist of small fragments of myxoma or blood clot, and, thirdly, general systemic effects such as loss of weight, fever, anaemia and a high sedimentation rate may result (Goodwin, 1963).

Confirmation of the diagnosis of left atrial myxoma depends upon echocardiography supplemented if necessary by angiocardiography. The latter will reveal a lobulated filling defect in the left atrium which often appears to move through the mitral valve into the left ventricle and back into the left atrium during various phases of the cardiac cycle (Goodwin *et al.*, 1962).

Treatment. In an emergency a change in the position of the patient may relieve the attack. Should the myxoma become impacted in the mitral orifice it is unlikely that the patient will survive long enough for it to be diagnosed and removed surgically. If partial obstruction increases, then the symptoms are likely to be those of acute pulmonary oedema. The only treatment is surgical removal.

Paroxysmal infundibular obstruction in the tetralogy of Fallot

Sudden episodes of extreme cyanosis and hyperventilation, leading to loss of consciousness, convulsions and even death, can occur from time to time in patients with the tetralogy of Fallot. The attacks are due to spasm of the infundibulum of the right ventricle, pulmonary blood flow being severely restricted and the right to left shunt greatly increased. The cause is uncertain, but sympathetic overactivity and hyperventilation may be factors. Attacks are recognised by rapid increase in cyanosis and disappearance of the pulmonary stenotic murmur.

Treatment. Place the child in the knee-chest position and give oxygen and a small dose of morphine (0·5 to 1 mg per 5 kg body weight). Further measures which may be needed are phenylephrine (Neophryn) (to increase systemic vascular resistance and reduce the right to left shunt) in a dose of 0·5 mg i v for an adult, 0·05 mg for a child of 2 years; propranolol (Inderal) to reduce sympathomimetic activity and over-ventilation, and an infusion of 1/6 molar sodium bicarbonate to correct metabolic acidosis. Propranolol by mouth may also be useful in preventing attacks. Urgent infundibular resection or a shunt operation may be needed.

J. F. GOODWIN

REFERENCES

BRAUNWALD, D. E. & MAROKO, P. R. Protection of the ischaemic myocardium. In *The Myocardium: Heart Failure and Infarction,* p. 329. New York: H.P. Publishing Co. 1974.

CHAMBERLAIN, D. A., WHITE, R. J., HOWARD, M. R. & SMITH, T. W. (1970). Plasma digoxin concentrations in patients with atrial fibrillation. *British Medical Journal,* 3, 429.

GOODWIN, J. F. (1963). The diagnosis of left atrial myxoma. *Lancet,* 1, 464.

GOODWIN, J. F. (1968). Acquired non-rheumatic mitral disease. *Journal of the Royal College of Physicians of London,* 3, No. 1, 61.

GOODWIN, J. F., HARRISON, C. V. & WILCKEN, D. E. L. (1963). Obliterative pulmonary hypertension and thrombo-embolism. *British Medical Journal,* 1, 701. Discussion, 777.

GOODWIN, J. F., *et al.* (1962). Clinical features of left atrial myxoma. *Thorax,* 17, 91.

JAMES, T. N. (1962). Arrhythmias and conduction disturbances in acute myocardial infarction. *American Heart Journal,* 64, 416.

KRIKLER, D. M. (1974). A fresh look at arrhythmias. *Lancet* 2, 51, 913, 974, 1034.

LEON-SOTOMAYOR, L. (1963). A clinical evaluation of the antiarrythmic properties of antazoline. *American Journal of Cardiology,* 11, 646.

LILLEHEI, R. C., LONGERBEAM, J. K., BLOCH, J. H. & MANAX, W. G. In *Cardiovascular Drug Therapy,* ed. Brest, A. N. & Moyer, J. H., p. 118. New York: Grune and Stratton. 1965.

MEDICAL RESEARCH COUNCIL (1969). Working party report on short-term anticoagulant administration in coronary thrombosis. *British Medical Journal,* 1, 335.

MELLANDER, S. & LEWIS, D. H. (1963). Effect of haemorrhagic shock on the reactivity of resistance and capacitance vessels and on capillary filtration transfer in cat skeletal muscle. *Circulation Research,* 13, 105.

ORAM, S., RESNEKOV, L. & DAVIES, P. (1960). Digitalis as a cause of paroxysmal atrial tachycardia with atrioventricular block. *British Medical Journal,* 2, 1402.

PERTROTH, M. G. & HARRISON, D. C. Medical therapy for shock in acute myocardial infarction. In *Progress in Cardiology,* Vol. 2, Ed. Yu, P. N. & Goodwin, J. F. Philadelphia: Lea & Febiger, 1973.

REPORT (1973). The urokinase pulmonary embolism trial. A national cooperative study. *Circulation,* **47,** supplement II.

ROSENBAUM, M. B. (1970). The Hemiblocks; diagnostic criteria and clinical significance. *Modern Concepts of Cardio-Vascular Disease,* **39,** 141.

RUBENSTEIN, J. J., *et al.* (1972). Clinical spectrum of the sick sinus syndrome. *Circulation,* **46,** 5-13.

SHILLINGFORD, J. P. (1965). The intensive care of the coronary crisis. *Proceedings of the Royal Society of Medicine,* **58,** 101.

SNOW, P. J. D. (1965). Effect of propranolol in myocardial infarction. *Lancet,* **2,** 551.

VAUGHAN WILLIAMS, E. M. In *New Perspectives in Beta Blockade.* Ed. Burley, D. M., *et al.* p. 11. Horsham: CIBA Laboratories. 1937.

ZOOB, M. & SHIRLEY SMITH, K. (1963). The aetiology of complete heart-block. *British Medical Journal,* **2,** 1149.

CHAPTER 11

Emergencies in Blood Diseases

As the history in blood diseases is very varied a blood and often a marrow examination is essential. When full facilities are not available much diagnostic information can be obtained from just a film and a haemoglobin estimation. In a haemorrhagic disorder a platelet count and coagulation screen (bleeding time, prothrombin time and a kaolin-activated partial thromboplastin time) should be done. If these three tests are normal it is unlikely that bleeding is due to a major defect in haemostasis. In severe anaemia and haemorrhage a blood sample must be sent immediately for grouping and arrangements made to ensure that compatible blood is ready for transfusion at short notice.

ANAEMIA

Anaemia from acute blood loss is considered under Haemorrhagic Shock (p. 9). In more gradual bleeding the plasma volume is maintained, shock does not occur and the condition does not present as an emergency. Chronic blood loss in itself does not constitute an emergency although it is by far the commonest cause of anaemia. When there is no obvious reason, such as menorrhagia, for an iron deficiency anaemia it is a matter of some urgency to identify the cause. Occult blood loss may be the only sign of a neoplasm of the large bowel which may be cured by surgery if the diagnosis is not too long delayed.

Megaloblastic anaemia

The megaloblastic anaemias are a group of disorders sharing a characteristic morphological and functional abnormality of the blood and marrow resulting from defective DNA synthesis due to deficiency of vitamin B_{12} or folic acid. The commonest variety seen in northern Europe is pernicious anaemia due to malabsorption of vitamin B_{12} but it can occur after gastric surgery and resection of the terminal ileum. Nutritional B_{12} deficiency is occasionally seen in strict vegetarians (vegans). Megaloblastic anaemia due to folate deficiency is seen in idiopathic steatorrhoea, pregnancy, haemolytic anaemia and in patients taking anti-convulsant drugs. It may also occur as a result of malnutrition. The anaemia in pernicious anaemia is often severe but because it develops insidiously it may produce

269

few symptoms until the haematocrit is very depressed. In very anaemic patients who may be elderly and in congestive cardiac failure, a bone marrow examination must be performed as a matter of urgency and blood sent immediately for vitamin B_{12} assay and for estimation of the serum and red cell folate levels. If the patient's condition gives cause for anxiety it is wise to give both vitamin B_{12} parenterally (200 μg twice weekly) and folic acid by mouth (5 mg daily) until the results of the assays are available. Blood transfusion is only rarely indicated but may have to be used if death is thought possible before haematological improvement can take place. It is not without risk since the danger of circulatory overload is considerable in patients who may already be in congestive cardiac failure and so should be given as packed cells and limited in the first instance to 500 ml over a six-hour period preceded by 40 mg of frusemide. The mortality rate in elderly patients with a haematocrit below 25 per cent is as high as 14 per cent. In some instances this is due to pulmonary oedema but in others it is associated with a dramatic fall in the serum potassium level shortly after the start of therapy.

Aplastic anaemia

This is characterised by pancytopenia due to hypoplasia of the bone marrow of unknown cause or due to toxins or ionising radiation. The stem cells of the marrow lose their capacity for normal cellular renewal. The clinical picture is one of severe anaemia with skin bruising, epistaxis and an increased susceptibility to infection. Physical examination is otherwise unremarkable. A palpable spleen is unusual and if found should cast doubt on the diagnosis. The primary objective in management is a supportive one aimed at keeping the patient active and comfortable until such time as remission occurs. An afebrile patient may remain ambulatory so long as the haemoglobin level is 7 or 8 g and transfusion is not needed unless it falls. Menstrual bleeding may be troublesome when the platelet count is very low and suppressive hormone therapy with an anovulatory agent such as norethynodrel (Enavid) may be required. If there is significant bleeding fresh blood should be transfused supplemented, if necessary, by infusions of platelet concentrate. These should be reserved for episodes of serious bleeding because the development of platelet antibodies makes them less effective as time goes by.

Infection in patients with aplastic anaemia can present urgent problems and its possibility in unusual areas such as the meninges or by unusual organisms (*Listeria, Aspergillus* and *Candida*) must be considered. A broad spectrum bactericidal antibiotic should be given until the results of bacteriological tests are available. Granulocyte concentrates are of some value if a cell separator is available.

Because of the risk of infection patients should be managed as far as possible on an out-patient basis. When admission to hospital is necessary special precautions should be taken to avoid infection in patients with very low neutrophil counts (below $2 \times 10^9/1$). Portable laminar air flow isolators are now available and make it possible to establish a sterile environment for the patient without imposing serious medical and nursing problems.

Androgens can induce remission in aplastic anaemia in children and current opinion is that oxymetholone (Anapolon 50 Syntex) 2 to 4 mg/kg per day by mouth is best. However, the outcome is influenced more by the severity of the initial insult than by the type of treatment. Complete recovery is achieved in only 10 per cent of cases and the five year mortality is around 70 per cent.

Haemolytic anaemias

The normal life span of the red cell (120 days) is shortened in haemolytic anaemia either because of an intrinsic abnormality—usually genetically determined, e.g. hereditary spherocytosis—or from an extra-corpuscular abnormality, usually acquired. Most haemolytic anaemias are chronic, the degree of anaemia depending on the balance between red cell destruction in the spleen and the increased output of the marrow. This delicate equilibrium may be suddenly upset in an 'aplastic crisis'. A period of erythroid aplasia in a patient whose red cell life is very short has a marked effect. There is a rapid onset of pallor and listlessness and a marked fall of haemoglobin. A preceding febrile illness due to respiratory or gastro-intestinal infection is common. Intravascular haemolysis may cause haemoglobinaemia and haemoglobinuria to present urgently in the following conditions: *Cl. welchii* septicaemia, blackwater fever (p. 451) and Oroya fever, favism and following eclampsia, burns, certain drugs and chemicals and after an incompatible blood transfusion.

Auto-immune haemolytic anaemia

Auto-immune haemolytic anaemia (AHA) though rare is the commonest variety seen in adults. It is usually caused by auto-antibodies of the warm type which are active against the patient's own red cells. The direct anti-human globulin (Coombs') test is positive. In something over half of all cases an underlying disorder such as malignant lymphoma or chronic lymphatic leukaemia is found but the condition is frequently idiopathic. An important variety is that seen in hypertensive patients on methyldopa (Aldomet).

Treatment

For urgent cases hydrocortisone 100 to 200 mg should be given i v in the first 24 hours, and prednisolone 75 mg daily by mouth started. Blood transfusion should be avoided if possible but if blood must be given for its temporary benefit packed cells should be used. It may accelerate haemolysis and in any case it may be impossible to find a compatible donor.

Sickle cell anaemia

This chronic haemolytic anaemia results from homozygosity for the sickle cell gene and it is seen almost exclusively in negroes. The sickling phenomenon is due to the presence in the red cells of haemoglobin S which crystallises out under conditions of reduced oxygen tension. The crisis is characteristic of the disease and is of two types—painful and aplastic. (A third hyper-haemolytic type with splenomegaly occurs in children but is very rare in adults.) The mechanism of the painful crisis is that crystal masses distort the red cells which then obstruct the micro-circulation in various organs and cause symptoms. Severe pain occurs in bones, the back and abdomen. Treatment is symptomatic and supportive. Transfusion is rarely indicated but when necessary the exchange method would seem logical. Painful crises are difficult to treat but i v fluid (dextrose 5 g/dl) may help. Powerful analgesics are often needed but there is a risk of addiction because of the recurrent nature of the problem. The patient should be told the nature of his condition and perhaps be advised to wear a Medic-Alert bracelet (p. 822) to protect him against possible misdiagnosis of a future crisis.

Glucose-6-phosphate dehydrogenase deficiency

This condition, inherited as a sex-linked recessive, occurs in negroes and people of the Mediterranean area and Far East. It results in a deficiency of reduced glutathione which renders the red cells liable to oxidative attack. In this condition, which superficially resembles blackwater fever (p. 541), many drugs such as sulphonamides, anti-malarials and analgesics, can cause haemolysis. The attacks of haemolysis are usually self-limiting.

Favism

In this condition an acute haemolytic anaemia with haemoglobinuria occurs in people from the Mediterranean areas who are sensitive to the common broad bean (*Vicia fava*) because they lack glucose-6-phosphate dehydrogenase. As not all those at risk develop haemolysis some other factor must be involved. The anaemia is acute and self-limiting and the treatment is on general lines.

POLYCYTHAEMIA

This is a consequence of an increase in red cell volume, i.e. more than 36 ml/kg in men and 32 ml/kg in women. It is either primary and purposeless (polycythaemia vera) or secondary to various hypoxic states as a consequence of increased erythropoeitin production resulting from renal hypoxia. The arterial oxygen tension in polycythaemia vera is normal (92 per cent or more). There is often a leucocytosis, an elevated platelet count and splenomegaly. Polycythaemia has also been described in association with renal tumours and cysts, uterine fibroids and cerebellar haemangioma when it is thought to be due to an inappropriate secretion of erythropoeitin. Spurious or 'stress' polycythaemia results from a reduction in plasma volume with a consequent relative increase in the haemoglobin concentration and haematocrit in the peripheral blood. The red cell mass is not increased. If polycythaemia is untreated vascular complications are common and to avoid these venesection (p. 746) is urgent. 500 ml of blood can be removed on alternate days to lower the haematocrit below 0·50. In emergency situations such as an impending stroke or in preparation for surgery more intensive venesection with return of the patient's plasma can be life-saving. Pruritus, weight loss and hyperuricaemia are indications for urgent treatment with a myelosuppressive agent such as ^{32}P (3 to 5 mCi i v initially). Treatment with ^{32}P is also necessary if the platelet count is over $750 \times 10^9/1$ or if venesection is needed too often.

LEUKAEMIAS
(For Di Gugliemo Syndrome see p. 471)

Chronic leukaemias rarely cause urgent symptoms but occasionally patients with chronic granulocytic leukaemia present with acute gout (p. 647), urinary stones (p. 385) and priapism (p. 145). When lowering of the white count is urgently needed the best agent is mustine hydrochloride 10 mg i v in a fast-running drip (p. 107) with allopurinol (Zyloric) 400 mg a day to prevent hyperuricaemia. Patients with chronic lymphatic leukaemia are particularly prone to respiratory infection which calls for prompt treatment with antibiotics.

Acute leukaemia occurs most frequently during the first and

after the sixth decades of life. Lymphoblastic leukaemia is commoner in children and myeloblastic leukaemia in adults. With modern treatment 90 per cent of patients with lymphoblastic leukaemia but less than 50 per cent of patients with myeloblastic leukaemia can be brought into remission. Patients commonly present with symptoms requiring urgent attention or develop them during remission induction. Severe anaemia requires transfusion but thrombocytopenic bleeding calls for infusion of platelet concentrate in addition (4 to 6 units on alternate days). Infections, including those due to Gram-negative organisms and fungi, are common and often bizarre. The severe neutropenia militates against pus formation and corticosteroids may mask the normal inflammatory response. Monilial infections require urgent treatment with amphoteracin B lozenges and also nystatin tablets. Meningeal involvement is a common acute complication of lymphoblastic leukaemia in children. Prednisolone is the only drug used in leukaemia which readily crosses the blood-brain barrier and so leukaemic meningitis is only apparent in most cases when they are in haematological remission. Routine CSF examination may show leukaemic meningitis before clinical signs appear. The condition is best controlled by intrathecal methotrexate 0·5 mg/kg every two or three days.

Complete remission, i.e. the absence of all evidence of leukaemia, is hard to maintain. To attain it we aim first at remission induction. In acute lymphoblastic leukaemia this is best attained by a combination of vincristine (2 mg per m^2 body surface per week i v) and prednisolone (40 mg per m^2 per day by mouth). In myeloblastic leukaemia the most effective combination is cytosine arabinoside (Cytarabine) 1 to 3 mg/kg i v daily for five days together with another agent such as 6-thioguanine (2 to 2·5 mg/kg daily by mouth). Treatment is best carried out at special centres.

MALIGNANT LYMPHORETICULAR DISORDERS

These do not usually present as emergencies but occasionally rapid enlargement of lymph nodes in Hodgkin's disease may cause acute superior mediastinal compression. The most effective treatment is quadruple chemotherapy using MVPP in the following regime : —

Nitrogen mustard	i v	6 mg/m^2	on days 1 and 8
Vinblastine	i v	6 mg/m^2	on days 1 and 8
Procarbazine	oral	100 mg/m^2	on days 1 to 14 inclusive
Prednisolone	oral	40 mg/m^2	on days 1 to 14 inclusive

Multiple myeloma may present urgently with severe pain or a pathological fracture. Paraplegia may occur. Prompt oral chemotherapy with melphalan or cyclophosphamide can do much to surmount these emergencies. Melphalan is given initially in a high dose of 8 to 10 mg daily for seven to ten days and then continued indefinitely in a dosage of 2 mg daily. Cyclophosphamide dosage begins at 200 mg daily for five to seven days and continues at 50 to 100 mg daily. Over-production of anomalous immunoglobulins often means decreased normal immunoglobulins and so bacterial infections are common. Occasionally patients with unusually high levels of monoclonal IgG present with the hyperviscosity syndrome which shows as circulatory impairment involving the brain and retina. Sustained plasma-pheresis, preferably by means of a cell separator, causes dramatic improvement.

AGRANULOCYTOSIS

This implies an absolute neutrophil count of $1·0 \times 10^9/1$ or less (a figure of $2·5 \times 10^9/1$ or less is referred to as neutropenia). It is usually drug-induced but other causes are acute leukaemia and infectious mononucleosis. Severe infective lesions occur in the mouth and throat and there is also septicaemia and liver damage. Aggressive antibiotic therapy and white cell infusions, if available, are indicated.

INFECTIOUS MONONUCLEOSIS

Although usually benign the presentation may on rare occasions be urgent with agranulocytosis, severe thrombocytopenia and haemolytic anaemia. Rupture of the spleen occasionally occurs necessitating urgent surgery covered by transfusions of blood and platelet concentrate (4 to 6 units).

HAEMORRHAGIC DISORDERS

Features which suggest the presence of a haemorrhagic disorder are spontaneous bleeding into the skin and mucous membranes, prolonged bleeding after surgery and trauma and the fact that bleeding is from more than one site. Haemorrhage is particularly liable to occur if more than one of the components of the haemostatic mechanism—vascular, platelet and coagulation—is defective.

VASCULAR DEFECTS usually cause mild haemorrhage confined to the skin and mucous membranes. There is sometimes an associated qualitative platelet abnormality as in uraemia, scurvy and the dysproteinaemias.

PLATELET ABNORMALITIES may be quantitative (thrombocytopenic) and qualitative. In thrombasthenia (Glanzman's disease), a familial disorder, the number of platelets is normal but they fail to aggregate in response to adenosine diphosphate (ADP). In thrombopathy, also familial, there is a functional abnormality involving platelet factor III. Similar defects occur in uraemia, scurvy, liver disease, dysproteinaemia and follow infusion of high molecular weight dextran and the ingestion of aspirin. No absolute relationship can be shown between the platelet count and the degree of bleeding but in general, bleeding is uncommon if the count is above $80 \times 10^9/1$. Thrombocytopenia may be idiopathic or secondary (Table 11.1).

Table 11.1. *Causes of secondary thrombocytopenia*

Common	Drugs and chemicals
	Leukaemia
	Aplastic anaemia
	Bone marrow infiltration (carcinoma, myeloma)
	Splenomegaly (Hypersplenism)
	Disseminated lupus erythematosus
Less common	Megaloblastic anaemia
	Infection
	Liver disease
	Massive blood transfusion
	Consumption coagulopathy
Rare	Thrombotic thrombocytopenic purpura
	Post-transfusion thrombocytopenia
	Post-partum thrombocytopenia
	Haemangioma

Haemorrhage from both thrombocytopenia and from platelet abnormalities can be controlled by infusion of platelet concentrate (p. 797) or by transfusion of fresh blood.

Idiopathic Thrombocytopenic Purpura (ITP)

This is an immune disorder most often seen in children and young people and is diagnosed by exclusion of known causes (Table 11.1). The chronic variety is only likely to present urgently after trauma such as dental extraction. In the acute variety the onset is abrupt and may be life-threatening, the main risk being intracerebral haemorrhage. Permanent recovery occurs in 80 per cent of cases irrespective of treatment. Oral steroid therapy is advised because of its beneficial effect on capillary permeability, although it is doubtful whether it shortens the duration of thrombocytopenia. In patients who relapse splenectomy is preferable to prolonged steroid therapy.

COAGULATION AND FIBRINOLYTIC ABNORMALITIES

These lead to a bleeding tendency or to intravascular coagulation or to a combination of both. The function of the coagulation system is to produce thrombin which has two effects. (1) It causes platelets to release adenosine diphosphate (ADP) and to form by aggregates a haemostatic plug. (2) It converts fibrinogen to fibrin and makes the plug stable. Both extrinsic and intrinsic prothrombin activators are concerned in fibrin production. Extrinsic activators are formed when tissue factor enters shed blood and intrinsic activators when blood comes into contact with a foreign surface. Both are necessary for efficient thrombin production (Figs. 11.1 and 11.2).

Table 11.2. *International nomenclature of coagulation factors*

FACTOR	SYNONYMS
I	Fibrinogen
II	Prothrombin
III	Tissue factor. Tissue thromboplastin
IV	Calcium
V	Labile factor. Proaccelerin
VI	(Not assigned)
VII	Stable factor. Proconvertin
VIII	Antihaemophilic globulin
IX	Christmas factor. Plasma thromboplastin component
X	Stuart-Prower factor
XI	Plasma thromboplastin antecedent
XII	Hageman factor
XIII	Fibrin stabilising factor

The function of the fibrinolytic system is to digest intravascular deposits of fibrin and the extravascular fibrin of haemostatic plugs and inflammatory exudates (see Fig. 11.3).

Plasminogen, a globulin thought to be synthesised in the liver, is converted by various activators into the fibrinolytic enzyme plasmin. The normal substrate for plasmin is fibrin but it can also, in pathological conditions, digest fibrinogen and various coagulation factors, particularly V and VIII. Plasmin is not normally present in the blood stream as it is rapidly inactivated by circulating anti-plasmins. Plasminogen activator is present in the tissues where it is localised in the vascular endothelium, in the plasma and in the urine (Urokinase). Tissue activator may be released into the circulation by various stimuli including ischaemia and exercise. When

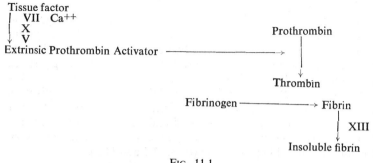

FIG. 11.1
Extrinsic coagulation system.

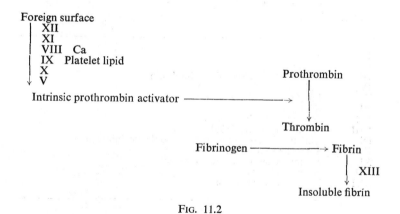

FIG. 11.2
Intrinsic coagulation system.

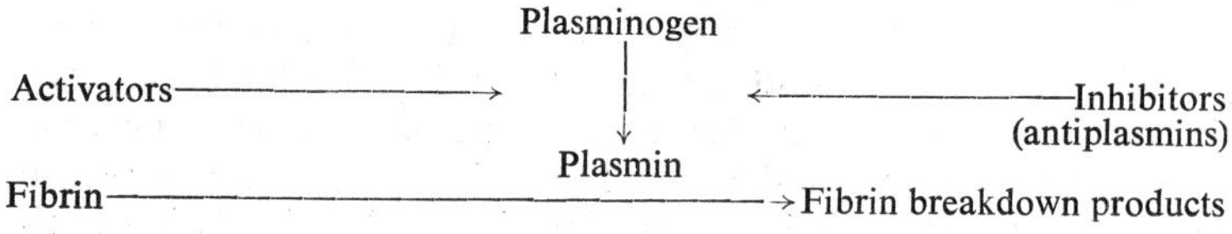

FIG. 11.3
The fibrinolytic system.

clotting occurs a small amount of plasminogen is absorbed on to the clot. Plasminogen activator is released locally from the vascular endothelium of traumatised tissues and diffuses into the clot where it converts plasminogen into plasmin. The plasmin is immediately adjacent to its substrate fibrin which it can digest before being inactivated by antiplasmin. Little or no fibrinolytic activity is found in the plasma under normal conditions since any plasmin which may be found by activation of plasma plasminogen is neutralised immediately by circulating antiplasmin.

A bleeding tendency may result from abnormalities in either the coagulation or fibrinolytic systems or from a combination of both. Defects of coagulation may result from deficiencies of coagulation factors or may be due to the presence of inhibitors. Increased fibrinolytic activity may lead to haemorrhage as a result of the digestion of fibrin in wounds and haemostatic plugs, the inappropriate digestion of fibrinogen and other coagulation factors and the anticoagulant effect of fibrin and fibrinogen breakdown products. Increased fibrinolytic activity is usually secondary to disseminated intravascular coagulation but may rarely be primary. Deficiencies in coagulation factors are summarised in Table 11.3.

Table 11.3. *Deficiencies in coagulation factors*

---

1. IMPAIRED SYNTHESIS
   a. Congenital
      Genetic causes usually lead to a deficiency of a single coagulation factor, e.g. Factor VIII in haemophilia; Factor IX in Christmas disease.
   b. Acquired
      A deficiency of vitamin K (or its antagonism by oral anticoagulants) and severe liver disease.

---

2. INCREASED UTILISATION
   a. Disseminated intravascular coagulation.
   b. Acute primary pathological fibrinolysis.

HAEMOPHILIA AND CHRISTMAS DISEASE
(For Haemophilia Centres see p. 791)

Haemophilia, the first haemorrhagic disorder to be recognised, is a hereditary bleeding disorder of males which is transmitted by healthy females. Classical haemophilia is due to a deficiency of Factor VIII and is about seven times as common as Christmas disease which is due to deficiency of Factor IX. The concentration of the clotting factor ranges from a complete deficiency to about 30 per cent. In severe haemophilics the concentration is usually less than 1 per cent. When it is between 1 and 3 per cent little trouble is usually experienced except following surgery or trauma.

Emergencies in haemophilia are common because of the tendency to bleed into joints and soft tissues either spontaneously or after minimal trauma. The most serious complications arise from pressure of blood on sensitive or vital structures. Compression of nerves is common and may result in paresis, hyperaesthesia or anaesthesia, the femoral nerve being the most frequently affected. A most serious complication is respiratory obstruction caused by blood spreading down the fascial planes after tooth extraction or following local trauma. Intracranial haemorrhage may follow trauma in children or occur spontaneously in adults. Gastrointestinal haemorrhage is seen as a complication of peptic ulceration or may result from alcohol or aspirin abuse. Complete intestinal obstruction may follow an intramural haemorrhage but this is fortunately rare. Bleeding into joints, which is the commonest complication of haemophilia, requires urgent treatment but this can often be managed on an outpatient basis.

Replacement of the missing factor is the cornerstone of treatment. The objective is to prevent or limit peripheral nerve and muscle damage, to arrest bleeding from wounds and mucous membranes and to reduce pain from bleeding into tissues and joints. Fresh whole blood is of limited value because it is not always readily available and because it is usually impractical to give enough to raise the Factor VIII level sufficiently to control bleeding.

Fresh frozen plasma is both effective and safe for most bleeding episodes in haemophilia. A dose of freshly thawed plasma (7 to 15 ml per kg body weight) is given i v over a period of half to one hour and repeated every 12 hours. Allergic reactions to plasma are sometimes seen.

Cryoprecipitate has largely replaced fresh frozen plasma in routine management of haemophilia, its small volume being a great advantage. Unfortunately the yield of Factor VIII in cryoprecipitate varies widely and as much as 50 per cent of the activity of the fresh plasma from which it is made may be lost in preparation. Accurate prediction of dosage is not always easy and, particularly with more severe bleeds, the dosage must be controlled by Factor VIII assay made immediately prior to an injection of cryoprecipitate. As a rough guide about 20 units of cryoprecipitate will be required every 12 hours in a 70 kg adult to raise the AHG level to 25 per cent.

Factor VIII concentrate is the agent of choice for those haemophilics who can undertake home treatment. It is used to supplement cryoprecipitate during and for the first few days after major surgery and is indicated for life-threatening haemorrhage when Factor VIII inhibitors are present. Animal Factor VIII concentrate is very potent being about 100 times purified as compared with human plasma but because it is antigenic it can only be used once in a patient's lifetime and usually then only for a maximum period of two weeks.

Patients with Christmas disease do not require fresh blood since Factor IX is stable but adequate blood levels cannot be achieved with whole blood. Fresh frozen plasma, prothrombin complex (Prothromplex) containing Factors II, IX and X and Factor IX concentrate are all available (see p. 795). Cryoprecipitate is useless in Christmas disease since it contains no Factor IX.

von Willebrand's disease

This haemorrhagic disorder is characterised by epistaxis, easy bruising and troublesome bleeding after tooth extraction. It is inherited in a Mendelian dominant manner and shows a prolonged bleeding time, a reduced level of Factor VIII and reduced platelet adhesiveness. It is usually mild and may be distinguished from haemophilia by the pattern of inheritance, by the prolonged bleeding time and by the Factor VIII level which is usually in the range of 25 to 30 per cent. However, in a small proportion of cases the Factor VIII level is much lower (1 to 5 per cent) and in these patients the resemblance to haemophilia may be close although haemarthroses are rare. Bleeding, spontaneous and after minor injuries, can usually be controlled by local measures but more troublesome bleeding requires the administration of cryoprecipitate or fresh frozen plasma.

Vitamin K deficiency

Fat soluble vitamin K is needed for the synthesis by the liver of prothrombin, Factor VII, Factor IX and Factor X. Deficiency occurs in haemorrhagic disease of the newborn (p. 402) and in conditions where fat absorption is impaired—obstructive jaundice, biliary fistulas, idiopathic steatorrhoea and pancreatic disease. The deficiency is rapidly corrected by oral or parenteral vitamin K, the i v or i m dose being 25 to 50 mg. When given i v it should be diluted with blood and given at a rate not exceeding 5 mg per minute. Deficiency of vitamin K is confirmed by showing that the prolonged prothrombin time returns to normal within 24 hours. If this does not occur liver disease should be suspected.

Liver disease

Since the vitamin K-dependent clotting factors are synthesised in the liver it is not surprising that low levels of prothrombin and Factors VII, IX and X and commonly found in patients with cirrhosis or severe hepatitis. The prothrombin time is prolonged and the defect is not corrected by vitamin K. Other haemostatic defects may also be present. Thrombocytopenia is common, particularly if there is associated portal hypertension; a decrease in Factor XIII occurs in about a third of patients and there may be evidence of increased fibrinolytic activity. Fibrinogen levels are only rarely depressed but there is evidence of increased fibrinogen turnover. This is thought to be due to intravascular coagulation rather than to increased fibrinolytic activity since the turnover is normalised in some patients by heparin and not by E-amino-caproic acid.

Despite the haemostatic defect bleeding in liver disease is usually only mild although severe bleeding may occur after liver biopsy (p. 59) or when there is a local cause such as varices or peptic ulceration (p. 150). In fulminating hepatitis, e.g. from paracetamol overdosage (p. 40) marked depression of fibrinogen and Factor V together with thrombocytopenia may occur in addition to depression of the vitamin K-dependent clotting factors. Diffuse bleeding into the skin and from mucous membranes is then common. The complex nature of the haemostatic defect makes the management of haemorrhage due to liver disease difficult. Large amounts of fresh plasma bring transient benefit which may be helpful before biopsy. Any benefit from plasma or concentrates of Factors II, IX and X (Prothromplex, p. 796) is likely to be short-lived. Platelet concentrate can be used to minimise thrombocytopenia.

Haemorrhage caused by oral anticoagulants

The coumarins and indanediones interfere with the vitamin K-mediated hepatic synthesis of prothrombin and Factors VII, IX and X. Orally administered coumarin is carried to the liver bound to plasma albumin. The clinical response depends upon intestinal absorption, body stores of vitamin K, degree of albumin binding, rate of detoxication and other as yet unknown factors so that the level after a standard dose varies widely. Barbiturates lessen the anticoagulant effect of coumarins by inducing synthesis of hepatic microsomal enzymes which metabolise the drug (p. 91). Other drugs such as phenylbutazone displace coumarin from its albumin binding site and thereby greatly enhance its anticoagulant effect (see also p. 92). A haemorrhagic state may result from giving phenylbutazone to a patient on an oral anticoagulant. Salicylates in high dosage may depress the vitamin K-dependent factors and potentiate the effect of coumarins. Reversal of the effects of coumarins and indanediones is achieved with parenteral vitamin K_1 a dose of 50 mg by slow i v injection restoring the prolonged prothrombin time to normal within six to twelve hours. For a more rapid effect fresh plasma or prothrombin complex (Prothromplex, p. 796) may be infused.

Haemorrhage following heparin therapy

Heparin inhibits the formation of thromboplastin and the action of thrombin. It is not absorbed from the gastro-intestinal tract and must be injected, the anticoagulant effect being immediate and lasting up to six hours. Up to 50 per cent of a large dose may be lost in the urine after conversion in the liver to a less active form. Heparin is best given i v by intermittent injection (5 000 to 10 000 units every four hours) or by continuous infusion (1 000 to 2 000 units hourly), the precise dose being monitored by the activated partial prothrombin time or thrombin time test. If intermittent injection is favoured then the test is made immediately before the next injection is due. Increased sensitivity to heparin may occur in patients with liver disease, renal disease and oliguria. Accidental overdosage may occur if the wrong strength of heparin is used. Bleeding during heparin therapy is treated by protamine sulphate (5 ml ampoules containing 10 mg per ml), one mg neutralising approximately one mg of heparin. The exact dose is best worked out by a protamine titration and this is the only method possible when heparin is given by continuous infusion. In an emergency 1 mg of protamine should be given for each 100 units of heparin if neutralisation is required at once, the dose being halved if neutralisation is required 30 minutes after injection and reduced by two-thirds if required after one hour.

Disseminated intravascular coagulation (DIC)

This condition (also called the defibrination syndrome and consumption coagulopathy) is a haemorrhagic disorder in which diffuse intravascular clotting results in haemostatic failure due to consumption of clotting factors and platelets. Chronic cases also occur. It is triggered by the release or entry of tissue factors which act as coagulants in the circulation. Extensive endothelial damage may also cause it. Coagulant substances are normally neutralised by naturally occurring circulating inhibitors and cleared by the reticuloendothelial system. When DIC is induced in animals by infusing thrombin, tissue extract or red cell lysate defibrination occurs with consumption of clotting factors and platelets. Fibrin is deposited diffusely throughout the microcirculation but is rapidly dissolved by the fibrinolytic mechanism. If the fibrinolytic inhibitor E-amino-caproic acid is given during DIC widespread thrombosis with necrotic infarction of various organs occurs suggesting that increased fibrinolytic activity is a secondary and protective mechanism. Fibrin breakdown products (FDPs) in the blood stream contribute significantly to the coagulation defect. FDPs exert a powerful antithrombin effect and also interfere with the polymerisation of fibrin.

Acute DIC occurs as a complication of obstetrical accidents such as septic abortion, abruptio placentae and amniotic fluid embolism (p. 185). It is seen also after prostatic surgery, procedures involving much handling of the lungs and when an extracorporeal circulation is used. It may be triggered off by Gram-negative and meningococcal septicaemia and a haemolytic transfusion reaction. Rarer causes are anaphylactic reactions and snake-bite poisoning (p. 629).

The clinical effects of DIC result firstly from the consumption of clotting factors (especially fibrinogen and Factors V and VIII) and platelets, and secondly from organ damage due to ischaemia with the kidneys and brain being the main target organs. In the more chronic forms of DIC as in disseminated carcinoma, a microangiopathic haemolytic anaemia may result. The diagnosis of DIC is confirmed by showing consumption of clotting factors and platelets and by detecting circulating FDPs. Damaged red cells and an increased reticulocyte count may be seen in the more chronic forms.

Management of DIC

The principles are the elimination of the cause, the replacement of missing coagulation factors and platelets and the inhibition of the clotting process by heparin. The precipitating cause may disappear (as after delivery in obstetrical patients) or may require treatment (antibiotics for septicaemia). Replacement therapy calls for fresh blood augmented by fresh frozen plasma and platelet concentrate. Fibrinogen should also be given if there is catastrophic bleeding. Heparin is indicated if there is evidence that the process of DIC is continuing or if there is organ damage and microangiopathic haemolytic anaemia.

Acute primary fibrinolysis

When a plasminogen activiator such as streptokinase is infused the thrombin time lengthens; fibrinogen and the levels of Factors V and VIII fall and a haemostatic defect may develop due to the accumulation of FDPs. These changes result from primary fibrinolysis, the circulating plasmin digesting fibrinogen and coagulation factors. Spontaneous primary fibrinolysis is very rare but does occasionally occur in liver disease. It may be differentiated from DIC by the platelet count (which is normal in primary fibrinolysis but low in DIC) and by evidence of enhanced systemic fibrinolytic activity (short dilute clot lysis time and euglobulin lysis time). In DIC with secondary fibrinolysis evidence of increased *in vitro* fibrinolytic activity is not usually found.

E-Amino-Caproic Acid (EACA) (See also pp. 185 and 548)

The use of EACA should be limited to the rare case of acute primary fibrinolysis or the rare patient with DIC in whom life-threatening haemorrhage is accompanied by laboratory evidence of marked secondary fibrinolysis. Unless one is sure that the intravascular clotting process is over it is safest to give heparin and EACA together. EACA given alone may precipitate acute renal failure due to cortical necrosis from deposition of fibrin in the glomerular capillaries. EACA can be given by mouth (5 g initially followed by 1 g hourly) or i v (5 g over the first hour followed by 1 g hourly). EACA is claimed to be of value in reducing postoperative bleeding following prostatectomy, in controlling menorrhagia and in helping to reduce bleeding after tooth extraction in haemophilics. In these conditions it is thought to act by neutralising local fibrinolytic activity and thereby allowing a firmer clot to form.

JOHN MACIVER

FOR FURTHER READING

Megaloblastic anaemia
LAWSON, D. H., MURRAY, R. M. & PARKER, J. L. W. (1972). Early mortality in the megaloblastic anaemias. *Quarterly Journal of Medicine*, **41**, 1.
Aplastic anaemia
WILLIAMS, D. M., LYNCH, R. E. & CARTWRIGHT, G. E. (1973). Drug-induced aplastic anemia. *Seminars in Hematology*, **10**, 195.
Haemolytic anaemias
DACIE, J. V. & WORLLEDGE, S. M. Auto-immune hemolytic anemias. In *Progress in Hematology VI*. Eds. Brown, E. B. & Moore, C. V. New York: Grune and Stratton. 1969.
WORLLEDGE, S. M. Immune drug-induced haemolytic anaemias. In *Blood Disorders due to Drugs and Other Agents*. Ed. Girdwood, R. H. Amsterdam: Exerpta Medica. 1973.
GUY, R. B. & ROTHENBERG, S. P. (1973). Sickle cell crisis. *The Medical Clinics of North America*, **57**, 1591.
ALLAN, N. C. Effects of drugs and other agents in erythrocyte enzyme deficiencies and haemoglobinopathies. In *Blood Disorders due to Drugs and Other Agents*. Ed. Girdwood, R. H. Amsterdam: Exerpta Medica. 1973.

Polycythaemia

MODAN, B. *The Polycythemic Disorders.* Springfield, Illinois: Charles C. Thomas. 1971.

Leukaemia

BEARD, M. E. J. & HAMILTON FAIRLEY, G. (1974). Acute leukemia in adults. *Seminars in Hematology,* **11,** 5.

SIMONE, J. (1974). Acute lymphocytic leukemia in childhood. *Seminars in Hematology,* **11,** 25.

Malignant lympho-reticular disorders

McELWAIN, T. J. (1974). Chemotherapy of the lymphomas. *Clinics in Haematology* **3,** 195.

FARHANGI, M. & OSSERMAN, E. F.. (1973). The treatment of multiple myeloma. *Seminars in Hematology,* **10,** 149.

BLOCH, K. J. & MAKI, D. G. (1973). Hyperviscosity syndromes associated with immunoglobulin abnormalities. *Seminars in Hematology,* **10,** 113.

Agranulocytosis

FINCH, S. C. Granulocyte disorders—benign quantitative disorders of granulocytes. In *Hematology.* Ed. Williams, W. J., *et al.* New York: McGraw-Hill Inc. 1972.

Infectious mononucleosis

FINCH, S. C. Clinical symptoms and signs of infectious mononucleosis. In *Infectious Mononucleosis.* Eds. Carter, R. L. & Penman, H. G. Oxford and Edinburgh: Blackwell Scientific Publications. 1969.

Haemorrhagic disorders

PRANKERD, T. A. J. Idiopathic thrombocytopenic purpura. In *Clinics in Haematology.* Ed. O'Brien, J. R. London: W. B. Saunders Company Ltd. 1972.

GYNN, T. N., MESSMORE, H. L. & FRIEDMAN, I. A. (1972). Drug induced thrombocytopenia. *The Medical Clinics of North America,* **56,** 65.

KWAAN, H. C. (1972). Disorders of fibrinolysis. *The Medical Clinics of North America,* **56,** 163.

KWAAN, H. C. (1972). Disseminated intravascular coagulation. *The Medical Clinics of North America,* **56,** 177.

DUTHIE, R. B., MATTHEWS, J. M., RIZZA, C. R. & STEEL, W. M. *The Management of Musculo-skeletal Problems in the Haemophilias.* Oxford: Blackwell Scientific Publications. 1972.

CHAPTER 12

Fits, Faints and Unconsciousness

IT is intended here to discuss in a general way the problem of the urgent call occasioned by a sudden illness in which consciousness is clouded or lost.

Cases fall into two groups:

1. Those in which the 'fit' or 'faint' is of short duration: 'episodic unconsciousness' due in most cases to epilepsy, hysteria or syncope.

2. Those in which unconsciousness is profound (i.e. coma) and relatively prolonged.

In general loss of consciousness from a faint is preceded by a period of lightheadedness and awareness of the impending episode, the vision failing first. Loss of consciousness from a fit may be preceded by a short aura whose nature remains constant for the particular patient. The dogmatic differentiation, however, which follows is not absolute for a prolonged syncopal attack may itself cause an epileptiform convulsion in a non-epileptic patient.

FITS AND FAINTS

Except when it occurs in hospital the attack is usually over or the patient obviously improving by the time the doctor arrives. Three questions should arise in his mind.

1. Is it a fit, i.e., neurological in origin?
2. Is it a faint, i.e., cardiovascular in origin?
3. Is it some other kind of attack?

Is it a fit?

This question may be easy to answer if there is a history of previous attacks competently observed. The occurrence of clonic movements, and not merely stiffness, suggests that the attack is a fit. Incontinence of urine, tongue biting, and injury in the attack also point strongly, though not conclusively, to epilepsy (but do not indicate its cause). Occasionally a daytime fit may bring the doctor to a patient whose previous nocturnal attacks were unrecognised. A history of waking with a headache and a bruised feeling in the limbs suggests convulsions during the night. Unequivocal evidence of organic nervous disease, such as cerebral tumour, suggests that the attack was a fit. The older the patient the more likely is a fit to indicate organic brain disease.

Minor epilepsy or petit mal as a cause of 'fainting' may be hard to diagnose since there are no clonic movements. Loss and recovery of consciousness are sudden, producing a mere hiatus in cerebration; postepileptic phenomena, automatism, etc. have special diagnostic value but they are relatively rare. In a cardiovascular 'faint' consciousness is more gradually lost and regained. It is generally preceded by dimness of vision since the retina is especially sensitive to hypoxia. Tongue scars and congenital epidermal defects suggest epilepsy. A convulsion in a child should only be classed as a 'febrile fit' if the child is off-colour and febrile and under 5 years old. It is rare in the first six months of life. The febrile convulsion is generalised and never focal.

Is it a faint?

In all the conditions of cardiovascular origin in which consciousness is lost the mechanism is that a period of cardiac systole or arrhythmia or of low blood pressure (< 50 mm Hg) affects first the cerebral cortex and releases the central reticular formation on which consciousness depends. A transient state of tonic rigidity may appear but there are no real clonic movements as in epilepsy and the EEG is normal. Pallor is somewhat in favour of syncope and is due to stimulation of the neurohypophysis by marked hypotension.

These cases may be placed in two groups.

1. Where there is clear evidence of heart disease, e.g., heart block, aortic incompetence.

2. Where there are no signs of cardiovascular disease, e.g., vasovagal attacks, and carotid sinus syncope. Cough syncope and fainting at stool come under this heading. Transient faintness after squatting and standing up as in gardening is really a normal phenomenon. The increased filling pressure of the heart from squatting causes reflex vasodilatation. Sudden erect posture in these circumstances may cause transient cerebral hypoxia. When fainting is caused by postural hypostatic hypotension the common causes are antihypertensive drugs and loss of vascular reflexes from ageing but a low serum sodium, often related to a hot climate and the use of diuretics, may play a part.

COUGH SYNCOPE. Syncope may follow a paroxysm of coughing in the same way as in Valsalva's manoeuvre where an attempt is made to breathe out against a closed glottis. Intrathoracic pressure raised by coughing impedes venous return and so leads to a decrease of cardiac output and a fall of blood pressure sufficient to cause cerebral hypoxia. Increased CSF pressure may also play a part by squeezing blood out of the cerebral vessels. As these are probably atheromatous in the patient subject to cough syncope he is abnormally intolerant of a fall in blood pressure. Sometimes an intracranial tumour has been present and so the symptom must not be too readily ascribed to haemodynamic changes.

The subject is rarely a woman but generally a middle-aged emphysematous and plethoric (but not hypertensive) man who, after a fit of violent coughing, and in rare cases after only a few coughs, becomes unconscious for a few seconds. Those who have much sputum rarely have syncope on coughing. In minor attacks there is simply giddiness and Charcot, who first described the condition, called it ' laryngeal vertigo '. The emergency soon rights itself and between attacks no special treatment is needed, though smoking which causes the cough should be avoided. The patient should try to cough gently as violence in coughing seems to be the important factor. When unconsciousness follows a single cough in a young adult it is thought that the condition is epilepsy with cough as the aura.

MICTURITION SYNCOPE. This may occur on rising to empty the bladder. Presumably powerful detrusor action causes a strong vagal stimulus. Recovery is rapid and complete. Loss of consciousness may follow rectal examination (PROSTATIC SYNCOPE) particularly in a dyspnoeic patient who has to stand and lean forwards. The left lateral position is safer and the patient should be relaxed and breathing through the mouth.

Is it some other kind of attack?

Two common ones should be considered.

1. Hypoglycaemia (see also p. 346). A clear history of insulin injected and not followed soon enough by a meal will usually point to the diagnosis but difficulties will arise if no witnesses are present. Search should be made for needle marks and a diabetic card, Medic-Alert bracelet (p. 822) or literature in the pockets. If in doubt, dextrose should be injected i v (p. 347). In a non-diabetic spontaneous hypoglycaemia is a rare cause of coma. Diagnosis may be difficult for the signs can be curiously focal. The history and other features such as sweating are useful clues.

2. Internal haemorrhage—as from a duodenal ulcer. There may be a history of dyspepsia. Increasing pallor, increasing rapidity of pulse, dyspnoea and restlessness should suggest that haemorrhage is the cause of the faint. Anaemia of similar degree but not due to acute blood loss does not cause syncope.

' Drop attacks '

The victim of the ' drop attack ' is nearly always a middle-aged woman whose legs suddenly ' give way ' while walking so that she falls without warning. Movement of the head plays no part in initiating the attack. There is no loss of consciousness and, while recovery is often immediate, loss of muscle tone may persist for some hours. Pressure on the soles or even moving the patient a little will often restore it. Falling is brought about by an interruption of the postural reflexes on which the erect position depends. Falling attacks of known origin are excluded, such as temporary brain stem ischaemia precipitated by certain movements of the head in patients with cervical spondylosis. A bruit over the mastoid or occiput points to an organic cause as does evidence of vestibular dysfunction. Attacks are liable to occur periodically over the years but spontaneous cessation is not unknown.

COMA

Here unconsciousness is more prolonged than in a fit or faint. There is nothing about unconsciousness which announces how it arose and diagnosis of the cause depends on the other fidings. A long list of causes, though valuable in discussion, is not as helpful when faced with a comatose patient as a plan of inquiry. The history from the relatives or the police will often point to the diagnosis and a Medic-Alert bracelet (p. 822) may provide the clue. A general and neurological examination should follow and be repeated over a period to enable a distinction to be made between toxic and localised (neurological) causes. The following inquiries are suggested. Is there a history of disease which might cause coma? e.g. diabetes (test the urine for ketone bodies and sugar); insulin coma (if this seems likely give dextrose 10 g i v or glucagon 1 mg i m); nephritis (test the urine for albumin); hepatic cirrhosis (look for spider naevi, red palms, a palpable spleen and hepatic fetor); malignant tertian malaria. (In persons reaching Britain by air from the tropics the first attack may occur here so take a geographical history, make thick and thin blood films and start treatment (see p. 449).

Does the immediate history point to the cause? Was there an injury? Do not too readily assume it is the whole cause. Consider poisoning, including alcohol, and have the urine or vomit examined for drugs (p. 25).

Are there any physical signs of a lesion in the central nervous system? In the case of an unresponsive patient without organic disease head movements cause conjugate movements of the eyes to the opposite side by the reflex mechanism which in an normal subject preserves ocular fixation despite head movement. Failure to show these 'doll's head eye movements' argues in favour of organic nervous disease. It may be necessary in a deeply comatose patient to fix the opened eyelids by tape. When eye tests are inconclusive an ear may be syringed with iced water. This normally causes conjugate deviation of the eyes towards the irrigated side. Failure to do this points to an organic lesion of the brain stem.

Unilateral lesions of the cerebral hemispheres unless very large and space-occupying rarely cause coma. Embolic infarction of the territory supplied by the middle cerebral artery in the dominant hemisphere may be responsible. When a tumour is suspected and other causes of unconsciousness are confidently excluded the patient should be moved to a unit where neurosurgery can be undertaken urgently if need be.

A rare pitfall in diagnosis is to mistake for coma the condition of a patient whose pontine lesion has made him quadriplegic and mute though alert and sentient. Some voluntary eyelid opening movements remain (the 'locked-in syndrome ').

Feigned or simulated unconsciousness. ' Psychogenic unresponsiveness.'

This phenomenon of escape from an intolerable situation is less common than it used to be. Detection rests on the fact that while the patient does not respond to stimuli ('Hysterical unconsciousness') all the reflexes are normal. There may be flickering of the eyelids and when the doctor tries to open them this is resisted. A light unexpected stroke of a finger on the eyelashes causes an obvious blink. Another sign is that when the vermilion border of the lips and the adjoining fine hairs are stroked with a wisp of cotton wool the facial muscles respond. Normal ' doll's head ' eye movements are present (see p. 729). Sometimes impressive signs such as simulated haemoptysis complicate the picture and there is a history of similar attacks and of admissions to many hospitals ('Munchausen syndrome'). The patient may be described in warning notices sent round to casualty departments.

Causes of coma

This list may help in considering a case of obscure coma. (For coma in the elderly see p. 619: for postoperative coma see p. 614.)

COMA WITH FOCAL SIGNS.

Supratentorial   Cerebral haemorrhage and massive infarction (p. 304).

                 Subdural and extradural haematoma (p. 300).

                 Cerebral tumour.

Brain stem   Pontine haemorrhage and infarction.

                 Cerebellar haemorrhage.

Diffuse   Encephalitis (pp. 313 and 441). Injury (p. 299).

                 Subarachnoid haemorrhage (p. 305).

                 Electric shock (p. 648).

                 Hypertensive encephalopathy (p. 232).

COMA WITHOUT FOCAL SIGNS

Diabetes (p. 337). Hypoglycaemia (p. 346). Injury.
Epilepsy (p. 308). Drugs (p. 27). Hepatic failure (p. 145).
Renal failure (p. 374).
Hypothermia (p. 361). Myxoedema (p. 363).
Simmonds's disease (p. 365). Adrenal cortical failure (p. 353).
Stokes-Adams attacks (p. 262).

EMERGENCY MEASURES FOR THE COMATOSE PATIENT

As well as treating the underlying cause attention must be directed to certain urgent aspects of any comatose patient.

1. Adequate oxygenation.

   The immediate need is to preserve the airway and to use artificial respiration if need be, i.e. if the rate and depth of breathing is no more than enough to clear the dead space so that cyanosis results (i.e. less than 4 litres a minute).

2. Position.

   The correct position lessens the risk of aspiration pneumonia and should be maintained until the patient can cough and swallow properly. Place the patient on his side with the foot of the bed raised 15 to 25 cm. Put pillows behind his back and between his knees but not under his head. Adhesive felt should protect the shoulder.

3. Fluid balance.

   An adult should receive 2 500 ml of fluid (dextrose 5 g/dl) and 4·5 g sodium chloride each day by intragastric or i v drip. A calorie intake of 1 500 should be aimed at.

C. ALLAN BIRCH

CHAPTER 13

Neurological Emergencies

THERE is a feeling of helplessness in the face of a neurological emergency based on the belief that damaged nerve cells do not regenerate and that the differential diagnosis is too difficult for all but the expert neurologist. Both of these beliefs are mistaken. When the nervous system, central or peripheral, is suddenly disturbed by physical disease or injury there is a temporary suspension of activity described as ' neuronal shock '. Though the nature of this arrest of function of nerve cells and their processes is unknown, recovery may be anticipated, leaving a permanent deficit of function due to loss of those neurones which were irreversibly damaged. It is therefore most important to preserve vital functions until the amount of recovery is seen. The emergency measures required depend on the site of the lesion rather than on its nature so that the question of rigorous diagnosis rarely arises. For this reason the following account will be based primarily on the disorders of function and their management.

Treatment aimed at the first cause is rarely possible, but a moment's reflection will show that this is also true of other organs. One does not fail to treat the disordered function of the failing heart or the effects of ischaemia of the myocardium because of ignorance of the cause of the disease or inability to reverse it. There is in fact as much therapy in the full sense for neurological disease as for disorders of other systems. It is not realistic to differentiate between medical and surgical emergencies of the nervous system. The physician will be responsible for advising on many aspects of head injuries and many agonising decisions must be taken in the home or medical ward regarding the necessity to decompress the brain or spinal cord surgically. Cerebrovascular disease is becoming a joint problem at a time when the role of the surgeon in treatment of subarachnoid haemorrhage is being re-examined. Tic douloureux is once again a ' medical ' disorder.

LOSS OF CONSCIOUSNESS

Few emergencies create such alarm as sudden loss of consciousness. Life is precarious and time wasted cannot be regained. It must be used with the right priorities.

Preservation of respiration

The first priority is to ensure a patent airway by removing mucus or foreign matter from the nasopharynx with a mechanical sucker and by pulling the tongue forward. The cleared airway is then maintained by placing the patient semiprone with the head lowered (see also p. 292). This posture encourages drainage of fluid from lungs and pharynx and has no harmful effects on the damaged brain. If it is possible to do so, a stomach tube should be passed and left in position. The stomach contents should be aspirated (p. 722) to remove a potential hazard to respiration (p. 601).

Do not be satisfied unless respiration is quiet and regular. Stertorous respiration is not a sign of cerebral damage but of respiratory obstruction. If this cannot be relieved by the simple measures described or if frequent suction is required it is necessary to pass an endotracheal tube if the depth of coma is sufficient for the patient to tolerate it. A cuffed tube is most satisfactory as it prevents aspiration while ensuring a patent airway but the cuff should be deflated every two hours (after sucking out the mouth and pharynx) to reduce the risk of pressure necrosis of the larynx.

Tracheostomy (p. 737) may be necessary if intubation is needed for more than 24 hours and if consciousness has not lightened. It may be considered earlier if a long ambulance journey is necessary. It is almost essential in cases of head injury complicated by fractures of the jaw. If in doubt, it is wise to make a tracheostomy earlier rather than later.

After the airway has been assured the respiratory excursion must be observed for a few minutes. Slow (10 to 12 per minute), shallow, periodic (Cheyne-Stokes type) or irregular breathing are all signs of medullary failure. Nikethamide Injection (4 to 8 ml) may be helpful but if respiratory failure is due to posterior fossa compression this must be relieved urgently as apnoea may supervene suddenly.

Neurological examination

The priority of safeguarding respiration is stressed since death may otherwise occur while diagnosis is being attempted. This is also important because of the contribution of cerebral hypoxia to the neurological picture. It is not uncommon for ' cerebral irritation ' or signs of decerebrate rigidity to disappear or even for consciousness to return when cerebral oxygenation is restored. Neurological examination is misleading if carried out before this is achieved.

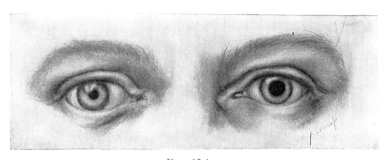

FIG. 13.1A

Hutchinson's pupils : second stage.
Opposite side to lesion : normal.
Side of lesion : dilated; reacts to light.

STAGE	PUPIL ON OPPOSITE SIDE TO THE LESION		PUPIL ON SIDE ON WHICH COMPRESSION COMMENCED	
1	Normal	●	Slightly contracted. Sluggishly reacts to light	●
2	Normal	●	Moderately dilated. Reacts to light	●
3	Moderately dilated. Reacts to light	●	Widely dilated. Does not react to light	●
4	Widely dilated. Insensitive	●	Widely dilated. Insensitive.	●

FIG. 13.1B

The four stages of Hutchinson's pupils.

The first stage is rarely seen. It is the second (Fig. 13.1A) and third stages that are of signal diagnostic importance. These changes are produced by initial irritation and subsequent paralysis of the third nerve, usually by subtentorial herniation of the hippocampal gyrus.

Facing page 295

At this stage the first decision to be made is whether coma is due to an intracranial lesion or to one of the many other causes (p. 292). The pupils should first be examined. Bilateral ' pin-point ' pupils suggest narcotic poisoning or a pontine lesion. Fixed dilated pupils may be found after an epileptic fit but if the patient has been unconscious for more than half an hour they indicate severe midbrain disturbance. This may be due to cerebral compression in its final stages. Less severe rise of intracranial pressure above the tentorium causes temporal lobe herniation with pressure on one oculomotor nerve (III), usually on the side of the expanding lesion. The pupil of the eye which it supplies contracts briefly then progressively dilates and fails to respond reflexly. With increasing pressure the other pupil is similarly affected until both are dilated and fixed (Hutchinson's pupils: Figs 13.1A and B). Other signs of oculomotor palsy such as ptosis and ophthalmoplegia are difficult to detect in the unconscious patient. Skew deviation of the eyes or dissociated rolling of the eyeballs indicate midbrain damage. Corneal reflexes may be tested now but rarely provide information unobtainable by less traumatic methods.

The ocular fundi should then be examined for papilloedema. Subhyaloid haemorrhage may be seen in subarachnoid haemorrhage, and the retinal signs of diabetes mellitus or renal failure may assist diagnosis. At this stage the important consideration is to identify raised intracranial pressure. If it is absent there is no need for emergency measures provided that respiration is controlled and diagnostic lumbar puncture may be considered when clinical examination has been completed. If there is papilloedema (other than the acute type associated with subarachnoid haemorrhage) lumbar puncture should not be carried out until a burr hole has been made in the skull to permit ventricular drainage if necessary. Papilloedema unaccompanied by the vascular signs of malignant hypertension normally indicates the presence of increased intracranial pressure which may require urgent treatment (p. 297).

The level of consciousness should now be assessed and findings written down in such a way that later observers can tell whether coma has lightened or deepened. Discussions about the difference between drowsiness, stupor, and precoma are tiresome. It is more important to record whether the patient can be roused to any sort of response and if so by what type of stimulus—a loud voice, shaking, slapping the face, stroking the soles of the feet, pinching the limbs, or pressure on a supraorbital nerve (an approximately ascending series of intensity of stimulus). The response should be observed since movement confined to one side of the body may indicate that the other side is paralysed. The same stimulus should be applied to symmetrical areas of each side of the body. Failure to respond to stimuli on one side only may indicate that that side is anaesthetic. (This test may be helpful in lateralisation of cerebral damage but should not be relied on as the sole sign.) If coma is not too deep the eyelids may blink in response to a feint by the examiner's hand. This should be repeated from each side as failure of response to a threat from one side only is valuable evidence of hemianopia. Spontaneous cough and swallowing should be noted if present.

The muscle tone should now be assessed. Any tendency of the head and eyes to turn to one side when the trunk is supine is noted. If there is recent cerebral damage the head and eyes tend to turn towards the damaged side. The limbs should be raised and allowed to drop. In deep coma all limbs are flaccid. If there is bilateral rigidity with extended legs, and upper limbs extended, adducted and hyperpronated with fists clenched, the signs indicate decerebrate rigidity due to midbrain damage which may be the result of a ' pressure cone '.

If tone is not symmetrical, the limb with greater tone tends to drop more slowly and in a less ' abandoned ' manner than its partner. Even though the pyramidal tract is damaged, in an acute lesion such as is likely to cause loss of consciousness the paralysed side is that with least tone. If tendon reflexes are present the decision is more difficult because the return of reflexes accompanies resumption of tone and with it the early signs of spasticity may appear. At that time the abnormal limb is the one with the greater tone. Plantar reflexes may not be helpful in deep coma as they may be absent or bilaterally extensor even in the absence of cerebral injury. Inequality of plantar reflexes is always a valuable sign. A unilateral extensor plantar reflex is the best possible indication of damage to the contralateral hemisphere (providing that the circumstances do not raise the possibility of concomitant spinal cord damage as in road accidents). A grasp reflex should be looked for as its presence on one side indicates a lesion of the opposite frontal lobe. This is tested for by drawing two fingers rapidly and firmly across the patient's palm. If it is positive the patient closes his hand and grasps the stimulating fingers firmly though involuntarily. Finally the patient should be examined for signs of meningeal irritation. Kernig's sign may always be sought, but neck stiffness should only be tested where circumstances exclude the possibility of cervical cord injury.

It should now be possible to decide on the presence of (1) raised intracranial pressure, (2) a unilateral cerebral lesion, (3) meningism.

If there is no evidence of compression or meningism and no lateral-ising signs the search should now be turned towards one of the many non-neurological causes of coma (p. 292). The most urgent question, if respiration is controlled, is now the management of intracranial hypertension.

INTRACRANIAL HYPERTENSION

High pressure within the skull is not necessarily dangerous to life although eyesight may be imperilled by chronic papilloedema. In the so-called benign intracranial hypertension states the patient is fully alert. It is not the pressure alone which is dangerous nor yet the ' compression ' of the cerebrum which is implied by the older terminology. The danger is greatest when pressure is unequal in the different compartments into which the cranium is divided by the falx and tentorium and in the spinal subarachnoid space. A gradient of pressure causes shift of brain substance from a high pressure compartment into a neighbouring lower pressure one. The herniated brain substance may compress other structures. The pupillary changes described above are due to the medial part of one temporal lobe herniating through the tentorial opening and compressing the oculomotor nerve. Other signs of ' tentorial cone ' are due to down-ward shift of the brain stem, probably causing traction on blood vessels with eventual petechial haemorrhages. As the unilateral pupillary dilatation occurs the patient becomes drowsy and there is progressive loss of consciousness. Decerebrate rigidity, brady-cardia, and reactive hypertension may occur.

These signs of acute tentorial herniation are now recognised more widely than they were. It is, however, easy to miss the slower type of chronic tentorial coning. The conscious level fluctuates with quite rapid changes from drowsiness to full alertness, conjugate upward gaze is depressed (often accompanied by bilateral ptosis) and there may be hemiplegic or hemianopic signs, both of which may fluctuate and appear on the ' wrong ' side for the supposed lesion.

When the pressure is greatest in the posterior fossa, the cerebellar tonsils tend to herniate through the foramen magnum (foraminal impaction or ' cerebellar cone '). The neck becomes stiff, the head tilted, and its backward movement causes tingling in the arms or sudden loss of consciousness. The disorders of respiratory rhythm described above occur with this type of pressure cone and death may occur suddenly.

In both types of brain shift, the condition may change rapidly from the chronic to the acute type if the patient is given a sedative or if respiration is impaired in any other way, or if a lumbar puncture is carried out despite the presence of papilloedema. In all unconscious patients the level of consciousness, judged by the response to verbal and painful stimuli, pupil size, respiration and pulse rate and the blood pressure should be recorded every half hour.

Treatment. The only certain method of reducing intracranial pressure rapidly and safely is by ventricular cannulation through a burr hole but this is effective only when there is some ventricular dilatation. If increased intracranial pressure is suspected, even without papilloedema, and lumbar puncture is deemed necessary a burr hole should be made so that a brain cannula may be inserted with the least possible delay. If this has not been done and the patient is already unconscious when seen, pressure may be relieved by dehydration therapy but the time gained must be used to prepare for urgent surgical treatment. On no account should a lumbar puncture be carried out in the presence of papilloedema unless there is strong evidence that this is due to meningitis, delay in treating which may jeopardise the chance of recovery.

The principle of dehydration therapy is to inject into the blood stream a slowly excreted crystalloid which will attract fluid from the tissues by increasing the osmotic pressure of the blood. A saturated (20 g/dl) solution of mannitol, stored in a warm cupboard to prevent crystallisation, may be given rapidly (up to 500 ml in 20 minutes). Frusemide 80 mg i v may be used instead of or before mannitol. These drugs are preferable to urea (30 g/dl in a 10 g/dl solution of invert sugar in a dose of 1·0 to 1·5 g per kg body weight). As urea is locally irritant the injection should take 10 to 30 minutes. This treatment dehydrates the brain in about 15 minutes by causing an osmotic diuresis and the pressure is reduced for four to six hours. Dextrose or sucrose 50 g/l is less effective and causes a rebound rise in pressure but 50 ml can be given by slow i v injection in an emergency. Corticosteroids are less valuable for urgent treatment but if a few hours delay is acceptable betamethasone may be used. The dose is 4 mg three times a day reducing to 2 mg three times a day after three days and continuing at 2 mg daily.

Dehydration therapy is used for the management of raised intracranial pressure when the duration of treatment is expected to be short, or to gain time so that essential investigations may be completed or preparations made for surgical operation. It should not be used for more that two days and its value must be weighed against the serious danger of dehydration of the body as a whole. In the conscious patient where recovery is anticipated and oral feeding is reasonably normal the treatment may be continued by the old-fashioned method of giving sufficient magnesium sulphate by mouth to keep the bowels loose. Enemas of concentrated magnesium sulphate are now used only in circumstances where improvisation is necessary (250 ml as a retention enema every six hours) (p. 728). If prolonged decompression is necessary the most suitable methods are surgical.

In the unconscious patient maintenance of fluid and electrolyte balance assumes increasing priority after the first day of coma. If further decompression is required it should be achieved by ventricular drainage or other surgical method. Standard nursing procedures for the care of the skin, paralysed limbs, bladder, bowel and body temperature must be instituted from the beginning. Failure to do so may cause pressure sores, hypostatic pneumonia, bladder distension, or 'frozen' joints which may take many months to cure but which are readily prevented (Simpson, 1974a).

The question of prophylactic antibiotic 'cover' is controversial. The present trend is against it and the appropriate antibiotic is only started if infection develops. There are sound reasons for this if illness is likely to be prolonged but for emergencies of comparatively short duration, such as head injuries and coma due to strokes, the prevention of unnecessary complications justifies prophylactic use. Such cover must not be a reason for relaxing nursing standards which must be of the highest.

HEAD INJURY

The management of the patient who is unconscious because of a head injury is essentially medical. Attention to respiration is particularly emphasised (p. 294). Traditionally or because of associated injuries, the treatment is commonly carried out in a surgical ward, although very few patients require neurosurgical intervention for intracranial complications. The importance of recognising these complications justifies this.

Immediate loss of consciousness after head injury ('concussion') is still not fully understood. In most cases full consciousness is regained within 24 hours. The management during this period should be as described above, no special measures being required. The later management is beyond the scope of this book and is well described by Potter (1965). The important point is that vigilance should not be relaxed when consciousness is seen to be returning because it may be lost again. Deteriorating conscious level is usually a sign of progressive cerebral ' compression ' and occasionally of meningitis. This progression may be continuous from the time of injury or after initial lightening of coma. If the patient has recovered consciousness and then lapsed into coma again the ' lucid interval ' is very evident but the changing level will only be noticed in the unconscious patient if the reaction to stimuli and other factors described by Potter (1965) are noted. The important point is that vigilance should be recorded at intervals not exceeding 30 minutes. This applies even during periods of apparent sleep during the first 24 hours. The nurse must attempt to rouse the patient every half hour. Restlessness may be equally significant, particularly if it persists after the bladder has been emptied. Cerebral compression may be due to an intracranial haematoma or to cerebral oedema.

Extradural haemorrhage

If the signs of intracranial hypertension are developing rapidly it is probable that there is a haematoma and this is likely to be extradural, particularly if there is injury in the temporal region. This is usually due to a fracture involving the middle meningeal artery. Haemorrhage is brisk and the extradural haematoma expands rapidly so that signs may be evident within an hour or so of injury. Most cases are diagnosed within 24 hours but this complication should be considered in all patients showing deterioration of consciousness within the first week. The site of the lesion may be suggested by soft tissue swelling in one temporal region, or X ray evidence of a temporal fracture. If the pupillary signs of tentorial herniation develop (p. 295), the dilatation first occurs on the side of the haematoma. A unilateral epileptic fit or neurological deficit may suggest the side involved but both sides should always be explored.

Treatment. Extradural haemorrhage is an emergency requiring immediate treatment and there is rarely time for the patient to be moved to a neurosurgeon. Any available surgeon must trephine the skull at the injured area or over the middle meningeal arteries to allow blood to escape (5 cm above the zygoma and 5 cm behind the posterior margin of the orbital crest). Once consciousness is lost, or the pupil dilates, or decerebrate rigidity and periodic breathing develop there may be only minutes left before it is too late (Jennett, 1970). Even asepsis may have to take a second place. The bleeding can later be stopped and evacuation of the clot completed by a neurosurgeon. As this may entail considerable blood loss the patient's blood should be grouped and cross-matched.

Subdural and intracranial haematoma

Slower development of signs of compression or negative exploration for extradural haemorrhage may be due to a subdural or intracerebral haematoma caused by ' cerebral laceration ' or tearing of subdural veins. These cases rarely present as medical emergencies but they may be acute. There is usually time to localise the lesion by electroencephalography, ultrasonography, and arteriography. The treatment is surgical. The main importance to the physician is their recognition as a cause of failure to improve after head injury or of persistent headache and mental changes.

Cerebral oedema

Brain swelling secondary to injury is difficult to diagnose as a cause of raised intracranial pressure and should only be accepted as the explanation if extradural haematoma has been excluded by exploratory burr holes and other haematomas by arteriography. Lumbar puncture is not helpful as some bleeding is invariable after injury and the rise in pressure is not in question. In view of the danger of precipitating a pressure cone (p. 297) it is best avoided.

If no haematoma can be demonstrated, dehydration therapy (p. 298) may be valuable. Steroids will reduce cerebral oedema but their action is too slow for use in an emergency (p. 298).

Cerebral irritation

This is the traditional term for the stage of restless and disorganised behaviour which is common in the transitional period between coma and regaining of normal consciousness after head injury. Contributory factors are blood in the subarachnoid space and discomfort due to a full bladder, but the restlessness and noisiness are mainly due to absence of normal inhibition.

In ideal circumstances the patient should be permitted to pass through this phase with only such physical restraints as may be necessary to prevent him from falling out of bed, and removing dressings or an oesophageal tube, or otherwise harming himself. Sedative drugs compromise the detection of relapse as the conscious level is artificially depressed. Depression of respiration and the cough reflex is undesirable. Mild sedation at night may be permitted and chlorpromazine (Largactil) 25 mg three times daily may be used from five days after the injury. Sedation is more often given for the convenience of the attendants and other patients. Suitable sound-insulated accommodation for the restless patient would be more rational.

11

WERNICKE'S ENCEPHALOPATHY

This is a syndrome due to thiamine (vitamin B_1) deficiency in which there is rapid onset of stupor, delirium, ataxia, nystagmus, ophthalmoplegias and pupillary disturbances caused by small vascular lesions in the midbrain. It is characteristically seen in chronic alcoholism and beri-beri but may accompany other causes of vitamin deficiency such as hyperemesis gravidarum and gastrointestinal disease. Wernicke's encephalopathy may be associated with polyneuropathy and Korsakoff's psychosis.

There may be dramatic resolution of mental and ocular signs within one to six hours after i v injection of thiamine, 2 to 5 mg. A convenient preparation is Parentrovite-HP. This treatment may also promote rapid return of consciousness from coma due to alcohol or hypnotic intoxication.

CEREBROVASCULAR CATASTROPHES

In considering the emergency problems of strokes it is necessary to think of the pathological state of the brain at the time the patient is seen by the doctor. It is too late to take action to preserve cerebral function if the patient has already recovered from a brief stroke or if the stroke is already complete and has destroyed cerebral tissue, either by infarction or by destruction from bleeding. Thus the problems of the doctor faced with a transient stroke or a completed stroke are the steps to be taken to prevent further attacks or to rehabilitate the brain-damaged patient. These are not emergency problems (Simpson, 1974a) except for the management of coma if present (p. 294).

Prevention of further attacks may, however, begin immediately. If there is strong evidence of embolism as a cause of cerebral infarction, heparin should be given as soon as possible, 10 000 units i v every six hours for 48 hours with warfarin 20 mg by mouth on the first day, 100 mg on the second, and thereafter according to the plasma prothrombin level.

The urgent problem is the stroke which is still progressing when seen by the doctor and the stroke which, though not advancing, has involved only part of the cerebral territory supplied by the damaged vessel (Marshall, 1968). If the neurological deficit is still progressing a few hours after the onset of the stroke it has been customary to make a diagnosis of cerebral infarction due to thrombosis of a cerebral artery. It is now certain that most of these are infarction due to stenosis or occlusion of an extracerebral artery (internal carotid or vertebral artery) and many to a slowly expanding intracerebral haematoma.

It is tempting to believe that viable brain tissue would recover if oxygen could be brought to the area of infarction within the first few minutes. Unfortunately the usual vasodilators do not dilate cerebral vessels; indeed their use may aggravate the condition by diverting blood from the brain to other parts of the body. Carbon dioxide is the only identified dilator of cerebral vessels. The CO_2 tension in an infarcted zone is already high and it is unlikely that there is any value in administering oxygen with added CO_2. It is possible to detect the onset of cerebral ischaemia within the first few minutes in patients who have recently had a carotid artery angiogram and in these circumstances oxygen with 5 per cent CO_2 may be given immediately. Oxygen inhalation may worsen the situation by provoking cerebral vasoconstriction and no benefit results from placing the patient in a chamber with oxygen at a pressure of two atmospheres.

Internal carotid stenosis

This is the probable cause of a slowly evolving stroke if the progress is 'stuttering' rather than regular. This diagnosis is also supported if the paralysis involves the face and arm but spares the lower limb and if there is evidence of carotid disease on the side of the affected hemisphere such as diminished pulsation, an audible bruit localised to the upper part of the carotid tree, or a slight Horner's syndrome (p. 713). The diagnosis is unequivocal if hemiplegia is accompanied or preceded by transient blindness of the opposite eye.

This is the most important indication for urgent anticoagulant therapy in cerebrovascular disease. Heparin and an oral anticoagulant should be started immediately with a view to limiting the infarction unless the patient has a diastolic blood pressure of 110 mm Hg or more.

Infarction of doubtful origin

There is no unanimity of opinion about the role of anticoagulant therapy in the evolving stroke without clear indication of a carotid lesion as advocated by Marshall (1968). In brain stem infarction it is not advisable. Minor haemorrhage in an area of infarction may be tolerable in a cerebral hemisphere but is obviously undesirable in the brain stem. Furthermore, the prognosis for the patient who has survived transient ischaemic attacks or small infarcts of the brain stem is reasonably good. For both of these reasons the indication for the use of anticoagulants in brain stem infarction (unless embolic) must be rare.

The incomplete stroke

A stroke may have completed its evolution when seen by the practitioner and yet the neurological deficit is less than would be expected from occlusion of the artery supplying the territory. Marshall (1968) reasonably points out that early use of anticoagulants may prevent subsequent spread of the lesion to the whole of that territory but it is possible that thrombosis has occurred in a small branch of the suspected vessel and there is no evidence that this is likely to spread back to the main stem if untreated. Cerebral oedema may account for a gradual or delayed increase of physical signs one or two days after the onset of a stroke. It may be treated by dehydration therapy (p. 298).

Intracerebral haemorrhage

As a cause of the slowly evolving stroke this is more common than is generally appreciated and consciousness need not be lost (McKissock et al., 1959). It is more likely to occur in the hypertensive patient or one who is having anticoagulant prophylaxis after an earlier stroke, but neither of these circumstances precludes infarction. Hypertension may be secondary to cerebral oedema after infarction but if the retinae show advanced hypertensive changes this is unlikely to be the explanation. The expert may observe that the signs of the stroke indicate a lesion involving more than the territory of a single artery. This distribution or the rapid development of signs of raised intracranial pressure would suggest haemorrhage rather than infarction.

If severe headache and vomiting persist and the level of consciousness deteriorates 24 to 48 hours after the onset of a stroke there is strong indication for angiography or pneumoencephalography to localise a haematoma with a view to washing it out through a trephine opening (Pennybacker, 1963). Surgical treatment is being increasingly used to reduce the residual disability by removal of a haematoma after a stroke with limited neurological deficit but it has little to offer in the management of the acute stroke with the possible exception of a cerebellar haemorrhage.

Hypotensive therapy (p. 232) may be used if there is evidence of hypertension in the malignant phase but it is otherwise without value in the treatment of intracerebral haemorrhage. No drug at present available will arrest bleeding and posture is without significant effect. There should be no hesitation in nursing the patient in the semiprone head-down position already recommended (p. 294) as the preservation of respiration is paramount and impaired respiration will increase the haemorrhage.

Hypertensive encephalopathy

The treatment has already been described (p. 232).

Subarachnoid haemorrhage

Sudden loss of consciousness associated with neck rigidity should always suggest subarachnoid haemorrhage. Kernig's sign may be absent. The majority of missed cases are referred to an isolation hospital as ' meningitis '. The diagnosis will also be considered in the patient who complains of sudden headache spreading rapidly to the neck even if consciousness is retained, but it is often overlooked in less severe cases where the only complaint is of pain in the neck and shoulders, sometimes associated with lumbosacral pain. The sudden rise of intracranial pressure with a major bleed causes acute papilloedema with haemorrhage near the optic discs. Subhyaloid haemorrhage is particularly helpful if present as this sign is virtually diagnostic. A previous history of headache with diplopia is useful confirmation of the presence of an aneurysm but the other main cause of subarachnoid haemorrhage, cerebral angioma, is usually clinically silent before rupture, though focal epilepsy may have been present. A migrainous history is of little diagnostic value unless the headache is confined to one side of the head when the possibility of a vascular anomaly is increased. Bleeding from either of these sources is more probable if blood pressure is raised.

If the diagnosis is in doubt it may be necessary to demonstrate blood in the cerebrospinal fluid (CSF). For differentiation of trauma and haemorrhage as causes of ' bloody tap ' (p. 710).

Treatment. Despite widespread belief, there is no surgical method of arresting subarachnoid haemorrhage. Bleeding from an intracranial aneurysm commonly recurs during the next two weeks and the place of surgery is to prevent what may be a fatal recurrence. After three weeks the chance is much reduced and after six weeks it is so low that surgical treatment is unnecessary. On the other hand, operation is dangerous in the first 48 hours after haemorrhage and if the patient is in coma it should rarely be considered.

The patient should be nursed as indicated for the unconscious patient (p. 292). Lumbar puncture is not necessary for treatment and need not be repeated after the diagnostic tap. Provided that respiration is assured the patient will survive unless the amount of brain lacerated by blood bursting into cerebral tissue is excessive. The only justification for surgery soon after haemorrhage is for removal of an expanding haematoma (p. 304). The evidence of increasing cerebral compression is exactly similar to that occurring after head injury and the management is the same (p. 298).

Once the patient has recovered consciousness, judiciously chosen operative treatment may prevent the second haemorrhage which is so likely to follow. Arteriography of both carotid and both vertebral arteries should be undertaken as soon as possible after the return of consciousness. If an aneurysm is demonstrated the appropriate surgical procedure should then be considered, bearing in mind that aneurysms are often multiple and that bleeding may be from another site than the aneurysm demonstrated. In particular cases (notably aneurysms of the anterior communicating artery) the technical hazards of the operation are equal to or greater than those of conservative management.

It will be apparent that the role of surgery is a preventative one in selected cases and for a period of less than one month. It is not good practice to transfer every case of subarachnoid haemorrhage to a neurosurgical centre forthwith. If this involves arduous transport with difficulty in controlling respiration or if the patient is in deep coma it is probably in his best interest not to move him but to continue management as described for intracerebral haemorrhage (p. 304). If the patient is within easy reach of a neurosurgical unit he should at least have the benefit of a consultation with a neurosurgeon at the earliest possible time.

The patient who is not submitted to operation should be kept in bed and as quiet as possible for four weeks. He may then be allowed out of bed for increasing periods and should then have a month's convalescence.

CEREBRAL TUMOUR

The inexorable progression of symptoms is of diagnostic value in cerebral tumour, but the tempo may accelerate rapidly with development of severe headache, vomiting, rapid deterioration of vision, and progressive loss of consciousness within a period of hours. This syndrome, which may simulate a stroke if the early neurological deficit has gone unnoticed, is due to abrupt rise of intracranial pressure caused by acute hydrocephalus. Herniation of brain tissue from one cranial compartment to another occurs as described in head injury (p. 299) producing the various types of ' pressure cone '. The brain shift obstructs the flow of cerebrospinal fluid between the ventricles or in the cranial cisterns so that the previously high pressure increases rapidly.

There is marked papilloedema. One of the pupils undergoes the sequence of changes described earlier (p. 295) and for similar reasons (pressure on a IIIrd nerve by herniation of the temporal lobe through the tentorium). Centres controlling respiration and circulation are endangered but bradycardia is an inconstant sign and its absence should not encourage delay. When this syndrome develops rapidly the emergency is extreme. Decompression of the supratentorial compartment must then be performed within half an hour if death is to be prevented. Dehydration therapy (p. 298) should be employed until a surgeon can trephine the skull and tap the ventricles. Decompressive surgery may be required after the emergency has been averted.

The experienced physician will not need to be reminded that emergency treatment of this nature should only be used if acute hydrocephalus develops before full diagnostic investigation has been completed. If it is known that the patient has a cerebral metastasis or malignant glioma it is bad practice to treat the terminal event in this way (p. 688).

INTRACRANIAL ABSCESS

Cerebral or subdural abscess may be a sequel to compound fracture of the skull, otitis media, sinusitis, bronchopulmonary infection, subacute bacterial endocarditis, and bacteraemia associated with cyanotic heart disease. Clinically it may present as acute or subacute encephalitis or as a chronic abscess with symptoms resembling cerebral tumour. Only the acute type is relevant to this chapter. Soon after head injury or otitis media (in which aural discharge may be temporarily suppressed) the patient develops headache, vomiting, and drowsiness passing to coma. Focal cerebral signs may be present and the temperature is usually raised.

The diagnosis may be confirmed by lumbar puncture, the pressure being raised and cells increased in the CSF (up to 100 per mm^3 (0.1×10^9/l), mainly lymphocytes). The protein may be raised to 2 g/l. Chloride and glucose content is normal and culture is usually sterile on culture unless there is accompanying meningitis. Lumbar puncture should be avoided if there is good clinical and EEG evidence of cerebral abscess unless there are marked signs of meningitis. If there is papilloedema or localising signs of a cerebellar lesion, or if the patient is drowsy, the lumbar puncture should not be attempted (see p. 58) until a cranial burr hole has been made to control the supratentorial pressure.

Cerebral abscess may prove fatal either by causing acute brain compression or by rupturing into a ventricle or the subarachnoid space.

Neurosurgical drainage is required urgently to control infection, minimise pressure effects and remove the danger of uncontrolled rupture. Electroencephalography is valuable in confirming the diagnosis and assisting localisation so that the cavity may be tapped for relief of pressure and instillation of crystalline penicillin and streptomycin into the abscess cavity. I m injection of benzyl-penicillin 2 mega units should be given immediately and followed by 1 mega unit four-hourly to control the suppurative encephalitis but this must always be ancillary to tapping of pus. Further therapy is guided by bateriological study of the pus.

ACUTE MENINGITIS

(See p. 436)

EPILEPSY

The seizure of major epilepsy is a dramatic occurrence which the layman expects to be treated as a medical emergency. It engenders great agitation in onlookers so that descriptions of an attack are rarely reliable and many transient disturbances of consciousness are reported as ' typical epileptic convulsions '. The drama of the event also makes the epileptic fit a suitable model for the hysterical patient desiring attention. It is therefore necessary to consider first the recognition of the hysterical and the epileptic fit.

The hysterical fit

This always has a purpose, even if it is only to gain sympathy, and usually follows an emotional crisis. If an attack occurs without a witness and if the patient sustains an injury the diagnosis is practically never hysteria. Indeed a true hysterical fit is now a clinical rarity in this country. More often the post-ictal state following a genuine epileptic seizure is considered hysterical, or the bizarre behaviour of some patients with temporal lobe seizures is not recognised.

The hysterical fit very rarely causes incontinence of urine and never incontinence of faeces. Movements are violent, not following the tonic-clonic sequence of grand mal epilepsy, and increase in proportion to any resistance offered to them. Despite their violent movements the threshing limbs are not injured. Corneal and tendon reflexes are retained and the plantar reflexes if they can be elicited are flexor. The attack continues as long as there is an audience to impress or it suddenly lapses into a tearful state but not a true post-ictal one. It may be followed by hysterical pseudocoma (p. 291). The closed eyelids flutter and surreptitious glances may be observed, but this is not the passive ptosis of true coma as attempts to open the eyelids are resisted. Strong and repeated pressure on the supra-orbital nerves usually rouses the patient. If it does not do so the patient 'wakens' rapidly if the nose and mouth are temporarily obstructed.

Syncope

True loss of consciousness of rapid onset and short duration may be syncopal or epileptic (p. 287). Syncope is the effect of temporary hypoxaemia of the brain and is usually caused by circulatory dysfunction (p. 227). There is usually a preceding sensation of sinking, faintness, nausea, tinnitus, visual blackout or of recession of voices. Loss of muscular tone is usually gradual so that the patient slumps to the ground.

The epileptic fit

The seizure of major epilepsy is sudden in onset. The patient falls sharply, sometimes emitting a harsh cry as he does so. Warning is either absent or insufficient to allow appropriate action. There is strong tonic contraction of muscles for about 30 seconds with apnoea causing cyanosis. The head and eyes may be turned to one side. Rapid but fine jerking begins rhythmically in all limbs. The rate of jerking slows and movements become more violent. Air is forced jerkily from the chest, frothing and expelling the unswallowed saliva. The tongue may be bitten if jaw closure does not precede extrusion of the tongue. If the bladder is full it may be emptied. The clonic phase lasts about 30 seconds then all muscle tone is relaxed. Tendon and corneal reflexes are absent but the plantar reflexes may be extensor. The patient may rapidly regain consciousness and resume normal activities. More often he wakens to a post-ictal state of confusion, drowsiness, and headache. Confusion and post-epileptic automatism may be mistaken for hysteria but if the epileptic patient is left to recover quietly he usually falls into a deep sleep. He wakens feeling quite well though his limbs and tongue may ache.

From the above it will be seen that 'typical' syncope and major epilepsy are readily distinguished. But this is not always so, for the epileptic fit is only the sign of spontaneous discharge of cerebral neurones and this may be induced by many causes, not least by hypoxia. Thus a prolonged attack of syncope may proceed to 'a genuine epileptiform convulsion'. The different types of seizure (major convulsion, petit mal 'spell', psychomotor attack, focal seizure, etc.) depend only on the site of the neuronal discharge. Unconsciousness is associated with an upper brain stem discharge and need not be present in other types of fit. The focus of origin is less important than the cause of the neuronal irritability. This may be genetically determined ('idiopathic') or acquired as the result of a lesion ('symptomatic'). It is unnecessary to give a comprehensive list of possible causes which may be found in any standard textbook (Simpson, 1971) but in principle any structural lesion of the brain can produce an 'epileptogenic lesion' provided that it damages a sufficient volume of neurones at one site without destroying their viability.

It is valuable for the later management of the case to have an accurate record of the first manifestations of the fit and its subsequent spread and any evidence pointing to a primary cause, be it neurological, circulatory, or metabolic, but these facts do not influence the emergency treatment unless there is severe hypertension (p. 232), asphyxia (p. 16 and 567), hypoglycaemia (p. 346), poisoning (p. 27), or pregnancy (p. 178).

Treatment of a fit. The emergency treatment expected by the layman is rarely necessary if the patient is protected from harm and his airway is assured. The traditional padded spoon may be inserted between the teeth if the onset of an attack is seen in a known epileptic. If the jaws are closed in the tonic stage it is not advisable to force them apart lest this breaks the jaw or loosens teeth which may be inhaled. It is best to wait until the stage of exhaustion. The tongue should then be withdrawn forward and the airway protected as in any other type of coma. Exceptions to this statement are fits occurring in young children and status epilepticus.

The danger of cerebral damage from hypoxia during a major seizure in childhood is considerable. The child should be placed in the semiprone position, secretions sucked out of the pharynx and a pharyngeal airway inserted as soon as there is adequate muscular relaxation. If the fit has not ceased by the time the airway has been assured, soluble phenobarbitone may be injected i m. A suitable dosage is 30 mg for a child under one month, 60 mg between one month and one year, 120 mg between one and three years, and 120 to 180 mg over three years of age. A common cause of fits in young children is acute meningitis and for this reason a child should be admitted to hospital if there is no previous history of convulsions. After 10 years of age it is unnecessary to arrange emergency admission to hospital unless status epilepticus develops.

Status epilepticus

Status epilepticus is the condition where one fit follows another without recovery of consciousness. It is commonly precipitated by abrupt withdrawal of anticonvulsant medication. Petit mal status is harmless and does not require emergency treatment other than protection of the patient from harm until he recovers consciousness. Grand mal status should always be treated in hospital except in quite exceptional circumstances. Several methods of treatment may be used, the choice depending on circumstances. Diazepam (Valium) is effective in children and in neurosurgical cases (cerebral abscess, head injury). It is less useful in status caused by irregular medication in chronic epileptics. Paraldehyde (p. 755) is a well-tried treatment still recommended for status in the chronic epileptic and in other types when treatment has to be given outside hospital. Whitty and Taylor (1949) recommend an initial dose of 8 to 10 ml for an adult (2 to 6 ml for children according to age). Further i m injections of 5 ml may be given every two hours. When there has been no fit for four hours the patient is allowed to recover consciousness but the regime is at once resumed if fits reappear before he has done so. In an emergency paraldehyde may be given by i v drip in a dosage of 0·05 to 0·1 ml per kg BW of a 10 g/dl emulsion in isosmotic sodium chloride solution (but see p. 86). The i m route is usually adequate and is easier in a convulsing patient. It has the disadvantage that it may cause a sterile abscess at the injection site and some of the pyrexia which is common after status epilepticus may be caused in this way.

Failing paraldehyde an i v injection of sodium phenobarbitone 120 to 140 mg or Phenytoin Injection BPC 250 mg may be used. Brown and Horton (1967) recommend thiopentone; an initial dose of 25 to 100 mg by slow i v injection being followed by infusion of one g of thiopentone in 500 ml of isosmotic sodium chloride solution at the minimal rate needed for control convulsions. Chlormethiazole (Heminevrin) may also be used in a dose of 1·2 to 1·6 g in 0·8 per cent solution by i v infusion also at the minimal necessary rate. Curarisation, intubation and artificial ventilation may be needed. If fits continue for more than two hours it may be necessary to correct water and electrolyte imbalance. If there is hyperpyrexia the patient should be sponged down and covered with a wet sheet over which air is played by an electric fan. If this is not sufficient to reduce the temperature to normal the skin should be rubbed vigorously with ice until vasodilation occurs. Penicillin may be given as a prophylactic if material has been aspirated (p. 601).

TETANY

Tetany may be mistaken for epilepsy and true epileptic seizures may occur in the hypocalcaemic patient. The treatment is described on p. 368.

ACUTE VERTIGO

(See also p. 217)

Dizziness or lightheadedness is a non-specific symptom of cerebral dysfunction without localising value. Vertigo, a sensation of rotation of the body, the brain within the head, or of the external environment is a symptom of disturbance of the vestibular apparatus. This includes the semicircular canals with their end-organs (e.g. Menière's disease), the vestibular division of the eighth nerve (vestibular neuronitis), the vestibular nuclei in the brain stem and their connections to the cerebellum (multiple sclerosis and brain stem infarction) and the temporal lobes of the cerebrum (a rare type of epilepsy). None of the diseases presenting as acute vertigo (see Table 9.1, p. 219) requires emergency treatment so their differential diagnosis need not be discussed, but severe vertigo is itself so incapacitating as to require immediate treatment and this does not differ with the various causes and sites.

Treatment. The patient should be put to bed and discouraged from moving the head. Injection of prochlorperazine (Stemetil) 12·5 mg, promethazine (Phenergan) 25 to 50 mg or triethylperazine (Torecan) 10 to 20 mg i m controls the associated vomiting and decreases the sensation of vertigo but it may be necessary to give a hypnotic drug in sufficient dose to ensure sleep. When vomiting stops one of the above drugs should be given orally until the attack subsides. A salt-free diet with restriction of fluid intake may limit recurrences in Menière's disease.

MULTIPLE SCLEROSIS

There is no treatment which has been shown to influence the long-term prognosis of multiple sclerosis and this is not surprising while its aetiology remains unknown. The symptoms are caused by plaques of demyelination scattered throughout the brain and spinal cord or in the optic nerve. The original lesion is inflammatory and it is currently postulated that it may be allergic in nature. Myelin breaks down in the inflamed area, interfering with conduction of impulses in nerve fibres. Recovery of function is possible unless the axon is destroyed by the acute lesion or by the resulting sclerosis.

Treatment. Steroid hormones have been suggested to combat the presumed allergic inflammation and to reduce the sclerotic reaction. Cortisone and its analogues have not shown convincing value but, for some unknown reason, corticotrophin may arrest an acute relapse and cause symptoms to subside more rapidly than usual. This is particularly valuable for acute retrobulbar neuritis. Spastic paralysis and sensory disturbances may also respond but ataxia, dysarthria and nystagmus are hardly affected by treatment. It is necessary to give high dosage for a week; 60 units of long-acting corticotrophin (ACTH) twice daily i m. The dose is then gradually reduced over a period of three to six weeks. If a symptom which had improved returns during this period of reduction the dose should be raised to the previous step and then reduced again more slowly. There is no evidence that the natural history of the disease is altered and neither long-term treatment with low dosage, nor administration at times other than acute relapses is recommended.

During the active stage of relapse rest is essential. As the sense of well-being returns vigorous exercise should be encouraged but fatigue must be avoided. Symptomatic treatment for vertigo is described on p. 218, and for paralysis of limbs and bladder on p. 318. The patient should be protected from irrational and quack remedies.

ACUTE DISSEMINATED ENCEPHALOMYELITIS

An acute demyelinating disease which resembles closely multiple sclerosis may occur spontaneously or in the course of infection with the causal virus of one of the exanthemata (measles, rubella, mumps, chickenpox) or after vaccination against smallpox or rabies. The spontaneous type may be related in the same way to respiratory infection. Direct viral invasion of the nervous system does not occur and it is believed that the myelin reaction is allergic. Various clinical syndromes occur according to the distribution of the lesion, e.g. encephalitis, transverse myelitis, bilateral optic neuritis or neuro-myelitis optica. Unlike multiple sclerosis with which it has many points in common, acute disseminated encephalomyelitis does not recur. Long-acting corticotrophin (ACTH) 80 to 120 units i m, or prednisone 60 mg daily, each for a week followed by a maintenance dose for two or three weeks may cause rapid resolution. If neurological signs persist after three weeks they are likely to be permanent and the continued administration of hormones is valueless.

Encephalitis due to direct viral invasion of the brain (polio-encephalitis, herpetic encephalitis and others) is not amenable to curative treatment. As injudicious use of steroid drugs may be deleterious it is important to distinguish between the two types of encephalitis and not to use hormones indiscriminately.

SPINAL CORD COMPRESSION

This rarely occurs as an acute emergency except in the case of injury to the spine, a subject beyond the scope of this chapter. Compression of the cord by a spinal tumour or in cervical spondylosis does not normally call for emergency treatment. But there is one circumstance in which the physician may have to take urgent action. If there is complete obstruction of the intraspinal flow of cerebrospinal fluid, removal of fluid from below the block may cause the spinal cord to shift caudally by the same mechanism of differential pressure which leads to pressure cones with cerebral tumours. This shift may prejudice the blood supply and cause irretrievable damage to cord tissue which is barely viable. For this reason lumbar puncture should not be carried out except for pre-operative myelography if the diagnosis of spinal tumour has been made on clinical grounds. If lumbar puncture reveals unexpected spinal block or if neurological signs hitherto absent develop within a day of this procedure it is necessary to obtain immediate neurosurgical advice as emergency decompression may be required to prevent irreversible loss of cord function. This is particularly important if the control of micturition suddenly deteriorates after lumbar puncture.

Spinal extradural abscess

Emergency treatment is always required for spinal cord compression and spreading thrombosis associated with extradural abscess of the spine. It should always be considered if paraplegia develops rapidly and is associated with root pains and local tenderness of the spine. Extradural abscess is a spread of infection from a small focus of osteomyelitis of a vertebra which usually follows a distant infection such as a staphylococcal skin lesion. The bone change can seldom be detected radiologically at this time and leucocytosis is inconsistent but the erythrocyte sedimentation rate is usually raised. Urgent laminectomy is required with local irrigation of the infected area by penicillin. A wide spectrum antibiotic should be given as soon as this disease is suspected.

ACUTE HERNIATION OF INTERVERTEBRAL DISCS

Chronic cervical and lumbar spondylosis are common causes of neurological syndromes but do not require emergency treatment. The secondary bony changes and postural deformities are more important than the degeneration of the intervertebral discs which provoke them. In the acute syndromes, however, herniation of the nucleus pulposus of a disc may cause sudden disorder of function of a nerve root or of the spinal cord according to its situation.

Acute lumbago/sciatica

The syndrome associated with protrusion of a lumbo-sacral or lower lumbar nucleus pulposus is well known. Rest in bed with wooden boards under the mattress is usually all that is required apart from analgesics. In most cases further orthopaedic or surgical measures should only be considered if rest in bed for three weeks fails to relieve symptoms but it is necessary that rest shall be complete. Sitting up for meals and ' toilet privileges ' are responsible for many of the failures of conservative treatment. Manipulation is often very effective in skilled hands but is not without its dangers. Epidural local anaesthesia has its advocates.

Central protrusions are more serious. They compress the cauda equina and cause bilateral sciatica and foot drop or more extensive paralysis of the legs and bladder. Operation should be the first choice in the treatment of these cases, preferably before paraplegia is established.

Acute brachialgia

This is often caused in a similar way to sciatica by protrusion of the nucleus pulposus of a cervical disc. Pain may affect one or both arms, commonly in the distribution of the C7 root, and there may be weakness of the triceps or other muscles. Rest is again the important principle of treatment. Bed-rest may be sufficient but intermittent neck traction by a physiotherapist is valuable. Between treatments the neck may be immobilised in slight flexion with a light metal or plastic collar and the arm supported with a sling. Analgesics are required as pain is severe. Acute central prolapse of a cervical disc is a cause of paraplegia of rapid onset which requires operation urgently. If skilled help is not available cervical traction should be maintained until it can be obtained.

ACUTE BRACHIAL NEURITIS

This condition must be distinguished from the cervical disc syndrome just described. Severe pain on one or both sides of the shoulder girdle spreads down the arm and persists for one to three weeks. On the second day paralysis develops, usually in muscles supplied by the fifth or sixth cervical roots (serratus anterior, spinati, deltoid and trapezius muscles). The paralysed muscles waste rapidly (' neuralgic amyotrophy ') but the condition may be distinguished from poliomyelitis by the usual presence of a small patch of diminished sensation over the insertion of the deltoid muscle and by the absence of pleocytosis of the cerebrospinal fluid.

Brachial neuritis may follow injection of a serum or vaccine (see p. 83) but it most often occurs without obvious cause or during convalescence from infection, injury, childbirth, or surgical operation. In the latter circumstance it may be mistaken for a traction injury of the brachial plexus. It is probably a limited form of the Guillain-Barré syndrome (see below) with an allergic aetiology. Prednisone in full dosage shortens the duration of pain and may hasten recovery but analgesics are needed while pain persists.

PERIPHERAL NEUROPATHY

Most of the peripheral neuropathies develop comparatively slowly. The causes have been reviewed by Simpson (1962). In three types emergency treatment may be needed—(1) Landry-Guillain-Barré syndrome, (2) acute porphyric polyneuritis and (3) toxic polyneuropathy—but in all cases ventilatory and circulatory failure may call for urgent attention.

Landry-Guillain-Barré Syndrome

The eponymous term is used instead of the current ' acute infective polyneuritis ' as there is little support for the suggested viral aetiology. It is probably an allergic neuropathy and occurs in circumstances similar to those in acute disseminated encephalomyelitis. Unlike other types of peripheral neuropathy the muscular weakness is commonly proximal in distribution and sensory loss may be minimal or absent. Calf tenderness is common. The diagnosis is confirmed by the presence of a raised protein level in the CSF (1 to 20 g/l) without cellular reaction.

Fifty per cent of cases show clinical improvement within three days of instituting treatment with steroids if these are given during the first two weeks. Prednisone may be used in a dose of 60 mg daily for two days, then 40 mg daily for two days, followed by 20 mg daily for as long as necessary (Graveson, 1961). In severe cases with bulbar and respiratory involvement treatment may be started with i v hydrocortisone hemisuccinate, 100 mg twice daily for two to three days before continuing by oral route.

Acute porphyric polyneuritis

The onset of acute motor or sensorimotor peripheral neuropathy associated with porphyrinuria is usually sudden. There is commonly a familial history of neuropathy or of the other manifestations acute abdominal pain (p. 123), confusional states, coma and convulsions. Attacks may be precipitated by alcohol, barbiturates and sulphonamides, which must be avoided if the aetiology is suspected. Diagnosis is confirmed by identification of haemato-porphyrin in the urine (see p. 123). Steroids, cyanocobalamin, neostigmine, and chelating agents have been advised for treatment but their value is uncertain. Vitamins are not indicated. Controlled respiration is essential as recovery is likely if this can be maintained.

Toxic polyneuropathy

A toxic origin should always be looked for, especially if more than one case of neuropathy occurs from the same environment. Careful and imaginative questioning about ingestion of unusual or adulterated foods or drugs, or exposure to domestic or industrial chemicals may reveal a cause. Further exposure to danger may be prevented but antidotes are rarely available. If a heavy metal is identified penicillamine should be tried (600 to 900 mg per day). Thiamine and other vitamins are of no value in this type of neuro-pathy. They are only indicated in nutritional neuropathies such as beri-beri and are rarely required for ' peripheral neuritis ' in this country. Corticosteroids are equally valueless in neuropathies other than the acute demyelinating type. Fortunately most cases undergo spontaneous remission if life can be preserved by artificial ventila-tion of the lungs. Respiratory failure may develop very rapidly. Function should be tested every hour until the spread of paralysis has ceased. Bedside tests which are convenient are (1) ability to count up to 30 or more on one breath and (2) Forced Expiratory Time (p. 193). Failure to perform these tests is an indication for assisted respiration. If swallowing is unimpaired a tank type of respirator may be used but if there is any evidence of involvement of the bulbar muscles it is essential to use intermittent positive pressure respiration through a tracheostomy (p. 737).

BELL'S PALSY

Unilateral facial palsy of rapid onset and not associated with disease of the ear or parotid gland has a good prognosis. It is probable that 70 per cent of cases recover without treatment. ACTH or corticosteroids may hasten recovery but it has not been proved that the incidence of incomplete recovery is reduced. In the writer's opinion electrical stimulation does not influence recovery and may predispose to contracture of the permanently paralysed face. There is therefore no satisfactory ' emergency treatment '. Splintage of the angle of the mouth by strapping may be used and the eye on the affected side should be protected from exposure keratitis.

EARLY MANAGEMENT OF THE PARALYSED PATIENT

The principles of management of the paralysed patient soon after the onset are the same regardless of the nature of the lesion or its site (upper or lower motor neurone or muscle). The same methods are used where applicable for restricted forms of paralysis such as that due to nerve injuries. In order of priority these are: (1) protection of respiration (p. 292), (2) avoidance of pressure sores by frequent turning and nursing on a bolster bed, (3) care of the neurogenic bladder (p. 319), (4) protection of paralysed limbs from later deformity and ankylosis.

The paralysed limb should be placed in that position which would be most favourable for function if no recovery were to take place. This position, which should avoid overstretching of paralysed limbs, may be maintained by sand bags or splints. Complete immobilisation is not required, indeed all joints should be moved passively through their full range of movements several times each day from the beginning until active movement returns. In the acute stage it does not matter whether the paralysis is due to an upper or lower motor neurone lesion. Later management is different and is described by Simpson (1974).

Extrapyramidal Disorders

There is little place for emergency treatment of Parkinsonism of the idiopathic or post-encephalitic type. Treatment with levodopa or anticholinergic drugs should be introduced progressively until the best clinical response is obtained. In acute dystonic syndromes caused by phenothiazine, reserpine and butyrophenone tranquillisers used in high dosage, rapid control may be achieved by i m injection of orphenadrine 20 to 40 mg or benztropine 1 to 2 mg followed by normal oral dosage. Similar treatment may be required for oculo-gyric crises in post-encephalitic Parkinsonism. Parenteral barbiturates or oral amphetamine may also be used.

PARALYSIS OF MICTURITION

Disease of the spinal cord or peripheral nerves may affect micturition in several ways. Urgency and precipitate micturition are due to failure of the inhibitory control of the brain because of a cord lesion (usually bilateral). They are not emergency problems and should be properly investigated before treatment. Hesitancy of micturition is a more important symptom which may herald complete retention. It is due to failure of the voluntary contraction of the pelvi-abdominal muscles and relaxation of the bladder sphincter (upper motor neurone paralysis). Retention may also be due to abolition of micturition reflexes by a lesion in the conus medullaris or cauda equina (lower motor neurone paralysis). Incontinence of urine may be due to overflow from a paralysed bladder.

Mismanagement of the paralysed bladder in the early stage is responsible for serious late complications. While the bladder must not be allowed to overdistend and back pressure on the kidneys must be avoided, sterility of the urine must be maintained. Catheterisation (p. 720) should not be embarked on without due consideration of the risk of introducting infection. Carbachol BP should be tried first. A test dose of 0·5 ml is injected subcutaneously. In the absence of ill effects such as a drop in blood pressure (p. 89) it may then be given in doses of 2 ml as required. If this is not effective catheterisation must be used with strict aseptic precautions (p. 720). It should be repeated three times a day for a week before an indwelling catheter is used so that the urethral mucosa may have time to harden. A fine polythene catheter is then inserted (or a self-retaining Foley type if leakage occurs) and led to a sealed drainage bottle. The important details of management to prevent infection are well described by Blandy (1965). A condensed account would be dangerously misleading but it is essential to emphasise this as chronic cystitis and respiratory paralysis are the most important causes of death from neurological disease and the damage may be preventable in the early days.

MYASTHENIA GRAVIS

Myasthenia gravis is not a rare disease. It is often missed because it is not considered in the diagnosis of muscular weakness, especially if the extraocular muscles are spared as they sometimes are. The characteristic increase of weakness with sustained or repeated effort is surprisingly rarely noted by the patient until specific inquiries about it are made. The onset of the illness may be quite sudden and is usually associated with an emotional disturbance, non-specific infection, or pregnancy, rather than with severe physical exertion. The course is characterised by variability amounting to complete remission at times. These features account for the fact that most cases are wrongly diagnosed as suffering from hysterical palsy or multiple sclerosis but the diagnosis is simple once the possibility has been considered. The patient should be asked to contract the affected muscles as strongly as possible for one minute. Progressive failure of contraction within this period (not a sudden relaxation) is very suggestive of myasthenia gravis and abolition of this response if the test is repeated one minute after injection of edrophonium is diagnostic (p. 321). The test is described below (for a fuller account see Simpson (1974)).

Myasthenic crisis

The treatment of a previously undiagnosed case of myasthenia gravis is rarely an emergency unless a dangerous degree of paralysis of respiration or swallowing is present. A myasthenic crisis is more likely to develop in a known case. The airway must be protected at once, pharyngeal secretion removed by posture or suction, and artificial respiration supplied by mouth-to-mouth breathing (p. 732) or by intubation and a ventilator according to principles described above. A tank respirator should not be used as dysphagia is almost invariable if respiration is affected.

When respiration is protected by intubation neostigmine may be given orally in a dose of 60 mg. If rapid response is essential, 2·5 mg should be given subcutaneously or i m. It acts in 15 to 20 minutes. Although the i v route gives a more rapid effect it is not recommended because of the danger of cardiac arrest. If it is selected it is essential to give atropine sulphate 0·6 mg with (or preferably 15 minutes before) the dose of neostigmine which should not exceed 1·5 mg. Many authorities give atropine with every injection of neostigmine, regardless of the route. It should be used with caution. In a myasthenic crisis thick stringy mucus streams from the mouth and chokes the patient. Atropine reduces the volume of saliva but increases its viscosity so that it may be more difficult to clear from the bronchi. When respiration is obstructed the secretion increases but failure to swallow is the main reason for the excessive amount in the mouth and pharynx. The correct treatment is postural drainage, suction and intubation by an endotracheal tube. Thymectomy should not be used as an emergency treatment. It is recommended for definitive treatment of early cases of myasthenia gravis but it is desirable to control respiration and stabilise the patient on anticholinesterase medication before operation.

The myasthenic crisis usually occurs in a patient who is already under treatment. Before resorting to parenteral medication the diagnosis must be very carefully considered to make quite certain that the cause of increasing weakness is not overdosage of drugs.

Edrophonium test

The short-duration antimyasthenic effect of edrophonium chloride (Tensilon) makes it very suitable for a diagnostic test. A syringe is loaded with 1 ml (10 mg) for i v injection. Initially 2 mg should be injected to detect abnormal sensitivity but if there is no response the remaining 8 mg is injected after 30 seconds. Within a half to one minute there is improvement if weakness is due to myasthenia gravis but the weakness returns in four to five minutes. As muscles may be differentially affected the response of the respiratory and bulbar muscles should be particularly observed if the test is used to distinguish between myasthenic and cholinergic crisis. In the latter the injection does not improve strength and may cause brief deterioration, even with the initial test dose. When the test is used to distinguish cholinergic crisis it should always be preceded by atropine and there should be resuscitation apparatus at hand. A negative or entirely subjective response must be interpreted as indicating overdosage in these circumstances (Simpson, 1974).

Cholinergic crisis

This term is used for the increasing paralysis due to overdosage with anticholinesterase drugs: neostigmine, pyridostigmine (Mestinon) and ambenonium (Mytelase). It is the likely cause of deterioration in any patient who is having more than 20 tablets daily of one or a combination of anticholinesterase drugs and may be the cause of weakness with much lower dosage.

If weakness of limb muscles or of respiration develops rapidly the exact time of onset should be determined. Onset 45 to 90 minutes after an oral dose of neostigmine (or earlier after injection) strongly suggests cholinergic crisis. Onset less than 30 or more than 120 minutes after oral dosage is more in keeping with myasthenic crisis, especially if there has been temporary improvement between these times. Parasympathomimetic signs (diarrhoea, colic, salivation, sweating, bronchospasm) and fasciculation of muscles are rare in myasthenic patients despite high dosage of anticholinesterase drugs. Their presence in a very weak patient is an indication of overdosage. The smooth muscle and glandular signs are suppressed if atropine is given routinely and for this reason it is not advised as it conceals the early warning of the cholinergic state. The muscarinic signs and fasciculation may be absent even if the motor endplates of the skeletal muscles are blocked with accumulated acetylcholine. Fortunately constriction of the pupils is invariable unless atropine is being used in exceptional dosage. If a collapsed myasthenic patient has pupils less than 3 mm in diameter in normal room lighting the diagnosis of cholinergic crisis is probable. Severe hypoxia with hypercapnia may cause a similar clinical picture. Neostigmine resistance is rare if indeed it exists. Further medication given in the mistaken belief that the patient has become resistant to neostigmine is likely to precipitate death.

Treatment of cholinergic poisoning. Respiration must be controlled by a positive pressure ventilator through a cuffed endotracheal tube and all anticholinesterase medication withdrawn until signs of myasthenic weakness with edrophonium responsiveness return. Atropine sulphate should be injected i v 2 mg every hour until signs of atropine toxicity develop (p. 140). Drugs of the oxime group are valuable in cholinergic poisoning due to organic phosphorus compounds (p. 467) but are of little value in overdosage with quaternary ammonium anticholinesterases. Personal experience is limited to pyridine-2-aldoxime methiodide (PAM) and its methane sulphonate (P_2S) but their latency has been found to be too long and their potency and duration of action inadequate for satisfactory treatment (see also p. 467).

PERIODIC AND INTERMITTENT PARALYSIS

Episodes of weakness or paralysis may be due to metabolic disease of muscle which may be inherited or sporadic.

Familial periodic paralysis

This type occurs in young adults after prolonged rest, especially if this is preceded by vigorous exercise. Other precipitating factors are a heavy meal or severe cold. The paralysis is flaccid in type. It spares the ocular muscles but respiration may be paralysed. It is associated with shift of potassium from the blood into muscle and liver cells. Hypokalaemia is present during an attack but the blood potassium level is normal at other times. The familial type and a similar sporadic type may both be associated with thyrotoxicosis. Similar attacks are due to primary hyperaldosteronism (Conn's syndrome). This disorder is associated with hypertension, alkalosis and hypernatraemia and the hypokalaemia persists between the attacks. Hypokalaemia with muscular weakness may also be due to potassium-losing nephropathy or prolonged administration of diuretics.

Recovery from attacks of paralysis of hypokalaemic type is hastened by oral administration of potassium chloride, 10 g in water. A further 5 g may be given in two hours if there has been no improvement. I v therapy is dangerous and rarely required (p. 604).

Adynamia episodica hereditaria

It must not be assumed without biochemical confirmation that all cases of periodic paralysis have hypokalaemia. In this familial type, which is often associated with myotonia, there is hyperkalaemia. Attacks of flaccid paralysis are brief (half an hour to two hours) and may be cut short by exercising the weak muscles. If this is not effective the attack may sometimes be terminated by i v injection of calcium gluconate (1 to 2 g).

Hyperkalaemia is usually iatrogenic (p. 604).

Normokalaemic periodic paralysis

This is a rare type in which attacks occur mainly at night and last for days or weeks. The blood potassium level is normal but attacks are induced or made worse by potassium. Large doses of sodium chloride are said to be beneficial and further attacks are prevented by taking a combination of 250 mg of acetazolamide (Diamox) and 0·1 mg of fludrocortisone daily. The disorder must be distinguished from Addison's disease (p. 353) as well as from other types of periodic paralysis.

Paroxysmal myoglobinuria (rhabdomyolysis) (see also p. 125)

This is a rare condition in which attacks of muscular weakness or paralysis lasting two to three days are accompanied by myoglobinuria. There is severe cramp-like pain and tenderness of the affected muscles. Renal damage may occur leading to anuria which may be fatal. It is sometimes familial and may be precipitated by exercise, acute infections and some rare toxic conditions. Myoglobinuria may complicate acute polymyositis and ischaemic muscle necrosis. During acute phases complete rest is required and the urine should be made alkaline.

HEADACHE

Headache is a symptom of many disorders. Most of these are benign (psychoneurosis, migraine, sinusitis, pyrexia, cervical spondylosis), some are due to lesions which may cause trouble at a later date (intracranial aneurysm, temporal arteritis, glaucoma), and only a few are disorders requiring urgent treatment (subarachnoid haemorrhage, p. 305; raised intracranial pressure, p. 297; meningitis, p. 436; and hypertensive encephalopathy, p. 232). Severe headache may be the only indication of a recent seizure (p. 309).

No drug more potent that aspirin or codeine compound should be used until the cause of headache has been determined. The powerful analgesics may cause serious depression of respiration if intracranial pressure is raised and this in turn leads to further rise of pressure. It is also undesirable to embark on habit-forming drugs if headache is due to migraine or other benign cause which is likely to recur frequently. Lumbar puncture to exclude subarachnoid haemorrhage and meningitis should be carried out in cases of sudden severe headache without previous history or if signs of meningism (p. 436) are present. Otherwise lumbar puncture is not required and it may be positively dangerous. It should never be done without taking expert advice if there is any question of papilloedema being present.

Migraine

Migraine, like epilepsy, may be idiopathic or symptomatic. Onset in late life with consistent recurrence on the same side of the head, or the presence of focal neurological signs are indications for further investigation to exclude intracranial aneurysm, angioma or atherosclerosis. Idiopathic migraine is often familial. It usually starts in early life and attacks are rarely confined to one side. Throbbing headache is preceded by symptoms of ischaemia of part of the brain, usually the visual or sensory cortex of one hemisphere or the brain stem. Ataxia, dysarthria, vertigo, tinnitus and bilateral dysaesthesia and disturbance of vision may precede occipital headache in the so-called ' basilar migraine '. With this type there is occasionally loss of consciousness. Nausea or vomiting, vertigo and severe prostration are common in migraine and may be the only symptoms of the attack.

Mild attacks are best treated with aspirin or Codeine Compound Tablets BP and the addition of an antiemetic such as prochlorperazine (Stemetil) 5 to 10 mg orally may be beneficial. If this is not effective ergotamine tartrate (2 mg) sublingually should be tried. It may be repeated in half an hour if necessary. Proprietary combinations with caffeine and an antiemetic such as cyclizine (Marzine) may be preferred. In severe attacks it may be necessary to give ergotamine tartrate by subcutaneous injection (0·25 to 0·5 mg) but this method is rarely used since the introduction of ergotamine tartrate for inhalation from a small nebulizer (Medihaler) which ensures rapid absorption of a measured amount of the drug (0·36 mg). Ergotamine is most effective when given at the earliest warning of the attack. It may have little effect when the headache is fully established. If it does not stop the attack it is better to give a quick acting hypnotic to make the patient sleep rather than proceed to morphine-like drugs.

In a few sufferers from migraine the symptoms do not progress beyond the phase of vasoconstriction. If this is prolonged it may cause cerebral infarction. A trial of nicotinic acid is worth while. An initial dose of 25 mg should be increased in successive attacks until a dose is reached which causes facial flushing. Inhalation of CO_2 may also be tried.

FACIAL PAIN

None of the causes of facial pain are dangerous to life. Successful treatment demands accurate diagnosis. Trigeminal neuralgia must be distinguished from pain referred from teeth or sinuses or temporomandibular joints, migrainous facial neuralgia, postherpetic neuralgia, temporal arteritis and 'atypical facial neuralgia' which is probably psychogenic. The diagnosis and treatment of these types are discussed by Simpson (1971). The same principles apply to the treatment of facial pain as to migraine. The embargo on potent analgesics may be less rigid as there is less danger of respiratory depression but the possibility of drug addiction is considerable in the psychogenic types.

Trigeminal neuralgia (Tic douloureux)

This name should be restricted to the syndrome characterised by brief attacks of lancinating pain confined to the territory of one or more branches of a trigeminal nerve. The attacks are triggered by stimulation of focal points on the face or gums and by chewing. There is no loss of sensation.

Simple analgesics may suffice in early attacks but the value of carbamazepine (Tegretol) is now well established and the response to the first dose is sometimes so striking as to justify inclusion of the drug on a chapter on emergency treatment. The initial dose is 100 mg twice a day by mouth, increased gradually to 400 mg three times a day. If this is not effective it is necessary to block the affected branch of the trigeminal nerve by injection of phenol or absolute alcohol or to cut the sensory root of the trigeminal nerve.

JOHN A. SIMPSON

REFERENCES

BLANDY, J. P. (1965). Catheterization. *British Medical Journal*, **2**, 1531.
BROWN, A. S. & HORTON, J. M. (1967). Status epilepticus treated by intravenous infusions of thiopentone sodium. *British Medical Journal*, **1**, 27.
GRAVESON, G. S. (1961). The use of steroids in the treatment of the Guillain-Barré syndrome. *Proceedings of the Royal Society of Medicine*, **54**, 575.
JENNETT, W. B. *An Introduction to Neurosurgery*. 2nd ed, London: Heinemann. 1970.

McKISSOCK, W., RICHARDSON, A. & WALSH, L. (1959). Primary intracerebral haemorrhage. Results of surgical treatment in 244 consecutive cases. *Lancet*, **2,** 683.

MARSHALL, J. *The Management of Cerebrovascular Disease,* 2nd ed. London: Churchill. 1968.

PENNYBACKER, J. (1963). The surgical aspects of strokes. *Proceedings of the Royal Society of Medicine,* **56,** 487.

POTTER, J. M. *The Practical Management of Head Injuries,* 2nd ed., London: Lloyd Luke. 1965.

SIMPSON, J. A. The neuropathies. In *Modern Trends in Neurology,* vol. 3. Ed. Williams, D. London: Butterworths, 1962.

SIMPSON, J. A. Diseases of the nervous system. In Davidson's *Principles and Practice of Medicine,* 11th ed. Ed. Macleod, J. Edinburgh: Churchill Livingstone. 1971.

SIMPSON, J. A. Diseases of the nervous system. In *Textbook of Medical Treatment,* 13th ed. Ed. Alstead, S. & Girdwood, R. H. Edinburgh: Churchill Livingstone. 1974a.

SIMPSON, J. A. Myasthenia gravis and myasthenic syndromes. In *Disorders of Voluntary Muscle,* 3rd ed. Ed. Walton, J. N. London: Churchill. 1974.

WHITTY, C. W. M. & TAYLOR, M. (1949). Treatment of status epilepticus. *Lancet,* **2,** 591.

CHAPTER 14

Psychiatric Emergencies

For psychiatric cases at sea see p. 481.
For methods of admission to a psychiatric hospital see p. 672.

PSYCHIATRIC emergencies differ from other medical emergencies in that they are brought on by their behavioural consequences and depend on the anxiety they cause in others. In a few instances admission to hospital for specific treatment is needed when the emergency is secondary to organic disease or when the patient cannot be looked after at home.

Psychiatric emergencies can be:

1. Patient-conditioned when the patient makes efforts to get help for intolerable symptoms.
2. Relative-conditioned when the patient's relatives are affected by his behaviour.
3. Social emergencies when the patient's behaviour makes others call for action.
4. Doctor emergencies when unwillingness or over-involvement makes him demand further action.

Examination of the patient

The doctor must make a full psychiatric and physical assessment. The pen is his chief tool but the sphygmomanometer and ophthalmoscope are also important. He should use a listening attitude and approach the emergency with calmness, empathy and understanding. Restraint frequently produces violence and is rarely necessary. A near relative or reliable informant should be interviewed. Subterfuge should never be used. The informant and the relative should be seen separately and the facts may be discussed with the family doctor.

The history should include present symptoms and their duration; any past history of psychiatric illness; family history; personal past history with special emphasis on the normal crisis situations of childhood, puberty and adolescence; the reaction to stressful events. An assessment of the previous personality must be made. Always inquire about suicidal threats and attempts.

The risk to the doctor

In most cases there is no risk but occasionally it is wise to have relatives or neighbours and even the police present at the examination. The doctor must be consistent in handling the situation. Tell the patient who you are, why you have come and what you intend to do. It is best to listen and to say as little as possible at first. The reality of the patient's experience must not be denied and the doctor should not argue with the patient about them. Only in the gravest emergency should a plan of action be implemented without the consent and understanding of the nearest relative. After the examination give the relatives your opinion preferably in the presence of the patient.

Drugs

These may be needed for the acute disturbances of behaviour in schizophrenia and mania. Ampoules of chlorpromazine (Largactil) 50 mg and haloperidol (Serenace) 5 mg should be on hand. They are contraindicated in patients with cardiac, respiratory and hepatic disease and should be used guardedly in the elderly because of the risk of hypotension and extrapyramidal side effects. The patient should lie down when they are injected. Biperiden (Akineton. Pfizer) 5 mg i m or procyclidine (Kemadrin) 10 to 12 mg i m will counter severe extrapyramidal side effects. Diazepam (Valium) 10 to 20 mg i v or i m is a safe drug when haloperidol and chlorpromazine are contraindicated. In the elderly thioridazine (Melleril) 50 to 100 mg by mouth is the safest of the phenothiazine drugs and chloral hydrate 0·5 to 1·0 g a useful and safe sedative, preferably given in the form of Welldorm (dichoral phenazone) 500 mg tablets or Triclofos 500 mg tablets which (like chloral itself) acts by yielding trichor ethyl alcohol in the body.

Chlormethiazole (Heminevrin) 500 mg tablets two to eight a day is very useful for alcohol and drug withdrawal states with the addition of diphenoxylate (Lomotil) 2·5 mg tablets one to six daily for heroin and methadone dependence. It is rarely necessary or advisable to give drugs to facilitate withdrawal for more than seven days because of the problems of dependency this might produce.

Family doctor emergencies

Most psychiatric emergencies encountered by the family doctor are associated with anxiety. Many reflect the interaction between disturbed individuals and their relatives. The major diagnostic psychiatric categories feature relatively infrequently averaging three to five referrals per year for each practice although the range for different practitioners varies from one to twenty per year (Littlemore Psychiatric Service). In a good general practice the family doctor is best equipped to deal with emergency situations because of his knowledge of the family and his empathetic understanding of their needs and interactions. However, Clyne (1961) stresses how readily general practitioners react adversely to emergency demands, especially at night, by resorting to medication and hospitalisation as the easiest way out. The salient features may be lost because the doctor does not take into account the background circumstances which precipitated the alerting process.

The commonest emergencies seen by the psychiatrist are:

1. Affective disorders.
2. Schizophrenic and paranoid states.
3. States of confusion and memory impairment in the elderly.
4. Behavioural problems associated with alcohol and drug dependence.
5. Personality disorders including histrionic episodes of acting-out behaviour.

These include concern about suicide, aggressive assault, homicidal threats and attempts as well as behaviour which causes anxiety or which is unacceptable because of the demands it makes on others.

States of tension and depression represent most of the cases diagnosed as affective disorder and only 10 per cent are patients suffering from a definite manic-depressive illness. Tension and depression during pregnancy, the puerperium and in relation to marital problems are not uncommon. Unwanted pregnancies which were totally unacceptable to the patient merit a psychiatric referral (see also p. 181).

Emergency admission to hospital

In cases needing emergency admission to hospital schizophrenia featured as the most prominent diagnosis. Unwillingness to accept treatment and unsettled living conditions were the factors necessitating admission in many cases. In patients living with relatives excessive demands were much more disconcerting than acts of violence or embarrassing behaviour (Grad and Sainsbury, 1963). The problem is to get the patient to take his drugs, and to cope with him when he does not go to work or stays in bed in the morning and is reluctant to help in the household.

When the patient has already been in hospital this may be a

signal indicating the possible need for readmission. Those schizophrenics living alone or drifting from place to place without adequate support are soon brought to the notice of the police or the social services and in this way constitute an emergency.

Suicide

In the affecive disorder the alerting factor frequently relates to anxiety about suicide. The threat or attempt is probably the commonest psychiatric emergency. A recent Edinburgh study of general practice (Kennedy and Kreitman, 1973) found the overall prevalence of attempted suicide to be one in 400 per year. It was one in 200 per year among women of 20 to 35 living in areas of high social pathology. Doctors should always take seriously an expression of suicidal intent. The risk of successful suicide is greatest in those with severe depressive states associated with delusional ideas of guilt, unworthiness and disease. Cancer phobia in particular points to a potential suicidal risk. Risks are also high in people who have attempted suicide or who have a family history of it and in those whose living situations seem intolerable and insoluble. Suicidal attempts by gassing, shooting, drowning, hanging and self-mutilation should lead to immediate action by the doctor. The acutely poisoned patient will need admission to a general hospital where the immediate management does not involve the psychiatrist although his assessment at a later stage is essential.

The taking of drugs in excess to escape from or to draw attention to an intolerable situation is a new behaviour pattern which has emerged in the last decade. Admissions to hospital because of overdosage during this period have increased tenfold. Only 20 per cent of men and 40 per cent of women in this group are suffering from a depressive syndrome. Many stress factors may precipitate this behaviour in those of relatively normal personality because of the ready accessibility of drugs. In 30 per cent of the men alcohol is also a factor.

Aggressive behaviour

Aggressive behaviour and loss of control is very effective in raising alarm and anxiety in others. The extent to which this might constitute a psychiatric emergency varies a great deal. In some settings such behaviour is more acceptable than in others. It may be considered a matter for the law and then much will depend on the sophistication of the Police Force and its concern to involve the Social Services Department. In few instances aggression has been the reason for referral but then it is usually a catastrophic happening often associated with alcoholism, psychosis, epilepsy or personality disorder. The fact that the patient may have seen a psychiatrist previously often influences the direction of the alarm.

Homicidal problems

Homicidal threats call for immediate action. The risk is greatest in those suffering from a schizophrenic illness or from morbid jealousy with associated delusional ideas about sexual infidelity. Severe depression with ideas of guilt and unworthiness may result in acts of self destruction and attempts to destroy the whole family. Similarly, when persecutory ideas focus on specific individuals there is a grave danger of violence. The doctor should not treat lightly any threatening letter and should seek the advice of a psychiatrist at once. Prompt legal action and consultation with the police may be necessary.

Infanticide

This is usually linked with acute depression in the mother. Arrangements will have to be made for someone to look after her baby or to admit mother and baby to a special unit if available. More difficult decisions arise in obsessional mothers who have thoughts of stabbing, strangling or drowning a member of her family. Here it is often difficult to assess the risk. If obsessional thoughts are accompanied by depression the case needs urgent consideration.

Casualty Department

The incidence of psychiatric emergencies in casualty departments has been variously reported as from 1·4 to 6·6 per cent. Whiteley and Dennison (1963) have shown that the casualty officer saw twice as many psychiatric patients as were seen in the psychiatric department of the same hospital over the same period of time. They were mainly problems of aggressive behaviour and overdosage. These occur in patients with personality disorders whose capacity for tolerating feelings is low and in whom acting-out behaviour is common and often explosive. People in states of panic with phobic and anxiety problems and in states of anxiety masked by somatic complaints also find their way to the casualty department. Hysterical dissociation and confusional symptoms of all kinds have been seen including fugues and amnesias, somnambulistic states, overbreathing, torticollis, paresis, aphonia, blindness and fits (Weir, 1972). Some patients because of their degree of hospital dependence have numerous investigations and operations. The symptoms simulated are of three types: abdominal, supposed haemoptysis or haematemesis and neurological symptoms such as faints, fits and stupor. This Munchausen syndrome is a severe form of hysterical dissociation with an associated personality disorder (Crown, 1972). Casualty departments are encountering more and more people with behavioural disturbances and confusional states associated with alcohol and drugs, sometimes complicated by head injury.

Management in the Casualty Department

There are many advantages in having a psychiatric firm linked with a casualty department but unfortunately this happens infrequently. It is important for the casualty doctor to try to get details from relatives and friends and social workers who accompany the patient. He should have sufficient time to listen to them and to assess the problem. A few beds for overnight stay are valuable especially for confusional states which may be complicated by alcohol and drugs. Most addicts who have manipulated casualty officers into providing drugs are discouraged when admission is suggested. Only those who are really interested in getting help will follow up these suggestions. Heroin and physeptone should not be given by casualty officers. Chlormethiozole (Heminevrin) and diphenoxylate (Lomotil) can be used successfully for drug withdrawal symptoms (see also p. 43).

Emergency Clinics

In the larger conurbations where many people do not know their family doctor well or where there are difficulties in getting an urgent psychiatric opinion, the emergency clinic is a useful intermediary. Brothwood (1965) has described the work of such a clinic at the Maudsley Hospital. Some of his patients had already received night sedation, antidepressants and phenothiazines before they attended the clinic. Out of 100 patients 70 were considered to be suffering from an affective illness which was predominantly associated with neurotic or personality problems and 22 were described as psychotic. The main reasons for treatment in this group included concern about the possibility of suicide and behavioural difficulties often related to delusional or hallucinatory preoccupations.

General Hospital

Psychiatric emergency problems in the general hospital tend to be related to medical disorders of a biochemical nature and to syndromes arising after anaesthesia and surgery. Toxic confusional states may appear in patients with cardiac, respiratory, hepatic or renal failure and in pyrexial and infective illnesses. Endocrine disorders are also more prone to complication by psychiatric disturbances—toxic confusional states or affective or paranoid syndromes occurring in a setting of clear consciousness. In obstetric units similar acute psychiatric disturbances may occur especially in the post-partum period. They are toxic confusional disturbances or more clear cut affective or schizophrenic psychoses requiring drugs like chlorpromazine or haloperidol.

Emergencies associated with alcohol and drugs (see also p. 41)

The sudden withdrawal of drugs or alcohol may precipitate a toxic confusional state characterised by agitation, confusion and disorientation, paranoid delusions and hallucinations of a visual and auditory nature. It usually responds to a general regime for drug withdrawal symptoms (p. 43). This includes the injection of sedative and anticonvulsant drugs such as chlormethiazole (Heminevrin) or the benzodiazepines, e.g. diazepam (Valium).

As a rule paraldehyde is unnecessary and chlorpromazine (Largactil) less satisfactory because of the danger of damaging side effects. Alcoholic emergencies are frequent and may need admission to hospital for ' drying out '. Delirium tremens, a toxic confusional state associated with alcohol excess or withdrawal is often self-limiting and rarely lasts more than seven days. A sedative, preferably chlormethiazole (Heminevrin) one to two capsules (500 to 1 000 mg) three times a day, will be needed. Parentrovite should be given in full doses. Nursing care and correction of electrolyte disturbances are important. Antibiotics are often life-saving. Alcoholic hallucinosis can be a terrifying experience because of the vivid auditory and visual hallucinations. Voices threaten the patient, call him obscene names, chastise him and may drive him to murder or suicide. It calls for urgent admission to hospital. The syndromes following anaesthesia and surgery may be confusional psychoses in a setting of clouded consciousness, or affective or paranoid states with consciousness unimpaired. States of excitement and aggressive behaviour cause much disorganisation of a hospital ward. Adequate sedation and a psychiatric opinion are required if the clamour for immediate removal is to be resisted. In some cases transfer to a psychiatric unit is the most appropriate way of management.

For erethism, a psychiatric syndrome of mercury poisoning, see p. 471.

Psychosomatic emergencies

In rare instances psychosomatic emergencies such as status asthmaticus and ulcerative colitis may be helped by psychiatric

12

intervention. Occasionally hypnosis can have dramatic results
(Leigh, 1965).

Psychiatric emergencies in the elderly

Most general practitioners see an increasing number of elderly
people and whilst some are specially interested in meeting their
needs and keep a register of them, many old folk are not known to
their family doctors. Crises may arise because of sudden emotional
situations such as bereavement and separation or because of the
outright rejection by a family whose tolerance of the demands of an
elderly relative is at a low ebb. In most cases there is a substantial
pathological basis such as cerebral thrombosis, pulmonary infection
or electrolyte imbalance to account for acute symptoms. In chronic
disorganised behaviour atherosclerosis and cerebral degeneration
frequently account for the dementing process. Aspects which are
specially disconcerting for relatives are faecal and urinary incontinence and restlessness and wandering at night with all the associated hazards of electricity, gas and fire.

To a lesser extent emergencies may be due to the onset of a
paranoid psychotic illness or an affective disturbance with concern
about the possibilities of suicide. Many of these problems present
initially because of pressures for disposal. Some elderly dementing
patients as well as some with psychotic illnesses need to have their
affairs looked after by a Receiver or by Power of Attorney. The
question of testamentary capacity may also be important. It is wise
to record memory impairments and delusional experiences which
may affect the patient's judgment and capacity to make a will.
When in doubt the advice of a solicitor and psychiatrist should be
sought.

In a general hospital, geriatric hospital or welfare home these
problems are not unlike those described in general practice. They
may be highlighted by behaviour disruptive to the other patients in
the ward or home which bring pressures to bear on the staff and
arouse anxiety. Appropriate assessment and advice about management is very necessary. Availability of side rooms may well determine whether advice will be acceptable or not. In psychiatric units
where patients are mobile and managed in groups with a regular
programme of occupation and recreation throughout the day, the
use of tranquillising drugs and sedatives is much reduced and the
extent of the disturbed behaviour is minimal.

Iatrogenic emergencies

Many drugs can cause psychiatric emergencies associated with a
toxic confusional syndrome or varied states of depression and

excitement with or without delusions and hallucinations. The drugs implicated include tricyclic compounds, mono-amine oxidase inhibitors, phenothiazines, sedatives and corticosteroids. The extrapyramidal side effects of phenothiazines and butyrophenones may cause states of akathisia and dyskinesia or dystonia which are sometimes misdiagnosed when presenting in the casualty department. Antihypersensitive drugs such as reserpine, guanethidine, methyldopa and clonidine have caused severe depression with the possibilities of suicide. These drugs must be used with caution in those who have a history of depressive episodes. The ready availability of drugs has led to a new syndrome which Kessel (1965) has called ' self-poisoning ' (p. 24) and which accounts for 10 to 15 per cent of medical emergencies admitted to hospital. This emphasises the need to assess carefully the role of drugs in treatment (Mandelbrote, 1972). In view of the accessibility of drugs and the dubious advantage of one sedative over another it is important to limit prescribing to less noxious drugs such as nitrazepam (Mogadon) and other benzodiazepams. Barbiturates and methaquinalone (Mandrax) are more hazardous and have resulted in suicide where perhaps it was not intended. The total number of successful suicides has dropped over recent years by about 20 per cent mainly as a result of the substitution of North Sea gas for coal gas. At the same time, the number of successful suicides from barbiturates has increased by about 100 per cent.

Facilities for dealing with psychiatric emergencies

Ideally a readily available psychiatric team to deal with emergencies on a 24-hour basis should be the aim of most psychiatric services. As an alternative, psychiatric expertise should be available to casualty departments, general hospitals and to the general practitioners. Where this is not practicable an emergency clinic is one way of meeting such needs. The doctor should be familiar with the emergency measures in his area for obtaining a psychiatric opinion. Voluntary groups may be contacted such as The Samaritans (p. 816) or Alcoholics Anonymous and the duty Social Service Worker involved if compulsory admission is required. For details of admission procedures see p. 672. Before initiating such procedures it is essential to discuss the position with the consultant on duty as admission is always dependent on acceptance by the hospital. The casualty officer should know that the request for admission under Section 29 should come from the nearest relative but can be completed by a member of the Social Services Department. The police have power to remove anyone who appears mentally ill to a place of safety under Section 136 but in the main it is preferable for them to link up with the Social Services Department and the psychiatric emergency facilities before invoking Section 136.

For those in despair and contemplating suicide but who refuse to see a psychiatrist the Rev. Chad Varah, Rector of St. Stephens Church, Walbrook, London E.C.4, and his band of helpers (Befrienders International (Samaritans Worldwide) 01–629 9000) are ready to offer advice at any time (see p. 816).

BERTRAM M. MANDELBROTE

REFERENCES

BROTHWOOD, J. (1965). The work of a Psychiatric Emergency Clinic. *British Journal of Psychiatry*, **111**, 631-634.

CLYNE, M. *Night Calls, a study in general practice*. London: Tavistock Publications. 1961.

CROWN, S. (1972). Psychiatry and the General Medical Service. Medicine. 10. *Psychiatric Disorder*, **2**, 661-671.

GRAD, J. & SAINSBURY, P. (1963). Mental illness and the family. *Lancet*, **1**, 544.

KENNEDY, P. & KREITMAN, N. (1973). An epidemiological survey of parasuicide ('Attempted Suicide') in general practice. *British Journal of Psychiatry*, **123**, 23-33.

KESSEL, N. (1965). Self poisoning (Milroy lectures). *British Medical Journal*, **11**, Part I, 1265-70. Part II, 1336-40.

LEIGH, D. *Asthma and the Psychiatrist: A Critical Review*. Book chapter 10. Psychological and allergic aspects of asthma. Illinois, U.S.A.: Charles C. Thomas. 1965.

MANDELBROTE, B. M. *Drugs and Psychiatry—Uses and Abuses*. Book chapter 2. Psychiatric aspects of medical practice. London: Staples Press. 1972.

WEIR, N. (1972). Casualty psychiatry. Medicine 9. *Psychiatric Disorder* **1**, 639-642.

WHITELEY, J. S. & DENNISON, D. M. (1963). The psychiatric casualty. *British Journal of Psychiatry*, **109**, 488.

CHAPTER 15

Medical Emergencies in Diabetes

EMERGENCIES in diabetes arise from three causes: (1) Precoma and coma due to uncontrolled diabetes. (2) Hypoglycaemia due to its treatment, and (3) the need to maintain control during situations of acute instability, e.g. surgical operations or intercurrent illness.

DIABETIC COMA

Coma strictly means loss of consciousness, but here the word is used to cover depression of consciousness (precoma) as well as its complete loss (coma) due to uncontrolled diabetes. The terms ' severe diabetic ketosis ' or ' ketoacidosis ' have often been used for the same clinical state but since diabetic coma is not always accompanied by ketoacidosis the terms are not synonymous. As we are concerned with a clinical state a clinical definition is preferable to a chemical one though less precise. Chemical findings such as plasma bicarbonate though exact are not closely related to the severity of the illness.

The clinical pattern of diabetic coma seems to have changed. It is now fairly common to see patients in coma without ketosis or acidosis (' aketotic diabetic coma ', ' hyperosmolar diabetic coma ', or ' diabetic coma without ketoacidosis ') whereas 15 years ago it was not. Why this peculiar syndrome should have apparently become so much commoner is unclear—perhaps we see it more often because it is now familiar rather than because its incidence has increased.

Diabetic coma and ketoacidosis

Diabetic coma with ketoacidosis is still the usual picture. The metabolic upset comes on gradually, is easy to recognise and can be corrected. Diabetic coma is therefore preventable. ' If preventable, why not prevented?'—this is usually because of ignorance or incompetence of the patient, or doctor, or both. But there are cases in which diabetic coma is unexpected and so swift to develop that it is upon the patient before it can be warded off.

The pathogenesis of diabetic coma is represented in Table 15.1, which shows the main clinical features and how they are produced.

The fundamental cause is lack of insulin. This leads to increase of blood sugar, dehydration, loss of electrolytes, ketosis and acidosis and eventually coma.

The condition is common. At King's College Hospital about 40 cases of diabetic coma are admitted in a year. In a diabetic clinic population about one patient per 100 per year will be admitted in

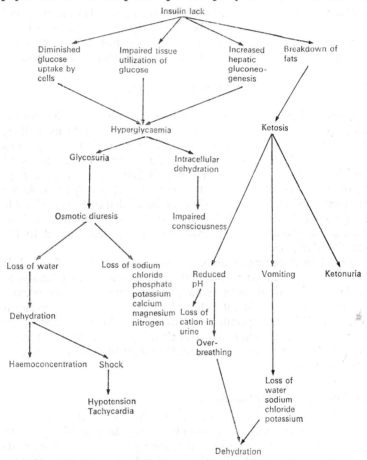

Table 15.1 *Physiological disturbances in diabetic ketoacidosis*

diabetic coma. That figure is for the whole group of diabetics; amongst the young, insulin-dependent the condition is much commoner than among older patients but no age is immune. A third of young-onset cases have at some time been in coma, but only a fiftieth of those diagnosed after 50. Although these figures show that in the diabetic diagnosed in middle-age there is only a small risk of coma, there is still some risk. An older diabetic may be insulin-dependent or, even if his diabetes is usually mild and controlled without insulin, the need for insulin may rapidly develop in the presence of an infection. A point which bears repeating is that diabetes starting in old age may be just as ' severe ' and demand insulin just as much as diabetes appearing in childhood. Since diabetic coma in the old is a dangerous illness this is an important lesson.

Coma is commoner in women than men. This is particularly true in adolescence and early adult life. The main reason is probably that at this age young women are more liable to emotional upsets which disturb their diabetes. It is asking a lot that an adolescent should never exploit (consciously or unconsciously) the unbeatable weapon for gaining attention which she always possesses—the ability at any time to become seriously ill. If a girl doesn't like school, cannot face an examination, has an argument with her boyfriend or doesn't get on with her parents—she always has a way out of her difficulties. She can precipitate an emergency by simply stopping her insulin—or by saying she has done so. Everyone then must rally round and she is assured of the intense attention of many people including those she holds to ransom. The psychiatric approach to the problem is singularly unrewarding, either because the problem is peculiarly intractable or the psychiatrists peculiarly unsuccessful.

The important conclusion is that difficult adolescents make bad diabetics; the cause of repeated episodes of diabetic coma is more likely to be found in the patient's character than in any inherent instability of diabetes. If a patient is admitted more than twice a year in coma look into his psyche and circumstances.

By contrast, a review of our patients who have had diabetes for 40 years shows what can be achieved. Over half of 92 patients had never been in diabetic coma—not once in 40 years. They show how well sensible patients can do.

Precipitating causes

Diabetic coma, being due to insulin lack, results from omission or reduction of insulin, failure to raise the dose in the presence of increased need, or unrecognised diabetes which can, but should not, present in coma. About a quarter of our cases fall into each of these three categories, the fourth quarter being unexplained.

1. The patient may stop or reduce his insulin out of perversity or emotional disturbance or, more commonly, because he believes, or his doctor tells him, that less is needed if he is ill and cannot eat. This is still a common and dangerous fallacy.

2. In an intercurrent infection the need for insulin usually increases, even though the patient may eat little. Vomiting is a particularly important feature. It may be a warning sign of impending coma and should always be taken seriously in an insulin-dependent diabetic. Few patients pass into precoma without starting to vomit. Intercurrent illness occasionally creates the need for insulin in a patient previously treated without it.

3. When a new case of diabetes presents in coma many days or weeks of thirst, polyuria and increasing illness must always have been concealed, ignored or misinterpreted by patient, family or doctor. Whereas coma may develop over as short a period as 12 hours in the established diabetic, it never does so in new cases.

Clinical features

The clinical picture is characteristic and easy to recognise. Onset is gradual, over 12-24 hours or longer, (more rapid in children than in adults) with increasingly severe symptoms of diabetes accompanied by vomiting, abdominal pain, overbreathing and drowsiness which, if still untreated, will progress to unconsciousness. The abdominal pain (p. 118) may be severe and occasionally leads to confusion with an acute surgical condition. Doubt can usually be resolved by treating the coma vigorously when, if diabetes is the cause as it usually is, the pain will subside. If it persists a surgical cause is likely. Abdominal pain cannot be ascribed to diabetes in the absence of precoma or coma.

The patient is dehydrated and over-ventilating. The rate of breathing may not be much increased, but the depth is, and for those with a sensitive nose the fruity smell of acetone in the breath is obvious. The patient is so dry that the skin is inelastic, the tongue parched and (a useless sign, always remembered!) the eyeballs soft. There is usually some degree of gastric and intestinal ileus; it may be so severe that a succussion splash may be elicited. In spite of the dehydration urine flow is plentiful.

When the illness is severe there may be signs of peripheral circulatory collapse—cold extremities, thin pulse, low blood pressure. Tachycardia is common and fever occasional. There may be signs of intercurrent illness which may have precipitated coma, especially respiratory, urinary or alimentary.

Diagnosis

Diagnosis is easy. It is made on the clinical picture and confirmed by finding glycosuria and intense ketonuria, elevated blood sugar and depressed bicarbonate (and pH). The characteristic story of deterioration in a known diabetic or progressive worsening of the usual symptoms in an unknown case, allow no alternative. Distinction from salicylate poisoning (p. 31) and advanced renal failure could lead to confusion but in practice does not. More often an intercurrent illness is overlooked or, if detected, may be thought to be the whole explanation for the clinical state.

Diabetic coma cannot be confused with hypoglycaemic coma except by those who read textbooks which list the features of both in a single table! Their pathogenesis and characteristics are totally different.

Treatment. All patients should be in hospital.

The following investigations are essential for the rational treatment of diabetic coma: Urine for sugar and ketones; blood for glucose, bicarbonate, sodium, potassium, urea.

The following tests are helpful: Urine for protein; blood for pH, ketones (by applying dilute serum to ketostix or by direct measurement); cardioscope or ECG for monitoring cardiac rhythm and early signs of hypokalaemia.

Other useful investigations are chest X-ray, urine microscopy and blood count (leucocytosis is common in coma and ESR, transaminase and amylase levels may also be raised in the absence of other disease).

The essential of any good treatment regimen is that it should be simple and effective. The scheme outlined here is both. The needs are: insulin, fluid replacement, aspiration of the stomach, electrolyte replacement and treatment of intercurrent illness.

Controversy concerning the treatment of diabetic coma centres on three aspects: 1. The dose and route of administration of insulin. 2. The time of starting potassium, and 3. The use of bicarbonate.

Insulin

All cases of diabetic precoma and coma need insulin. The need is urgent, though not immediate. One can usually safely wait to establish the diagnosis, admit the patient to hospital and measure the blood sugar before starting insulin, but it is sensible to set up a saline infusion without delay. The blood sugar will fall from rehydration even before insulin is started.

The insulin treatment of a diabetic coma has recently been simplified. The best method is to give soluble insulin by continuous i v infusion (Page *et al.*, 1974; Kidson, *et al.*, 1974; Semple *et al.*, 1974). The advantage of the i v route is that one can be certain that the insulin is entering the circulation; even with very small doses effective blood levels are obtained. Insulin must be infused continuously as it rapidly disappears from the circulation having a half life of only four minutes. Intermittent i v injections are therefore only briefly effective.

The method requires an infusion pump* (Fig. 15.1). Adding insulin to the saline infusion bottle is not satisfactory because the rate of administration is uncertain and adsorption of insulin to

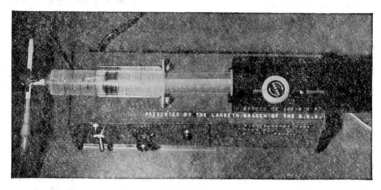

FIG. 15.1

Constant-rate infusion pump attached by four-way tap to i v line.
The pump is set to deliver 5 ml hourly containing 6 units of insulin.
The rate of infusion is independent of the speed of flow of the saline.
(*With kind permission of Blackwell Scientific Publications.*)

plastic may at this dilution be a significant factor. The pump is attached by a four-way tap to the i v infusion line. Insulin is thus administered at a constant rate whatever the speed of the saline infusion. In the concentration we use, insulin does not adhere to the plastic of syringe or tubing, so it is not necessary, as had been thought, to add human albumin to prevent adsorption.

Technique. We give 6 units insulin/hour (but even smaller doses seem to be effective). 24 units of soluble insulin (i.e. 0·6 ml of 40 u/ml strength or 0·3 ml of 80 u/ml strength) are drawn up into a 1 ml syringe and injected into a 20 ml syringe which is then filled with isosmotic sodium chloride solution. This syringe is laid on the

* Constant-rate infusion pumps may be obtained from : —
 (1) Dylade Company, Brindley 45, Astmoor Industrial Estate, Runcorn, Cheshire.
 (2) Rocket (London) Ltd., Imperial Way, Station Estate, Watford, Herts.
 (3) Charles F. Thackray Ltd., 67 Weymouth Street, London W.1.
 (4) Harvard Apparatus Co. Inc., 150 Dover Road, Millis, Mass., 02054, U.S.A.

pump which is adjusted to deliver 5 ml (=6 units insulin) an hour (Fig. 15.1). If the infusion needs to be maintained for more than four hours, the syringe is recharged (or a new syringe used). The pump has a light or sound signal so that it is easy to see that it is working. In children under the age of about 10, 3 u/hour of insulin are given. In older children the dose is the same as for adults.

The biochemical response is satisfactory and consistent. Blood sugar and ketone levels fall steadily and plasma bicarbonate rises, although sometimes more slowly. Biochemical monitoring is necessary and blood sugar and electrolyte determinations must be repeated after two hours, and thereafter as required. In most cases the blood sugar level falls by about 5·5 mmol/l (100 mg/100 ml)/ hour but, if the response is inadequate, the rate of infusion can be doubled or trebled by adjusting the infusion pump.

When the blood sugar has fallen to 8·25-11·0 mmol/l (150-200 mg/100 ml) the insulin infusion is stopped (although the saline is usually continued) and subcutaneous injections given four hourly according to urine or blood tests. In most cases insulin infusion needs to be maintained for 4-8 hours. There seems to be no advantage and some danger, from hypokalaemia or cerebral oedema, in attempting more rapid correction of the biochemical abnormalities.

This technique, so simple and satisfactory, depends upon having an infusion pump. If this is not available insulin should be given by hourly i m injections—a priming dose of 10-20 units (according to the severity of the illness) and then 5-10 units hourly. This technique is even simpler and seems to be almost as effective as the continuous infusion method.

When the blood sugar has been brought under control a suitable regime of four-hourly injections of soluble insulin according to urine tests is:

if urine glucose is + + + or + + + + with ketonuria give 32-40 units
+ + + or + + + + with little or no
ketonuria   16-32 units
+ or + +   8-16 units
0 or trace   0- 8 units

After a day or two it is usually possible to go over to a regular twice daily regime of soluble insulin injections. In cases of diabetic coma without ketoacidosis we give 3 units hourly of soluble insulin instead of 6 as these patients seem to be relatively sensitive to insulin.

FLUID

All patients in diabetic coma need large quantities of fluid, which is always best given by i v infusion. A patient who has not vomited may be able to take large amounts of water by mouth, but in any seriously ill patient attempts to give fluids this way are usually a waste of valuable time and may be dangerous. If in doubt, set up a drip.

There is disagreement about the best type of fluid to use. However, isosmotic sodium chloride is safe and as effective as any other. We use sodium bicarbonate only in severely acidotic patients, giving 100-200 mmol if pH is less than 7·1, or bicarbonate less than 5 mmol or if there is no clinical improvement in two hours, or if the serum potassium on admission is over 6·5 mmol/litre.

The volume of fluid needed is large. The first one or two litres are run in within an hour unless the patient is elderly or has been in heart failure, when the rate is reduced to about one litre in one to two hours and a close watch kept on the jugular venous pressure, if necessary with a central venous pressure line (p. 751). After about two hours when two to three litres have been given the rate can be slowed, but a total infusion of six to twelve litres is likely to be needed.

ASPIRATION OF THE STOMACH

In any ill diabetic there is likely to be gastric dilatation, probably caused by intracellular potassium depletion. In the semiconscious or unconscious patient there is a danger of inhalation of vomit, so the stomach should always be emptied via a nasogastric tube.

ELECTROLYTES

As blood sugar falls potassium re-enters the cells and the serum level, which is usually normal at the onset, falls, sometimes dangerously. I v potassium is therefore needed in all except mildly ill patients. We prefer to wait for two hours to see the response of the serum potassium to treatment before adding potassium 2-4 g per litre of saline, to the infusion. If for any reason there is delay in finding the blood level, or if there are ECG indications of hypokalaemia (flattening or inversion of T waves) (p. 603) and provided the admission level was not raised and the urine flow is adequate, potassium can be added ' blind ', and should be if the original level is less than 4 mmol/l.

As an indicator of *change* in serum potassium a cardiac monitor is invaluable (although it is possible to have a normal ECG in the presence of hypokalaemia).

A total dose of potassium chloride of 4 to 20 g will usually stabilise the serum level. If sodium bicarbonate is given serum potassium may fall quickly and a close watch on the level is therefore essential.

INTERCURRENT ILLNESS

In a quarter of cases of coma, infection is the precipitating factor. Don't forget to look for it. Give antibiotics if in doubt. Cardiac infarction, precipitating or resulting from ketoacidosis, can easily be missed in an ill patient.

Peripheral vasomotor collapse usually responds to fluid replacement. Cardiac irregularities are fairly common and not serious, but occasionally they are dangerous and require treatment on the accepted lines (p. 249). Urine flow is usually ample because of osmotic diuresis but severely ill patients may show oliguria soon after admission. If this does not rapidly respond to fluid therapy frusemide (Lasix) is often effective.

Prognosis depends upon the level of consciousness, age, and the presence of complications, such as cardiac infarction, severe infection or vascular occlusion. The young, conscious patient should always recover, the elderly unconscious patient has no better than an even chance of doing so. Overall mortality is about 5-10 per cent. Occasionally dysphagia may persist for a few days but there are no permanent sequelae of diabetic coma.

Diabetic coma without ketoacidosis

This type of coma is being seen increasingly often in Britain, especially among coloured immigrants. The differences from the 'ordinary' coma are:

1. Patients are often older and may not previously have been known diabetics.

2. Dehydration is extreme, but ketosis and acidosis (as shown by overbreathing, ketonuria, reduced plasma bicarbonate and pH) are slight or absent. Although urine tests for ketones may be positive they are not strongly so, and plasma bicarbonate is usually not below 15 mmol/l and pH is 7·3 or more.

3. The patients are relatively sensitive to insulin presumably because of the lack of ketosis and acidosis; recovery has even been described in a patient treated without insulin.

4. After recovery the patient can, in about half of the cases, be managed without insulin, a rare situation after ketoacidotic coma.

The cause of the condition is not known, nor is the greater tendency of black people to develop it. Drinking large amounts of sugar-containing fluid in an attempt to quench increasing thirst has been suggested but hardly explains all cases. However, the distinction between the two types of diabetic coma is not absolute and a patient may at different times suffer from each.

Treatment differs from that of ketoacidotic coma. The need for fluid is just as great but that for insulin less. We give insulin in *half* the dose we use in ketoacidotic coma, and we use *half*-strength isosmotic sodium chloride solution. Special risks include arterial thrombosis. The prognosis is not as bad as has been claimed (50 per cent mortality) but the condition is still dangerous.

HYPOGLYCAEMIA

This can result from (1) injected insulin, (2) sulphonylurea drugs, (3) spontaneous causes, especially islet-cell tumours of the pancreas.

Minor hypoglycaemic episodes are common in diabetics treated by insulin and do not present as emergencies, but more serious hypoglycaemia can develop from overdosage, omission or delay in taking food, unusual exercise and from unknown causes.

The known causes are self-explanatory. Overdosage may be the fault of the doctor, e.g. not appreciating the common tendency to improvement in the diabetic state which may occur in the early weeks after diagnosis, or attempting to get postprandial urine tests free of sugar, or of the patient who may have raised his insulin dose inappropriately, or even deliberately. The blood sugar-lowering effect of exercise in diabetics is variable. The patient should be warned to proceed carefully, to carry glucose tablets always and if necessary to take extra carbohydrate before or during unusual exertion. Hypoglycaemia is usually preceded by warning but the early symptoms may be misinterpreted by the patient or others, perhaps because of mental slowing induced by the hypoglycaemia itself. Some patients, particularly longstanding diabetics, may pass into hypoglycaemic coma abruptly.

Hypoglycaemia presents as an emergency only if its onset is sudden. If it comes on gradually it is easily dealt with. The features are: (1) Rapid onset of unusual or aggressive behaviour or unconsciousness in a diabetic on insulin, probably at a time of maximum insulin action and minimum food absorption, i.e. before lunch or during the night, but it can occur at any time whatever the insulin regime. (2) Sweating, tachycardia with strong pulse, and pallor, due mainly to autonomic responses to the hypoglycaemia. (3) There may be odd neurological signs including extensor plantar responses and even hemiparesis, which clear rapidly on treatment. (There is, of course, no dehydration and no overbreathing.)

The diagnosis should always suggest itself in any diabetic on insulin (or on sulphonylurea) who behaves oddly, becomes confused or drowsy, or loses consciousness. Children may become fractious or miserable.

Diagnosis here, unlike in diabetic coma, may be difficult. There may be no history and it may not even be known that a patient is a diabetic on insulin. The condition can be confused with any other causing rapid change in behaviour or loss of consciousness, e.g. alcohol ingestion (which may itself provoke hypoglycaemia), epilepsy, cardiac arrhythmia or stroke. The distinction from alcoholic intoxication is particularly important, clinically and medico-legally. The fact that a man has been drinking does not prove that his coma is due to alcohol. If suspected, the diagnosis can easily be made or refuted. Testing the urine may be no help, as it may contain sugar secreted earlier, but the blood will always show a low blood glucose level; if it does not, and the test has been properly done, the diagnosis is excluded. The simple paper test dextrostix is very useful; although not precise it is accurate enough for this purpose. In cases of hypoglycaemia it will indicate a blood sugar value of 2·20 mmol/litre (40 mg/100 ml) or less.

If the diagnosis is in doubt and cannot be rapidly determined, give glucose by mouth if the patient is conscious, otherwise inject i v 20-50 ml of dextrose 50 g/dl. This will usually restore consciousness within a minute or two, unless the patient has been unconscious for a long time when recovery will be slower and may even take days.

Very severe hypoglycaemia lasting for many hours can lead to disastrous brain damage or even death. The rule therefore is in any case of unconsciousness in a diabetic, the cause of which is not certain, give i v glucose, preferably after taking blood for glucose determination. This will do no harm even if the patient is in a diabetic coma. Prompt recovery makes the diagnosis, but failure does not exclude hypoglycaemia. On recovery from hypoglycaemic coma the patient must take further carbohydrate by mouth, in both a rapidly absorbed and more slowly absorbed form to maintain the blood sugar level, since if he has had any long-acting insulin this may tend to fall again.

The right treatment for hypoglycaemia is glucose 20 to 30 g by mouth if the patient is conscious or 20 to 50 ml of 50 g/dl solution i v if he is unconscious. If sterile glucose solution is not available glucagon 1 mg i m will be effective although more slowly. If this too is not at hand Adrenaline Injection BP (1 in 1 000) 0·5 to 1·0 ml subcutaneously is perhaps a little better than nothing.

Hypoglycaemia due to sulphonylureas

As sulphonylureas act principally by stimulating the islets of Langerhans they can cause hypoglycaemia. In practice hypoglycaemia due to these drugs rarely presents as an emergency, but it can so easily be missed and as its consequences can be so serious the condition is important. Chlorpropamide is probably the sulphonylurea which most often leads to serious hypoglycaemia, mainly because of its long action. Elderly patients, especially those living alone, who have recently started sulphonylurea treatment are most at risk. When they are found after being unconscious for a long period the cause may not be apparent. With or without neurological signs, a cerebrovascular episode may be the obvious diagnosis and the hypoglycaemia may be missed. Every unconscious patient, whether diabetic or not, in whom a diagnosis is not certain should have his blood sugar estimated.

The risk of hypoglycaemia from sulphonylurea can be greatly reduced by (1) not putting diabetics on to these drugs unless the need is proved by failure to respond to diet alone, (2) using shorter-acting drugs in the elderly, e.g. tolbutamide (Rastinon), acetohexamide (Dimelor), or tolazamide (Tolanase), rather than chlorpropamide (Diabinese), or glibenclamide (Euglucon), (3) keeping the dose as low as possible, e.g. 500 mg of tolbutamide twice a day, or 250 mg once a day of tolazamide, and no more than 375 mg if chlorpropamide is used. (4) Taking the same dietary precautions as with insulin treatment to prevent hypoglycaemia, and in particular a late night snack.

As chlorpropamide has a very long action (half life 30 hours) patients severely hypoglycaemic from this drug should always be admitted to hospital and their blood sugar level monitored for 3-4 days.

MANAGEMENT OF DIABETES DURING INTERCURRENT ILLNESS OR SURGICAL OPERATION

For diabetes and pregnancy see p. 180.

Intercurrent illness

The insulin requirement is often increased by infections, even when accompanied by loss of appetite. The urine should be tested and if there is intense glycosuria the usual dose of insulin increased by 4-8 units and even more if there is severe ketonuria. The urine is tested four-hourly and if necessary extra doses of soluble insulin are given. If symptoms persist, and especially if vomiting starts, the patient is best admitted to hospital. Soluble insulin should be given four-hourly according to urine tests thus:—

If urine glucose is $+++$ or $++++$ with ketonuria	32-40 units
$+++$ or $++++$ with little or no ketonuria	16-32 units
$+$ or $++$	8-16 units
0 or trace	0- 8 units

If on the other hand, during an infection tests show only moderate glycosuria the normal dose of insulin is given. If the patient cannot eat and there is no glycosuria the normal dose is reduced by about 20 per cent, *but insulin is not stopped.*

Carbohydrate intake should be maintained. If the patient cannot eat, glucose can usually be retained if given in soda water and drunk slowly. The following drinks contain 10 g of carbohydrate: Lucozade 60 ml, Ribena 15 ml, milk 200 ml, orange juice 120 ml (1 teaspoonful=5 ml; 1 tablespoonful=15 ml). If feeding is impossible the patient should be sent to hospital as an i v drip will probably be needed.

In any case of severe diabetic upset due to illness, accident, or *prolonged* operation we now use the constant-rate i v infusion technique (p. 342). In labour we give soluble insulin at the rate of 2 units an hour covered by i v glucose infusion (10 g hourly).

Surgical operation

The management of diabetes during surgery depends upon (1) type of diabetic treatment, (2) whether the patient is adequately stabilised, and (3) whether operation is urgent or elective.

The hazards are hypoglycaemia which, though acute, can easily be treated, and ketoacidosis, which is gradual in onset and infrequent, but serious.

If a patient is on diet only or treated with biguanides (Phenformin) the risk of hypoglycaemia is nil; if he is on a long-acting sulphonylureas there is a very slight risk and it is wise to test the urine for sugar before operation. If there is no glycosuria give 10-20 ml of glucose 50 g/dl iv (unless a blood test indicates a level of over 100 mg per 100 ml (5·5 mmol/l)).

For the patient on insulin there is some risk of hypoglycaemia. Insulin is therefore best omitted in the six to eight hours before operation. This will seldom lead to a great rise of blood sugar and insulin can be resumed after operation according to four-hourly urine tests. It is an advantage to arrange operations on diabetics at a definite time and preferably early in the morning. If the patient normally takes only soluble insulin the normal dose is given on the previous evening and the morning dose omitted. If he takes long-acting insulin that is omitted on the previous day and a soluble preparation is substituted and a small evening dose of soluble insulin given.

It is essential always to do a preoperative urine test. If this shows no sugar a blood test (dextrostix) is done and if this indicates a low level (4·5 mmol/1 90 mg per 100 ml or lower) 10-20 ml 50 g/dl glucose is given i v (*never by mouth* within four hours of operation). It is seldom necessary to do more than this. The blood sugar may rise during operation, especially if a long procedure, but the rise is hardly ever serious and control can easily be re-established after operation.

STATE OF STABILISATION

In practice it is extremely rare for a diabetic to need an emergency operation at a time when his diabetes is seriously out of control. If the operation is not urgent a few hours or a day or two can be spent regaining diabetic control with a sliding scale of insulin dosage and then the operation performed. If he is in precoma or coma treatment for this is started (p. 341) and as soon as considerable improvement has been achieved the operation is done. In less severe cases of diabetic upset, it is desirable to postpone operation for a few hours while the diabetes is controlled, but if this is impossible an i v drip is set up, insulin is given, operation started and blood glucose monitored. In practice, this type of crisis hardly ever arises.

HOW URGENT?

Questions of surgical urgency are considered in the two previous sections.

Provided reasonable vigilance is maintained operations on diabetics are safe. Disasters occasionally happen because of careless-ness, such as failure to notice and act upon a serious deterioration of urine tests or even of the clinical state. (For management of diabetes in pregnant patients see pp. 180 and 562.)

DAVID PYKE

FOR FURTHER READING

ALBERTI, K. G. M. M., HOCKADAY, T. D. R. & TURNER, R. C. (1973). Small doses of intramuscular insulin in the treatment of diabetic ' coma '. *Lancet*, **2**, 515.
HOCKADAY, T. D. R. & ALBERTI, K. G. M. M. (1972). Diabetic coma. *British Journal of Hospital Medicine*, **7**, 183.

HOCKADAY, T. D. R. & ALBERTI, K. G. M. M. (1972). Diabetic coma. *Clinics in Endocrinology and Metabolism*, **1**, 751.
KIDSON, W. *et al.* (1974). Treatment of severe diabetes mellitus by insulin infusion. *British Medical Journal*, **2**, 691.
McCURDY, D. K. (1970). Hyperosmolar hyperglycaemic non-ketotic diabetic coma. *Medical Clinics of N. America*, **54**, 563.
OAKLEY, W. G., PYKE, D. A. & TAYLOR, K. W. *Diabetes and its Management*, 2nd edition, p. 102. Oxford and London: Blackwell. 1975.
PAGE, M. McB. *et al.* (1974). Treatment of diabetic coma with continuous low-dose infusion of insulin. *British Medical Journal*, **2**, 687.
PYKE, D. A. (1969). Diabetic ketosis and coma. *Journal of Clinical Pathology*, **22**, suppl. (*Ass. clin. Path.*), 2, 57-65.
SEMPLE, P. F. *et al.* (1974). Continuous intravenous infusion of small doses of insulin in treatment of diabetic ketoacidosis. *British Medical Journal*, **2**, 694.
SHELDON, J. & PYKE, D. A. Severe diabetic ketosis; precoma and Coma. In *Clinical Diabetes and its Biochemical Basis*, p. 420. (Oakley, W. G., Pyke, D. A. and Taylor, K. W. eds). Oxford and London: Blackwell. 1968.
WINEGRAD, A. I. & CLEMENTS, R. S. (1971). Diabetic ketoacidosis. *Medical Clinics of North America*, **55**, 899.

CHAPTER 16

Medical Emergencies in Other Endocrine Disorders

ADRENAL CORTEX

URGENT symptoms may occur in both hyper- and hypo-adrenocorticalism.

HYPERADRENOCORTICALISM

Cushing's syndrome

Over secretion of cortisol may lead to complications such as hypertension, heart disease with cardiac failure or renal disease with uraemia, the emergencies of which will require treatment along conventional lines. Hypokalaemia may cause urgent symptoms, particularly in those cases associated with corticotrophin-secreting tumours of non-endocrine tissues such as carcinoma of the bronchus. The diagnosis in such cases may not be immediately apparent since the condition tends to be comparatively rapid in onset and to occur before the more florid manifestations of Cushing's syndrome appear. Patients will present with pronounced muscular weakness and this symptom should always lead to an estimation of the serum potassium. Therapy is with potassium chloride. Initially i v doses of 1 g are given at intervals of four hours for 24 hours. At the same time 1 g should be given four-hourly by mouth. A watch should be kept on the serum potassium and the dose adjusted appropriately. Subsequently surgical measures must be taken to remove the source of excessive cortisol production, either by excision of an adrenal tumour or total or partial bilateral adrenalectomy.

Hyperaldosteronism (Conn's syndrome)

Aldosterone-secreting tumours may cause urgent muscle weakness from hypokalaemia: they may also present as hypertension with cardiac and renal manifestations.

The differential diagnosis of primary hyperaldosteronism is more difficult than was originally thought. Hypokalaemic alkalosis was once considered diagnostic. However, idiopathic malignant hypertension may lead to secondary hyperaldosteronism with a similar biochemical picture, and indeed this is now considered the commoner cause of hypokalaemic alkalosis. Renin assays, if available, will help to establish the diagnosis, since levels are raised in secondary and depressed in primary hyperaldosteronism. Adrenal aerograms and arteriograms may also help. Another condition which may cause difficulty is that of ' salt-losing nephritis '. Various renal disorders, notably chronic pyelonephritis, may by renal tubular damage cause loss of sodium and potassium and acid base disturbances with hyponatraemia, hypokalaemia and acidosis. The attempt to conserve sodium leads to nitrogen retention with uraemia. Other causes of hypokalaemia, including the rare Bartter's syndrome (Bartter *et al.*, 1962; Takayasu *et al.*, 1971) might also need consideration.

Immediate treatment will consist in correction of the metabolic disturbance. Sodium and potassium deficiencies must be rectified, and disturbances of the acid base balance corrected—chloride infusions for alkalosis, and sodium lactate or bicarbonate for acidosis. Thereafter the correct diagnosis must be established and appropriate action taken.

HYPOADRENOCORTICALISM

Acute adrenal deficiency may show in several ways.

Adrenal crisis in Addison's disease

This may appear in a previously undiagnosed patient, or may follow infection, accident or operation in a known case. The patient will present with increasing weakness, abdominal pain and vomiting or mental disturbance. Hypotension will be found. Pigmentation of the skin and mucous membranes is usually pronounced, though on occasion it can be minimal, probably when the onset of the disease process has been rapid. Hyponatraemia, raised blood urea and sometimes hypoglycaemia may be found. If untreated, prostration, stupor, coma and finally death will supervene.

Salt-losing nephritis can present real difficulty in diagnosis. Weakness, vomiting, hypotension, perhaps minimal pigmentation, hyponatraemia and uraemia closely simulate Addison's disease. The absence or minimal presence of pigmentation, hypokalaemia and acidosis should suggest the possibility. Estimation of plasma cortisol (send plasma from 10 ml of blood) will help greatly since it is very low in Addison's disease. The true diagnosis may only emerge following initiation of treatment.

Treatment. This consists in dextrose saline infusion, hydrocortisone and fludrocortisone. Two to three litres of dextrose saline should be given i v over the first 24 hours, the first litre being given fairly rapidly. Hydrocortisone should be added and infused at the rate of 100 mg eight-hourly. Fludrocortisone 2 mg can be given by mouth to patients who are not vomiting. Alternatively deoxycortone acetate (DOCA) 10 mg should be given by i m injection. Any precipitating factor such as infection should be dealt with appropriately. After the first 24 hours it will usually be possible to give all drugs by mouth. Dosage should be controlled as far as possible by estimation of serum metabolites. Approximately 50 mg cortisone six-hourly and a single 1 mg dose of fludrocortisone will be needed on the second day. Dosage is then reduced fairly rapidly until daily maintenance levels are reached by about the end of a week. These will be around 25 mg for cortisone and 0·1 mg for fludrocortisone.

Stress states in patients on corticosteroid therapy

Adrenal response to stress tends to be impaired, sometimes severely, in patients who are taking or who have taken corticosteroids. Serious infections or accidents and surgical operations may lead to collapse with lowered blood pressure which if untreated will be fatal.

Steps should be taken to prevent the onset of adrenal failure where possible as, for example, in the preparation of patients for operation. Cortisone 100 mg should be given i m 12 hours before and just before operation, and then for three doses at six-hourly intervals. Thereafter it will usually be possible to change to oral therapy with cortisone or other steroid in equivalent dosage (25 mg cortisone—5 mg prednisolone phosphate—0·5 mg betamethasone phosphate). Dosage can be reduced fairly rapidly until usual maintenance levels are reached by about the end of one week.

The recovery of responsiveness to stress following cessation of corticosteroid therapy has been studied by Livanou, Ferriman and James (1967) using plasma cortisol response to insulin hypoglycaemia and by Plumpton, Besser and Cole (1969) using the plasma cortisol response to surgery. Recovery is affected by the dose of corticosteroid employed, possibly by the duration of treatment and almost certainly by an important individual factor. The evidence does not clearly establish how soon it is *perfectly* safe to operate without steroid cover in patients who have been taking corticosteroids. Most will have recovered full responsiveness within two or three months after stopping treatment and all by the end of a year. As a general rule it will be safe to operate without steroid cover two months after stopping treatment. Some authorities say it is safe in as short a time as two weeks. All patients should be monitored after operation for any sign of hypotension or collapse and appropriate hydrocortisone therapy started should this appear

(100 mg hydrocortisone immediately by i v injection followed by i v hydrocortisone infusion at the rate of 100 mg every eight hours for the first 24 hours.

If staffing problems make detailed monitoring difficult it would be reasonable to give corticosteroid cover to all patients who have operations within two years of discontinuance of corticosteroid therapy.

Fludrocortisone will not be needed in this type of patient. Underlying factors such as infections must be dealt with vigorously. Drugs to raise blood pressure such as metaraminol (Aramine) may be used but are of doubtful value.

Miscellaneous causes

Acute adrenal failure may also occur in various severe stress conditions such as septicaemia (not necessarily meningococcal) with haemorrhages into the skin and elsewhere, including the adrenals (Waterhouse-Friderichsen syndrome), after difficult labour or abortion or in the rare condition of idiopathic adrenal apoplexy (with haemorrhage into one or both adrenals). It has been suggested that features of the Waterhouse-Friderichsen syndrome previously attributed to adrenal failure are related to the Schwartzman reaction, a complex, ill-understood response involving capillary damage by bacterial endotoxins (Taichmann, 1971). The condition should be suspected if there is collapse, hypotension and perhaps stupor under any of these circumstances. The diagnosis of adrenal apoplexy is particularly difficult but the association of pain in one or both renal angles associated with collapse may be a pointer. Estimation of plasma cortisol may be of help (send 10 ml of blood with heparin). An i v infusion of hydrocortisone should be set up at a dosage of 100 mg eight-hourly. Hydrocortisone is of undoubted value in the Waterhouse-Friderichsen syndrome but this may be due to a beneficial effect on capillary damage in the Schwartzman reaction rather than to a correction of adrenocortical deficiency.

Congenital adrenal hyperplasia (see also p. 412)

This rare condition manifests itself early in life. It is due to enzyme deficiencies in the synthesis of cortisol and other adrenal steroids. Danger arises when defects in the synthesis of salt-conserving steroids are present. Anorexia, vomiting, loss of weight, failure to thrive and hypotension with circulatory failure will be shown by infants of both sexes. Ambiguous external genitalia are an assistance towards diagnosis in female infants. Hyponatraemia, raised blood urea, and a markedly raised level of 17-ketosteroid (oxosteroid) excretion with characteristic steroid anomalies on chromatography complete the diagnosis. Initial treatment consists of 30 ml isosmotic sodium chloride solution per kg body weight, four-hourly i v, cortisone 50 to 100 mg in 24 hours by mouth or i m if vomiting is present, and 1 mg fludrocortisone by mouth or 5 mg deoxycortone acetate i m. If sufficiently severe 100 mg hydrocortisone should be given by i v drip in the first eight hours. Thereafter dosage must be controlled by estimation of serum metabolites. Eventually daily maintenance dosage will be reached in the neighbourhood of 4 to 6 g sodium chloride orally, cortisone 25 mg by mouth, and fludrocortisone 0·1 to 0·2 mg by mouth. It must be remembered that for some reason this condition is more difficult to keep under control than is that caused by simple absence of adrenals. It may be that there is excess production of some (unknown) factor with salt-losing properties. Infections readily precipitate crises and increases in dosage become urgently necessary. It greatly assists management of these cases if the diagnosis is firmly established at the onset. Every effort should be made to collect urine prior to treatment, provided the infant's condition is not so desperate as to call for immediate therapy. As little as 20 ml of urine may be sufficient; this should be placed in deep freeze while arrangements are made for expert assay of steroid metabolites.

THE ADRENAL MEDULLA

Phaeochromocytoma

PHYSIOLOGICAL CONSIDERATIONS. Adenomas and carcinomas of the adrenal medulla secrete noradrenaline and adrenaline in varying proportions, and the dominance of one or other will determine the clinical presentation. Noradrenaline acts on α-receptor sites leading mainly to constriction of blood vessels throughout the body and a rise in blood pressure. Adrenaline acts on β-receptor sites leading to constriction of skin vessels and dilatation of those in muscle, the effect on blood pressure depending upon a balance between these two effects. It also causes tachycardia, sweating, tremor, a sense of anxiety or even fear, fever and perhaps glycosuria.

CLINICAL PRESENTATION. The condition may present broadly in one of three ways. The first is with bouts of paroxysmal hypertension. It must not be forgotten that the commonest cause of paroxysmal hypertension is essential hypertension, but if the attacks are accompanied by palpitation (fast or slow), severe throbbing headache, marked sweating, a corpse-like pallor, perhaps fever or glycosuria, and are short lived (five minutes or so), suspicion of the diagnosis should be aroused. A tumour may sometimes be palpated in the loin or at sites in the abdomen where chromaffin bodies are located, and palpation may lead to hypertensive paroxysms. A second mode of presentation is with sustained hypertension, perhaps with superimposed exacerbations. The diagnosis here will be from all other causes of hypertension, though the characteristic features of paroxysmal palpitation, throbbing headaches, sweating and pallor or palpable tumours may provide a clue. In both these forms the patient may present with hypertensive complications such as acute left-sided cardiac failure with dyspnoea, tightness in the chest or frank pulmonary oedema, hypertensive encephalopathy, and in the sustained form with features of malignant hypertension such as retinitis or uraemia. The third and least common presentation is with collapse and normal blood pressure or even hypotension (Richmond *et al.,* 1961; Steiness, 1961; Hamrin, 1962). This occurs if adrenaline secretion is dominant, when dilatation of muscle vessels may outweigh the effect of constriction of cutaneous vessels. This type presents a peculiarly difficult diagnostic problem, though again a history of paroxysmal attacks with headaches, sweating and pallor and possibly a palpable tumour may provide a clue.

AIDS TO DIAGNOSIS. If time permits estimation of the excretion of catechol amines or vanilyl mandelic acid will sometimes, but not invariably, provide a diagnosis. I v pyelography and adrenal aerograms or arteriograms may help. Alternatively, a test which might also prove therapeutic would be to see if an i v injection of 5 to 10 mg of phentolamine (Rogitine) had an hypotensive effect.

Treatment. Hypertensive patients, including those with phaeochromocytoma, present at times in dangerous crises with pulmonary oedema, requiring immediate use of hypotensive agents. Luckily those in common use are effective irrespective of the cause. Ansolysen (pentolinium) should be given as a slow i v injection or drip at the rate of 1 mg per minute until an effect is obtained. This usually occurs after 2 to 8 mg have been given. Guanethidine (Ismelin), methyl dopa (Aldomet) and bethanidine (Esbatal), however, sensitise vessel walls to noradrenaline and may exacerbate the situation in phaeochromocytoma; they should be avoided in the emergency treatment of paroxysmal hypertension where the cause is unknown.

Once the diagnosis is established phentolamine (Rogitine) can be used in 5 to 10 mg doses i v. The effect is short-lived, however, and the injection would be needed at approximately four-hourly intervals. A better preparation is phenoxybenzamine (Dibenyline) since its action lasts longer and it is effective by mouth. A trial dose of 10 mg should be given. This can then be increased up to 10 to 30 mg three or four times a day until the hypertension has been brought under control. If cardiac arrhythmia is also present then a beta-adrenergic blocking agent propranolol (Inderal) may be needed to control the (beta) stimulating effects of the catecholamines. Operative removal of the tumour must be arranged as soon as possible. It is usual to replace phenoxybenzamine by phentolamine two or three days before operation since the prolonged effect of phenoxybenzamine will block the action of noradrenaline should this be needed following operation. Immediately before operation the patient is well sedated and an i v drip is set up so that phentolamine (in doses of 2 to 10 mg) can be injected if the blood pressure shows any tendency to rise as it may when the tumour is handled. In the past hypotension followed tumour removal and was attributed to delay in recovery of other chromaffin cell activity suppressed by the tumour. Noradrenaline was employed in correction (4 ml of 1 in 1 000 solution in 0·5 litres of isosmotic sodium chloride solution being infused at a rate sufficient to bring the blood pressure up to normal levels). It is now realised that the hypotension is due to hypovolaemia caused by the intense vasoconstriction. After removal of this by phenoxybenzamine the hypovolaemia corrects itself. If time is allowed for this to take place and blood loss from these very vascular tumours is replaced by transfusion, postoperative hypotension can be avoided and noradrenaline should rarely be necessary.

So far we have been discussing treatment where hypertension has been a presenting feature, noradrenaline the dominant secretion and therapy has been with α-adrenergic blocking agents. The situation must now be considered where hypotension is a presenting feature and adrenaline the dominant secretion. This must be a singularly difficult condition to diagnose or even suspect. Luckily treatment for the hypotension is likely to be with noradrenaline since this will counteract the action of adrenaline on muscle vessels and may prove effective. If the correct diagnosis can be made or seriously suspected a β-adrenergic blockading agent should be successful, though the author knows of no case in which this has been tried. Propranolol (Inderal) 5 to 10 mg should be given i v at the rate of 1 mg per minute until the desired effect is obtained followed by 20 to 30 mg three to four times a day by mouth (Black et al., 1964; Paul, 1969).

THE THYROID GLAND

HYPERTHYROIDISM

This may present urgently as a thyroid crisis or 'storm', malignant exophthalmos, acute thyrotoxic bulbar palsy or as a psychosis or a case of cardiac arrhythmia with congestive failure.

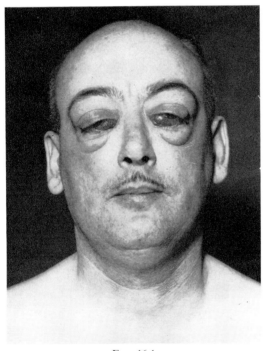

Fig. 16.1
Malignant exophthalmos.

Facing page 358

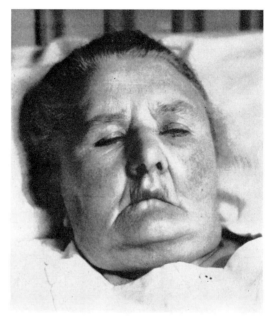

FIG 16.2
Accidental hypothermia.

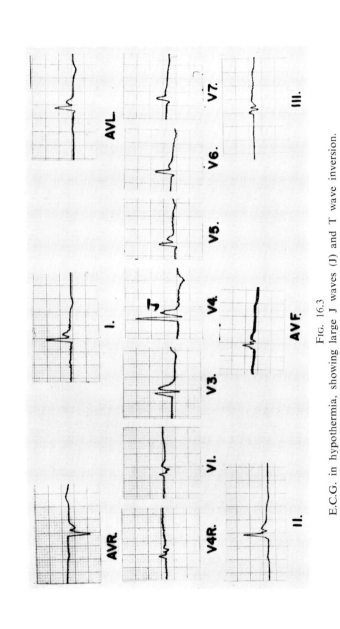

Fig. 16.3

E.C.G. in hypothermia, showing large J waves (J) and T wave inversion.

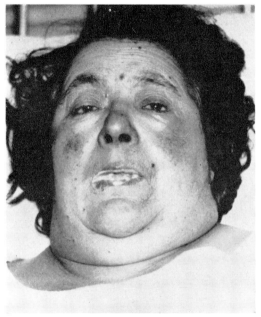

FIG. 16.4
Myxoedema coma.

Thyroid crisis

Years ago a thyroid crisis was a serious hazard of surgery in hyperthyroidism. Preoperative anti-thyroid drugs have now made it rare. It is usually seen when undiagnosed hyperthyroidism is complicated by operation, accidents and infection or by an emotional disturbance. A poor nutritional status may be a factor. The patient, usually a woman, presents with signs and symptoms of hyperthyroidism but many are present in an exaggerated form. She is very restless, irritable and apprehensive. Sweating and loss of weight are often pronounced. The pulse rate may increase up to 200 per minute. Fever is present and the temperature may rise as high as 41°C. Acute left-sided heart failure with pulmonary oedema can develop. The patient may become delirious and collapse may occur with a pale, cold, clammy skin, coma and death. Some patients, particularly the elderly, present with apathy instead of restlessness and anxiety.

Treatment. This must be vigorous and prompt. An initial dose of 500 mg sodium or potassium iodide should be given i v, together with 100 mg carbimazole by mouth. Thereafter 500 mg sodium or potassium iodide and 15 mg carbimazole should be given orally at six hour intervals. The dosage of these drugs should be reduced slowly, since it takes some time to bring the condition under control.

Sedation may be required; 200 to 400 mg doses of sodium amytal given i m and repeated as may be necessary will usually be sufficient. Chlorpromazine (Largactil) is a useful alternative and should be given in a dosage of 25 mg i m or 50 mg orally three times a day. Morphine 10 mg or pethidine 50 mg may be needed in exceptional cases. Hyperthermia must be vigorously controlled. Salicylates may be used; alternatively, cold sponging can be employed in mild cases or a wet sheet and a fan in more severe forms. Tachycardia needs urgent attention and here the effect of propranolol (Inderal) is dramatic; 5 to 10 mg should be given at the rate of 1 mg per minute until the desired effect is obtained followed by 20 to 40 mg three times a day by mouth (Turner, 1969). Digoxin may be needed for atrial fibrillation or heart failure and if none has been received before should be given by the intensive method. It has been suggested that adrenal function may be inadequate in this condition and value has been claimed for corticosteroid therapy particularly if hypotension is present. Hydrocortisone should be infused in 5 per cent dextrose at the rate of 100 mg eight-hourly for the first 24 hours; thereafter cortisone can be given by mouth, 200 mg on the second day reducing slowly to discontinuance in about one week.

Other measures which have been recommended are an ample nourishing diet with added B vitamins. A useful preparation is high potency Parentrovite, one pair of ampoules being given daily for three to four days by i m injection, thereafter Tab. Aneurin Co. or Aneurin Co. Forte one to two three times a day can be given by mouth.

Malignant exophthalmos (Fig. 16.1)

Proptosis, periorbital oedema, chemosis and paresis of external ocular muscles are not uncommon in thyrotoxicosis. In a few cases proptosis reaches serious dimensions with corneal ulceration leading to perforation, panophthalmitis and loss of an eye. Mild exophthalmos is treated with eye drops containing neomycin 0·5 per cent and betamethasone phosphate 0·1 per cent (Betnesol-N Glaxo) and by dehydration therapy: salt-restricted diet, frusemide (Lasix) 40 mg twice daily and potassium chloride 1 g three times a day. Steroids in high dosage (prednisone 120 mg daily) have helped some severe cases. Deep X-ray therapy to the orbits has been advocated. Failing satisfactory control by medical measures, a lateral tarsorrhaphy on each side will preserve corneal integrity. In the rare cases where this is insufficient, decompression may be needed if there is deterioration in visual acuity. This should be watched for and any falling off should lead to prompt reference for an expert opinion.

Psychosis

Thyrotoxicosis sometimes presents as a psychosis (in the author's experience usually paranoid) or as a mental disturbance verging on the psychotic. Management of such cases can be very difficult. Surgery is refused and antithyroid drugs are taken irregularly or not at all. The patients can usually be persuaded to accept a dose of radioactive iodine, and 15 mCi should be given without hesitation. If hypothyroidism develops it can be controlled much more readily than the preceding hyperthyroidism.

Acute thyrotoxic bulbar palsy

This is a very serious condition with paralysis involving bulbar as well as limb musculature. It is rare and its aetiology is uncertain; however, it is possibly due to thyrotoxicosis superimposed upon some other muscular disorder such as the related auto-immune disease of myasthenia gravis in a latent form. The effect of edrophonium (Tensilon) should be tried; 2 mg are injected i v followed 30 seconds later by a further 8 mg provided no reaction has occurred. If effective, treatment with neostigmine in appropriate dosage is instituted (p. 319). Failing a response, the serum potassium should be estimated in case some hypokalaemic disorder is present.

Congenital thyrotoxicosis

In this rare condition a thyrotoxic child is born to a mother who is or has been thyrotoxic. It is believed to be due to the placental transfer from the mother of long-acting thyroid stimulator (LATS) or the more recently discovered long-acting thyroid stimulator protector (LATSP) (Adams *et al.*, 1974) and is therefore self-limiting. Prognosis has been poor in the past but need not be so if treatment is prompt and vigorous. Carbimazole 1 to 2 mg and sodium or potassium iodide 25 mg should be given, both three times a day. Symptomatic treatment should be used as indicated (Zaidi, 1965). A prophylactic approach to the problem is highly desirable. This presents little difficulty in the clinically toxic patient since anti-thyroid drugs readily cross the placenta and the baby will be well controlled at birth by treatment given to the mother. Difficulties arise in patients who have been treated by partial thyroidectomy and while euthyroid, still have high titres of LATS in their blood. Clinical pointers to this possibility are the presence of marked eye signs, pretibial myxoedema and a history of suspicious neonatal deaths. LATS assays should be obtained if possible in such patients since they confirm the potential dangers. Mothers with known or suspected high LATS titres should receive carbimazole 5 to 10 mg three times a day during pregnancy. Babies born to such mothers should be treated from birth without waiting for thyrotoxic features to appear since these develop with alarming rapidity. Dosage should be reduced very slowly but can probably be abandoned within six to twelve weeks from birth.

HYPOTHYROIDISM

The hypothermia of myxoedema coma may present with many features common to accidental hypothermia in non-myxoedematous patients and so both conditions will be considered here.

Accidental hypothermia (Fig. 16.2) (see also pp. 69, 404 (newborn) and 620 (the elderly)).

Exposure to cold is the over-riding cause but endogenous factors are important. These include cerebrovascular accidents, confusional states, conditions causing vascular collapse such as myocardial infarction, immobility, severe infections such as pneumonia and drugs with hypothermic effects such as phenothiazines, barbiturates and alcohol.

Hypothermia produces various secondary pathological changes which have an important bearing on the clinical picture and its management, and on prognosis. It leads to slowing of the circulation and impaired oxygen saturation. The resultant hypoxia damages the capillaries and plasma escapes into the tissues causing oedema. Haemoconcentration causes multiple arterial thromboses resulting in myocardial infarction, gastric erosions and pancreatitis. The serum amylase has been found significantly raised in some of these patients. The lungs are damaged and pneumonia, if not already present, may supervene. Impaired pulmonary ventilation may lead to carbon dioxide retention and respiratory failure (Buckle and Garfield, 1969). The intense vasoconstriction of skin vessels may cause peripheral gangrene.

CLINICAL ASPECTS. Patients present with mental retardation, confusion, stupor or even coma. Plantar responses may be extensor. The skin is cold, pale, dry, and corpse-like. A little oedema is present; this includes the face and at first glance suggests hypothyroidism though the appearances are never so pronounced as in the hypothyroidism of myxoedema coma (Fig. 16.4). Bradycardia is present, sometimes with an arrhythmia such as atrial fibrillation. Respiration is slowed, and the blood pressure is lowered. The ECG may show characteristic changes with prolongation of the Q R S interval, and inverted T deflections; a J wave at the junction of the Q R S and ST segment in left chest leads is characteristic (Fig. 16.3). Muscular rigidity is usual and the voice may be croaking. There may be slight epigastric tenderness due presumably to pancreatitis. Gangrene of toes may appear. The temperature is low (by definition) but many cases will be missed unless the practitioner is alive to this condition (see p. 69) and uses a low-reading thermometer (G. H. Zeal Ltd., 8 Lombard Road, London, SW19 3 UU) or a Temtake device. Hypothermia is considered to start at 32·2°C but its severity has an important bearing on prognosis. From 26·7 to 32·2°C the outlook is quite good with proper treatment, but thereafter the lower the temperature the more likely is a fatal outcome.

Treatment. Active rewarming is known to be harmful. The usual explanation given is that it leads to dilatation of cutaneous vessels, drawing blood away from more vital organs such as the heart and brain. Patients are therefore best covered by a single blanket and nursed in a warm room. The optimal temperature is not known for certain, but a figure of 26·7 to 32·2°C has been suggested.

Steps should be taken to restore blood volume. An i v infusion of dextrose 5 g/dl should be set up and this should be warmed to normal body temperature. The use of a plasma expander such as Rheomacrodex—a low molecular weight dextran—has been suggested. Care should be taken not to overload the circulation (p. 106); a slow infusion of 500 ml of a 10 g/dl solution in dextrose or isosmotic sodium chloride solution is suggested initially.

Tri-iodo-thyronine seems to be of no particular value in this condition unless associated hypothyroidism is definite (see p. 364) and is best avoided since elderly persons may have myocardial disease which could be adversely affected. On the other hand, hydrocortisone is useful and 100 mg should be given eight-hourly in the first 24 hours by i v drip; this should be replaced by oral corticosteroids subsequently. A broad spectrum antibiotic such as tetracycline 250 mg. six-hourly should be given as a prophylactic against pulmonary infection. It can be given by drip with advantage in the first 24 hours when absorption via the gastrointestinal tract may be impaired.

Hypoxia and acidosis call for urgent consideration. Arterial blood gas analyses (pH, PaO_2, $PaCO_2$) should be undertaken. If hypoxia and acidosis are present the patient should be intubated and treated by intermittent positive pressure respiration.

For further consideration of treatment see Rosin and Exton-Smith, 1964; McNichol and Smith, 1964; British Medical Association Special Committee, 1964.

Myxoedema coma

Much of what has been said about accidental hypothermia applies to myxoedema coma and only the features peculiar to myxoedema will be considered here.

Myxoedema and accidental hypothermia though presenting similarities can usually be distinguished on clinical grounds. The puffiness of the face, thickening and dryness of the skin and croakiness of the voice are usually more pronounced in the hypothermia of myxoedema (Fig. 16.4). Frank alopecia and features of the case history may also point clearly to the diagnosis of myxoedema. Laboratory studies are rather unhelpful. Radioactive iodine uptake studies are impracticable, and serum cholesterol, serum protein bound iodine and labelled T3 resin uptake measurements are of doubtful validity owing to the various blood changes already described. Moreover, treatment is a matter of urgency and must follow on clinical diagnosis without awaiting results of investigations. Since it is useful in retrospect to have some objective evidence of the diagnosis, a clinical photograph should be taken.

Treatment. A thyroid hormone is required, but a course must be steered between tardiness in restoring thyroid status and imposition of undue stress upon the heart. It must be remembered that the myocardium is directly involved by the myxoedematous process and indirectly through ischaemic changes from gross coronary atheroma. Over-enthusiastic use of thyroid hormone may precipitate acute cardiac failure and death. Thyroxine is too slow in action, taking a week before it exerts any significant effect. Tri-iodi-thyronine acts quickly—within a matter of hours—but dosage is critical. A slow i v drip will have been set up and the author adds trio-iodo-thyronine to this, infusing at the rate of 5 μg every eight hours. The rate of delivery must be regulated carefully (pp. 107 and 342) since it is imperative not to overload the circulation. At the same time thyroxine 0·1 mg daily is started by mouth, and this will be ready to take over from tri-iodo-thyronine in a week's time. It is important to discontinue the latter drug as soon as possible, since the danger of precipitating acute cardiac failure persists for some time.

Corticosteroid therapy is particularly desirable. The use of thyroid hormone will increase the metabolic requirements for hydrocortisone which the adrenals, affected by hypothyroidism, may not be able to supply.

Hydrocortisone should be added to the i v drip in a dosage of 100 mg eight-hourly for 24 hours. Cortisone 200 mg should be given by mouth on the second day and the dose reduced slowly thereafter to nil by the end of a week.

A severe case of hypothyroidism should be treated with respect, even though not in stupor. Mildly hypothermic patients with myxoedema may lapse into stupor after admission. Moreover, the same caution must be exercised with regard to the dose of thyroid hormones in such cases, since the cardiac condition is just as serious.

THE PITUITARY GLAND

NEUROHYPOPHYSIS

Diabetes insipidus

A variety of lesions may disturb hypothalamic centres or the pituitary stalk controlling water metabolism and lead to impaired secretion of antidiuretic hormone (ADH). Patients present with gross polyuria, polydipsia and loss of weight. The condition must be distinguished from psychogenic and nephrogenic polyuria. Characteristic biochemical features are a high blood and a low urine osmolality with a much lower urine/blood osmolality ratio than the normal one of 2:1. A six-hour fluid deprivation test may be employed, the polyuria failing to respond to deprivation resulting in a worsening of the urine/blood osmolality ratio. This test must be used with discretion since the patient's condition may deteriorate seriously. It should be terminated if there are any signs of distress. The polyuria fails to respond to hypertonic saline but does so to an injection of pitressin. Give 1·5 mg pitressin in oil i m followed by daily injections or intra-nasal insufflations of 15 to 25 mg of posterior pituitary snuff (Di-Sipidin) at four-hourly intervals. Chlorpropamide (Diabenese) 250 mg by mouth twice daily is sometimes very effective in milder cases.

Inappropriate secretion of anti-diuretic hormone

This condition is due to the ectopic over-production of ADH by a neoplasm, usually a bronchial carcinoma. Patients present with general malaise, debility, anorexia and perhaps confusion, the significance of which may be missed through attribution to the underlying carcinoma. The possibility must be kept in mind since correct treatment will bring relief. Biochemical studies reveal hyponatraemia with a low blood and high urine osmolality and a higher than normal urine/blood osmolality ratio. Radio-immune assays will reveal high blood levels of ADH. Since the hyponatraemia is due to water retention and not sodium loss, treatment must be by fluid restriction; saline infusions are contraindicated.

Hypopituitarism (Simmonds's disease)

The two common causes of pituitary failure are post-partum necrosis and tumours above the sella turcica, both of which destroy the gland. The post-partum cases are sometimes called Sheehan's syndrome and the others Simmonds's disease. This can occur in both sexes.

There is usually a story of lactation failure following a difficult labour and this is an important diagnostic feature. The patient complains of tiredness, lethargy and amenorrhoea or scanty menstruation. She is characteristically pale (but not anaemic) and her normally pigmented areas such as the areolae lose their pigment. Body and sexual hair is scanty. Undue sensitivity to cold causes the patient to huddle in front of the fire and so to show *erythema ab igne* in her legs. The blood pressure is low. Often on admission to hospital the patient is stuporose or comatose and hypothermic.

Essentially these patients are suffering from defective secretion of thyroxine and cortisol. Both the thyroid and adrenal glands are, however, capable of some autonomous activity, and the severity of the hypothyroidism and hypoadrenocorticalism is not individually as severe as in the primary disorders of these glands, although

13

their combined effect can be serious. Treatment to be successful therefore need not be pursued with quite such vigour. Hypercholesterolaemia and atheroma are either absent or mild, and the complicating factor of cardiac disease present in primary hypothyroidism does not arise.

Treatment. The hypothermia should be treated as in myxoedema coma (p. 363.) Hydrocortisone should be added to an i v dextrose saline drip and run in at the rate of 100 mg every eight hours for the first 24 hours. Thereafter cortisone should be given orally; 50 mg six-hourly at first, reducing fairly rapidly to a maintenance dose of 25 to 50 mg per day by the end of the week. Fludrohydrocortisone will not be needed. Over-enthusiastic corticosteroid therapy may lead to ‘water intoxication’ with fluid retention, cerebral oedema, convulsions and coma. Costicosteroids should then be temporarily suspended and measures taken to reduce cerebral oedema (pp. 298 and 728). Thyroid compounds must be avoided in the early stage since the increased metabolism makes demands on an hypoplastic adrenal cortex which cannot be met. Thyroxine 0·1 mg daily may be started after a few days.

Pituitary apoplexy

A very serious condition may follow haemorrhage into a pituitary adenoma. The patient usually complains of sudden severe headache. This is followed rapidly by signs of pressure on structures outside the sella turcica with loss of sight and oculomotor palsies. The resulting acute failure of adrenocortical secretion can be serious with hypotension and acute circulatory collapse with hyponatraemia. Escape of blood into the cerebrospinal fluid may lead to signs of meningeal irritation with neck stiffness, somnolence, confusion or even coma. Pressure on the hypothalamus may account for other features such as polyuria or water retention, thermal disturbance and hypoglycaemia.

The most urgent question which arises in treatment is whether to relieve pressure on the optic nerve by operative measures. Decision may turn on the degree of visual loss. It is said that operation will be ineffective if perception of light has been lost by the time the patient is seen. With lesser degrees of visual defect, operation may hold some hope of retaining some visual capacity. Evidence of adrenal failure should be treated by hydrocortisone i v, followed by oral cortisone; this is important since lives have probably been lost in the past owing to unawareness of this complication. Fludrohydrocortisone is not required, nor is thyroxine at this stage. Other features such as polyuria, or hypoglycaemia, should be treated appropriately. (For further reading see Jefferson and Rosenthal, 1959.)

THE PARATHYROID GLANDS

Hyperparathyroidism

This may present as an emergency through one of its complications, e.g. a fracture, renal colic (p. 385), haematuria (p. 386) and uraemia (p. 375), and these conditions must be dealt with appropriately.

Acute hyperparathyroidism (see also p. 126)

This purely endocrine complication has serious emergency aspects and may arise *de novo*, or be superimposed upon a long history suggestive of hyperparathyroidism. The patient presents with abdominal pain, vomiting, constipation, oliguria, loss of weight, lassitude, weakness and confusion which may pass on to coma and death. The symptoms do not immediately suggest the diagnosis, but a chance radiograph may reveal bone changes or nephrocalcinosis. A very high level of serum calcium will be found, together with evidence of uraemia and haemoconcentration. Immediate treatment is to reduce viscosity of the blood and bring down serum calcium levels. An i v infusion of isosmotic sodium chloride solution and 5 per cent dextrose should be set up and given at a rate of three to four litres in 24 hours. Phosphate is an effective agent for lowering calcium (Dent, 1962). A preparation containing Na_2HPO_4 (Analar) 46·6 g $NaH_2PO_42H_2O$ (Sodium Acid Phosphate BP) 15·2 g in 500 ml water has been used in Professor C. R. Dent's unit at University College Hospital (details provided by Mr A. R. Williams). It is supplied in 10 ml ampoules and one of these should be given slowly over 10 minutes by i v injection. These neutral phosphate solutions (Martindale, 1972, p. 1723) are not available commercially and cannot be prepared in a hurry. Physicians liable to be confronted with this problem should see to it that their hospital pharmacies have a small supply of suitable ampoules available for use in an emergency. Thereafter effervescent phosphate tablets (Phosphate-Sandoz) should be given by mouth one or two three times a day. Each tablet provides the equivalent of 500 mg elemental phosphorus. Hypocalcaemia may develop but responds readily to calcium therapy. Calcitonin is ineffective in this condition. Infusion of sodium sulphate has been used (Chakmakjian and Bethune, 1966) but is not always effective and needs to be given in a rather large volume (3 litres of isotonic solution infused over nine hours). The chelating agent sodium versenate reduces serum calcium but is intensely irritating locally and probably nephrotoxic; it is not recommended. Haemodialysis should be effective, but the author has no experience of its use. A low calcium diet should be instituted, at least avoiding milk, cheese and ice-cream. Treatment should be biochemically controlled and the parathyroid adenoma should be removed as soon as the patient is fit to withstand operation. (For further reading see Bradlow and Segal, 1956; Thomas *et al.*, 1958; Payne and Fitchett, 1965). Severe hypercalcaemia is sometimes found in sarcoidosis. It responds readily to oral cortisone 50 mg three times a day.

Hypoparathyroidism

The classical emergency in hypoparathyroidism is that of tetany. This has a number of causes, and the problems it presents are essentially those of differential diagnosis, modes of presentation and management.

CAUSES. The commonest cause of hypoparathyroidism is surgical removal of the glands at partial thyroidectomy. A severe but transient episode follows removal of a parathyroid adenoma with associated bone disease. Tetany due to hypocalcaemia may also occur in rickets and osteomalacia (and then usually after initiation of treatment with vitamin D when increased uptake by the bones leads to a temporary fall in serum calcium), malabsorption syndromes, renal dysfunction and the rare hereditary disorder of brachymetacarpal dwarfism (pseudohypoparathyroidism).

Tetany also occurs in alkalotic states caused by persistent vomiting, excessive ingestion of soluble alkalies or hyperventilation.

MODES OF PRESENTATION. A mild case may present with muscle spasms, notably carpopedal, but more severe symptoms can occur with laryngisimus stridulus, convulsions and drowsiness which may progress to coma and death. Papilloedema may be found. Mental symptoms can dominate the picture with depression, confusion, delusions or paranoia. Various skin lesions such as eczema or impetigo herpetiformis may be prominent, with other ectodermal manifestations—alopecia, nail dystrophy and cataract. Peripheral nerves are hypersensitive to percussion, forming the basis of Chvostek's and Trousseau's signs.

BIOCHEMICAL CHANGES. Hypocalcaemia will be found in calcium deficiency but not in alkalotic states. Normal levels lie around 2·1 to 2·6 mmol/litre (8·5 to 10·5 mg/100 ml). Magnesium levels may be low (normal 0·6 to 1·0 mmol/l (1·5 to 2·5 mg/100 ml)).

Treatment. This is based upon administration of calcium salts and vitamin D. Choice of route and dosage depends upon severity and likely duration of the underlying disturbances. Treatment should be controlled by daily serum calcium estimations tempered by clinical assessment of the patient's state.

In an emergency a calcium salt should be given i v. Calcium chloride may be used, but the gluconate is preferable, being less irritant and so less likely to cause thrombosis; 20 ml of a 20 per cent solution should be given over a period of 10 minutes. This can be repeated once or twice daily, but is usually unnecessary provided oral therapy is started immediately. Sedatives may be needed if convulsions occur.

The most difficult hypocalcaemic situation to treat is that following removal of parathyroid adenomas with associated bone disease. Oral therapy appropriate for this will be described; dosage can be scaled down for less severe conditions. Sandocal effervescent calcium tablets (Sandoz) are particularly suitable. They are palatable and less apt to cause diarrhoea than other preparations. Each tablet contains 4·5 g calcium gluconate. Vitamin D in some form must also be prescribed. Calciferol 8 mg may be given on the first day, followed by 4 mg daily for two days, and then 2 mg daily; final adjustments will be made in the light of serum calcium estimations. A more potent compound—dihydrotachysterol—is given in a dose approximately half that of calciferol. I m injections of calcium salts are liable to cause necrosis and are best avoided. Parathormone 50 mg as an initial i m injection has been employed in the past, but has been largely replaced by oral vitamin D.

Attention has been focused recently on the possible contribution to the symptomatology made by hypomagnesaemia in hypoparathyroidism and also in other states such as malabsorption syndrome, removal of parathyroid adenomas, renal tubular disease in chronic pyelonephritis and alcoholism, diabetic ketosis and following large electrolyte infusions in children with diarrhoea. The possibility should be considered and the magnesium level measured (normally 0·6 to 1·0 mmol/litre or 1·5 to 2·5 mg/100 ml). Treatment is by 2 to 4 ml of magnesium sulphate (p. 728) every four hours until normal blood levels are restored.

Alkalosis due to persistent vomiting or the excessive ingestion of alkalies is corrected by i v infusions of isosmotic sodium chloride solution; considerable amounts may be needed in the order of 5 to 10 litres given over the course of 24 to 48 hours. Hyperventilation tetany usually occurs in hysterical girls; inhalation of 5 per cent carbon dioxide has been recommended for it but most patients respond readily when instructed to breathe normally.

D. Ferriman

REFERENCES

Adrenals

BARTTER, F. C., PRONOVE, P., GILL, J. R. & McCARDLE, R. C. (1962). Hyperplasia of the juxtaglomerular complex with hyperaldosteronism and hypokalaemic alkalosis. *American Journal of Medicine,* **33,** 811.

LIVANOU, T., FERRIMAN, D. & JAMES, V. H. T. (1967). Recovery of hypothalamopituitary-adrenal function after corticosteroid therapy. *Lancet,* **2,** 856.

MARGARETTEN, W. & McADAMS, A. J. (1958). An appraisal of fulminant meningococcaemia with reference to the Schwartzman phenomenon. *American Journal of Medicine,* **25,** 868.

MONTGOMERY, D. A. D. Adrenogenital syndrome. In *Genital Anomalies.* Ed. Rashad, M. N. & Norton, W. R. M. Springfield, Illinois: Thomas, 1969.

PLUMPTON, F. S., BESSER, G. H. & COLE, P. V. (1969). Corticosteroid treatment and surgery. *Anesthesia,* **24,** 3 and 12.

TAICHMAN, N. S. *Inflammation, Immunity and Hypersensitivity,* 479. (Ed. Movat, H. Z.) New York: Haper and Row. 1971.

TAKAYASU, H., ASO, Y., NAKAUCHI, K. & KAWABE, K. (1971). A case of Bartter's syndrome with surgical treatment followed for four years. *Journal of Clinical Endocrinology,* **32,** 842.

Phaeochromocytoma

BLACK, J. W., CROWTHER, A. F., SHANKS, R. G., SMITH, L. H. & DORNHORST, A. C. (1964). A new adrenergic beta-receptor antagonist. *Lancet,* **1,** 1080.

HAMRIN, B. (1962). Sustained hypotension and shock due to an adrenaline-secreting phaeochromocytoma. *Lancet,* **2,** 123.

RICHMOND, J., FRAZER, S. C. & MILLAR, D. R. (1961). Paroxysmal hypotension due to an adrenaline-secreting phaeochromocytoma. *Lancet,* **2,** 904.

STEINESS, I. (1961). Hypotension due to an adrenaline-secreting phaeochromocytoma. *Lancet,* **2,** 1149.

Thyroid

ADAMS, D. D., KENNEDY, T. H. & STEWART, R. D. H. (1974). Correlation between long-acting stimulator protector level and thyroid 1_{131} uptake in thyrotoxicosis. *British Medical Journal,* **2,** 199.

THOMSON, J. A., DIRMIKIS, S. M., MUNRO, D. S., SMITH, B. R., HALL, R. & MUKHTAR, E. D. (1975). Neonatal hypothyroidism and long-acting thyroid stimulator protector. *British Medical Journal,* **2,** 36.

TURNER, P. (1969). *Clinical Aspects of Autonomic Pharmacology,* 150. London: Heinemann. 1969.

ZAIDI, Z. H. (For Mortimer, P. E.) (1965). Congenital thyrotoxicosis with hepatosplenomegaly and thrombocytopenia. *Proceedings of the Royal Society of Medicine,* **58,** 390.

Hypothermia

BRITISH MEDICAL ASSOCIATION, SPECIAL COMMITTEE (1964). Accidental hypothermia in the elderly. *British Medical Journal,* **2,** 1255.

BUCKLE, R. M. & GARFIELD, J. (1969). Myxoedema coma complicated by respiratory failure. *Proceedings of the Royal Society of Medicine,* **62,** 38.

McNICOL, M. W. & SMITH, R. (1964). Accidental hypothermia. *British Medical Journal,* **1,** 18.

ROSIN, A. J. & EXTON-SMITH, A. N. (1964). Clinical features of accidental hypothermia with some observations on thyroid function. *British Medical Journal,* **1,** 16.

Pituitary

JEFFERSON, M. & ROSENTHAL, F. D. (1959). Spontaneous necrosis in pituitary tumours. *Lancet,* **1,** 342.

Parathyroids

BRADLOW, B. A. & SEGAL, N. (1956). Acute hyperparathyroidism with electro-cardiographic changes. *British Medical Journal*, **2**, 197.

CHAKMAKJIAN, Z. H. & BETHUNE, J. E. (1966). Sodium sulfate treatment of hypercalcaemia. *New England Journal of Medicine*, **275**, 862.

DENT, C. E. (1962). Some problems of hyperparathyroidism. *British Medical Journal*, **2**, 1495.

MARTINDALE. *The Extra Pharmacopoeia*. London: Pharmaceutical Press. 1972.

PAYNE, R. L. & FITCHETT, C. W. (1965). Hyperparathyroid crisis. *Annals of Surgery*, **161**, 737.

THOMAS, W. C., WISWELL, J. G., CONNOR, T. B. & HOWARD, J. E. (1958). Hypercalcaemic crisis due to hyperparathyroidism. *American Journal of Medicine*, **24**, 229.

CHAPTER 17

Medical Emergencies in Renal Disease

ACUTE OLIGURIA AND ANURIA
(For hazards of dialysis see pp. 71 and 72)

EARLY diagnosis of this lethal emergency is important for the patient's survival. There are three types:
1. **Obstructive** (Post-renal).
2. **Pre-renal.**
3. **Renal** (Acute renal failure. Glomerulonephritis and vascular lesions).

OBSTRUCTIVE OR POST-RENAL OLIGURIA AND ANURIA

The exclusion of urinary obstruction as a cause of oliguria or anuria is not always easy. A full bladder from outlet obstruction is usually palpable but catheterisation may be required to exclude it. The commonest causes of supra-vesical obstruction are primary or recurrent uterine, rectal or urothelial neoplasms, stone in a ureter or a sole functioning kidney, hydronephrosis, ureteric stenosis, retroperitoneal fibrosis and ureteric obstruction by a sloughed renal papilla or by crystals (urates after anti-tumour treatment) or rarely acetylated sulphonamides.

Fortunately a drip IVP of 45 g/dl Hypaque (2 ml/kg body weight) with tomography will nearly always confirm or exclude obstruction, define its site and often its nature and will thus obviate the need for retrograde urological investigations. *Absolute* anuria alternating with periods of profuse diuresis is characteristic of obstructive uropathy.

Treatment.—If the blood urea exceeds 33·2 mmol/1 (200 mg/100 ml) and the patient is hyperkalaemic or acidotic he is not fit for surgical decompression under general anaesthesia. Occasionally a period of drainage of the better kidney through an indwelling ureteric catheter or by needle nephrostomy under local anaesthesia (Ogg *et al.,* 1969) may render the patient fit for definitive surgery. Usually it is better to transfer such a patient to a urological centre equipped with dialysis facilities (p. 805).

Occasionally relief of chronic obstruction results in a tremendous diuresis. This requires appropriate fluid and electrolyte replacement by the i v route.

PRE-RENAL OLIGURIA

This is caused by excessive falls of cardiac output, blood pressure or volume, dehydration or electrolyte depletion (particularly of sodium) and is often accompanied by infection. Usually these factors act in concert producing ineffective renal perfusion and thus oliguria. Early recognition and correction may prevent the full evolution of Acute Renal Failure (ARF). The potentially reversible ingravescent phase lasts from as little as one to forty-eight hours. During this period the urine/plasma osmolality ratio will usually be greater than 1·5, the urine/plasma urea ratio greater than 10 and the urine specific gravity greater than 1 015. With rare exceptions (particularly burns) the urine output will fall below 150 ml per six hour period.

Treatment. Fluid repletion should commence by peripheral vein as soon as the condition is recognised. A central venous pressure (CVP) line (p. 751) is inserted, its position checked radiologically and the CVP raised to plus 5-10 cm saline by fluids designed to correct the underlying abnormality, i.e. blood for blood loss; dextrose 5 g/dl for pure dehydration; isosmotic sodium chloride solution or twice this strength with or without potassium chloride for electrolyte depletion and sodium bicarbonate 2 g/dl for acidosis and plasma for burns. Half the estimated fluid deficit should be given within the first four hours but the remainder more slowly over 12-16 hours. Over-rapid normalisation of the internal chemical environment may lead to tetany, fits and cardiac arrhythmias.

The induction of a diuresis by means of i v mannitol or frusemide (Lasix) during the stage of pre-renal oliguria or ingravescent Acute Renal Failure helps to prevent the full evolution of established ARF. Mannitol 20 g/dl solution 2·5 ml/kg dry body weight may be safely given i v as a bolus with 80 mg frusemide, unless the patient is overhydrated. In that case only frusemide in a dosage of 125-500 mg should be given, the larger dose over 20 minutes. Temporary catheterisation with a 6 or 10F gauge Gibbon catheter is permissible to obtain an early and accurate measurement of any diuretic response which is indicated by a diuresis of at least 100 ml within an hour. A diuresis thus obtained may be maintained by the hourly infusion of 10 ml of mannitol 20 g/dl for at least 24 hours or until a urine flow of at least 60 ml per hour is maintained spontaneously, with replacement of fluid and electrolytes lost in the urine. Nevertheless a daily blood urea check is essential as partial ARF frequently results even when the urine flow is thus maintained.

Blood and urine should be cultured and appropriate antibiotics given if septicaemia is suspected, together with an initial single dose of gentamicin 2·0 mg per kg body weight. Failure to induce a diuresis by the above measures indicates that the patient has developed ARF and must be treated accordingly, with particular reference to fluid restriction and cessation of potassium therapy.

ACUTE RENAL FAILURE (ARF)

Definition. This is a sudden cessation of renal excretory function after a short ingravescent potentially reversible phase. After this anuric or oliguric phase which varies from a few to fifty days, a diuretic phase occurs during which renal excretory function gradually returns towards normal. Residual renal damage is usually unimportant.

Etiology. The pathology of ARF has been much debated, but there has always been agreement on the basic importance of inadequate renal blood flow brought about by hypovolaemia, hypotension and low cardiac output. The only kinds of renal failure in which these extra-renal circulatory factors do not play a part are those caused by nephrotoxins (e.g. mercuric chloride), excessive use of dextran and sucrose or transfusion of incompatible blood.

The cortex particularly is rendered ischaemic when intra-renal cortical vasospasm, perhaps mediated by renin, is the mechanism. Recently the intravascular deposition of fibrin has also been implicated. The kidney is particularly sensitive to the effects of ischaemia in pregnancy and during bacterial infections, hyponatraemia and obstructive jaundice.

Diagnosis. This is based on the demonstration of rapidly progressive nitrogen retention, usually—but not always—with a daily urine volume of less than 500 ml resistant to i v frusemide. Absolute anuria suggests obstruction, glomerulonephritis, cortical necrosis or occlusion of the renal arteries.

In established ARF the urine/plasma osmolality ratio is less than 1·05, the urine/plasma urea ratio is less than 10, the urinary urea concentration is less than 800 mg/100 ml (133·6 mmol/l) and the specific gravity is less than 1 013. The daily urine volume is usually between 50-300 ml.

A high index of suspicion should guard against delayed diagnosis in oliguric patients. This commonly results in iatrogenic overhydration in an attempt to relieve non-existent fluid depletion.

Prognosis. Even in expert hands ARF still carries a mortality of 10-50 per cent depending on the cause. Early transfer to the nearest Haemo-dialysis Unit (see Appendix 7, p. 805) is therefore advised as soon as the diagnosis is established. A good airway and a safe potassium level (p. 605) must be assured prior to transfer.

Death in ARF is usually due to:

1. The condition responsible for the ARF.

2. Pulmonary oedema due to overhydration and hypoprotein-aemia.

3. The biochemical derangements of uraemia, in particular hyper-kalaemia.

4. The haemostatic defects of uraemia resulting in gastrointestinal haemorrhage.

5. Pyogenic and fungal infections.

6. Prolonged recumbency resulting in pressure-sores, phlebo-thrombosis and pulmonary embolism.

It should be noted that half the deaths occur during the diuretic phase, particularly those due to infection and pulmonary embolism.

As all deaths except those in group 1 are potentially preventable, improved results will be obtained if due attention is paid to the following principles:

1. ' Prophylactic' dialysis, applied before the patient becomes clinically uraemic.

2. Provision of adequate and appropriate nutrition.

3. Avoidance of overhydration.

4. Avoidance of immobility and provision of active physiotherapy to chest and limbs.

5. Prophylactic anti-monilial therapy.

6. Prevention, early recognition and treatment of pyogenic infections.

MANAGEMENT OF ESTABLISHED ACUTE RENAL FAILURE

Treatment appropriate to the underlying cause must continue, modified if necessary to take account of the oliguric state. Gross fluid and electrolyte deficiencies should be partly corrected. Conservative (i.e. non-dialytic) therapy should be considered for a limited period only, in young, previously fit and non-hypercatabolic patients. Adequate calorie intake without excessive fluid is best assured by giving 500 ml dextrose 500 g/1 and 30 units soluble insulin by central venous line each 24 hours together with a small, dry diet containing 35 g protein. Fluids entering the mouth should be limited to 300 ml per day (plus mouthwashes) but if none is given i v the oral intake can be increased to 800 ml daily. The blood sugar, urea and electrolytes should be monitored at least once a day.

Though conservative therapy was sometimes successful before dialysis became available, it is not normally used nowadays except in partial ARF, i.e. patients with a rising blood urea and a urine output exceeding one litre per day, or on a trial basis, as above.

Once dialytic therapy is decided upon, there is no need to practice the strict fluid and protein restriction necessitated by conservative therapy, since fluid is removed by dialysis. The diet may consist of 1 g/kg body weight of protein (or more in post-traumatic cases likely to run a prolonged course) and should produce 3 000 to 4 000 non-protein calories. This may be achieved with the aid of plenty of salt-free butter, double cream, Caloreen* (a glucose polymer mixture) and Hycal† (a demineralised highly concentrated syrup based on glucose). No salt must be used in the cooking, or added during the meal, and fluid should be restricted to 1 litre/day plus the volume of any unusual non-urinary losses.

Whereas haemodialysis is available only in special centres, peritoneal dialysis (PD) can be performed in any hospital. It must be stressed, however, that dialysis constitutes only a small aspect of the total treatment of ARF which is usually best conducted in a special unit. The apparent simplicity of PD constitutes a temptation which should be resisted unless the doctor concerned with the treatment has had appropriate training. The method is described on p. 716.

In most cases of ARF either Haemodialysis (HD) or PD can be used. HD will be preferred in hypercatabolic cases and when surgical abdominal drains would make aseptic PD difficult, but these do not constitute an absolute bar as outflow of the PD fluid can take place through surgical drains. Indeed, peritonitis may be treated in this manner by including an appropriate antibiotic in the fluid. Areas denuded of peritoneum lead to excessive fluid absorption and after recent intestinal anastomoses HD is preferable. PD will be preferred in patients with active peptic ulcers and with uraemic pericarditis where heparin required for HD might result in gastrointestinal or pericardial haemorrhage.

As HD is performed in special centres, the details will not be further discussed except to say that short daily treatments are preferred to longer, spaced-out treatments which increase the risk of bleeding.

PD with the 'Trocath' catheter‡ (p. 716) is used continuously until the blood urea can be kept below 25 mmol/l (150 mg/100 ml) by intermittent dialysis. Most adults can tolerate hourly two

---

* Caloreen—Scientific Hospital Supplies Ltd., 38 Queensland Street, Liverpool L7 3LE. Tele. No. 051-709 3588.

† Hycal—Beechams Research Ltd., Great West Road, Brentford, Middlesex. Tele. No. 01-560 5151.

‡ 'Travenol', Baxter Laboratory, Caxton Way, Thetford, Norfolk. Thetford (0842) 4581.

litre exchanges. Subsequently smaller exchanges may suffice. Automatic machinery* using 10 litre vats of PD fluid (Boots) is available. If commercial PD fluid in one litre containers is used only the strictest aseptic precautions, using Betadine or Weak Iodine Solution BP for all connections, will prevent iatrogenic peritonitis.

Four solutions containing dextrose 1·36 g/dl and 6·3 g/dl with 130 and 141 mmol/l sodium respectively are available† (i.e. four different solutions in all). Normally the low dextrose and sodium solution is suitable, but hyponatraemia is best corrected with the 141 mmol/l sodium solution. Its prolonged use will, however, cause hypernatraemia. The low dextrose fluid will result in the desirable loss of 1-2 litres of fluid/day, thus making room for an acceptable oral fluid intake.

Pulmonary oedema is best treated by simultaneous use of the high and low dextrose solutions, but soluble insulin, 30-60 units daily, will be required to keep the blood sugar below 250 mg/100 ml (13·75 mmol/l).

Potassium is normally added only after 24-48 hours of PD in a concentration of 4 mmol/l, best given as 1 g potassium chloride to every third or fourth litre.

One thousand units heparin may be added to each litre to prevent fibrin deposition in the cannula. Antibiotics are not used prophylactically. To treat suspected or established peritoneal infections gentamicin 4 to 6 mg/litre for 48 hours then 4 mg/litre for a further three days may be used. Peritonitis (abdominal tenderness, pain, fever, and a cloudy effluent) should be confirmed by microscopy and culture of the fluid and bacterial sensitivity patterns determined.

PD needs to be continued for several days after the urine output has reached two litres per day and is then tailed off gradually. The peritoneal catheter may be left *in situ* for a further two days in case treatment needs to be resumed. Prior to its withdrawal 40 mg gentamicin is given through the catheter. Accumulation of fluid in the flanks or pubic region suggest multiple peritoneal punctures or insufficient depth of insertion of the catheter. Whilst on treatment, the patient should be encouraged to lift his head and shoulders off the bed, to walk around the bed several times a day and, while holding on to the foot of the bed, to practice standing on tip toe and doing knee bending exercises.

---

* Sterimed Ltd., Atlantic Industrial Complex, Dunningsbridge Road, Bootle, Merseyside, L30 4UZ. 051-525 6206.

† 'Dialaflex', Allen & Hanbury, Bethnal Green, London E2 6LA. 01-739 4343.

Prophylactic heparinisation is indicated in subjects predisposed to pulmonary embolism by previous prolonged immobility, age and heart disease. A daily weight loss of 300 to 500 g is appropriate, constant weight implying fluid retention.

SPECIAL ASPECTS

Infection

Dialysed patients are predisposed to oral, oesophageal and intestinal thrush with resultant dysphagia and diarrhoea. Preventive treatment with oral nystatin, 100 000 units four times a day, should be given.

A daily aerobic and anaerobic blood culture gives early warning of infection. Urine, sputum and any other discharges should also be cultured frequently.

Bladder catheterisation is required only for diagnosis. Once ARF has been confirmed a bladder wash-out with isosmotic sodium chloride solution can be given, leaving 250 000 units of penicillin with 250 mg streptomycin in the bladder prior to withdrawal of the catheter.

Antibiotic therapy

Apart from anti-thrush treatment and special situations, such as post-partum ARF or that associated with diabetes or extensive muscle injuries, antibiotics should be reserved for the treatment of established infections. Most antibiotics normally excreted through the kidney are also dialysable to varying degrees. When possible, those antibiotics which are least harmful when the therapeutic blood level is exceeded should be used. These include penicillin and penicillanic acid derivatives, erythromycin and chloramphenicol, which still has a place if the offending organism is not known or if facilities for measuring antibiotic blood levels are not available. Even with 'non-toxic' antibiotics, the therapeutic blood levels should not be greatly exceeded and their estimation is therefore desirable. Unfortunately, one of the most useful drugs for Gram-negative infections, gentamicin, causes irrecoverable inner ear damage if too high a blood level is maintained. Though dosage formulae in renal insufficiency have been developed, inner ear damage can be avoided only if a blood level of 4 to 10 μg per ml can be ensured by regular estimations. The maximum level can be estimated from a blood sample taken two hours after giving the drug and the minimum level from blood taken immediately before the next dose is due. In oliguric patients on haemodialysis 0·5 to 1·0 mg per kg body weight at the end of dialysis only will usually maintain therapeutic blood levels. In patients on PD the drug is best added to the PD fluid in a concentration of 6 mg per litre. Cephaloridine and tetracycline and its derivatives being potentially nephrotoxic should not be used in patients with reversible renal failure. Septrin and Bactrim (Co-trimoxazole) should not be used for more than four days.

Anaemia

Patients with ARF invariably become anaemic, haemoglobin levels of 7-9 g/dl being usual. Failure of the haemoglobin to fall after a few days implies haemoconcentration. Except in elderly subjects or those with heart disease, the temptation to transfuse should be resisted unless the haemoglobin falls below 6·5 g/dl.

Human albumin should be given in doses of 60 g per day if the serum albumin falls below 3 g/dl as this predisposes to pulmonary and other infections. (Low salt human albumin is supplied by the Blood Transfusion Service as a dry powder and is made up, in double or triple strength if need be, with sterile water.) Plasma has been discarded in favour of plasma protein fraction (PPF) which avoids the risk of hepatitis. Human albumin heat-treated to 60°C for 10 hours is said not to carry the risk of transmitting hepatitis (Maycock, 1972) (see p. 91).

Overhydration

Iatrogenic overhydration often unnecessarily precipitates an emergency in patients with ARF. It usually occurs through continued administration of i v fluid before the diagnosis of ARF has been established, or insidiously thereafter, through a combination of excessive oral or i v fluid intake as well as endogenous hypercatabolism. Life-threatening pulmonary oedema is most rapidly corrected with hypertonic PD using a mixture of the 13·6 and 63 g/l glucose peritoneal dialysis solutions.

As fluid can be abstracted more quickly from the vascular tree than it is replaced from the extra-cellular space, a careful watch needs to be kept on the blood pressure and circulation whilst using this mixture. Orthodox 13·4 g/l glucose PD fluid results in the loss of 1·0 to 2·0 litres of fluid/24 hours. Similar amounts can be removed during a six hour HD treatment using appropriate physiological conditions.

Hyperkalaemia

The rate at which extra-cellular potassium accumulates in ARF varies with the type of underlying disease but is predictable. Blood transfusion accentuates hyperkalaemia which should be anticipated by twice daily electrolyte estimations once the potassium level reaches 5 mmol/l. Dialysis should be started before the level reaches 6 mmol/l. Cardiac arrhythmias and a hyperkalaemic ECG (p. 605) are late changes and call for urgent treatment by the i v administration over 15 minutes of the following mixture which may be life-saving for a few hours:

100 ml 50 g/dl dextrose (2·78 mol/l)
30 units soluble insulin
100 ml 8·4 g/dl sodium bicarbonate (1 mol/l)

Fifty ml of calcium gluconate 10 g/dl should be given i v over a period of 10 minutes. (It cannot be added to the above mixture as it would precipitate out.)

This will enable urgent preparations to be made for dialysis treatment or transfer to a renal unit. The protective action of the above mixture can be prolonged by the use of Resonium-A (Winthrop), 30 g given eight-hourly for 24 hours, as an enema made up with Sterculia 0·75 g and water to 150 ml. Alternatively give 15 g eight-hourly by mouth. This resin exchanges sodium for potassium and the patient will therefore become sodium overloaded if such treatment is continued too long. Twelve hours of effective PD or four hours haemodialysis will remove the hyperkalaemia from the emergency category.

SPECIAL FORMS OF ARF

Mercuric chloride poisoning

This has a sinister reputation as it may be complicated by torrential haemorrhage from mercurial colitis for which an emergency total colectomy may be required. Dimercaprol (BAL) is probably useful within a few hours of the ingestion of the poison but is not helpful once ARF has set in. A suggested dosage scheme for early cases is 5 mg/kg body weight i m followed by two injections of 2·5 mg/kg after four and eight hours. The urine should be kept alkaline to encourage excretion of the chelated mercurial product. BAL in excess is itself nephrotoxic.

Incompatible blood transfusion (see also p. 103)

This may cause fever, backache, asthma and collapse in conscious patients, and incoagulability of the blood may be recognised under general anaesthesia. The initial urine will be pink or brown and the centrifuged blood specimen shows a pink plasma. Even following transfusion of massive volumes of incompatible blood ARF can

be averted by immediate i v frusemide-mannitol therapy, adjusted
to maintain a urine output of 500 ml/hour in the first few hours
and then less, until haemoglobinuria ceases. If preventive treatment
is applied too late the case should be treated on routine ARF lines.

Paraquat poisoning (pp. 38 and 468)

Forced diuresis and perhaps dialysis may save the patient if there
has not been any lung damage.

Uric acid crystalluria

This may cause blockage of the renal collecting ducts, pelves and
ureters during the course of advanced neoplastic disorders and particularly following their treatment with cytotoxic drugs or radiation.
Prophylactic allopurinol with a high fluid intake and alkalinisation
of the urine to pH 8 should prevent this. Allopurinol potentiates
the action of azathioprine and cyclophosphamide. Washing out
the renal pelves with 1 per cent sodium bicarbonate through ureteric
catheters together with diuretics, may result in a resumed urine flow
in early obstruction. Late cases are treated with dialysis and allopurinol.

Renovascular ARF

Thrombotic or embolic renal artery occlusion of a sole functioning kidney is usually diagnosed too late for effective therapy, which,
in the first few days would be by surgical disobliteration. Multiple
peripheral renal emboli may result in early oliguria, with late
recovery being sufficiently frequent to make a prolonged period of
dialysis worthwhile. The prognosis for malignant hypertension with
a slowly progressive rise of the blood urea is poor unless the uraemia
has been precipitated by excessive hypotensive therapy, prolonged
gastro-intestinal fluid losses or starvation. In that case, a trial of
dialysis with continuous heparinisation may be worthwhile. If subsequent transplantation or regular haemodialysis is available then
dialysis may be justifiable provided the brain has not been damaged
too much.

Hepato-renal failure (p. 144)

Hepatic failure with jaundice sensitises the kidney to ARF.
Special care therefore needs to be taken to avoid additional predisposing factors when operating on heavily jaundiced patients and
mannitol prophylaxis is generally indicated (Dawson, 1965).

The combination of parenchymatous liver failure and secondary
ARF is highly lethal. When the cause is likely to be virus hepatitis

special precautions to protect the staff during HD and PD are essential (see also p. 91). Passive immunisation may be used (pp. 748 and 800).

Other points in the management of ARF

At all times a free airway must be maintained as respiratory obstruction may lead rapidly to hyperkalaemic cardiac arrest. At all stages of the disease the patient should be kept mobile. Failing ambulation, twice daily physiotherapy to the chest and limbs will help to prevent pneumonic and embolic complications. Patients with ARF presenting acute respiratory problems are best treated on an intensive care unit. In prolonged ARF a patient's life may depend on accessible veins. Entry points of i v drips should be protected by neomycin-bacitracin ointment. Disruption of an i v drip by a confused patient is predictable and therefore preventable, using careful strapping with elastoplast (not crepe bandages). Thrombophlebitis in peripheral veins can be delayed by 5 mg hydrocortisone in each bottle of i v fluid (see p. 54). In obstetric ARF the i m administration of testosterone is thought to delay involution of the genital tract and thus to slow down the rate at which the urea rises. It is not of proven value in other forms of ARF.

In ARF following major fractures early unconsciousness may be due to cerebral fat embolism (p. 653) rather than uraemia. ARF of uncertain aetiology may be associated with acute pancreatitis (p. 113).

Oliguria or anuria in association with the nephrotic syndrome may be due to severe acute glomerulonephritis with a poor prognosis, or be part of a ' minimal change ' (steroid responsive) nephritis with an excellent prognosis. Micro- or macrohaematuria is always seen in the former, whereas red cells are scanty or absent in the latter. The oliguria of ' minimal change ' nephritis usually responds to intensive diuretic therapy (frusemide up to 500 mg four times a day orally or i v). The patient may require a period of haemodialysis during which expert help should be obtained. Convulsions in patients with ARF are usually of hypertensive origin, except in terminal uraemia. They will yield to treatment with i v diazepam 10 mg or paraldehyde 6-10 ml i m (using a glass syringe) or sodium phenobarbitone 200-300 mg i m (see p. 310) repeated as necessary until the underlying hypertension is controlled. The hypertension is associated with a sodium and fluid overload and is most rapidly brought under control with i v diazoxide (Eudemine) 300 mg given as a bolus. Alternatively, hydrallazine (Apresoline) 20 mg iv may be given. These can be repeated after a few hours whilst awaiting the effects of oral diazoxide (Eudemine) 100 mg four-hourly, until the diastolic pressure has been reduced to 100-110 mm. This maintenance treatment may be supplemented with oral diuretics, reserpine and aldactone-A. Once blood pressure control has been achieved, diazoxide can often be replaced by methyldopa or propranolol.

Another factor precipitating fits in uraemia is a very low serum calcium level. It is treated with repeated i v doses of 10 to 20 ml of calcium gluconate 10 per cent whilst the serum phosphate is lowered by oral Aludrox 15 ml four times daily. Occasionally hyponatraemia (sodium less than 125 m mol/l) contributes to convulsions. Depending on acid-base status, the sodium is best elevated to 130 mmol/l with i v hypertonic saline or sodium bicarbonate.

Amblyopia

In uraemia this is usually associated with hypertension but hypertensive retinopathy in renal failure may occur with diastolic levels of only 110-125 mm Hg if the onset of the illness has been rapid (Eclampsia, Acute Glomerulonephritis). Vision returns within a few days of lowering the blood pressure (p. 232). Other causes of blindness are retinal vessel thrombosis and retinal detachment by oedema, which may respond to dehydration. Skilled advice should be sought.

PREVENTION OF ACUTE RENAL FAILURE

The doctor should regard the supervention of ARF in a patient under his care as a nurse regards a pressure sore, i.e. as a somewhat discreditable occurrence which could have been prevented by better care.

Adequate and early treatment of hypotension, dehydration, electrolyte depletion and sepsis, particularly in surgical patients, will prevent ARF in most cases. Prophylactic mannitol therapy should be given in eclampsia and during and after surgery in heavily jaundiced patients.

Daily inspection of the fluid chart together with estimation of the plasma urea and electrolytes, should lead to the detection of threatened ARF during the early ' pre-renal ' phase during which suitable emergency treatment may avert its full evolution with consequent saving of life.

URINARY TRACT INFECTIONS

These only rarely give rise to much diagnostic or therapeutic difficulty: pus cells and bacteria can be seen on urine microscopy except in certain ' closed ' infections and when some treatment has already been given.

Severe and persistent loin pain, high fever and rigors persisting more than two days after beginning antibiotic therapy should lead to suspicion of resistant organisms or stone or other obstruction to the flow of urine.

Treament. Whenever practical, urine—and blood in cases with rigors—should be obtained for culture before beginning antibacterial therapy. The ' Uricult ' method may be useful in remote areas.

Alkalinisation of the urine to a pH 7-8 with three to five level teaspoons of sodium bicarbonate daily gives symptomatic relief of bladder pain. Analgesics may also be required. A fluid intake of at least three litres per day helps to combat infection mechanically.

Antibacterial treatment should normally be given for one week, urine cultures being repeated soon after the end of treatment and a month later to confirm sterilisation of the urinary tract. Patients of all ages, except perhaps those with mild coitus-related cystitis, should have one urological investigation to exclude underlying structural abnormalities of the urinary tract.

In cases mild enough to be treated at home one of the following drugs will generally prove effective (all four times a day):

> Ampicillin 250 mg.
> Nitrofurantoin 75-100 mg.
> Nalidixic acid 1 g.
> Erythromycin 250 mg.

Severe cases of pyelonephritis, those commencing in hospital and infections complicating obstruction of the urinary tract are best treated with Septrin (Co-trimoxazole) 2 tabs. twice daily or one of the cephalosporin group of drugs, 250 mg four times a day. Alternatively, gentamicin 1 mg per kg may be given systemically three to four times daily provided a serum creatinine level of more than 1·5 mg per 100 ml (132·6 μmol/l) does not indicate a reduced dose. For dosage in renal failure see p. 388.

The correct choice of drug is confirmed or otherwise by laboratory demonstration of the bacterial sensitivity pattern. In all cases, therefore, treatment may need revising in the light of bacteriological findings.

When using potentially ototoxic or nephrotoxic drugs, regular monitoring of their level in the blood is mandatory, especially when renal function is—or may become—impaired. Oliguric patients with pyelonephritis should be referred to the nearest renal centre as emergencies, preferably before they are desperately ill and hyperkalaemic. When dealing with recurrent or severe infections, the possibility of underlying tuberculosis, neoplasm and analgesic nephropathy should be borne in mind and obstruction excluded by radiological investigation.

GRAM-NEGATIVE SEPTICAEMIA

Urethral manipulations, cystoscopy and prostatic surgery occasionally give rise to septicaemia by Gram-negative organisms which may result in shock and acute renal failure. Prophylactic insertion of a urethral antiseptic (chlorhexidine) jelly will minimise these risks. The urine should be sterile before planned urological surgery.

Clinically septicaemia should be suspected and treated in a case of otherwise unexplained post-operative collapse, which only rarely proves to be due to myocardial infarction.

Emergency treatment consists of taking a blood culture, inserting a central venous pressure line (p. 751), administration of i v fluids and of an immediate dose of gentamicin 2 mg/kg body weight.

Acute renal failure can usually be prevented by maintaining a urine flow of at least 60 ml/hour with mannitol 25-40 g, and/or frusemide 40-80 mg i v. The latter drug may be repeated if necessary. Hydrocortisone 0·5 to 1 g i v may be helpful when shock remains resistant to the above measures.

RENAL COLIC

This is severe spasmodic pain in the flank with frequent reference to the groin, testicle or labium. Nausea and vomiting occur at the height of the pain spasms, leaving the patient with residual pain and loin tenderness.

The most important differential diagnoses include abdominal emergencies such as perforations, inflammations and torsions which necessitate urgent surgery. Such conditions should be excluded as far as possible before analgesics are given. In renal colic the urine will often give a delayed positive test for blood on testing with Hemastix. In doubtful cases a plain X ray of the abdomen may show a radio-opaque stone, or an emergency IVP delayed function with a distended collecting system on the side of the pain.

Treatment. Severe cases obtain quick relief from 50-100 mg of pethidine i v or 10-15 mg of morphine with or without 0·6 mg of atropine. Patients should be investigated after recovery.

Repeated and otherwise unexplained attacks of renal colic and abacterial ' cystitis ' may occur in patients with hyperuricaemia.

Treatment by an increased fluid intake and sufficient allopurinol to normalise the serum uric acid level will prevent further attacks.

RENAL INJURIES

Post-traumatic haematuria may be of renal origin. The source of the bleeding can generally be inferred from the nature and location of the injury. An emergency IVP should be done, however, as soon after admission to hospital as possible to help assess the extent of any renal damage or urinary extravasation, to establish the integrity of the lower urinary tract and the presence of two functioning kidneys. Major renal lacerations may be further delineated by an emergency per-femoral renal arteriogram.

Though surgical exploration may be required, even with severe renal injuries only uncontrollable internal haemorrhage should lead to nephrectomy as the results of conservative therapy are generally excellent. Absolute bed rest should be enforced until the urine contains no visible blood. Prophylactic antibiotics should be given. A high urine output should be aimed at, using diuretics if necessary. This will reduce the risk of acute renal failure from coincidental shock. A diuresis will also reduce the chance of painful ' clot colic '.

NON-TRAUMATIC HAEMATURIA

This should be investigated whilst bleeding is still going on. First confirm that the colour is due to haemoglobin with Labstix (Ames) and also the degree of proteinuria. Ensure by urine microscopy that excessive red cells are present to exclude haemoglobinuria. The important practical question is whether a urothelial tumour is present.

A thorough history with particular reference to smoking and the use of analgesic tablets as well as to occupational exposure to carcinogens should be taken. Does haematuria occur early during micturition (urethral and bladder-base lesions), late (bladder lesions), or is it ' total ' (of supra-vesical origin)? Is micturition painful?

Proteinuria in excess of 3 g/l is highly suggestive of glomerulonephritis. Surgical disorders of the urinary tract usually show proteinuria of 1 g/l or less. Urinary blood clots usually indicate a surgical lesion. In doubtful cases urine cytology is useful after the bleeding has stopped.

An emergency IVP is carried out. This may show the source of the bleeding but blood clot must not be confused with tumour. A thorough urethroscopy and cystoscopy is next done, preferably by a urologist so that any tumour discovered may be treated endoscopically at the same session. Retrograde pyelography may be necessary but usually adds little to the information obtained from a good IVP. If at this stage a diagnosis has not been reached, two early morning specimens of urine should be examined and cultured for tubercle bacilli.

Haematuria occurring repeatedly within 48 hours of the onset of an upper respiratory infection is usually due to benign focal haemorrhagic glomerulonephritis. This diagnosis may be confirmed by renal needle biopsy. Haematuria with some nitrogen retention and a radiologically normal urinary tract is likely to be caused by renal disease. Most patients with haematuria will need cystoscopy to exclude a tumour even if a medical cause of bleeding is thought likely.

ACUTE GLOMERULONEPHRITIS

The diagnosis is based on the combination of oliguria, fluid retention, hypertension (often mild), proteinuria and haematuria. Rare cases without urinary abnormalities undoubtedly occur. The patient should receive systemic penicillin (one mega unit twice a day for 10 days) in case there is an underlying streptococcal infection. Fluids should be restricted only to keep the daily weight constant and protein to keep the blood urea below 80 mg/100 ml (13 mmol/l). Adequate non-protein calories must be given (30 cal/kg weight) when the blood urea is rising. Hycal and Caloreen (p. 376) are suitable supplements (p. 6). Until body weight and blood pressure have stabilised or are falling, salt must be rigorously restricted.

Excessive fluid retention may be overcome with frusemide 40-500 mg orally or i v). The blood pressure should be kept below 170/100 mm Hg by appropriate drugs (p. 232) unless the patient was previously hypertensive. In the defervescent stage strict bed rest is no longer indicated. Severe cases with complications should be referred to a renal unit, as dialysis may be required.

PRINCIPLES OF ANTIBIOTIC USE IN RENAL FAILURE

1. Preferentially use a drug eliminated other than by the kidney (A) or one with little toxicity if therapeutic blood levels are exceeded (B).

	Therapeutic blood level μg/ml
(A) Erythromycin	1- 4
Fusidic acid	10-20
(Chloramphenicol not more than 5 days)	4-10
(B) Nalidixic acid	20-50
Sulphonamides	40-80
Penicillin G	1- 5 i v

2. Do not use tetracycline, cephaloridine or nitrofurantoin.

3. The following may be life-saving with Gram-negative infections, but are highly toxic if therapeutic blood levels are exceeded.

	Therapeutic blood level μg/ml
Cephalexin	10-20
Colistin	4-12
Rifampicin	3- 5
Vancomycin (weekly or fortnightly only)	10-20
Kanamycin	10-20
Streptomycin	10-25
Gentamicin	4-10

The initial dose of Group 3 drugs should be full and unmodified. If serum creatinine is less than 4 mg/100 ml (353·6 mmol/l) give further $\frac{2}{3}$ dose over 12 hours but if more than 8 mg/100 ml (707·2 mmol/l) after 24 hours (Bennett *et al.*, 1974).

Take blood for antibiotic level estimation two hours after the second injection and immediately prior to the projected third injection and thereafter once daily before each injection.

Maximal and minimal blood levels thus measured will give a safe indication of future dosage and frequency. Do not forget to inform the laboratory if any other antibiotics have been given during the previous 10 days, as this will affect the test organism used.

H. J. GOLDSMITH

REFERENCES

BENNETT, W. M., SINGER, I. & COGGINS, J. (1974). A guide to drug therapy in renal failure. *Journal of the American Medical Association,* **230,** 1544-1553.

DAWSON, J. L. (1965). Post-operative renal function in obstructive jaundice; effects of a mannitol diuresis. *British Medical Journal,* **1,** 82-86.

MAYCOCK, W. D'A. (1972). Hepatitis in Transfusion Services. *British Medical Bulletin,* **28,** 2, 163.

OGG, C. F., SAXTON, H. M. & CAMERON, J. S. (1969). Percutaneous needle nephrostomy. *British Medical Journal,* **4,** 657-660.

CHAPTER 18

Medical Emergencies in Infancy and Childhood

PAEDIATRIC emergencies are particularly liable to cause panic. This often leads to pressure on the family doctor for vigorous and dramatic action. He is not capable of rational activity, however, until he has made a diagnosis. Symptomatic treatment based on a hurried clinical impression is often ill-directed and may be harmful. An example is the traditional but discredited hot mustard bath for the convulsing child. Diagnosis implies an understanding of the sequence of events which has led to the emergency. This is specially difficult in the newborn because the physiology, pathology and symptomatology peculiar to this period differ from those of older infants. Yet 70 per cent of all deaths in the first year of life occur in the first month. Moreover, the present low mortality rate in the period from one month to one year could be further reduced were some emergencies of infancy better recognised as being different from those of later childhood. We shall consider separately, therefore, the paediatric emergencies of the neonatal period, of infancy, and of childhood.

NEONATAL PERIOD
(Birth to 1 month)

A major part of neonatal mortality is attributable to disorders of respiration. There may be an initial failure of the respiratory apparatus to function at birth, or subsequent respiratory difficulty.

ASPHYXIA NEONATORUM

Failure of the infant to establish spontaneous respiration at birth resutls in progressive hypoxia (lowered arterial PaO_2) and hypercapnia (raised $PaCO_2$). This is asphyxia neonatorum, and it is in most instances the result of preceding fetal (intrapartum) hypoxia. Unfortunately we have no reliable clinical methods of detecting fetal hypoxia. Alterations in the fetal heart-rate or meconium staining of the liquor amnii are highly significant observations during labour but severe fetal anoxia can exist in their absence. While the likelihood of asphyxia neonatorum can often be foreseen from the course of labour the attendants must be prepared to deal with this emergency at every delivery. A considerable advance in recent years has been the measurement of the pH of blood taken from the fetal scalp during labour (Beard *et al.*, 1966). A pH level of below 7·2 is clear evidence of fetal hypoxia and an indication for appropriate obstetric interference. This technique has also prevented many unnecessary Caesarean sections by showing that dangerous fetal hypoxia was not in fact present in spite of clinical suspicions to the contrary. Even when the infant has failed to establish respiration within one minute of birth it is frequently difficult to assess the severity of the asphyxial state. In severe asphyxia marked bradycardia is usually associated with a few spontaneous but feeble gasping efforts. Muscle tone and the response to cutaneous stimuli are poor or nonexistent. The colour varies from deep cyanosis to deathly pallor (fetal shock). In some asphyxiated infants there is complete apnoea after delivery but it is then impossible to be certain whether this is the stage of ' primary ' apnoea which (in the experimental animal at least) is always followed by spontaneous gasping, or whether the infant has, in fact, already passed the stage of the last gasp and is showing the ' terminal ' apnoea which immediately precedes death. The clinician clearly cannot wait until the situation becomes clear lest the infant's condition rapidly deteriorates. His treatment must be prompt and effective.

Treatment

Chilling must be avoided. The infant should be placed with head lower than feet and the pharynx and nostrils thoroughly sucked clear of secretions with a mucus extractor or low-pressure suction pump. The part of the apparatus for insertion into the infant's mouth or nose must be of soft rubber with a square-cut open end. Mucus extractors must incorporate a suitable trap between the infant and the operator, and suitable disposable models are now available. When the airway has thus been cleared a stream of pure oxygen should be directed by plastic or rubber funnel over the infant's face. Alternatively, a suitable face-mask may be fitted and intermittent short puffs of oxygen administered from the anaesthetic machine. In most cases these simple measures are sufficient to establish respiration. Thereafter, the infant's head should be raised to a level higher than feet to avoid pressure on the diaphragm. If cyanosis is slow to clear from the face and extremities he should be placed in an atmosphere of 35 to 40 per cent oxygen for a few hours. When slowness to initiate respiration may be due to the effects of pethidine or morphine administered to the mother late in labour, 0·5 to 1·0 mg nalorphine or naloxone (Narcan) should be injected into the umbilical vein proximal to a clamp placed a few centimetres from the infant and the cord should then be ' milked ' towards the infant. Analeptics such as nikethamide and ethamivan (Vandid) are of very doubtful value. They are not free from risk and are best eschewed.

On the other hand, it has been increasingly recognised that severe asphyxia is associated with progressive metabolic acidosis correction of which considerably improves the chances of recovery. When the heart rate is below 60 per minute sodium bicarbonate should be given into the umbilical vein in a dose of 10 to 15 mmol (10 to 15 ml of 8·4 g/dl solution (see p. 727)). This is frequently followed by gasping and a rise in heart rate.

When such conservative and non-traumatic measures have failed to establish respiration within three to four minutes, and sooner if there is severe bradycardia and shock, the standard and extremely effective method of resuscitation is tracheal intubation and intermittent positive pressure inflation of the lungs (Barrie, 1963). The larynx is exposed with an infants' size laryngoscope, and a close-fitting plastic tube is inserted. The trachea and bronchi are sucked clear using a fine tracheal catheter and intermittent positive pressure breathing is commenced. Various types of apparatus are available for this purpose, such as the Resuscitaire (Vickers Medical), but the maximum permissible inflationary pressure is 30 cm water. When the heart has stopped or remains very slow or irregular external cardiac massage, using the fingers to depress the sternum 1 to 2 cm, should also be tried. Tracheal intubation and positive pressure inflation requires a skilled operator and in unskilled hands it is not free from the risks of interstitial emphysema and pneumothorax.

The author and his colleagues have reported their favourable experience with hyperbaric oxygen (p. 814) as a method of resuscitation (Hutchison and Kerr, 1965). The infant is placed in a small pressure chamber capable of compressing pure oxygen to 4 atmospheres absolute in just under five minutes, so that there is a steep gradient of 3 000 mm Hg (400 kPa) between the environment and the infant's hypoxic tissues. This method is completely atraumatic, simple to operate and free from toxic effects. It has been criticised, principally on the grounds that it is much less effective than tracheal intubation in experimental animals which have been asphyxiated beyond the stage of the last gasp. In the human situation this is extremely rare and in any event not often susceptible to any method of resuscitation. In the author's experience hyperbaric oxygenation can prevent the death from asphyxia of infants who are born alive and it is a method which can always be immediately available in hospitals at all hours. Controlled trials of hyperbaric oxygen versus intermittent positive pressure breathing have failed to reveal a statistically significant difference in effectiveness between the two methods (Hutchison *et al.*, 1966) and measurements of tissue oxygen tension have shown a rapid rise with both methods (Rodger *et al.*, 1968).

In dire emergency outside hospital where special apparatus is not available mouth-to-mouth breathing should always be tried (p. 732). The attendant takes a deep breath and then places his lips so as to enclose the infant's nose and mouth in an effective seal. He then blows air into the infant *using only his cheeks as a source of pressure*. He then removes his mouth from the infant's face to allow expiration. This is repeated about 20 times per minute. He should also during this manoeuvre press the infant's trachea backwards with his fingers to lessen the danger of blowing up the infant's stomach. The infant successfully resuscitated by this method is, of course, at some risk of infection from the attendant, and it is wise to protect him for a few days by the i m administration of cloxacillin and ampicillin, each in a daily dose of 50 mg per kg.

ACUTE RESPIRATORY DISTRESS IN THE
FIRST WEEK OF LIFE

Four-fifths of all neonatal deaths are preceded by obvious respiratory difficulty.

The respiratory distress syndrome of the newborn. This syndrome which is also called the pulmonary syndrome of the newborn, or hyaline membrane disease, is a frequent cause of death in the first week of life. It is characterised by resorption atelectasis and intense pulmonary congestion. In fatal cases an eosinophilic hyaline membrane is found lining the dilated alveolar ducts, and in some there is intra-alveolar haemorrhage. The hyaline membrane is composed largely of fibrin and it is thought to arise from the plasma. This disease is seen only in infants who have breathed and survived for at least one hour but its aetiology remains obscure. There is a demonstrable lack of the normally complete lung-lining film which continuously prevents the occurrence of atelectasis in healthy lungs but the reasons for its deficiency in this syndrome are as yet unknown.

This lung-lining film or surfactant is a lipoprotein composed mainly of dipalmitoyl lecithin. It has been shown that if the ratio in liquor amnii of lecithin to sphingomyelin is over 2·0 the infant will not develop hyaline membrane disease (Whitfield *et al.*, 1972).

This relatively simple test can be performed on liquor obtained by amniocentesis in selected cases. Hyaline membrane disease is sometimes prevented by delaying the birth of the baby for a week or two. A ratio of less than 1·5 almost invariably indicates the development of neonatal respiratory distress.

Hyaline membrane disease is occasionally seen in full-time infants but it is essentially a disease of the premature. There is a significant association with Caesarean section, maternal diabetes mellitus and ante-partum haemorrhage. In some cases the infant appears normal for a few hours after birth but most are in poor condition at birth with limpness, diminished response to stimuli and irregular grunting respirations. *Tachypnoea with a respiratory rate above 50 per minute and which persists for longer than two hours after birth should always be taken seriously. It is likely to herald some disorder of the lungs, and it is a good practice to chart the respiratory rate hourly in every infant who shows any delay in the initiation of respiration.* Respiratory distress, once present, progresses until there is marked inspiratory indrawing of the lower sternum, subcostal margins, intercostal spaces and suprasternal notch. Tachypnoea is associated with audible expiratory grunting. Cyanosis is invariable in severe cases and auscultation reveals very poor air-entry into the lungs. Oedema and jaundice frequently develop after 12 hours. Pulmonary haemorrhage is sometimes revealed by the presence of frothy blood-stained mucus in the mouth and pharynx. There may be signs of cerebral hypoxia such as wakefulness, a shrill cry or convulsive twitchings. Radiographs reveal a characteristic reticulogranular mottling throughout the lung fields and the main bronchi appear excessively well outlined—an air bronchogram.

The blood chemical changes include a lowered PaO_2, raised $PaCO_2$ (respiratory acidosis), diminished plasma standard bicarbonate (metabolic acidosis) and hypoglycaemia. Hyperkalaemia with abnormalities in the ECG (p. 605) is common after the first 12 hours. Death is due to respiratory failure because the large functional dead space in severe cases approaches the tidal volume.

Pneumonia. This has been increasingly recognised as a cause of death in the first week of life since autopsies have been routine in stillbirths and neonatal deaths in several maternity units. Clinical diagnosis is extremely difficult. The infection is usually acquired *in utero* and its incidence is significantly higher in infants born more than 48 hours after rupture of the membranes. Infection in the mother at the time of birth increases the risk. So do Caesarean section and complicated vaginal delivery. Histological diagnosis must be based on the presence of an inflammatory exudate, usually polymorphonuclear, in the air spaces and interstitial tissues of the lungs.

The infant born with pneumonia usually shows some asphyxia at birth with delay in the initiation of respiration. Thereafter there is likely to be persisting or increasing tachypnoea, expiratory grunting and cyanosis. Crepitations and rhonchi may be heard and sometimes bronchial breath sounds. Radiographs may show a widespread consolidation which is quite different from the miliary mottling of hyaline membrane disease. Signs of cerebral irritation are also common.

Intracranial birth trauma. Such trauma occurs in both full-term and premature infants. Most commonly there is a tear of the tentorium cerebelli involving the straight sinus or the great vein of Galen. Next in frequency is a tear of the falx cerebri with damage to the sagittal sinus or cerebral veins. Signs of intrapartum asphyxia are present in other tissues. In premature infants hyaline membrane or intrapulmonary haemorrhage is often coexistent.

High maternal age, multiple pregnancy, long labour, forceps delivery, breech delivery and antepartum haemorrhage should all suggest the possibility of birth trauma. In full-time infants obvious cerebral signs are usually present. These include extreme irritability or lethargy, a shrill cry, spasticity, a tense fontanelle, inability to suck and convulsions. However, respiratory distress is almost always present, and in premature infants this may be the only feature.

Intraventricular haemorrhage. Intraventricular haemorrhage is peculiar to premature infants and characterised by massive haemorrhage into one or both lateral ventricles. Most affected infants also show evidence of the respiratory distress syndrome of the newborn.

It is not possible to differentiate the respiratory distress of intraventricular haemorrhage from that of uncomplicated hyaline membrane disease. Cerebral signs are as frequently seen in both conditions. Indeed, intraventricular haemorrhage is the consequence of asphyxia and frequently develops in the premature infant who already has hyaline membrane disease.

Meconium aspiration. This condition occurs most frequently in dysmature infants when placental insufficiency has produced fetal hypoxia with the passage of meconium *in utero*. It is rare in premature births.

Marked respiratory distress with grunting breathing and sternal recession is present from birth. Crepitations may be heard. Hypoxia may give rise to signs of cerebral irritation. Radiographs often show emphysema and a coarse interstitial streaking which fans out from the hila. Spontaneous pneumothorax (p. 202) or mediastinal emphysema (p. 599) may complicate the picture. This condition should be suspected when the infant shows such features of dysmaturity as widespread desquamation, loose skin especially over the thighs and buttocks, and nails which may be stained yellow.

Oesophageal atresia. Oesophageal atresia occurs in several anatomical variations, of which the commonest is a blind upper oesophageal pouch while the lower segment of oesophagus enters the trachea about the level of its bifurcation. Rarely there is a fistula without atresia. In all forms of this anomaly respiratory distress is a presenting feature. Hydramnios is a common association.

The infant appears healthy at birth but soon two characteristic signs appear. Firstly, there is excess accumulation of mucus in the mouth and oropharynx, and oesophageal atresia should be suspected in every infant who requires repeated suction after birth. Secondly, as soon as a feed is given the infant develops acute respiratory difficulty and becomes cyanosed. At first normal respiration and colour return between spasms but if the diagnosis is delayed aspiration atelectasis and pneumonia cause persistent difficulty in breathing. Radiographs show atelectasis, most often of the right upper lobe. Successful treatment is dependent on early diagnosis before the lungs become extensively damaged. Careful search should be made in such patients for other congenital abnormalities, especially in the heart.

Diaphragmatic hernia. Herniation through a large defect in the posterolateral muscular segment of the diaphragm permits the stomach, small intestine, transverse colon and spleen to enter the left hemithorax with consequent collapse of lung and mediastinal displacement.

In 90 per cent of cases the infant shows severe respiratory difficulty and cyanosis from shortly after birth. The percussion note over the left side of the chest may be dull or tympanitic. Breath sounds are often absent and intestinal gurgling may be heard. The diagnosis is readily established by radiography.

Congenital lobar emphysema. This condition arises as the result of a check-valve type of obstruction of a primary bronchus which prevents the egress of air during expiration while allowing its free entry during inspiration. In consequence, the affected lobe becomes grossly over-distended with mediastinal displacement towards the opposite side. The cause is probably hypoplasia of the bronchial cartilage.

The infant appears normal at birth but within a few days is in acute respiratory difficulty and may have cyanotic attacks. The affected side of the chest may bulge visibly. The percussion note is hyper-resonant while the breath sounds are absent or distant. There may be an audible wheeze. Radiographs show increased translucency of the affected lobe which may, indeed, herniate across the midline anteriorly. The mediastinum is displaced to the healthy side.

Differential diagnosis

Accurate differential diagnosis between the respiratory distress syndrome of the newborn, birth trauma, pneumonia, intraventricular haemorrhage and meconium aspiration is often difficult. The respiratory distress syndrome of the newborn is usually seen in the small premature infant. Intrauterine pneumonia is commoner in the full-term infant and should be suspected if the membranes were ruptured longer than 48 hours before delivery, if the mother has fever or other signs of infection, and in all difficult deliveries. Meconium aspiration is characteristically seen in the low birth weight ('light-for-dates') infant exhibiting the signs of dysmaturity. On the other hand, accurate diagnosis of the various congenital abnormalities is always possible and particularly important because they are all amenable to complete surgical correction, provided diagnosis is not too long delayed. A No. 8 rubber catheter should be passed into the oesophagus of every infant who produces excess mucus after birth. If the catheter fails to enter the stomach the diagnosis of oesophageal atresia is confirmed. It should always be possible to reach this diagnosis before the infant has been offered his first feed provided the attendants are sufficiently alert to the significance of excess mucus in the mouth and pharynx. The examination may be repeated by the surgeon in the X ray room using a radio-opaque catheter. Diaphragmatic hernia and congenital lobar emphysema are readily confirmed by plain radiographs. When possible, ill newborn infants should be X rayed with portable apparatus to reduce handling to the minimum.

Treatment. (For immediate management at birth see p. 578.)

The newborn infant in respiratory distress can only be efficiently treated in hospital. In many instances the difficulties can be foreseen and confinement in hospital should be advised. This is obviously indicated when there is antepartum bleeding, toxaemia, hydramnios and multiple pregnancy and for diabetic mothers and primigravidae over the age of 35. When an infant born at home shows signs of disordered respiration his transfer to a nearby paediatric unit should be arranged. Many maternity hospitals will now send out a trained nurse with a portable battery-operated incubator, oxygen and suction apparatus to collect the infant. Failing this he is all too likely to arrive having suffered a disastrous fall in temperature (See Cold Injury, p. 404).

Infants shown to have congenital anomalies must be operated upon as soon after diagnosis as possible. They should be transferred to a centre which specialises in this type of neonatal surgery.

Infants with respiratory difficulty from any cause are likely to exhibit some degree of cyanosis in room air and should be placed in an incubator in oxygen, high humidity (80 per cent) and an ambient temperature of 32 to 35°C. In most cases of pneumonia, and in the less severe degrees of hyaline membrane disease or meconium aspiration, the cyanosis can be abolished in an oxygen concentration of 35 to 40 per cent. This should invariably be monitored with a paramagnetic oximeter because there is a risk of retrolental fibroplasia in premature infants who are exposed needlessly to higher concentrations. Oxygen should, however, be withdrawn as soon as the infant's respiratory distress has subsided. A useful initial measure is gastric aspiration by rubber catheter and 20 ml syringe. This lessens the risk of aspiration of gastric contents into the lungs and serves also to exclude oesophageal atresia. In all infants with respiratory distress, and certainly in those in whom intrauterine pneumonia seems probable, broad spectrum antibiotic cover is advisable, preferably by the i m route. The objective must be to deal with possible penicillinresistant staphylococci and Gram-negative organisms in an acute situation where bacteriological diagnosis from nose and throat swabs may be uncertain and relatively time-consuming. Cloxacillin and ampicillin, each in a dosage of 50 mg/kg/day make an effective combination. A suitable single antibiotic is cephaloridine, 50 mg/kg/day.

When the respiratory distress is of such severity that cyanosis is not abolished in 40 per cent oxygen, a situation most often due to hyaline membrane disease, more sophisticated measures are required. These are likely only to be obtainable in a few specialised units for the sick newborn. The first essential is a concentration of oxygen in the incubator sufficient to achieve a satisfactory arterial PO_2 level, if possible over 50 mm Hg (6·65 kPa). This may necessitate enclosing the infant's head in a plastic hood within the incubator to achieve oxygen concentrations above 90 per cent. In those circumstances it is essential to catheterise an umbilical artery and to measure the arterial PO_2 at frequent intervals. It is important to prevent the PaO_2 level exceeding 120 mm Hg (16 kPa) to prevent

14

retrolental fibroplasia. Concurrently it is important to correct the metabolic acidosis usually present with i v sodium bicarbonate or THAM (tris-hydroxymethylaminomethane), and to replenish the depleted glycogen stores with i v fructose or dextrose solutions. This type of regime requires the use of the Astrup apparatus (or equivalent) on which blood PaO_2, pH, $PaCO_2$ and plasma standard bicarbonate and base excess values can be estimated on small volumes of arterial blood. The author's practice (Hutchison *et al.*, 1964 is to administer sodium bicarbonate 8·4 g/dl (1ml=1 mmol) (see p. 727) and 20 per cent fructose solutions via an umbilical arterial or venous catheter. Between injections the umbilical arterial catheter is filled with heparin solution (10 units per ml). The dose of bicarbonate is derived from the base excess (a negative value in metabolic acidosis) (see p. 11) and calculated upon the assumption that the extracellular fluid space is 35 per cent of the body weight. The dose of sodium bicarbonate 8·4 g/dl in ml (or mmol) is given by the formula base excess in mmol/1 × body weight in kg × 0·35. In this way the base excess value is used as the unit for titration of the infant with sodium bicarbonate. The object is to raise the blood pH and plasma standard bicarbonate towards normal. The blood gases and acid/base status are checked at hourly or two-hourly intervals, and further ' topping up ' doses of bicarbonate are usually required to replenish that which enters the acidotic cells and the losses in the urine. Meantime the total daily fluid intake is brought up to 60 ml/kg with hourly injections of 20 g/dl fructose. This regime is continued until the arterial PaO_2 can be satisfactorily maintained in less than 40 per cent oxygen and the acid/base equilibrium can be maintained without further doses of sodium bicarbonate when oral feeds are started. It places a heavy load upon medical and nursing staff but the results are often gratifying. In the author's hands the mortality rate in severe cases of hyaline membrane disease has been reduced from about 45 per cent to under 15 per cent. In some centres the alkali and carbo-hydrate replenishment is preferably given by continuous infusion via scalp veins.

There are, however, cases in which the regime outlined fails. These are associated with low arterial PaO_2 levels despite very high inspired oxygen concentrations (largely due to large right-to-left shunts of blood), and high $PaCO_2$ values. It is in such cases that mechanical ventilation through an endotracheal tube has been em-ployed (Tunstall *et al.*, 1968). The indications for this stressful and hazardous method of treatment are not firmly established and it must be remembered that many infants with severe abnormalities in their blood gases, and acid/base status survive without mechanical ventilation. It may be that the clearest indication is the apnoeic attack with severe bradycardia which does not respond to peripheral stimulation within three minutes (Adamson *et al.*, 1968). An increased survival rate can now be achieved if the infants are ventilated at low peak airway pressures, slow respiratory frequencies, and high inspiration:expiration ratios (Reynolds and Taghizadeh, 1974).

Others have attempted to ventilate such infants by means of intermittent negative pressure (as in the Isolette Respirator). More recently the institution of continuous positive airways pressure (5 to 12 cm H_2O) either by means of a specially designed head box or via an intratracheal tube has been recommended for infants with hyaline membrane disease (Gregory *et al.*, 1971). Alternatively a continuous negative pressure may be applied to the chest wall (Cherwick and Vidyasagar, 1972). The author has used both techniques more freely than he now uses mechanical ventilation but their value is difficult to assess in this unpredictable situation. All that can be said is that in well staffed intensive care units for neonates better results are obtained than in special care baby units where only an occasional case of the respiratory distress syndrome is handled.

Symptomatic Hypoglycaemia of the Newborn

The importance of hypoglycaemia in the newborn infant has been increasingly realised in recent years (Cornblath and Schwarz, 1966). Unrecognised and untreated it is likely to leave behind severe brain damage. It is particularly prone to develop in the ' small for dates ' or dysmature infant, especially the infant who is more than two standard deviations below the mean weight for his gestational age. The incidence is higher in male infants and in the second born of twins. Pre-eclamptic toxaemia also increases the risk. The aetiology is not quite clear but poor glycogen stores in association with the well developed glucose-dependent brain of the dysmature infant probably play a part in causing the hypoglycaemia, which develops from a few hours to a few days after birth.

The symptoms are protean and, unfortunately, may occur in other unrelated disorders. They include excessive jitteriness, lethargy and reluctance to suck, apnoeic attacks, or frank convulsive twitching. The signs of dysmaturity such as low weight with long thin body and relatively large head, dry cracked skin, and meconium staining of nails may be obvious.

Diagnosis

Any infant who develops the manifestations described above should have the true blood glucose level estimated without delay. A figure below 20 mg per 100 ml (1·1 mmol/l) is a clear indication for emergency treatment. Indeed, it is good practice to check the blood glucose levels of all dysmature infants at six hourly intervals with Dextrostix strips (Ames & Co.). If the Dextrostix fails to record a colour change (lowest reading 45 mg per 100 ml (2·5 mmol/l)) the blood glucose level should be estimated in the laboratory. It has been suggested that while hypoglycaemia (blood glucose below 20 mg per 100 ml (1·1 mmol/l) with symptoms in the newborn is an undoubted cause of brain damage, the presence of hypoglycaemia without overt manifestations may be relatively harmless. Screening all 'at risk' infants with Dextrostix will reveal a fair number of cases without symptoms, and it is now the author's practice to treat *all* babies in whom the blood glucose falls below 20 mg per 100 ml (1·1 mmol/l) in the belief that some cases of permanent brain damage are thereby prevented (Campbell *et al.*, 1967).

Treatment

As soon as the diagnosis has been confirmed 50 g/dl dextrose in water is syringed into a scalp vein in a dose of 2 ml/kg body weight. A continuous infusion of dextrose 10 g/dl in water is then set up into a scalp vein at a rate of 60 to 75 ml/kg/day. If the infusion has to be continued for longer than 24 hours to maintain satisfactory blood glucose levels the fluid should be changed to 10 per cent dextrose in quarter strength isosmotic sodium chloride solution to prevent water intoxication. The longer the duration of symptoms before treatment the more difficult it sometimes proves to correct the hypoglycaemia, and the greater the risk of brain damage. In such cases glucocorticoids or corticotrophin have been added to the therapeutic regime, with doubtful benefit. Finally, it is a good plan to estimate the serum calcium level in all convulsing infants because hypocalcaemia (see below) can occasionally coexist with symptomatic hypoglycaemia and require concurrent treatment.

CONVULSIONS IN THE NEWBORN

Convulsive twitchings in the newborn are common and precise diagnosis is often difficult. Some are related to infections such as meningitis, pneumonia and pyelonephritis, and some to gross congenital abnormalities of the brain, heart or kidneys. Hypocalcaemic tetany is not rare and is probablyl related to the high phosphate content of cow's milk preparations used for artificial feeding. It does not occur in the wholly breast fed baby. Symptomatic hypoglycaemia has already been considered. Kernicterus due to the hyperbilirubinaemia of haemolytic disease or prematurity may be associated with convulsions. However, in most cases the convulsions are the consequence of intrapartum hypoxia which can lead to intracranial haemorrhage, cerebral oedema or venous congestion. Fever is not a cause of convulsions in the neonatal period.

Convulsions due to birth trauma and hypoxia should be suspected when the infant has been difficult to resuscitate at birth, and especially in association with high maternal age, antepartum haemorrhage, prolonged labour and difficult delivery. A tense fontanelle within 48 hours of birth indicates intracranial bleeding. Respiratory distress is usually marked and in premature infants is often due to concomitant hyaline membrane disease. Cerebral agenesis should be suspected if the head is too small, if there is an unusual facial configuration and if the convulsions are violent and uninfluenced by anti-convulsant drugs. Neonatal tetany develops between the fifth and seventh days of life. It takes the form of generalised convulsive twitchings, and is always to be suspected when the infant has been born after an uneventful labour and has seemed healthy during the first four days. Confirmation will be found in a serum calcium level below 8 mg per 100 ml (2 mmol/l), whereas the phosphate level is often abnormally high. Convulsions due to infection are more common after the first week of life. The infant looks grey and anxious, loses weight abruptly, goes off his feeds and may be dyspnoeic. Fever is often absent. In pyogenic meningitis, usually due to *E. coli*, the fontanelle may be tense and bulging, but nuchal rigidity is not to be expected. Lumbar puncture should always be performed if an infant suddenly becomes lethargic, reluctant to feed or has twitchings after the first week of life.

Treatment

Respiratory distress should be treated as already described. Suitable anti-convulsant drugs are sodium phenobarbitone 8 mg six-hourly by mouth or Triclofos 50 to 100 mg every four hours (the BPC elixir contains 500 mg in 5 ml). In severe convulsions the phenobarbitone may be given by the i m route. Infections should be treated with broad spectrum antibiotics, preferably under laboratory control. Neonatal tetany can be quickly abolished by the production of a metabolic acidosis with calcium chloride, 300 mg four-hourly by mouth for three to four days. Lumbar puncture is essential if meningitis is suspected, but its value as a therapeutic measure is doubtful. In the rare instance in which anticonvulsant drugs prove ineffective it is worth trying pyridoxine, 5 to 10 mg i m, because a few infants with convulsions have a metabolic error which results in much greater pyridoxine requirements than normal. In these rare cases permanent administration of pyridoxine is indicated. The prognosis in infants who have had neonatal convulsions should always be guarded because there is an appreciable incidence of mental or physical handicap in the survivors. The exception is hypocalcaemic tetany which is rarely followed by neurological sequelae.

Haemorrhage in the Newborn

The newborn infant is peculiarly susceptible to haemorrhage. It may complicate many disorders such as sepsis, hypoxia, liver damage, congenital thrombocytopenic purpura and leukaemia. However, haemorrhage in itself only constitutes an emergency when it is severe enough to endanger life. Rarely the infant is dangerously anaemic at birth as a result of fetal bleeding into the maternal side of the placenta (feto-maternal transfusion). In this circumstance fetal erythrocytes can be identified in the maternal blood by techniques of differential agglutination, or more simply by staining blood films from the mother after they have been treated with an acid buffer at pH 3·4 which leaves only the fetal erythrocytes able to react with haemoglobin stains whereas the adult erythrocytes appear as ' ghosts ' (Zipursky *et al.,* 1959). The infant's blood contains large numbers of erythroblasts indicative of marrow hyperplasia as a response to haemorrhage. Very rarely one fetus bleeds into its twin so that at birth one is deathly pale while the other is polycythaemic. Fetal bleeding may also arise from rupture of a blood vessel on the fetal side of the placenta. This should be suspected if bright red blood flows from the mother's vagina during labour. Its fetal origin can be confirmed by chemical tests based on the fact that fetal haemoglobin is alkali-resistant. Fetal bleeding has also occurred from incision of the placenta during lower segment Caesarean section. Haemorrhage after birth may arise from the umbilical cord due to a loose ligature, trauma or infection. The commonest cause is **haemorrhagic disease of the newborn** in which spontaneous bleeding, most often melaena but often also from stomach, umbilical cord, nose and genito-urinary tract, occurs between the second and seventh days of life. The precise nature of this disease is not fully understood but affected infants show deficiencies in several clotting factors including factor

VIII (proconvertin), factor IX (Christmas factor) and factor X (Stuart-Prower factor). A variant of haemorrhagic disease of the newborn is the massive subaponeurotic haemorrhage which may occur under the scalp of the infant born by vacuum extraction and which may exsanguinate an infant within a few hours (Ahuja et al., 1969). The whole scalp looks swollen and either pits on pressure or feels tight and tense. Congenital afibrinogenaemia is a rare hereditary defect in the synthesis of fibrinogen. Bleeding often appears in the neonatal period and recurs throughout the patient's life. The blood is completely incoagulable. Haemophilia and related disorders rarely cause trouble in infancy.

Diagnosis

Fetal bleeding should always be suspected when an infant is born in a state of extreme pallor. It differs from asphyxia pallida in that the apnoea and slow heart rate of severe hypoxia are absent. The anaemic infant's respiration is usually established without initial difficulty. External bleeding is obvious and most often due to haemorrhagic disease. Occasionally the haemorrhage in this disease is solely internal, e.g. subcapsular haematoma of the liver. In this event the signs of shock and marked pallor, perhaps a palpable intra-abdominal mass, are indications enough of an emergency. Treatment to save the infant's life is imperative. There is time enough later for the special laboratory tests necessary for diagnosis of the less common causes of bleeding. The physician must, however, beware of mistaking altered blood in the stools, which the infant has swallowed from a crack in the mother's nipple, as an indication of haemorrhage. A simple test for the absence or presence of fetal haemoglobin will resolve the issue when there is any doubt.

Treatment

Most cases of haemorrhagic disease are mild. An i m injection of vitamin K_1 (phytomenadione) 2 to 5 mg is sufficient treatment. When the infant is pale, shocked and restless blood transfusion (20 to 30 ml per kg body weight) is urgently required whatever the cause of the haemorrhage. The blood may be given via the umbilical vein during the first three or four days of life, or after this period, into a scalp vein or by a ' cut-down ' over the long saphenous vein at the ankle. It is now the author's practice in all infants born by vacuum extraction to forestall severe subaponeurotic bleeding with a transfusion of fresh frozen plasma 10 ml per kg body weight if the Thrombotest gives a level of 10 per cent or less.

COLD INJURY (HYPOTHERMIA)
(See also p. 361)

Death from exposure to cold is not at all uncommon in young infants (Arneil and Kerr 1963; Bower *et al.*, 1960). Unfortunately, the typical clinical appearances are often overlooked by parents and doctor until it is too late. The cause is body chilling at or after birth. It is seen most frequently during the winter months when the temperature of rooms in many British homes is considerably below 18°C. The ordinary coal fire is apt to go out in the early morning hours with a dangerous drop in room temperature. The ritual daily bath is a particularly hazardous thing for the newborn infant. This emergency is not confined to poorer homes; many a well-appointed house remains uncomfortably cold in winter.

Cold injury occurs in infants of all birth weights although premature infants are at greater risk. The infant is usually healthy at birth but later, as his body temperature falls, he becomes apathetic and lethargic, disinclined to feed, and his cry becomes an infrequent whimper. His skin feels very cold although the significance of this is often overlooked. The infant's breath on the physician's cheek is also strikingly cold. The face, hands and feet develop a characteristic lobster-red colour, associated with a misleadingly placid appearance, which is often misinterpreted as indicating well-being. Subsequently the subcutaneous tissues, especially over the cheeks, buttocks, thighs and calves, develop a palpable hardening and thickening. Tachycardia in the early case is replaced by bradycardia as the body temperature falls below 32·2°C. In some cases the presence of massive intrapulmonary haemorrhage is revealed by blood-stained frothy mucus in the mouth and pharynx. Bleeding from stomach and bowel and into the skin may also occur. Hypoglycaemia is a constant biochemical finding. Infection is not infrequently superimposed. The mortality rate in cases reaching hospital is over 40 per cent.

Treatment

Preventive. Cold injury should never be allowed to happen. Doctors and midwives must insist that no infant is to be delivered or kept in a room with a temperature below 18°C. Adequate body covering and a suitably warmed cot are essential. The infant's temperature should be recorded daily throughout the neonatal period. For this purpose the usual clinical thermometer is valueless. Temperatures should be taken rectally with a low-reading thermometer (range 29·4 to 43·3°C) (p. 362) which is essential equipment for all family doctors and district midwives. The daily bath is unnecessary and could, with advantage, be abandoned. If it is necessary to transfer a newborn infant to hospital a portable incubator should be used.

Curative. Re-warming must be gradual and is best done in an incubator. A start should be made with an incubator temperature of 26·6 to 29·4°C and a slow rise to 35°C should take 36 to 48 hours. An intragastric drip of 20 per cent glucose in water is thought by many to be valuable. When the blood glucose level is below 20 mg per 100 ml (1·1 mmol/1 it is better to give 10 g/dl dextrose in water by continuous i v infusion, 60 ml per kg per day. Milk feeds can be started if the infant survives for 48 hours. Infection must be combated with i m cloxacillin and ampicillin.

HYPERBILIRUBINAEMIA

The elucidation of the normal pathways of bilirubin metabolism has been followed by the development of practical measures for the treatment of hyperbilirubinaemia in the neonatal period. Its frequent association with severe brain damage (kernicterus or nuclear jaundice) has long been recognised and is now preventable.

Bilirubin, which is derived from haemoglobin breakdown, circulates in the plasma loosely bound to albumin. It is fat-soluble but not water-soluble. It gives an indirect van den Bergh reaction and is not excreted in the urine. If the serum level of ' indirect ' bilirubin rise above 20 mg per 100 ml (342 μmol/1) it may enter the brain and cause kernicterus, which is irreversible. In normal people ' indirect ' bilirubin is conjugated in the liver with glucuronic acid to form bilirubin diglucuronide (' direct ' bilirubin) and it then passes into the intercellular bile canaliculi and is excreted in the gut. ' Direct ' or conjugated bilirubin is water-soluble and may be excreted in the urine, but as it is fat-insoluble it does not enter the brain even in the presence of high serum levels. The conjugation of bilirubin in the liver is dependent upon the presence of adequate amounts of the enzyme glucuronyl transferase. The adult liver has a large reserve capacity for the conjugation of ' indirect ' bilirubin. In the newborn, this function is immature and readily overwhelmed by an increased rate of red cell breakdown, such as occurs in haemolytic disease of the newborn, with resulting high serum levels of ' indirect ' bilirubin. In the premature infant, in fact, functional immaturity of the transferase enzyme system may be so marked that dangerously high levels of ' indirect ' bilirubin in the serum may be reached in the absence of excess haemolysis and when the rate of red cell destruction is entirely normal. These facts explain why the newborn infant has, in the past, been so vulnerable to the effects of jaundice, whereas in the older person even severe haemolytic processes are rarely associated with brain damage. In obstructive types of jaundice such as biliary atresia and viral hepatitis the circulating bile-pigment is, of course, in the conjugated or ' direct ' form which being fat-insoluble, cannot enter the nerve cells. It is, on the other hand water-soluble and freely enters the urine.

Clinical features

Hyperbilirubinaemia is most often due to Rhesus incompatibility (when jaundice appears within a few hours of birth), to ABO in-compatibility (maternal blood group O, infant's group A or B, when jaundice appears during the first or second day), or to prematurity (when severe jaundice may develop during or after the second day of life) (Mollison, 1959). In certain parts of the world such as Greece, Singapore and Sardinia hyperbilirubinaemia in the early days of life appears frequently to be due to a sex-linked inherited deficiency of the red cell enzyme glucose-6-phosphate dehydro-genase (see p. 272). In this type of haemolytic disease the preponder-ance of males is marked. Hyperbilirubinaemia must be distinguished from ' physiological ' jaundice which is due to mild temporary im-maturity of the liver enzyme system. This occurs in otherwise healthy infants about the second or third day and disappears in seven to 10 days. Haemolytic disease due to Rhesus incompatibility should be foreseen by finding a rising titre of antibodies in the mother's serum during pregnancy; confirmation of the diagnosis should be based on a positive Coombs' test in cord blood obtained at the time of delivery. Haemolytic disease due to ABO incompatibility, and to other rare factors, should be suspected when a healthy infant develops jaundice of unusual severity during the first or second day of life. Confirmation should be sought by the demonstration in the mother's serum of immune antibodies specific for A or B antigen. Every small premature infant should be carefully watched for the appearance of jaundice; if it appears the serum bilirubin level should be estimated daily until it starts to fall. In all these conditions the serum bilirubin is in the ' indirect ' form. A high serum level of ' direct ' bilirubin will be associated with bile in the urine and indicates obstructive jaundice in which there is no danger of kernic-terus.

If kernicterus develops the infant becomes lethargic and refuses to suck. He may show twitching, rolling of the eyes, hypertonicity and head retraction. When this happens it means that the physician has failed to realise that a state of emergency existed, or if he did, that he has failed to deal with it. The damage to the brain will leave the child mentally handicapped, athetotic and partially deaf, a high price to pay for lack of watchfulness.

The probable severity of haemolytic disease can now be accurately predicted by spectrophotometric examination of the liquor amnii obtained by amniocentesis from the twenty-eighth week of pregnancy or earlier (Liley, 1961). Common indications for this test are a history of a previous stillbirth or severely affected infant, or an indirect Coombs' antibody titre which exceeds 1:8 by 32 weeks gestation. When this examination suggests the likelihood of a moderately severely affected infant labour is usually induced at 36 weeks. If the analysis of the amniotic fluid suggests a severely affected fetus with the probability of intrauterine death or the birth of a hydropic infant the use of intrauterine transfusion is recommended (Liley, 1965). In either situation exchange transfusion soon after birth is likely to be required.

Treatment (of children of Jehovah's Witnesses: see p. 660)

In haemolytic disease due to Rhesus incompatibility dangerous levels of bilirubin in the serum must be prevented by timely replacement transfusion via the umbilical vein. It may have to be repeated on several occasions in the most severely affected infants. The purposes of the early exchange transfusion are: (1) to remove damaged red cells from the circulation, (2) to remove red cells which are susceptible to the circulating Rhesus antibodies, (3) to remove unfixed antibodies, (4) to correct anaemia. The indications for early replacement transfusion are: (1) a haemoglobin level in umbilical cord blood below 15 g per 100 ml (15 g/dl), (2) a bilirubin level in cord blood above 5 mg per 100 ml (85·5 μmol/l), (3) a history of a previously affected infant, (4) premature birth; (3) and (4) to be regarded as imperative indications irrespective of (1) and (2). On the other hand, the sole purpose of delayed or repeated exchange transfusions is to remove ' indirect ' bilirubin from the tissues and the circulation. The indication for this manoeuvre in haemolytic disease of the newborn is a serum bilirubin level of 20 mg per 100 ml (342 μmol/l) during the first five days of life. In the hyperbilirubinaemia of prematurity the peak level in the serum is usually reached somewhat later, fifth to eighth day, and the danger of exchange transfusion is greater in the feeble low birth weight baby. It is probably safer to avoid exchange transfusion until and unless the serum bilirubin exceeds 24 mg per 100 mg (410 μmol/1) (Wishingrad *et al.*, 1965). The risks of replacement transfusion such as cardiac failure, hyperkalaemia, alkalotic tetany and sepsis are small in experienced hands, but they tend to be high in hospitals where cases are too few to allow of adequate mastery of the technique.

In recent years two other methods of combatting hyperbilirubin-aemia in the newborn have been introduced. One is the use of phenobarbitone as an ' enzyme inducer '. To be effective it must be started at birth and before icterus develops. It is given i m in a daily dose of 8 mg per kg as two twelve-hourly injections (Carswell *et al.*, 1972). The other is phototherapy by which the infant is exposed to blue or white light (wave length 420-480 nm) for periods of 12 to 48 hours, the eyes being carefully protected (Tabb *et al.*, 1972). This method is used once jaundice has appeared and reduces the serum bilirubin by photo-oxidation to biliverdin or other intermediate products. Both methods may reduce the number of exchange transfusions in haemolytic disease and in premature infants but their precise value and possible dangers have not yet been fully ascertained. In some neonatal units i m phenobarbitone is now used in all small pre-term infants from the day of birth.

It is of practical importance to note, also, that menaphthone (vitamin K analogue), novobiocin and sulphafurazole (Gantrisin) have been shown to increase considerably the risks of kernicterus in premature infants. They should, therefore, no longer be used. Vitamin K_1 (phytomenadione), however, does not carry this risk.

CARDIAC FAILURE IN EARLY INFANCY

Cardiac failure in the neonatal period, or shortly after, is due most often to paroxysmal supraventricular tachycardia (p. 250), congenital anomalies such as large ventricular septal defects, patent ductus arteriosus and coarctation of the aorta (often combined), transposition of the great vessels, and, less commonly, to endocardial fibroelastosis. A rare cause is acute myocarditis due to Coxsackie virus.

Diagnosis is more often delayed by a lack of awareness on the part of the doctor than by any difficulties in the mode of presenta-tion. Dyspnoea develops in an apparently healthy infant some days or weeks after birth. This is associated with disinclination to suck, restlessness, and there may be vomiting. The infant has a greyish colour and may be cyanosed. Oedema is a late sign and frequently first seen in the face, later spreading to legs, genitalia and lumbo-sacral area. An early sign is hepatomegaly but venous overdisten-sion is difficult to appreciate. Crepitations heard over the lungs may be misinterpreted as infective in origin; indeed, respiratory infection frequently precipitates overt cardiac failure in these infants. The heart will be found to be enlarged by both clinical and radiological examination. In paroxysmal tachycardia its rate approaches 300 per minute. In the congenital defects loud murmurs are heard, but are usually absent in endocardial fibroelastosis. The electrocardiogram is always abnormal but the findings will obviously vary with the cause. It is often of considerable value in the future management. Precise diagnosis is often difficult but this can be achieved with such ancillary methods as cardiac catheterisation and angiocardiography after the cardiac failure has been brought under control.

Treatment

The results of treatment of cardiac failure in infancy are often gratifying and in most cases the immediate emergency can be overcome. Dyspnoea, restlessness or cyanosis should be relieved by placing the infant in an oxygen tent or incubator with the head raised above the level of the feet. While dyspnoea is marked, feeds may be given by tube and the daily fluid intake should be restricted to 150 ml per kg body weight. The mainstay of treatment is rapid digitalisation. Digoxin is available in liquid form for infants (Lanoxin paediatric elixir, 1 ml containing 0·05 mg). The initial dosage should be 0·08 mg per kg body weight per day in four divided doses. In a severe emergency the first one or two doses may be given i m. After 24 to 36 hours, depending upon the response as measured by heart rate and electrocardiogram, the maintenance dosage should be in the region of 0·02 mg per kg per day in two or four divided doses. If oedema is marked or fails to disappear with digitalisation chlorothiazide, 25 mg per kg per day, should be given in two or four doses, or frusemide, 5 mg per kg per day in a single dose. On these drugs it is necessary to monitor the serum potassium level every few days. It may be necessary to prescribe potassium chloride 500 mg twice daily or potassium gluconate as Katorin (Boots) 5 ml twice daily. In paroxysmal tachycardia of the young infant the long-term prognosis is excellent as the heart is usually structurally normal. It is, however, essential that a maintenance dose of digoxin be continued for six months to ensure against recurrence. When the cardiac failure is due to a congenital defect the infant should be transferred to a centre which specialises in the cardiac surgery of infancy as soon as he is fit to be moved. Cases of endocardial fibroelastosis have a less happy prognosis and recovery is rarely seen.

INTESTINAL OBSTRUCTION IN THE NEWBORN

In recent years the results of major surgery in the newborn have greatly improved. Indeed, the newborn withstands major surgery remarkably well, provided his electrolytes and acid-base balance have not been too severely disordered by the effects of intestinal obstruction. Early diagnosis is, therefore, imperative. It should always be suspected when there is a history of hydramnios during the pregnancy. The obstruction may be complete as in duodenal or ileal atresia, and meconium ileus; or it may be partial and intermittent as in obstruction of the duodenum by the root of the mesentery due to malrotation of the caecum, in annular pancreas, and in Hirschprung's disease. Precise diagnosis of the cause is often not possible but this is relatively unimportant as operation is always necessary.

The presenting symptom is vomiting from or soon after birth. The vomit is usually bile-stained. *Bilious vomiting in the newborn infant should always be assumed to indicate intestinal obstruction until the contrary is proved.* When the duodenum is obstructed abdominal distension is at first absent. Later the stomach may distend the epigastrium and peristalsis may be visible, until vomiting again empties the stomach. In ileal or colonic obstruction abdominal distension is marked. When the obstruction is complete there is absolute constipation. When it is partial, meconium may be passed normally. In Hirschprung's disease the abdominal distension and vomiting may be coincidental with spurious diarrhoea due to colitis. The site of obstruction can be defined by radiographs taken with the patient in both supine and erect positions, and then determining the position at which the dilated loops of bowel containing fluid levels cease. In some cases especially in meconium ileus, the bowel may perforate before birth and then seal itself off again. This results in meconium peritonitis when, in addition to distension, radiographs will reveal the presence of intra-abdominal calcification. In difficult cases additional information can be obtained by fluoroscopy after the introduction by tube of lipiodol into the stomach or of barium into the lower bowel.

Treatment

Bile-stained vomiting always indicates the need for admission to hospital. As i v fluid therapy is necesary when operation on intestinal obstruction is planned the infant is best admitted to a paediatric centre accustomed to the correction of electrolyte disturbances in young infants. This is a situation which can go disastrously wrong in inexpert hands.

For urgent skin conditions in the newborn see p. 548.

INFANCY

(1 month to 1 year)

ACUTE DEHYDRATION

It is well known that infants become more quickly dehydrated than adults. This is due to the different distributions of body water. In the infant, water constitutes about 80 per cent of the fat-free weight, whereas the comparable figure in the adult is 70 per cent. In the newborn the extracellular fluid, of which the main cation is sodium and the anions chloride and bicarbonate (4 : 1), comprises 35 per cent of the body weight, whereas the adult percentage is only 20. On the other hand, the infant's intracellular fluid compartment amounts to 45 per cent of body weight, and contains potassium and phosphate as the principal cations and anions. In the adult the intracellular fluid amounts to 50 per cent of body weight.

Modern methods of rehydration have reduced the death rate to small proportions but they are very demanding of time and effort. Their successful application requires a sound knowledge of the mechanisms of fluid, electrolyte and acid-base balance. Good laboratory facilities are very helpful but not absolutely essential.

Causes and biochemical consequences

It is important to recognise that dehydration may arise in different ways with different biochemical and functional consequences. **Hypertonic dehydration** occurs when the loss of body water, mostly from the intracellular compartment, exceeds the loss of electrolytes. This can develop very quickly in the young infant who goes off his feeds because of any infection in which a reduced fluid intake is combined with an increased insensible loss of water through the skin and lungs. Vomiting and diarrhoea may aggravate the situation. It must never be forgotten that the ill, fevered baby, unlike the adult, cannot ask for more fluids. Hypernatraemia has also occurred in infants because they have been given feeds of excessively high electrolyte concentration. This can occur when a mother in reconstituting a dried milk preparation uses heaped up measures of the milk powder instead of levelled-off measures as instructed by the manufacturers. Even at the correct concentration cow's milk preparations contain several times the electrolyte concentrations

as human milk. The recently introduced low solute milk preparations should reduce the risks of hypernatraemia in young infants.
*It cannot be overemphasised that the infant's fluid intake must be
assured at all times and particularly when he is ill or anorexic.* In
hypertonic dehydration there is hypernatraemia (a known cause
of permanent brain damage), hyperchloraemia, raised blood urea,
raised serum osmolality, and, often, metabolic acidosis. On the other
hand, haemoconcentration, oligaemia and peripheral circulatory
failure do not commonly occur.

In **hypotonic dehydration** the losses of electrolytes from vomiting, diarrhoea or into the urine exceed the loss of body water, while
in **isotonic dehydration,** from much the same causes, the losses of
water and electrolytes, are proportional. These types of dehydration may develop in pyloric stenosis, intestinal obstruction, gastroenteritis, paralytic ileus and severe burns or scalds. A rare but
important cause is the type of congenital adrenal hyperplasia in
which there is excessive loss of sodium chloride into the urine so that
an adrenal crisis occurs (see p. 355). These infants are often called
' salt losers '. In hypotonic and isotonic dehydration with marked
losses of electrolytes the plasma volume must be reduced to maintain
the osmotic pressure of the body fluids. The resultant oligaemia may
cause fatal peripheral circulatory failure, and haemoconcentration
will be reflected in high levels of haemoglobin (in the absence of
preceding anaemia), packed cell volume and serum proteins. On
the other hand, the haemoconcentration so distorts the serum electrolyte levels that they cannot reliably reflect the extent of the losses
from the body. Diminution in the glomerular filtration rate results
in a raised blood urea. The acid/base status in these types of
dehydration varies with the cause. In pyloric stenosis the high loss
of chloride ions from the stomach results in a metabolic alkalosis,
whereas in infantile diarrhoea with large losses of sodium (and
potassium) in the stools metabolic acidosis is common. In low
intestinal obstruction and paralytic ileus large amounts of potassium are lost into the distended bowel and there is often a hypokalaemic alkalosis. In all these causes of dehydration there are
excessive losses of potassium from the cells and *after* the dehydration has been corrected the serum potassium level will frequently
be found to be low with concomitant electrocardiographic changes.
In contrast to these causes, the ' salt loser ' with adrenal hyperplasia
shows a high urinary excretion of chloride with a low serum chloride
but raised serum potassium levels. Indeed, an adrenal crisis should
be suspected in any markedly dehydrated infant whose urine
contains abundant chlorides. The next steps must be to look for

hyperkalaemia and the characteristic effect of this upon the electro-cardiogram (see p. 605).

Clinical features

The earliest signs are an anxious expression, restlessness, sleep-lessness, thirst, red lips and dry tongue. Fluids are taken eagerly but may be vomited. Weight loss amounts to $2\frac{1}{2}$ to 5 per cent of body weight. Later the eyes become sunken, the anterior fontanelle is depressed and normal skin turgor disappears. A constant wailing cry, dry tongue and pale or cyanosed lips complete the picture. Weight loss increases to 10 to 15 per cent of body weight. When peripheral circulatory collapse develops the infant lies limp and apathetic, with an ashen pallor, deeply sunken eyes and fontanelle, scaphoid abdomen and no further ability to suck or to cry. The body skin is cold to the touch although the rectal temperature may be high. The infant may be semiconscious and the eyes are often rolled upwards, the cornea being glazed and the conjunctiva injected. At this stage death is imminent and resuscitation is urgently re-quired. In hypertonic dehydration, however, where the loss of water is mainly from the intracellular compartment, the external signs of dehydration are often misleadingly slight.

Tachycardia is a constant sign. Respiration varies with the state of the acid-base balance. In alkalotic states respiration is slow and shallow to conserve free CO_2. In acidosis there may be rapid, sigh-ing, pauseless breathing (air-hunger). In some infants with high fever there may be rapid shallow 'canine' breathing. Oliguria is marked. Albuminuria and casts are frequently found. The urinary chlorides are usually diminished, especially in pyloric stenosis. A striking exception is seen in the salt-losing adrenogenital syndrome where they are greatly increased. This syndrome is readily diag-nosed in female infants whose genitalia show masculinisation. In male infants, however, the cause of the profound dehydration and collapse will not be obvious until the high level of chloride is demon-strated in the urine. It is important to obtain a specimen of urine from every dehydrated infant at the first opportunity (see p. 355).

Biochemical assessment

While it is not possible to measure the losses from the body of water or electrolytes by estimations of the individual levels in plasma or serum such measurements are a useful guide to treatment of severely ill infants. In *hypertonic dehydration* the serum levels of sodium and chloride are raised. The higher the serum sodium, osmolality and urea the more common are depression of conscious-ness and convulsions, and the greater the risk of brain damage

(Morris-Jones *et al.*, 1967). In *hypotonic or isotonic dehydration* haemoconcentration and shifts of sodium and potassium between the intra- and extracellular fluid spaces confuse the picture. Sodium levels in the serum are variable save in an adrenal crisis when hyponatraemia is common. Large losses of body potassium will not be reflected in hypokalaemia because of the haemoconcentration, although the serum potassium often falls to low levels *after* the initial correction of dehydration. There will then be present characteristic changes in the electrocardiogram. In an adrenal crisis, on the other hand, hyperkalaemia is the rule with corresponding electrocardiographic abnormalities. Severe metabolic acidosis will produce a low blood pH, low plasma standard bicarbonate and marked base deficit (Astrup technique). In metabolic alkalosis the blood pH and plasma standard bicarbonate are raised and there is a base excess. It will be apparent, therefore, that while the biochemical findings in the severely dehydrated infant must be interpreted with caution they can provide the clinician with valuable information for the planning of therapy.

Treatment

When there is pyloric or intestinal obstruction surgical relief is imperative, but it must be preceded by rapid correction of the dehydration. In gastroenteritis milk feeds must be withdrawn for a period, during which vomiting and diarrhoea usually subside. They should be restarted in carefully graduated amounts or concentrations when the dehydration has been corrected, usually after 24 to 48 hours.

The correction of the dehydration itself has long been an area of therapeutics in which there is controversy, and a large number of multi-electrolyte solutions have been devised. To a large extent these differences in practice merely reflect the fact that, provided kidney function is not seriously impaired, the glomerular filtration and tubular reabsorption mechanisms can compensate for widely varying intakes of water and electrolytes, and so return the composition of the body fluids towards normal. Mild degrees of dehydration can usually be corrected in the home by offering the infant quarter-strength isosmotic sodium chloride solution (1 teaspoonful of salt to two and a half litres of water). This is given by mouth in small volumes at two-hourly intervals to a total daily intake of 200 ml per kg. A palatable alternative is Electrosol.* One tablet in 125 ml of water makes a solution which should be given in a daily amount of

* McCarthys Ltd., Chesham House, Chesham Close, Romford, Essex, RM1 4JX. Romford 46033 (STD 0708).

200 ml per kg. *It is much more urgent to ensure an adequate fluid intake for the ill anorexic infant than to prescribe an antibiotic.* If this proves impossible because of vomiting or reluctance to suck, or if the baby is already severely dehydrated, immediate admission to hospital is required for i v fluid therapy. This is a demanding regime best carried out in specialised paediatric units under biochemical control. Too much water with too little electrolyte can result in water intoxication, convulsions and brain damage; whereas an excess of electrolyte can aggravate acidosis and loss of potassium, or lead to oedema.

In hypertonic dehydration the high serum sodium and chloride levels must be reduced slowly. Too rapid a rehydration may result in cerebral oedema and convulsions. A suitable regime is the continuous i v infusion of dextrose 50 g/l of quarter-strength isosmotic sodium chloride solution, 100-150 ml per kg per 24 hours. For hypotonic or isotonic dehydration, in which serum sodium and chloride levels are normal or low, suitable i v fluids are 5 per cent dextrose in half-strength isosmotic sodium chloride solution, and equal parts of citrated plasma and dextrose 100 g/l of water. If dehydration is very severe and there are signs of peripheral circulatory failure (' oligaemic shock ') the most useful solution for rapid reconstruction of the plasma volume is the citrated plasma/dextrose water mixture given rapidly by syringe in a dose of 45 ml per kg. Thereafter a continuous infusion of the plasma/dextrose solution followed by dextrose 5 g/dl of half-strength saline can be continued at a rate of 150 to 200 ml per kg per 24 hours. Severe metabolic acidosis is best corrected by periodic i v doses of 8·4 per cent sodium bicarbonate (1 ml=mol) controlled by frequent esimations of the blood pH, $PaCO_2$ and base excess on the Astrup apparatus (or equivalent). A suitable formula for calculation of the dose of sodium bicarbonate has already been given on p. 398. *In the newborn infant it is important to give i v fluids in much smaller quantities than those previously mentioned, the daily intake not to exceed 65 ml per kg.* It is also safer to avoid stronger concentrations of saline than quarter-strength isosmotic sodium chloride solution because of the relative inefficiency of the newborn infant's kidneys.

When dehydration of any type has been overcome the severe losses of intracellular potassium in stools and urine are likely to be reflected in a reduced serum potassium level and electrocardiographic changes. At this stage in treatment, but never in the initial stage of dehydration, hypokalaemia can be corrected by adding potassium chloride to the infusion fluid in a concentration of 10 to 20 mmol per litre (1 g potassium chloride = 13 mmol). I v potassium therapy must only be instituted when there are facilities for frequent serum estimations and electrocardiograms. In their absence, it is safer but less rapid to give potassium chloride 1 to 2 g daily by mouth. Milk is also a useful source of potassium once oral fluids are tolerated. Where there is concomitant anaemia blood transfusion (20 to 30 ml per kg) may be required after initial rehydration. The successful treatment of dehydration depends upon meticulous attention to detail such as charting the fluid intake and losses by the various routes. Daily weighing gives a very reasonable assessment of the state of fluid balance in the young infant. The author has not found any significant advantage from the use of some of the more complex multi-electrolyte solutions which have been devised for parenteral therapy.

When dehydration is due to gastroenteritis antibiotics may be prescribed, e.g. oral neomycin 50 mg per kg per day or colistin 150 000 units per kg per day. Their value, however, in infantile diarrhoea is doubtful and much less important than the prevention or correction of dehydration. When there is severe circulatory collapse it is common practice to give hydrocortisone, i m or i v, in doses of 50 mg six-hourly for 48 to 72 hours. Its value is only undoubted in the salt-losing syndrome due to adrenal hyperplasia. Indeed, in this condition permanent steroid therapy will be necessary to suppress adrenal over-activity and to maintain salt balance. A mineralocorticoid will also be required such as deoxycorticosterone acetate, 1 mg i m twice or thrice daily, until the acute adrenal crisis has been overcome. Finally, the value of oxygen in severely shocked or dehydrated infants should never be forgotten.

ACUTE BRONCHIOLITIS IN INFANCY

An earlier generation of physicians called this capillary bronchitis or bronchopneumonia. The term bronchiolitis serves to distinguish it from the bacterial pneumonias, of which the most common nowadays is staphylococcal. In bronchiolitis there is no massive consolidation detectable clinically or radiologically, and suppuration in the form of lung abscesses and empyema does not occur. Most cases are caused by the respiratory syncytial (RS) virus (Elderkin et al., 1965; Medical Research Council, 1965) although it is likely that several viruses can cause this type of lower respiratory tract infection. Certainly none of the antibiotics are to be expected to cause any rapid improvement.

Clinical features

The disease is seen only in infants, in whom it produces a distinctive clinical picture. It is most common in the winter and early spring, and in some recent years has proved a heavy burden in the wards of paediatric and isolation hospitals. The infant often has signs of upper respiratory catarrh for a few days before the sudden onset of acute respiratory difficulties which are aggravated by a frequent spasmodic cough. Dyspnoea is the most striking clinical sign. It is associated with pronounced inspiratory indrawing of the lower chest wall and of the suprasternal notch. However, expiration is often even more distressing and prolonged. Hypoxia may produce an extreme agitated restlessness. Greyish cyanosis is common. Consolidation is not clinically demonstrable although radiographs may reveal segmental or lobar atelectasis. The usual picture is of hypertranslucency and depression of the diaphragm and this is often associated with hyper-resonance to percussion. Auscultation reveals prolongation of expiration, often with many rhonchi. Numerous inspiratory crepitations are also common. Fever is usually slight (37.7 to 38·3°C), but tachycardia may be severe. Dehydration may develop from the summation of several factors, e.g., increased insensible water loss from tachypnoea, inability to take fluids because of dyspnoea, and vomiting caused by the spasms of coughing. In severe cases it is common to find evidence of a respiratory acidosis in the form of a fall in the blood pH and a rise in the $PaCO_2$. Considerable falls in the arterial PaO_2 (obtained by femoral or radial artery puncture) (see also p. 745) are also common.

Treatment

Even the most severely ill infants usually recover with adequate treatment. Skilled nursing is at a premium and rarely to be found outside good hospitals. Affected infants are usually more comfortable when propped up. Frequent suction of the pharynx is often required, for which purpose an electric suction pump is a great advantage. Infrequently, bronchoscopic suction, or even tracheal intubation with intermittent positive pressure respiration and periodic aspiration of mucopus has been life-saving. Cyanosis, restlessness and sleeplessness are frequently abolished rapidly, even dramatically, by placing the infant in a cool, humid and oxygen-rich atmosphere. Suitable apparatus is the Oxymist (Vickers Medical) or Croupette (Air Shields, Inc.). It has been increasingly recognised that the administration of oxygen to dyspnoeic infants has in the past been too haphazard. It is not infrequent to find oxygen running into a tent at too low a flow rate, or with the sides of the tent inadequately secured so that the concentration of oxygen within the tent is not much greater than that in the room air. The concentration of oxygen in the tent should be maintained at not less than 40 per cent and periodically checked with a paramagnetic oximeter. In severely dyspnoeic infants it is extremely helpful to monitor the PaO_2 and $PaCO_2$ levels periodically on arterialised capillary blood (Doig, 1971). The PaO_2 should be maintained above 70 mm Hg (9·3 kPa) by adjusting the oxygen concentration in the tent. There is no danger of CO_2 narcosis in these infants. Indeed the indication for instituting intermittent positive pressure ventilation is a $PaCO_2$ which rises above 70 mm Hg (9·3 kPa). An adequate fluid intake is important. If milk is not tolerated glucose 50 g/l of quarter strength isosmotic sodium chloride solution may be given by mouth or in rare cases, by i v infusion (150 ml per kg of body weight per day). Antibiotics have little effect and the infant begins to recover spontaneously after 7 to 10 days. The author tends to prescribe them only if the chest radiograph shows pneumonic consolidation which is exceptional. In the worst cases hydrocortisone may be given i m, 100 mg in the first 24 hours and in diminishing doses over the next few days, but it is difficult to assess its value in this situation.

CHILDHOOD

(1 year to puberty)

ACUTE STRIDOR (see also p. 224)

Acute laryngeal obstruction in this country today is most often due to acute laryngo-tracheitis. This is probably a viral infection in most cases, although in some, laryngeal swabs have yielded bacteria such as *Haemophilus influenzae*, haemolytic streptococci, pneumococci and coagulase-positive staphylococci. In some of the most fulminating cases the pathology is limited to an acute epiglottitis. In these cases *Haemophilus influenzae* can be cultured from both larynx and blood. Acute stridor may occur in measles before the appearance of the rash. Less common causes of stridor are laryngeal diphtheria, papillomata of the larynx, inhaled foreign body and acute retropharyngeal abscess. Laryngismus stridulus due to hypocalcaemia has disappeared together with rickets.

In acute laryngo-tracheitis the onset may be abrupt or it may follow upon a few days of mild fever, malaise and hoarseness. Thereafter the main features are increasing inspiratory difficulty with an audible wheeze or crow, the use of the accessory muscles of respiration, and severe inspiratory indrawing of the suprasternal notch and the supraclavicular fossae. The child looks frightened. Hypoxia produces restlessness and sleeplessness, and later, overt cyanosis. Fever is usually high. There may also be signs of bronchitis. In diphtheria fever is usually slight and the child often has a grey toxic look. The child with a large pyogenic retropharyngeal abscess (p. 223) may have stridor but he is not hoarse. He sometimes adopts a characteristic posture with neck fully extended, elbows on a table and chin supported in his hands. A fluctuant mass can be palpated arising from the posterior pharyngeal wall. Inhalation of a foreign body may happen in the absence of an adult observer. Stridor may be extreme but fever is absent. In papilloma of the larynx there may be recurring attacks of stridor without fever. Indeed, stridor of sudden onset without fever is an indication for immediate direct laryngoscopy.

Treatment

Every child with laryngeal obstruction associated with fever should be given 24 000 units of diphtheria antitoxin i m, irrespective of a history of active immunisation. Thereafter he should be placed in an atmosphere which is cool, humid and rich in oxygen, such as can be achieved with an Oxymist or Croupette. This is much more effective than the traditional steam tent. Antibiotic therapy should depend on the results of cultures but ampicillin given i m (50 mg per kg per day) is the drug for initial treatment as it is effective against *H. influenzae*. Severe or increasing stridor is an indication for tracheostomy. The necessary apparatus should be immediately available and it should be performed before the child is obviously cyanosed. Postoperative care demands skilled nursing, night and day. An inhaled foreign body must be removed through the laryngoscope or bronchoscope before it can set up severe inflammation or oedema. Papillomata may require prolonged treatment, sometimes including tracheostomy, by a laryngologist.

CONVULSIONS

The causes of convulsions in early childhood are legion. They include organic intracranial disease such as pyogenic and viral meningitis, intracranial neoplasms, head injury, subdural haematoma, encephalitis and the hypertensive encephalopathy of acute nephritis. The term epilepsy is usually reserved for a state in which recurring convulsions or lapses of consciousness occur without obvious precipitating cause. Nowadays hypocalcaemic convulsions (tetany) are rare after the neonatal period. By far the commonest type of convulsion to which doctors are called in emergency is the so-called 'febrile convulsion' which seizes an apparently normal child at the onset of some acute infection. This is rare before the age of 6 months, nor should such a reassuring explanation be lightly accepted after the age of 5 years.

The most common variety of convulsion is the generalised tonic and clonic major seizure, but the fit may vary from a few myoclonic jerks to sudden loss of consciousness without rigidity or twitching. A febrile convulsion may herald the onset of any kind of infection, e.g., upper respiratory inflammation, acute pyelonephritis or bacillary dysentery. It seems to be related more to the speed and height of the rise in body temperature than to the causal organism. It is usually a solitary fit of short duration. Most paediatricians think that the solitary febrile convulsion is only rarely a precursor of established epilepsy, and that a reassuring prognosis is justifiable. A convulsion of long duration (over half an hour) or repeated convulsions in the course of an infection warrant a much more guarded prognosis. An electroencephalogram is of limited usefulness in this situation because prolonged anti-convulsant therapy is rarely indicated on the strength of a single convulsive episode, and an abnormal EEG does not invariably imply recurrence of convulsions. Nonetheless, a gross abnormality in the EEG does indicate a greater likelihood of recurrence.

Management (see also p. 310)

It is wise to give the alarmed parents something to do before the doctor can reach the patient. The traditional hot mustard bath can only further raise the body temperature and is contraindicated. A tepid sponge is a rational method of lowering the temperature. The doctor's first duty is to look for evidence of organic disease, intracranial or extracranial, on the basis of the history of the events leading up to the fit and careful physical examination, which should include inspection of the throat, ears, and ocular fundi. By this time the convulsion will often have ceased spontaneously. A prolonged convulsion in a young child carries with it the risk of causing asphyxial sclerosis in the temporal lobe and subsequent temporal lobe epilepsy (Falconer, 1968). It must therefore be stopped as quickly as possible. The drug of choice for this purpose is now diazepam (Valium) 2 to 10 mg by i m or slow i v injection. It is also important to maintain a clear airway and to give oxygen if there is cyanosis. Paraldehyde 0·15 ml per kg, sodium phenobarbitone 5 mg per kg and phenytoin sodium 50 to 100 mg may be given i m in a grand mal seizure or in status epilepticus but they are less effective. Sulphonamides and antibiotics should always be withheld until an accurate diagnosis has been made. It is easy to mask serious meningeal infections or to make successful cultures and sensitivity tests impossible by the unnecessarily hasty administration of antibacterial drugs. Many infections are viral and unresponsive to such drugs. When the convulsion has ceased and the child has been made comfortable the doctor can well spend some time in explanation and reassurance for the parents, who may, indeed, be as much in need of a sedative as the patient. Multiple, severe and prolonged convulsions call for a careful review and special investigations.

INTESTINAL BLEEDING (see also p. 157)

The sudden appearance of severe melaena is not very uncommon in older infants and young children. The most common source of such bleeding is a peptic ulcer which has developed in the presence of acid-producing heterotopic gastric mucosa situated in a Meckel's diverticulum or in a duplication of bowel. Haematemesis and melaena may both occur, as in the adult, from a duodenal ulcer. This is less rare than has been thought in the past. Bleeding may also come from oesophageal varices produced by portal hypertension arising from such causes as hepatic cirrhosis, thrombosis of the splenic or portal veins, or congenital malformation of the portal vein in the porta hepatis. Intestinal bleeding may also complicate disorders of the blood and capillaries such as thrombocytopenic and anaphylactoid purpuras, leukaemia and clotting deficiencies. A rare cause is polyposis of the duodenum and jejunum (Puetz-Jeghers syndrome). This is unrelated to the better known familial polyposis of the colon and it is not premalignant.

Severe intestinal bleeding will produce the usual signs of pallor, restlessness, cold clammy skin, tachycardia and hypotension. The source of the haemorrhage is not usually immediately obvious and investigations will often have to await replacement of blood loss by transfusion. Duodenal ulceration can be visualised by fluoroscopy after a barium drink. Typical ulcer symptoms with ' hunger-pain ' are unusual in childhood, but there is frequently a preceding history of recurring attacks of generalised abdominal pain, nausea and vomiting. Portal hypertension is associated with a firm and enlarged spleen. Oesophageal varices may be demonstrated by a barium swallow or by oesophagoscopy. It is rarely possible to visualise a Meckel's diverticulum or duplication of bowel by radiography and a tentative diagnosis must depend on a process of exclusion, to be confirmed by laparotomy. Blood diseases usually produce other signs of their presence such as skin haemorrhages and abnormalities in the peripheral blood. In anaphylactoid purpura the typical rash distributed over the buttocks and extensor aspects of the limbs, the frequent joint pains, and the severe abdominal pain serve to differentiate from other causes of intestinal bleeding which are usually painless. The Peutz-Jeghers syndrome is associated with a characteristic distribution of small areas of pigmentation, like freckles, over the lips and the mucous membrane of the mouth.

Treatment

Blood transfusion is urgently required for the exsanguinated, shocked, restless child. When bleeding is less rapid the indications for transfusion are a haemoglobin level below 5 g/dl, and a falling blood pressure with rising pulse rate, both of which should be recorded hourly. It is perfectly safe to carry out a barium meal soon after haemorrhage. If the findings are negative, and bleeding continues or recurs, a laparotomy is indicated as the only means to confirm and treat a Meckel's diverticulum or duplication. Surgical treatment such as partial gastrectomy or vagotomy combined with a drainage procedure, should be avoided as long as possible in the child with a duodenal ulcer. The parents should be instructed that such a child must never be given aspirin in any form. The results of portocaval shunts in young children have been dismal. Cases of portal hypertension have a better chance of survival from repeated blood transfusions, at least until adolescence has been reached. In thrombocytopenic purpura and acute leukaemia remissions may be most rapidly obtained by steroids, e.g., prednisolone 15 mg six-hourly, the dose being gradually reduced at 10 day intervals. Splenectomy as an *emergency* operation in purpura is probably never necessary nowadays. There is no specific treatment available for anaphylactoid purpura but complete recovery is the rule if haemorrhage is adequately treated.

CYCLICAL VOMITING

Cyclical vomiting is one of the manifestations of the ' periodic syndrome '. This condition, which has no recognised organic basis, is most often encountered in nervous, over-protected children of good intelligence. They are not infrequently only children. A family history of migraine can often be obtained, and indeed, the child who is a victim of cyclical vomiting may also complain of headaches. The condition has often been referred to as ' acidosis '. This is unfortunate. A state of metabolic acidosis with diminished plasma bicarbonate is only found in the most severe cases, and it should be realised that although ketonuria is present in every case this is not evidence of acidosis. Nevertheless, a severe attack of cyclical vomiting is an emergency which can be very worrying for the physician who has to differentiate it from the other more dangerous causes of intractable vomiting such as high intestinal obstruction and diabetic precoma.

The condition is rare before the age of 3 years. The attacks of vomiting may each last several days. They are periodic and irregular rather than cyclical. Some seem to be precipitated by minor infections, some by emotional upsets, but many have no obvious cause. After a short period of nausea and anorexia, in which the child looks pale and drawn and may pass a pale stool, vomiting starts. It is frequently repeated and even sips of water may be returned. Soon the vomit is bile-stained and it may contain altered blood. Constipation is often severe. Rarely there is diarrhoea. Generalised abdominal discomfort and tenderness on palpation are mainly due to the persistent retching. In severe attacks the child becomes markedly dehydrated with dry tongue, sunken eyes and scaphoid abdomen. Metabolic acidosis with deep, rapid, pauseless and acyanotic air hunger is, in fact, quite rare. A sweet smell of acetone from the breath is constant and associated with marked ketonuria.

Differential diagnosis

It is sometimes extremely difficult to exclude high intestinal obstruction. This may be due to volvulus of a malrotated intestine so that the third part of the duodenum is obstructed by the root of the mesentery, and it too can be recurring and periodic. If it does not undo itself spontaneously within a short time only surgical intervention can save the patient's life. Acetonuria and ketosis may also develop in high intestinal obstruction as a consequence of starvation. A useful clinical indication of possible high obstruction is the presence of slow shallow breathing which is due to metabolic alkalosis. This can be quickly confirmed on the Astrup apparatus by the finding of a raised blood pH, elevated plasma standard bicarbonate and considerable base excess.

A first attack of severe cyclical vomiting with acidotic breathing and ketonuria may simulate diabetic pre-coma. However, the blood sugar level, which is always above 300 mg per 100 ml (16·65 mmol/l) in the child with untreated diabetes mellitus, will serve to differentiate it from cyclical vomiting. It should be remembered that if urine from a child with cyclical vomiting is only obtained after treatment with i v glucose solutions it will reduce Benedict's solution. The author has, on several occasions, seen unnecessary alarm produced by this finding.

Treatment

During the period of vomiting sips of glucose 50 to 100 g/l of half-strength isosmotic sodium chloride solution should be given frequently. Chlorpromazine or promazine by injection in doses of 25 mg on one or two occasions, followed by oral administration for a few days, is often a most effective anti-emetic measure. It must, however, never be prescribed if the slightest doubt exists as to the correctness of the diagnosis. When dehydration is marked dextrose 50 g/l of half-strength isosmotic sodium chloride solution should be given by continuous i v infusion, after withdrawing blood for the estimation of serum electrolyte levels and assessment of the acid/base status.

Between attacks the regular administration of phenobarbitone, 30 mg twice or thrice daily, is often effective in reducing their frequency and severity. Few paediatricians, however, are willing to accept this observation as supporting the concept of ' abdominal epilepsy ' (p. 125) which has been advanced. The limitation of dietary fat, high carbohydrate diets, and the use of sodium bicarbonate have often been advised but they are of no value. In the author's view psychiatric treatment is contraindicated.

ACUTE ENGORGEMENT OF THE MOTHER'S BREASTS

This develops early in puerperium and may cause lactation to fail. The breasts become tense and painful and they feel lumpy. Prevention may be achieved by the patient massaging her breasts 12 times a day during pregnancy with both hands from the chest wall towards the areola.

Treatment

A firm brassière should be worn and analgesics given. Heat should not be applied but ice bags are comforting. The infant should be taken off the breast. He cannot obtain milk and may crack the nipple and so increase the risk of mastitis. The breasts must be emptied manually by massage and then rhythmic expression applied between the thumb and forefinger just behind the areola. The mother may manage to do this herself after instruction. Manual expression is more effective and less disturbing than the use of a breast pump. The expressed milk can be fed to the infant from a bottle after sterilisation by boiling. When expression is not tolerated temporary suppression of lactation may be achieved by one single dose of frusemide (Lasix) 40 mg. Drugs like stilboestrol and bromocroptine are not usually advisable. When the breasts are again soft and comfortable three-hourly feeds should be started. Sucking will usually re-establish lactation and on this occasion smoothly.

J. H. HUTCHISON

REFERENCES

Asphyxia neonatorum

BARRIE, H. (1963). Resuscitation of the newborn. *Lancet* **1**, 650.

BEARD, R. W., MORRIS, E. D. & CLAYTON, S. G. (1966). Foetal blood sampling in clinical obstetrics. *Journal of Obstetrics and Gynaecology of the British Commonwealth*, **73**, 562-570.

HUTCHISON, J. H. & KERR, M. M. (1965). Treatment of asphyxia neonatorum by hyperbaric oxygenation. *Annals of the New York Academy of Sciences*, **117**, 706-712.

HUTCHISON, J. H., KERR, M.M., INALL, J. A. & SHANKS, R. A. (1966). Controlled trials of hyperbaric oxygen and tracheal intubation in asphyxia neonatorum. *Lancet*, **1**, 935.

RODGER, J. C., KERR, M. M., RICHARDS, I. D. G. & HUTCHISON, J. H. (1968). Measurements of oxygen tension in subcutaneous tissues of newborn infants under normobaric and hyperbaric conditions. *Lancet*, **2**, 232.

The respiratory distress syndrome of the newborn

ADAMSON, T. M., COLLINS, L. M., DEHAN, M., HAWKER, J. M., REYNOLDS, E. O. R. & STRANG, L. B. (1968). Mechanical ventilation in newborn infants with respiratory failure. *Lancet*, **2**, 227.

CHERNICK, V. & VIDYASAGAR, D. (1972). Continuous negative chest wall pressure in hyaline membrane disease: one year experience. *Pediatrics*, **49**, 753.

GREGORY, G. A., KITTERMAN, J. A., PHIBBS, R. H., TOOLEY, W. H. & HAMILTON, W. K. (1971). Treatment of idiopathic respiratory distress syndrome with continuous positive airway pressure. *New England Journal of Medicine*, **284**, 1333-1340.

HUTCHISON, J. H., KERR, M. M., DOUGLAS, T. A., INALL, J. A. & CROSBIE, J. C. (1964). A therapeutic approach in 100 cases of the respiratory distress syndrome of the newborn infant. *Pediatrics*, **33**, 956.

REYNOLDS, E. O. R. & TAGHIZADEH, A. (1974). Improved prognosis of infants mechanically ventilated for hyaline membrane disease. *Archives of Disease in Childhood*, **49**, 505.

TUNSTALL, M. E., CATER, J. I., THOMSON, J. S. & MITCHELL, R. G. (1968). Ventilating the lungs of newborn infants for prolonged periods. *Archives of Disease in Childhood*, **43**, 486.

WHITFIELD, C. R., CHAN, W. H., SPROULE, W. B. & STEWART, A. D. (1972). Amniotic fluid lecithin:sphingomyelin ratio and fetal lung development. *British Medical Journal*, **2**, 85.

Hypoglycaemia

CAMPBELL, M., FERGUSON, I. C., HUTCHISON, J. H. & KERR, M. M. (1967). Diagnosis and treatment of hypoglycaemia in the newborn. *Archives of Disease in Childhood*, **42**, 353.

CORNBLATH, M. & SCHWARTZ, R. *Disorders of Carbohydrate Metabolism in Infancy*, chap. 5. Philadelphia: Saunders. 1966.

Convulsions

FALCONER, M. A. (1968). The significance of mesial temporal sclerosis (Ammon's horn sclerosis) in epilepsy. *Guy's Hospital Reports*, **117**, 1-12.

Haemorrhage

AHUJA, G. L., WILLOUGHBY, M. L. N., KERR, M. M. & HUTCHISON, J. H. (1969). Massive subaponeurotic haemorrhage in infants born by vacuum extraction. *British Medical Journal,* 3, 743.

ZIPURSKY, A., HULL, A., WHITE, F. D. & ISRAELS, L. G. (1959). Fetal erythrocytes in the maternal circulation. *Lancet,* 1, 451.

Cold injury

ARNEIL, G. C. & KERR, M. M. (1963). Severe hypothermia in Glasgow infants in winter. *Lancet,* 2, 756.

BOWER, B. D., JONES, L. F. & WEEKS, M. M. (1960). Cold injury in the newborn. *British Medical Journal,* 1, 303.

Hyperbilirubinaemia

CARSWELL, F., KERR, M. M. & DUNSMORE, I. R. (1972). Sequential trial of effect of phenobarbitone on serum bilirubin of preterm infants. *Archives of Disease in Childhood,* 47, 621.

LILEY, A. W. (1961). Liquor amnii analysis in the management of the pregnancy complicated by rhesus sensitization. *American Journal of Obstetrics and Gynaecology,* 82, 1359.

LILEY, A. W. (1965). The use of amniocentesis and fetal transfusion in erythroblastosis fetalis. *Pediatrics,* 35, 836.

MOLLISON, P. L. (1959). Factors determining the relative clinical importance of different blood-group antibodies. *British Medical Bulletin,* 15, 92.

TABB, P. A., INGLIS, J., SAVAGE, D. C. L. & WALKER, C. H. M. (1972). Controlled trial of phototherapy of limited duration in the treatment of physiological hyperbilirubinaemia in low-birth-weight infants. *Lancet,* 2, 1211.

WISHINGRAD, L., *et al.* (1965). Studies of non-hemolytic hyperbilirubinemia in premature infants. I. Prospective randomized selection for exchange transfusion with observations on the level of serum bilirubin with and without exchange transfusion and neurologic evaluations one year after birth. *Pediatrics,* 36, 162.

Dehydration

MORRIS-JONES, P. H., HOUSTON, I. B. & EVANS, R. C. (1967). Prognosis of the neurological complications of acute hypernatraemia. *Lancet,* 2, 1385.

Acute bronchiolitis

DOIG, W. B. (1971). Value of arterialized capillary blood gas analysis in lower respiratory tract infection in childhood. *Archives of Disease in Childhood,* 46, 243.

ELDERKIN, F. M., GARDNER, P. S., TURK, D. C. & WHITE, A. C. (1965). Aetiology and management of bronchiolitis and pneumonia in children. *British Medical Journal,* 2, 722.

MEDICAL RESEARCH COUNCIL (1965). A collaborative study of the aetiology of acute respiratory infections in Britain 1961-64. Report. *British Medical Journal,* 2, 319.

CHAPTER 19

Emergencies in Infectious Diseases

General Considerations

Nowadays patients with infectious diseases are usually admitted to an infectious disease unit of a general hospital rather than to a separate hospital. This is because they require hospital investigation and treatment and are or *may be* infectious. Virtually all admissions are urgent but even when not clinical emergencies, urgent public health decisions may be required. Apart from treating the patient, the physician has constantly to consider whether he can suggest any line of action which may limit the spread of illness in the community, an aspect of his work which requires a detailed family and social history.

Emergencies in infectious diseases, therefore, fall clearly under the headings of diagnosis, treatment and prevention.

DIAGNOSIS

The best opportunities for successful therapy may have passed before a final diagnosis is possible. Many severe and life-threatening infections have a common symptomatology on the first day or two of illness—non-specific febrile and toxic symptoms dominating the clinical picture. In such cases as well as in those in whom localisation of signs or symptoms are beginning to suggest a probable as opposed to a certain diagnosis, material for certain basic investigations should be collected as soon as practicable, the specimens for culture being taken before antibiotic therapy is begun. The necessary specimens are:

1. *Blood-culture.* (Consult the microbiologist about media.)

2. *Blood from which serum is extracted and kept in a refrigerator.* Should need arise later for the examination of paired sera for a rising antibody level, there is then available a specimen of serum taken early in the illness. Enteric fever, as well as many viral and rickettsial diseases, are examples in which such a specimen may later prove helpful in diagnosis.

3. *Cultures from appropriate sites.* The specimens taken will clearly depend on the symptoms. They may include swabs and serum-coated swabs from the nose, throat or rectum, or any discharge, stool or urine specimens and so on. Scrapings from rashes

will on occasion give an immediate rapid diagnosis. Meningococci may be seen in material from the roseolar papules or petechiae of a meningococcal rash. Material from smallpox spots is likely to give valuable help within two to three hours (p. 699).

4. A *total and differential white cell count with a report on the film.* The need for the latter cannot be too strongly emphasised as in many severe pyogenic infections, such as staphylococcal septicaemia, the total white cell count may be normal but in most such cases there will be a preponderance of polymorphs with a marked ' shift to the left ', indicating the presence of many young cells in the polymorph series. Although the white cell count is of great help in distinguishing pyogenic infections from other acute febrile illnesses due either to enteric organisms, viruses or collagen diseases, it can be equivocal.

The above investigations are the minimal essentials in any severe febrile illness of unknown nature. Others, for example lumbar puncture or a chest X-ray, may well be appropriate in a given patient. Throat and nose specimens for virus studies must be kept moist, either by breaking the end of the swab at the bedside into special transport media-containing bottles, or by taking washings. They must be taken to the virus laboratory as quickly as possible in a vacuum flask containing ice. Lower temperatures lessen the chance of recovering certain respiratory viruses. Faecal specimens for virus, on the other hand, can be safely stored in a deep freeze at temperatures down to $-70°C$ and transported at convenience in dry ice. Enteroviruses are very resistant to cooling. For instructions on how to send a specimen by post see p. 698. Telephoned clinical details can often materially assist the virologist.

TREATMENT

Symptomatic emergencies fall into three main groups: (1) bacteraemic shock (2) severe dyspnoea, (3) purpura fulminans.

Bacteraemic shock

This can best be defined as shock occurring in a patient with bacteraemia. Occasionally only bacterial products (endotoxins) rather than viable bacteria are present in the blood. This is known as ' endotoxic shock '. Such a distinction is rather artificial as it normally means merely that the organisms have not been recovered on blood culture from a patient with the clinical picture of bacteraemic shock. The commonest organisms are staphylococci and Gram-negative bacilli (' Gram-negative shock ').

Although first described following surgical operations it is now realised that ' Gram-negative shock ' often complicates renal and biliary tract infections, generalised peritonitis and pelvic sepsis. The onset is sudden and severe with rigors, sweats, mental confusion, tachycardia, hypotension and a cold, clammy, mottled skin. The central venous pressure is usually normal which is not the case in pulmonary embolism, myocardial infarction or sudden hypovolaemia from internal haemorrhage—all conditions which may lead to confusion (see also p. 610).

It is not possible here to discuss the disturbed physiology in bacteraemic shock which in any event is imperfectly understood. At the present time treatment, which is of great urgency, should be along the following lines:

1. *Restoration of effective circulating blood volume by i v infusion.* Provided urine is still being secreted a low molecular weight dextran (Dextran 40, Rheomacrodex) up to a maximum of one litre can be used after starting with glucose and one fifth strength isosmotic sodium chloride solution. If, however, there is any question of serious renal dysfunction dextran preparations are better avoided.

2. *Antibiotics.* Two bactericidal drugs should be used until the aetiology is known. If staphylococcal infection is likely cloxacillin 4 g per day should be combined with ampicillin 4 g per day while awaiting bacteriological findings. If a staphylococcal etiology is confirmed sodium fusidate (Fucidin) 500 mg orally three times a day should be substituted for ampicillin. When gram-negative organisms are probable gentamicin (Genticin) 5 mg/kg/day i m or i v should be combined with cephalothin (Keflin) 150 mg/kg/day in divided doses. This combination may be nephrotoxic and also carries the risk of damage to the eighth nerve. With *pseudomonas* infections carbenicillin (Pyopen) up to 24 g a day should replace ampicillin. Penicillins in high concentration render gentamicin inactive and so these antibiotics should never be mixed in the same drip. They can, however, be given separately since when diluted in body fluids inactivation does not occur. Serum levels of potentially toxic drugs must be monitored. This is mandatory if there is any renal impairment. An adequate therapeutic level of gentamicin is between 4 and 10 μg per ml. Clindamycin (Dalacin C) is the best antibiotic before surgery in Gram-negative anaerobic (*Bacteroides*) infection.

3. *Oxygen.* Continuous oxygen is required to compensate for excess wastage due to the slow capillary flow.

15

4. *Steroids.* The value of steroids is debated (see p. 756). Circulatory levels of hydrocortisone are usually normal or raised so steroids are not required as replacement therapy. If it is decided to use steroids massive doses of hydrocortisone (50 mg/kg/day) (i.e. 400 mg three-hourly i v for an average adult), should be given for 24 hours. After this time the dose can be rapidly reduced.

5. *Avoidance of vasopressors.* The circulatory deficiency in most patients is due to reduced cardiac output and peripheral arteriolar tone is normal or increased.

6. *Digitalis.* This is indicated if there is a rise in the central venous pressure.

7. *Reduction of temperature.* Reduction of temperature is usually achieved by simple measures with or without steroids. In the desperate case which shows no improvement with the treatment described, hypothermia should be considered. A low reading thermometer is essential (p. 362). The temperature is reduced to about 32·2°C (not below 30·5°C) by the combined use of ice, fans and i v chlorpromazine, pethidine and promethazine 50 mg of each. The effect of one dose should last from four to eight hours.

Specific toxaemia from known toxins are dealt with under the appropriate disease (diphtheria, p. 433, tetanus, p. 637, botulism, p. 136).

Severe dyspnoea

Dyspnoea accompanying infectious disease is most likely to be due to one of the following causes:

1. Mechanical obstruction (pp. 225 and 418) from spasm, oedema and exudation (usually infective but sometimes allergic or traumatic).

2. Paralysis of respiratory muscles as in diphtheritic neuritis, poliomyelitis or by spasm as in tetanus.

3. Pulmonary diseases (e.g. pneumonia and bronchiolitis).

4. Metabolic disturbances. Ketosis in infections may accompany dehydration, uraemia or diabetes.

Measures for dealing with urgent dyspnoea resulting from laryngotracheitis (p. 418), bronchiolitis (p. 416) and pneumonia (p. 199) are described on the pages indicated (oxygen therapy, p. 740).

Paralysis of the diaphragm and/or intercostal muscles of acute onset is best treated in a cabinet type respirator *providing the swallowing musculature is normal and there has been no accumulation of secretions in the lower respiratory tract before artificial respiration is started.* If there is any suggestion of pharyngeal pooling or swallowing difficulty or of excess bronchial secretions, the patient should be intubated and connected to a breathing machine until a tracheostomy can be performed and a cuffed James or similar tube inserted. Respiration is then continued by intermittent positive pressure. There are many machines available (p. 730). The management of these cases is such that it is best carried out at a special centre (p. 790). The basic principles are concerned with the prevention of pulmonary infection by two-hourly posturing, intensive chest physiotherapy, aspiration of secretions, and proper care of the cuff together with maintenance of satisfactory ventilation as evidenced by minute volume, pulse, blood pressure and PCO_2 recordings.

CROUP. The syndrome of hoarse voice, croupy cough and stridor constitutes croup. Most cases are infective (for causes see laryngeal diphtheria, p. 433), para-influenza 1 being the virus most frequently incriminated. Four clinical stages can be recognised:

Stage 1. Hoarse voice perhaps progressing to aphonia; croupy cough; inspiratory stridor when disturbed but absent at rest; fever.

Stage 2. Continuous stridor; retraction of lower ribs and soft tissues of the neck; use of accessory muscles of respiration; respiration laboured especially when disturbed.

Stage 3. Signs of hypoxia and/or carbon dioxide retention, i.e. restlessness, anxiety, pallor, sweating and increase in respiratory rate.

Stage 4. Cyanosis, either intermittent or permanent; cessation of breathing.

Treatment. Only Stage I cases may be managed safely at home as Stage 2 may progress to Stage 4 in a matter of hours.

Having excluded diphtheria, the patient should be nursed in a steam tent and given amoxycillin 125 mg eight-hourly for a child. Antibiotics are mandatory in case the laryngitis is due to *Haemophilus influenzae*. Some physicians prefer chloramphenicol (100 mg/kg/day) but in a condition in which the vast majority of cases are viral in origin and unaffected by antibiotics it seems wiser to avoid a potentially toxic drug. If signs of hypoxia develop (Stage 3) oxygen should be added to the steam by using an apparatus such as an Oxymist, prednisolone 40 mg given i m and the child kept under continuous observation. Response to steroids may be dramatic and they should be continued in much reduced dosage to finish in two or three days. All Stage 4 patients and those in Stage 3 not responding to conservative treatment require a tracheostomy.

Sedatives are dangerous and must not be used in Stage 3 cases when the restlessness is a symptom of hypoxia. Chloral hydrate in the form of Triclofos Elixir BPC (1 ml for a child up to 1 year and 5 ml (500 mg) after 5 years) is sometimes useful in the nervous child with Stage 2 croup but should only be used if he can be kept under continuous observation.

Purpura fulminans

Severe infections with certain viruses such as measles, chicken pox and smallpox may be complicated by a bleeding tendency with spontaneous haemorrhages which tend to become gangrenous. Such cases are usually fatal. Similar haemorrhagic manifestations may complicate septicaemic illnesses of which fulminating meningococcal septicaemia is perhaps the best known. The haemorrhages are the result of disseminated intravascular coagulation. In any severe infection the appearance of purpura in association with a sudden fall in the ESR and platelet count suggests haemorrhagic necrosis due to consumptive coagulopathy. As this syndrome develops the kaolin cephalin clotting time is lengthened, fibrin degradation products increase markedly and coagulation factor VIII and others fall. Treatment is with fresh whole blood or fresh frozen plasma as appropriate. The value of heparin is now uncertain and if used should be given in low dosage (500 units per hour). Antibiotic and supportive treatment is mandatory.

SPECIAL URGENT FEATURES OF CERTAIN INFECTIONS

Scarlet fever

Scarlet fever is now so mild that it is only rarely an emergency when complicated by mastoiditis or anuric nephritis (p. 387). These complications should be very rare even in severe attacks if penicillin is given early. The need for i v serum even in the rare hypertoxic case is now doubted and massive parenteral penicillin is indicated instead. A special advantage of penicillin is that it rapidly eliminates haemolytic streptococci from the throat and so allows release from isolation in 7 to 10 days. Occasionally the post-streptococcal state ensues with evidence of carditis or renal damage. A persistently raised sedimentation rate is an indication for long continued penicillin.

Sore throat

Diphtheria, agranulocytosis (p. 275) and acute epiglottitis (p. 434) are rare but important causes of sore throat, because of the urgent need for specific treatment. Chemotherapy is urgent but if possible nose and throat swabs, and a blood culture too if epiglottitis is suspected, should be taken first.

Diphtheria

Immunisation has made diphtheria a rare disease. Outbreaks still occur, however, and some recent ones have followed the arrival of a member of the family from abroad (e.g. Cyprus). Antitoxin should be given immediately in silent, obstructive states in which adherent exudate, usually off-white or creamy, but occasionally brownish from the presence of altered blood, is present on the tonsils or pharyngeal wall. It should also be given forthwith when adherent exudate is present on both tonsils, especially if it has spread to the palate or uvula. The decision to withhold antitoxin in the presence of probable diphtheria is one which must only be taken by a physician familiar with the disease. Mild tonsillar and nasal cases require 5 000 to 10 000 units of antitoxin i m, moderate invasions 10 000 to 25 000 units and late, malignant attacks will require 100 000 units or more, at least half of which should be given i v (p. 745). The dose is related to the duration of illness, the extent of the membrane and the clinical assessment of toxaemia. It is virtually unaffected by age. All patients should be given erythromycin. A high calorie, easily assimilated diet is required. Adequate fluids (by mouth, nasal catheter or parenterally, if vomiting, are essential in all severe cases. The amounts and concentrations depend on requirement as revealed by the presence of oedema and changes in plasma protein and electrolyte levels. I v therapy must be very carefully supervised in the presence of an active myocarditis because of the danger of precipitating heart failure. Digitalis is inadvisable on account of the frequency of heart block of varying degree in diphtheritic myocarditis but must be used, together with diuretics if congestive heart failure develops. Restlessness, insomnia and distressing praecordial pain may require morphine, or methadone (Physeptone) for complete relief.

Acute circulatory collapse in diphtheria results from a combination of peripheral circulatory failure and myocarditis. *Complete rest* together with nursing flat or with the foot of the bed raised to maintain an adequate cerebral circulation if there is severe hypotension, are essential measures. Hypertensive agents such as metaraminol (Aramine) should be avoided if possible in the presence of an active myocarditis.

Laryngeal diphtheria

Most cases of laryngitis are caused by respiratory viruses, a few by bacteria such as *H. influenzae* or haemolytic streptococci and a very few by diphtheria. A toxic appearance, offensive breath, enlargement of cervical lymph glands and a sanguinous nasal discharge suggest the latter. Treatment consists in giving antitoxin (20 000 to 40 000 units) and erythromycin and in nursing the patient in an atmosphere of steam. When relief of obstruction is indicated (Croup, p. 418) a tracheostomy is generally preferable to intubation.

Acute epiglottitis (see also p. 418)

This rare but severe form of ' croup ' is a real emergency which may kill within 24 hours of the first symptom. It causes a rapidly increasing dyspnoea with inspiratory stridor, a red, beefy epiglottis and marked toxaemia due to invasion with *H. influenzae* which is invariably present in the blood as well as in the throat. Chloramphenicol in full dosage is the drug of choice until sensitivity tests are available. Death is more usually due to toxaemia than airway obstruction but a tracheostomy may be required.

Measles

The prodromal or pre-eruptive stage of measles may be accompanied by alarming symptoms of laryngeal obstruction ('croup') (p. 418) and by considerable toxaemia; indeed, it is usual for the patient to feel better as the rash appears. Most cases are due to the measles virus but as secondary bacterial infection with streptococci or *H. influenzae* is always possible, ampicillin should be used routinely. (Routine chloramphenicol is *not* indicated as even in those few cases due to superinfection with *H. influenzae* there is no septicaemia as with epiglottitis). Steam, oxygen, sedation under strict observation and ephedrine (30 mg) are indicated as in croup due to other causes. There is as yet insufficient evidence of the value of steroids in the acute invasive stage of measles. Their use should, therefore, be avoided unless it is considered they may be life-saving.

Mumps

Orchitis is a common complication in post-pubertal males, appearing any time up to 10 days after the onset. Rapid relief of pain and tenderness is achieved by giving two doses of 100 mg of corticotrophin with a 24 hour interval between, *provided* the first dose is administered within a day of the onset of testicular pain. Resolution of the swelling is little affected. It is important to reassure patients that neither impotence nor sterility will follow.

Whooping cough

This remains a disease in which emergency situations occur. The severe bouts of coughing (p. 210) may be helped by Codeine Linctus Paediatric BPC 5 ml up to 4-hourly for a child, or dihydro-codeine (Dicodid) 30 mg by mouth for an adult, or pheno-barbitone 15 mg twice daily in a mixture, but the variety of drugs recommended is a good indication of their therapeutic inadequacy. For the baby who vomits repeatedly after spasms of coughing, liquid atropine methonitrate (Eumydrin) 1 to 2 drops of a 0·6 per cent solution in 90 per cent alcohol given four times a day before meals is of real value in lessening the vomiting although it has little effect on the spasms. One drop contains 0·2 mg. Two Eumydrin lamellae are approximately equivalent to 1 drop; each lamella containing 0·085 mg.

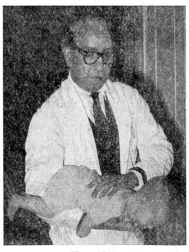

FIG. 19.1
Resuscitation from apnoeic attack in whooping cough.

Chlorpromazine (Largactil) 0·5 to 1·0 mg/kg three times a day is sometimes very useful.

Reports on broad spectrum antibiotics suggest that they may have a permanent place in treatment, at least in preventing respiratory complications. Ampicillin or amoxycillin are effective against the *Bordetella pertussis* (minimum inhibitory concentration 0·5 micrograms per ml) only if given in the catarrhal stage but it is a useful prophylactic in young babies. Bronchopneumonia complicating whooping cough is always accompanied by atelectasis and calls for prompt antibiotic treatment with ampicillin or amoxycillin together with physiotherapy. Convulsions (p. 419) may be due to hypoxia, intracranial haemorrhage or encephalopathy. In the *apnoeic attack* of whooping cough, the infant, usually under six months, fails to breathe after a paroxysm of coughing. He may be pale or cyanosed; his muscles are limp and he may have a convulsion. In a severe case as many as a dozen attacks can occur in a day. Any baby under 12 months of age with a severe attack of whooping cough or under 6 months of age while spasms are developing, must be under constant supervision. Oxygen and a suction apparatus must be available at the cotside. As recovery from an apnoeic attack always follows prompt treatment, this is listed in detail (Fig. 19.1).

1. Place the infant prone across your right fore-arm with one leg on either side of your elbow. Put your right index finger in the mouth and pull the tongue forwards. Steady the baby by putting your left hand on his back.

2. Having established an airway, give artificial respiration by rocking him on the fore-arm. Assist expiration in the ' down ' position by pressing the back with your left hand.

3. Give oxygen, if necessary, by nasal catheter and remove mucus by suction.

Meningitis

All forms of meningitis cause severe headache which may be accompanied by some clouding of consciousness. The headache progressively worsens and there may be pain in the back of the head. The patient lies curled up, resentful of interference and avoiding the light. Repeated vomiting is usual and convulsions may occur, especially in children.

Physical examination shows evidence of meningeal irritation (neck rigidity, rigidity of the paraspinal muscles and a positive Kernig's sign). There may be retinal congestion but papilloedema of more than mild degree in the presence of meningitis, suggests an underlying intracranial abscess. Once the possibility of meningitis has arisen, a lumbar puncture must be performed and this will confirm or refute the diagnosis or reveal another cause for the symptoms (e.g. subarachnoid haemorrhage). Meningitic signs accompanied by a normal cerebrospinal fluid (meningism) calls for a search for infection elsewhere. Although any severe infection *may,* on occasion, cause meningism, the common causes are tonsillitis, cervical adenitis, pneumonia (apical or central), acute pyelonephritis, salmonella gastroenteritis and viral respiratory infections such as influenza.

Pyogenic meningitis

Investigations include blood culture and examination of cerebrospinal fluid and of smears obtained from scraping any petechiae. In older children and adults, 20 000 units of crystalline penicillin G should be instilled intrathecally at the diagnostic lumbar puncture when a turbid fluid is removed. The dose is 5 000 units for those under 3 months and 10 000 units for those aged 3 months to 2 years.

The maximum dose of sulphadiazine i v or i m together with 1 mega unit of penicillin i m should be administered *as soon as the culture material is taken* and before the results are available. Further definitive treatment depends on the bacteriological diagnosis.

It is unfortunately common, nowadays, for patients with pyogenic meningitis to have received antibiotics before admission to hospital. This can make the diagnosis very difficult as the cerebrospinal fluid may resemble that from a case of aseptic meningitis, organisms being neither seen nor cultured. In pyogenic meningitis the protein is likely to be more raised. The decision whether to treat the case as one of ' partially treated pyogenic meningitis ' or to withhold treatment and observe, is one which can only be taken on all the facts in an individual case.

Sulphadiazine and penicillin is the combination of choice for meningococcal infection in the UK where sulphonamide-resistant meningococci remain uncommon. The daily amount of sulphadiazine in divided dosage four-hourly is as follows:

```
 0 to  2 years 3   g daily, reducing after 48 hours to 2   g daily
 3 to  5 years 4·5 g daily, reducing after 48 hours to 3   g daily
 6 to 10 years 6   g daily, reducing after 48 hours to 4·5 g daily
11 to 15 years 7·5 g daily, reducing after 48 hours to 6   g daily
16 upwards     9   g daily, reducing after 48 hours to 7·5 g daily
```

A high, preferably alkaline, urinary output is important.

Penicillin 1 mega unit four- to six-hourly should be given routinely as well. In patients known to be allergic to penicillin chloramphenicol is the drug of choice. This can also be used to replace sulphadiazine in countries, such as USA, where most meningococci are now sulphonamide resistant. Rifampicin is a useful alternative but unfortunately resistance develops quickly.

Meningitis due to *H. influenzae* (influenzal meningitis) requires sulphadiazine and chloramphenicol, the starting dose of the latter being 200 mg per kg per day, up to a maximum of 4 g per day. Infants under 4 weeks should be given 50 mg per kg and neonates 25 mg per kg. A course of 10 to 14 days is necessary to prevent relapse. If response is satisfactory, the dose can be reduced after 48 hours.

Pneumococcal and streptococcal meningitis require massive treatment with i m penicillin for a minimum of 10 days together with intrathecal penicillin for 7 to 10 days and oral sulphonamides for a week. Staphylococcal meningitis should be treated with cloxacillin 4 to 6 g daily with 40 mg intrathecally (until the organism is proved to be penicillin sensitive). In addition 40 mg should be given intrathecally to an adult every day. As these forms of meningitis are commonly secondary to foci elsewhere, an intensive search of the ears, sinuses, lungs and spine must be made. If there is an intracranial or extradural spinal abscess, neurosurgical help must be sought. Otherwise primary foci of infection can be left alone until the meningitis is cured. Return of temperature, vomiting, coma or convulsions after initial improvement suggests the development of an abscess or subdural effusion or the onset of hydrocephalus. Neurosurgical investigation is indicated.

A high cerebrospinal fluid protein or a very high cell count (greater than 30 000 cells per cu.mm) or the appearance of fresh focal signs are indications of excessive exudate and indicate steroid therapy.

In patients with pyogenic meningitis of unknown aetiology, i.e. with a sterile cerebrospinal fluid, treatment should consist of penicillin, sulphonamides and chloramphenicol.

Fulminating meningococcal septicaemia (Waterhouse-Friderichsen syndrome)

The onset of sudden vomiting followed rapidly by collapse with peripheral circulatory failure and a rapid respiratory rate, together with a spreading purpuric eruption is one of the greatest medical emergencies. Although rarely due to other organisms such as *H. influenzae,* therapy is directed at the meningococcus as by far the most likely cause. Death is probably inevitable once the adrenal cortices are destroyed and can occur within 4 to 24 hours. It should be noted however that the cortisol levels are normal. Therapy must therefore precede investigation other than the taking of blood for culture the same needle being used to give 4 mega units of penicillin and 80 mg of prednisolone 21 phosphate. If the veins are collapsed i m injection should be used. The hospital should be telephoned to say the patient is on the way. Treatment is continued with sulphadiazine in doses indicated under pyogenic meningitis (p. 436) together with penicillin, prednisolone and continuous oxygen. As the essential pathology seems to be widespread intravascular coagulation urgent heparinisation should be considered (see Purpura fulminans, p. 276). In those who survive, the prednisolone can rapidly be tailed off to finish within a week.

Enteric fever

Typhoid and paratyphoid fever require the same treatment. Whereas typhoid used to be a serious disease with a mortality of over 10 per cent, deaths are now exceptional when optimal therapy starts within a fortnight of onset. Chloramphenicol remains the drug of choice and should be given in a dosage of 75 mg/kg BW per day for a week followed by 50 mg per kg per day for a second week (maximum daily dose 4 g per day). No loading dose should be given. With a shorter course relapses are more frequent. Prednisolone 40 mg per day, rapidly reducing to finish in a week, is indicated in toxic cases and produces dramatic symptomatic improvement in most patients. Without steroids the temperature usually takes four to five days to fall to normal. Although the organism may be sensitive to ampicillin *in vitro,* clinical results have not been as good as with chloramphenicol. Co-trimoxazole (Bactrim, Septrin) is a useful alternative to chlorampenicol if this is contra-indicated. A high calorie (p. 376), low residue diet should be given but rigid dietary restriction is no longer necessary.

Haemorrhage, which without chemotherapy used to occur in up to 10 per cent of cases, is now rare. It varies from mere oozing to the sudden loss of several pints of blood, manifested by pallor, rapid, thready pulse, sighing respiration and a fall of temperature. There may be dull pain or a sensation of something giving way in the abdomen. If the patient is constipated, blood may be passed as tarry stools only after a long interval. Treatment is on the usual lines by morphine and blood transfusion.

Perforation (p. 121) is nowadays a rare emergency in typhoid because the improved dietetic regimen has almost eliminated severe meteorism, but it may ocasionally complicate an apparently satisfactory case. The usual onset is with sudden pain, followed by tenderness and rigidity of the lower abdomen, but these features may be masked by severe toxaemia. After a brief fall in temperature and apparent improvement following the initial shock, the temperature rises with the onset of generalised peritonitis. Increasing distension, rapid respiration and the Hippocratic facies appear. As perforations are often multiple, the results of medical treatment with continuous gastric suction, parenteral fluids and an increased dose of chloramphenicol are as good as, if not better than, those of surgery. Surgery should be considered, however, when perforations complicate the non-toxic case.

Dysentery-salmonella infections

Salmonellae are sometimes acutely invasive and can cause a severe septicaemic illness with peripheral circulatory failure. A few offensive stools at the onset suggests the diagnosis. When invasive salmonellosis is suspected, the treatment should start immediately with chloramphenicol in large doses (1 g six-hourly for an adult) together with measures for acute toxaemia. Symptomatic treatment is described on p. 136.

It is best to avoid antibiotics in the management of the ordinary case of gastroentertitis due to Shigella or Salmonella. Such drugs upset the normal bowel flora; they play little part in speeding recovery and they may increase the duration of the excretor state in convalescence. In the toxic case in which invasion is considered possible, though unlikely, ampicillin is the drug of choice while awaiting the result of blood culture. If it is felt that antimicrobial treatment must be used, whether in the acute or carrier stage, and the organism is sensitive to it, nalidixic acid (Negram) can be tried. This has the merit over other antibiotics that, should drug resistance develop, it will not be transferred to other organisms in the gut, i.e. nalidixic acid resistance is not infectious.

Varicella-zoster

This is a serious and sometimes fatal illness when it occurs in immunologically deficient patients, i.e. those with Hodgkin's disease or taking steroids. Cytosine arabinoside (Cytabarine) 100 mg a day should be given subcutaneously for three days. Specific immunoglobulin normally for prophylaxis (p. 801), might be given in high dosage for treatment as a last resort.

Smallpox (see also p. 757)

Smallpox has been introduced into Great Britain on numerous occasions. Modified smallpox with scanty lesions may be disregarded by patients and unrecognised by doctors but can spread and cause malignant attacks in the unvaccinated, the source of which may not be readily traced. Influenzal symptoms, with severe backache followed by a few papules, usually on the face, but which may commence on the trunk and may not pustulate, should be regarded with suspicion. (For laboratory diagnosis of smallpox see p. 699.)

In the treatment of malignant attacks, characterised by prostration and vomiting, i v dextrose saline and plasma should be employed, together with appropriate antibiotic therapy to combat the effects of secondary bacterial infection. Methisazone (Marboran, Burroughs Wellcome) is active against smallpox virus but, although it may have an effect in the incubation period, is of no value in treatment of the established disease. Gentian violet and hibitane, 1 or 2 per cent as creams, are valuable in controlling skin sepsis, both being bland and stable with little tendency to cause sensitisation.

Lassa fever

This highly contagious virus disease was first recognised in 1969 in West Africa. It is thought to be spread by the rat *Mastomys natalensis* and has a maximum incubation period of 17 days. The symptoms are largely toxic and non-specific but pharyngitis with membrane formation is suggestive. Renal, cardiac and neurological involvement may occur together with a haemorrhagic rash. The mortality in Europeans has been high. The strictest precautions are necessary by all who attend on the patient and by the pathologist who examines the body of a fatal case. Admission should only be to a hospital providing high risk accommodation. The disease may be imported by air and any doctor seeing a possible victim should at once contact a Tropical School (see Appendix 19, p. 827). Convalescent serum offers the only hope of specific treatment.

Leptospirosis

Some strains of Leptospira cause severe illness in human beings —complete or incomplete forms of Weil's syndrome. The incidence in men working in contact with sewage or water contaminated by rat's urine is now low. Farming folk are the commonest group to be infected nowadays. The illness begins with fever, muscular pains and conjunctival injection. Jaundice appears later and there may be meningeal involvement. Urgent symptoms are gross haemorrhage (haematemesis and haemoptysis) and acute renal failure. Treatment is by conventional supportive measures, blood transfusion and early recourse to haemodialysis or peritoneal dialysis. Antibiotics (penicillin, erythromycin) may be given though their efficacy when treatment is started later than the seventh day is doubtful. The disease is notifiable. Advice can be obtained from the Leptospirosis Reference Laboratory, rear of Colindale Hopital, Colindale Avenue, London NW9 5DX (01.205 6144).

ENCEPHALITIS COMPLICATING INFECTIOUS FEVERS

The usual times of onset of encephalitis complicating specific infections are:

Measles. Third to fourteenth day of illness, as temperature falls and rash is beginning to fade, i.e. about third post-eruptive day.

Rubella. Three to six days after the appearance of the rash.

Vaccinia. Five to 23 (usually 9 to 13) days after the vaccination.

Smallpox. One to 28 (usually eight) days after the appearance of the rash.

Whooping cough ' encephalitis '. Two to seven weeks after onset.

Mumps. Within one week of the parotitis.

Chickenpox. Five days after the rash appears.

Neurological complications of virus diseases may be infective (due to invasion of the central nervous system by a neurotropic strain of virus) or post-infective when the reaction is allergic and truly an encephalopathy or an encephalo-myelopathy rather than an encephalitis. The infective types cause symptoms early in the illness, are usually febrile and more often accompanied by a pleocytosis in the cerebrospinal fluid. Both conditions are notifiable. If the history suggests neurological invasion by the causal virus, rather than a post-infective allergy, steroids are better avoided. In certain cases, however, such as when optic neuritis develops, the chance of saving the patient's sight by the anti-inflammatory action of steroids may outweigh the theoretical danger of spreading the primary infection.

Herpes simplex encephalitis

Encephalitis due to Herpes simplex virus is usually a rare manifestation of a primary infection but it occasionally occurs in persons who have suffered recurrent ' cold sores ' in the past. Herpes group viruses are sensitive to a number of anti-viral drugs of which cytosine arabinoside (Cytarabine) is currently the most promising. For any hope of success with specific treatment early diagnosis is essential. This requires specialised techniques of fluorescent microscopy, comparative CSF/serum complement fixation tests and viral culture. Many cases need cerebral decompression and brain biopsy. This is best undertaken in units familiar with the problem. In spite of theoretical dangers dexamethasone should also be used as it may lessen cerebral oedema dramatically.

Post-infective meningo-encephalitis

This type of encephalitis is not related to the severity of the primary illness and often follows a mild attack. The onset is marked by headache, vomiting and rapidly increasing drowsiness. Occasionally retention of urine is the first symptom. Any type of paralysis may appear, hemiplegia, transverse myelitis or peripheral neuritis arising separately or together. The cerebrospinal fluid shows an increase in protein and perhaps a few cells but it may well be normal.

Treatment. There is as yet no clear evidence from controlled investigation in humans that steroids are of benefit. On theoretical grounds supported by animal experiments, however, corticotrophin, and to a lesser extent prednisolone or dexamethasone, aid the chances of recovery. Early treatment probably matters and the following scheme is suggested for severe cases which present with a sudden onset of encephalitic symptoms (e.g. hemiplegia, myelitis, recurrent fits or gross disorientation): either corticotrophin 100 units daily reducing after five to seven days or prednisolone 80 mg daily i m rapidly reducing after two to three days to finish in about 10 days. In cases in which the signs of encephalitis are mild it is justifiable to withhold steroids for 24 hours. In severe cases which fail to respond to steroids and show evidence of cerebral oedema, with or without hyperpyrexia, hypothermia (p. 728) should be considered.

EMERGENCY ASPECTS OF PROPHYLAXIS

The Community Physician and his staff play an essential part in the prevention of infectious disease. Whether they could help to lessen spread of an infection should always be considered and notification of infectious diseases should by no means be restricted to the officially notifiable diseases. In addition, the need for urgent protection against infection may, in the young or debilitated, constitute an emergency.

Smallpox (see also p. 757)

Once a diagnosis of smallpox is considered and cannot be excluded, the Community Physician *must* be notified by telephone. He will see the case and if need be he can call for help from the Panel of Smallpox Opinion (telephone Department of Health and Social Security, Room A 319 01-407 5522, Ext. 6850). A patient with suspected smallpox must be kept where he is first seen until examined by an expert. *He must never be sent to a hospital or other institution for diagnosis.* Advice on further procedure is given in detail in *Memorandum on the Control of Outbreaks of Smallpox* (1964) published by the Department of Health. The principles involved are isolation and vaccination together with daily surveillance of the primary contacts and vaccination of secondary contacts. Mass vaccination is to be avoided.

Diphtheria

The diagnosis of diphtheria nowadays calls for isolation of the patient and search for carriers and unrecognised cases by examination and nose and throat swabbing of family and school contacts. Absentees from school must be visited at home. If these investigations reveal more cases or carriers, the rest of the class are protected by active or combined passive and active immunisation as indicated by their previous immunisation history. Second swabs must be taken from all close contacts as false negatives are not uncommon. Schick testing has little part to play in modern management of a diphtheria outbreak but it may be useful in an individual swab positive case to decide whether he is a carrier or a mild case.

PROTECTION BY IMMUNISATION

Active immunisation with living vaccines can be used to produce rapid herd immunity and terminate an outbreak. This particularly applies to poliomyelitis. It will probably also apply to measles in the future. Passive immunisation provides only short-term protection and is available for the following diseases:

Diphtheria. 2 000 to 5 000 units of diphtheria antitoxin i m should be given according to age (see p. 433). This may be combined with active immunisation by giving 0·5 ml of toxoid in the other arm followed four weeks later by 1·0 ml. One of the more bland preparations, e.g. TAF, should be used.

Scarlet fever. If protection is desirable in particular circumstances, phenoxymethyl penicillin (Penicillin V) may be given by mouth for as long as necessary. The use of antitoxin, which only protects against the rash and not against the infection, has been abandoned.

Measles. Human normal immuno-globulin of known measles antibody content (p. 798) is to be preferred to unaltered serum because it is more stable and its effective dose is smaller. It is also virtually free from the risk of transmitting the virus of hepatitis. For dosage see pp. 798 and 800.

Rubella. Because of the risk to the fetus, a woman in the first trimester of pregnancy who has no neutralising rubella antibodies and who has been in contact with a case, should be protected with human normal immuno-globulin (p. 799) or preferably high potency human immuno-globulin, prepared from convalescent rubella serum, as early in the presumed incubation period as possible. Antibody studies must be repeated in four to six weeks to exclude a symptomless attack in the interval (see also p. 176).

Chickenpox. Susceptible contacts such as neonates born of non-immune mothers and others with impaired resistance whether due to drugs (e.g. steroids) or lympho-reticular disease should receive hyper-immune immunoglobulin (p. 779). This may not prevent infection but it is likely to modify it considerably.

Infective hepatitis. A small dose of human normal immuno-globulin (see p. 798) will prevent or modify virus A (epidemic) hepatitis if given early in the incubation period. Although not of wide application, human normal immunoglobulin can be used to terminate an epidemic under certain conditions, as, for example, in a partially closed community. Human specific immunoglobulin from Australia antigen positive convalescents is now under trial for the prevention of virus B hepatitis for which human normal immunoglobulin is of value (p. 800).

Tetanus. Immediate passive protection is given by human anti-tetanus immunoglobulin (Humotet) 250 to 500 international units. If the patient is known to have had tetanus vaccine (toxoid) in the past, a booster dose of vaccine should be used instead of tetanus antitoxin.

Mumps. Human normal immunoglobulin and convalescent serum are ineffective in preventing mumps. There is an effective living vaccine available.

ISOLATION AND QUARANTINE

(For Infectious Diseases in General Wards see p. 698)

The recognised rules of quarantine have been considerably relaxed in recent years and no useful purpose can be served in trying to formulate new ones to meet all contingencies.

Up to date recommendations regarding isolation and quarantine of patients in hospital and their discharge stress that particular circumstances must govern the appropriate action whether it affects the individual or the group. Legally, contacts and carriers cannot be controlled or their liberties restricted apart from the prohibition of the handling, preparation and cooking of foodstuffs by carriers of intestinal pathogens.

Generally speaking, the patient is not infectious during the incubation period and no restrictions on movements are commonly applied. (Infectivity, however, has been shown to occur, occasionally, in the later stages of the incubation period of such diverse diseases as chickenpox, enteric fever and poliomyelitis, and may conceivably occur similarly in other infections.) The quarantine period, rarely applied in strict form nowadays, is the maximum incubation period with one or two days added in case the initial phase of the attack was overlooked.

Contacts may contract the disease early in the supposed incubation period because they had been exposed to an undetected case or carrier before the first recorded case. Smallpox is the classical example of the official policy of surveillance combined with strict isolation in quarantine, used with constant success, to prevent spread of a serious disease.

For the ' inevitable ' diseases of childhood, isolation within the home is impracticable and quarantine seldom advisable. Susceptible child contacts of mumps, chickenpox, rubella, measles, whooping cough, scarlet fever and dysentery should be allowed to go to school. This causes little risk in others, *provided* isolation at home is carried out at the first suggestive symptom. Family contacts of cases of diphtheria and enteric fever should be swabbed, the advisability of their continuing at school or work depending on the circumstances but usually it would be preferable to keep them at home until the first swab results were available. Contacts of meningococcal infection should receive sulphadiazine for 24 hours and need not then be quarantined. Contacts of poliomyelitis should be kept at home until the whole situation, including immunisation history and degree of risk, can be properly assessed.

G. DONALD W. MCKENDRICK

REFERENCES

MCKAY, D. G. & MARGARETTEN, W. (1967). Disseminated intravascular coagulation in virus diseases. *Archives of Internal Medicine,* **120,** 129-152.

MILLAR, J. W., SEISS, E. E., FELDMAN, H. A., SILVERMAN, C. & FRANK, P. (1963). In vivo and in vitro resistance to sulphadiazine in strains of *Neisseria Meningitidis. Journal of the American Medical Association,* **186,** 139.

FOR FURTHER READING

CHRISTIE, A. B. *Infectious Diseases: Epidemiology and Clinical Practice,* 2nd edition. Churchill Livingstone. 1974.

KRUGMAN, S. & WARD, R. *Infectious Diseases of Children and Adults.* 5th ed. St. Louis: Mosby. 1973.

CHAPTER 20

Emergencies in Tropical Medicine

(For where to seek advice about tropical diseases see
Appendix 18, p. 19)
(For Ackee poisoning see p. 135)
(For snake-bite in the tropics see p. 631)

THIS chapter is largely written from the point of view of practitioners in temperate climates who may occasionally encounter examples of tropical diseases. It is important to bear in mind that most travellers from the tropics arrive by air. This allows ample time for them to disperse to their destinations within the incubation period of most of the infections that they may have acquired during the last days of their residence abroad. Most tropical parasitic diseases are easily cured in their early stages and serious emergencies would seldom arise if a prompt diagnosis were made in every case. The clue to the diagnosis of most illnesses lies in the history and an affirmative reply to a routine enquiry about visits abroad should alert the physician to the possibility that he is dealing with an exotic disease.

MALARIA

The four species of malaria parasite which affect man are *Plasmodium vivax*, *P. ovale*, *P. malariae* and *P. falciparum*. The first three of these cause infections which are not emergencies in the sense that they are dangerous to life, though from the patient's point of view they are unpleasant enough to demand rapid diagnosis and treatment. Untreated *P. falciparum* infections in Europeans can be quickly fatal.

Visitors to malarial countries should take regular prophylactic drugs from a few days before entering the area until three or four weeks after leaving it. This precaution will generally ensure complete protection against *P. falciparum* infections. The other types of malaria will be suppressed so long as the drug is taken but will become manifest after stopping it. This usually happens within a few weeks but may rarely be delayed for a year or more. The prophylactic drugs are proguanil (Paludrine) (100 to 200 mg daily), chlorproguanil (Lapudrine) (20 mg weekly), pyrimethamine (1 tablet weekly) and chloroquine (150 mg twice weekly) and amodiaquine (Camoquin) (200 mg twice weekly). All these drugs are satisfactory and free from harmful effects in the recommended doses. However, strains of *P. falciparum* resistant to some or all of these drugs have emerged in various parts of the world so that there is no one drug which can be guaranteed to give total protection everywhere. Most falciparum malaria occurs in Africa and so far no strains resistant to chloroquine or amodiaquine have appeared in that continent so that either of these can be used there with complete confidence. Chloroquine resistant strains occur in South East Asia and in tropical S. America and in these areas dapsone with pyrimethamine (Maloprim) one tablet weekly is perhaps the most reliable prophylactic as resistance to proguanil is also common in these areas.

Benign tertian malaria (*P. vivax*) is the usual form of malaria in most countries except Africa (Fig. 20.1). If the primary attack is inadequately treated relapses may occur at intervals for one and a half to two years before the infection dies out naturally. In the primary attack the temperature chart is often irregular for a few days before settling into the characteristic intermittent pattern, with fever occurring every 48 hours. As the temperature mounts the patient is cold and shivery, at its height he is hot and flushed and as it falls he sweats. Headache and vomiting are common during the rigor.

P. ovale infections resemble those due to *P. vivax*. Malaria of the benign tertian type acquired in West Africa is usually due to *P. ovale*, but the distinction between the two parasites is an academic one of no practical importance.

The parasite of quartan malaria (*P. malariae*) has a wide geographical distribution, but is everywhere rather uncommon. It is better adapted than are the other species to the human host, in whom it can survive for many years causing few or no symptoms. It occasionally comes to prominence in the recipient of a blood transfusion from a donor in whom the presence of the infection was quite unsuspected. When it does cause overt symptoms the bouts of fever occur at 72-hour intervals.

Though malignant tertian malaria (*P. falciparum*) occurs throughout the tropics it is mostly found in tropical Africa, where it accounts for over 90 per cent of cases. It should always be considered as the first cause of fever in Africa or within a few weeks of departure therefrom. It has two dangerous features: the parasites may multiply unchecked in susceptible people (broadly speaking non-African) until life is destroyed; and by its mimicry it may simulate many other illnesses so that the correct diagnosis is missed. The pattern of fever in falciparum malaria is less characteristic than in the other forms.

The spikes of fever have a broader base and tend to merge giving a remittent or continuous appearance to the temperature chart. Headache and vomiting are severe. Diarrhoea is not uncommon. Jaundice may occur after the first week; it is usually slight, but sometimes considerable. Mental confusion, stupor and coma may supervene at any time. Various combinations of these symptoms may suggest influenza, gastroenteritis, meningitis or infective hepatitis.

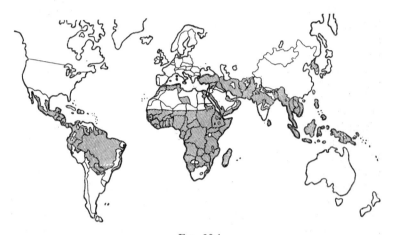

FIG. 20.1

Countries where it is still possible to catch malaria. From DHSS Health Protection Leaflet by permission of HMSO.

To diagnose malaria other than by demonstrating the parasites in blood films is to indulge in guesswork. Therefore blood should be taken routinely from any person in whom the possibility of malaria arises. Once this is done specific treatment should not be delayed. Unless the practitioner is accustomed to making thick and thin blood films he will do better to send 1 or 2 ml of venous blood in a sequestrene bottle to a laboratory. (See Appendix 19, p. 827). If he has to rely on his own inexpert microscopy the fact that he cannot find parasites in the peripheral blood should not make the doctor delay treatment when the clinical picture is that of cerebral malaria.

Treatment. The treatment of the uncomplicated case of malaria is straightforward. In falciparum malaria an initial dose of 800 mg of chloroquine (Nivaquine, Avlochlor, Resochin) followed by 200 mg eight-hourly for three days will eradicate the infection, save in the relatively rare cases of chloroquine-resistant malaria from South

America and South-east Asia. Either of the other available 4-amino-
quinolines (amodiaquine, Camoquin; hydroxychloroquine, Pla-
quenil) can be substituted for chloroquine in the same doses. The
same regime will abolish the parasitaemia in the other forms of
malaria but will not prevent relapses. This can usually be done by
a course of primaquine 7·5 mg twice daily for 14 days, begun concurrently with the chloroquine.

Chloroquine resistant strains of *P. falciparum* are designated RI,
RII and RIII according to degree. The first is the commonest. In it
there is a normal initial response to a standard course of chloroquine
followed by a recrudescence of parasitaemia. In the last there is
no marked reduction in parasitaemia. The second form is intermediate. A satisfactory treatment for such cases is quinine 600 mg
twice daily for two or three days followed by a single dose of
sulphadoxine (Fanasil) 1·5 g and pyrimethamine (Daraprim) 75 mg.

Serious complications are confined to malignant tertian malaria
and should be treated in hospital. Apart from blackwater fever,
which is in a category of its own, they occur in the second or third
week of an untreated attack in a person with little or no immunity.
In such cases the infection is always heavy, up to 20 per cent of
the red cells being parasitised. The clinical effects are a consequence
of massive red-cell destruction and localised ischaemia, particularly
of the brain, due to obstruction of internal capillaries by aggrega-
tions of parasites (Fig. 20.2). They include mental confusion passing
into coma, peripheral circulatory failure and renal failure and
jaundice. Though such cases have often passed beyond the point
where they can be cured with a few tablets, it is obviously the first
step to get a sufficient amount of anti-malarial drug into the blood
stream. Thereafter the necessary measures must be taken to support
life and allow the damaged organs to recover their function. The
chemotherapy is simple. An ampoule of chloroquine (200 mg in 5
ml) should be injected i v. Thereafter, if the patient is able to
swallow and retain tablets, chloroquine can be given by mouth as
set forth above. If he is unconscious or vomiting the injection can
be repeated i v or i m at six-hourly intervals.

The supportive measures vary according to the needs of the case.
An i v saline drip should be set up in the patient who is unconscious
or shows signs of peripheral circulatory failure. Hydrocortisone 1 g
should be given in the drip and repeated if necessary at the rate of
1 g daily.

It is advisable to measure the urinary output in all complicated
cases of malaria, if necessary collecting the urine from an indwelling catheter. Renal failure is indicated when the 24 hour

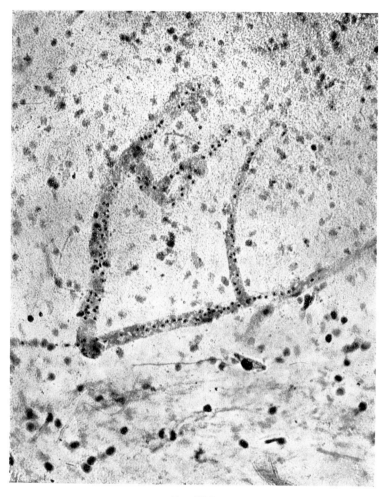

FIG. 20.2

Photo-micrograph of brain section from a fatal case of malignant tertian malaria. The capillaries are distended and obstructed by parasitised red cells. The heavy black dots in the vessels represent malarial pigment. × 400.

Facing page 450

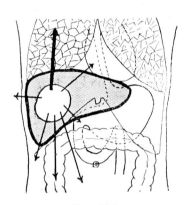

FIG. 20.3
Directions in which an amoebic
liver abscess may burst.
(*After Cope.*)

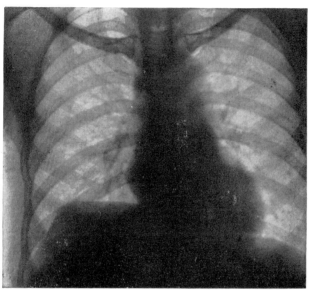

Fig. 20.4

A liver abscess causing deformity and elevation of the right
dome of the diaphragm.

(*Dr. Carmichael Low, by courtesy of Sir P. Manson-Bahr.*)

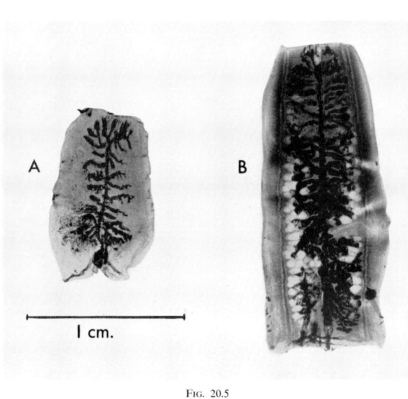

Fig. 20.5

Mature segments of *Taenia solium* (A) and *Taenia saginata* (B). The uteri
have been injected to show 6 to 12 primary branches on each side in *T.
solium* and more than 15 in *T. saginata*.

urinary volume is less than 500 ml, when the blood urea exceeds 100 mg per 100 ml (16·7 mmol/l) and the specific gravity of the urine is under 1 016. In such a case renal function may be restored by the i v infusion of 30 g mannitol with 20 mg frusemide (Lasix). Should this fail peritoneal dialysis (p. 716) should be started and maintained until kidney function is resumed. If the accompanying jaundice is intense (serum bilirubin over 40 mg per 100 ml (684 μmol/l)) exchange transfusion may be necessary.

BLACKWATER FEVER

Of this complication it has been said that malaria loads the gun and quinine pulls the trigger. It virtually disappeared with the replacement of quinine by synthetic anti-malarials but the appearance in recent years of strains of *P. falciparum* resistant to chloroquine and related drugs, notably in South-east Asia, has revived the use of quinine there with its associated risk of provoking blackwater fever. The illness consists of a series of waves of severe haemolysis, each one accompanied by fever. The urine passed in each paroxysm is first dark red from oxyhaemoglobin, later dark brown from methaemoglobin. The chief danger is renal failure, which can be satisfactorily treated by peritoneal dialysis. Anaemia is often profound enough to require transfusion. The underlying malarial infection, always due to *P. falciparum,* is light and can be dealt with by any anti-malarial except quinine.

GLUCOSE-6-PHOSPHATE DEHYDROGENASE DEFICIENCY

This condition in which the enzyme deficiency allows haemolysis to occur resembles blackwater fever clinically. For further details see p. 272.

AMOEBIASIS

Amoebic liver abscess

This is the commonest complication of intestinal amoebiasis to which it is always secondary. The intestinal ulceration may never have been sufficient to cause symptoms, though a history of dysentery is obtainable in about half the cases. The abscess, which is usually single and in the right lobe, is formed by amoebae which have reached the liver as emboli from the colonic ulcers via the portal vein and have contrived to survive and multiply. The abscess extends centrifugally and if untreated will burst in one of the directions indicated in Figure 20.3, the usual way being through the diaphragm into the lung.

An amoebic liver abscess may develop at any time after the original intestinal infection, sometimes many years later. There is much variation in the rate at which symptoms appear, no doubt corresponding to the site and speed of growth of the abscess. Pain is almost always present and is usually felt beneath and behind the right lower ribs anteriorly. When the upper part of the right lobe is affected referred pain in the right shoulder is usual. There is usually irregular remittent fever but apyrexial cases are sometimes seen. Moderate neutrophil leucocytosis (total count about $15 \times 10^9/l$) (15 000 per mm^3) is to be expected. Examination will reveal a swollen tender liver often with a point of maximal tenderness in the hypochondrium or lower right intercostal spaces. Later obvious bulging in one or other of these sites indicates the position of the abscess. Jaundice is most unusual. Radiography will often show that the right side of the diaphragm is elevated and fixed (Fig. 20.4).

The association of these signs and symptoms allows a clinical diagnosis of amoebic liver abscess to be made with some confidence and treatment to be started without delay. There is now no doubt that metronidazole (Flagyl) is the best treatment for liver abscess and other invasive forms of amoebiasis. It is given by mouth, 800 mg three times a day for five days. Emetine hydrochloride and chloroquine are also effective in hepatic amoebiasis and used together give better results than either singly. Emetine is given subcutaneously 60 mg daily for 10 days. Chloroquine is given orally 600 mg initially and then 200 mg twice daily for 10 days. Although these drugs can be depended on to destroy the amoebae in the liver they will not necessarily eradicate the underlying infection in the intestine. This must be treated subsequently with either diloxanide furoate (Furamide) 500 mg three times a day for 10 days or tetracycline 250 mg six-hourly for seven days. Failure to respond to treatment usually indicates a wrong diagnosis, primary carcinoma of the liver being the commonest source of confusion.

Aspiration. Although one or other of these chemotherapeutic regimes is essential in hepatic amoebiasis, it is necessary, when the abscess is large, to aspirate it. This has the advantage of confirming the diagnosis and of relieving the patient of much discomfort. The site for aspiration is usually indicated by a localised bulging or point of maximal tenderness in an intercostal space. The technique is to inject local anaesthetic into the chosen area and to advance the needle through which it has been given into the liver, as the abscess is often very superficial and a little of its contents can be withdrawn into the syringe which contained the local anaesthetic. Having located the abscess in this way, a longer wide-bore needle should be introduced and as much pus as possible aspirated with a two-way syringe. When, as often happens, the volume of pus aspirated is large (in excess of 1 litre) it may be necessary to repeat the procedure a day or two later.

Rupture of an amoebic liver abscess into the lung is followed by the coughing up of large amounts of reddish-brown sputum in which amoebae can often be found. Much less often the abscess will discharge into the pleura, causing sudden pain, shock and respiratory distress. This must be treated by immediate aspiration of the pleura repeated every 48 hours, together with the usual chemotherapy. Rupture into the peritoneum initially simulates an ' acute abdomen ', followed in a few hours by the signs of intra-peritoneal fluid. The diagnosis is usually made at operation, when the pus should be aspirated and medical treatment begun.

Pericarditis

Amoebic pericarditis is due to an extension of an abscess from the left lobe of the liver. The development of a frank suppurative pericarditis may be heralded by a pericardial rub, in which case the rupture into the pericardium must be prevented if possible by aspiration or surgical drainage of the liver abscess. Suppurative amoebic pericarditis, which is often fatal, is best treated by repeated aspirations (p. 714) and chemotherapy.

Amoeboma

An amoeboma is a granulomatous thickening of an area of the large intestinal wall consequent on a deeply penetrating amoebic ulcer. It presents as a palpable tumour, often associated with fever and partial obstruction of the bowel. Amoebomas are often mis-taken for carcinomas and are unnecessarily resected, as they will usually resolve satisfactorily with the ordinary medical treatment. The distinction between amoeboma and carcinoma is not easy, but if there is any history of dysentery, or if microscopy of the stools shows the presence of *Entamoeba histolytica,* the effect of chemo-therapy should be tried before embarking on surgery unless the indications for the latter are urgent.

TRYPANOSOMIASIS

Trypanosomiasis is prevalent in a number of fairly well defined rural areas of tropical Africa. In its earlier stages it is characterised by irregular fever, tachycardia, swollen cervical lymph nodes and transient circinate erythemata of the trunk. At this stage trypanosomes can be found in blood films and in material obtained by lymph gland puncture. The brain is involved later in the disease and the first indication that this has happened is usually the development of peculiarities of behaviour. The disease is seldom seen outside Africa, but should always be considered in persons from sleeping-sickness areas in whom symptoms suggestive of mental disturbance develop. Trypanosomes may not be demonstrable in the later stages, but the increase in cellularity and protein content of the cerebrospinal fluid is sufficiently characteristic. In early cases of the disease, with normal cerebrospinal fluid, six weekly i v injections of suramin 1 g are curative. Patients with evidence of nervous involvement should be given melarsoprol (Arsobal), 5 ml of the 3·6 g/dl solution in propylene glycol i v daily for four days. The course is repeated two weeks later. For prophylaxis see p. 703.

HELMINTHIC INFECTIONS

Cestodes

The only tapeworm of serious medical importance is *Taenia solium,* whose eggs are infective to man as well as to the pig, which is the usual intermediate host. Persons swallowing the eggs of this tapeworm, whether derived from an adult worm in their own intestine or from elsewhere, will develop cysticercosis. The cysticerci are distributed generally in the muscles and subcutaneous tissue where they cause no particular trouble. Unfortunately, however, the brain is often involved, causing epilepsy. It follows that, as a person harbouring *Taenia solium* is a danger to himself and to others, the parasite should be dislodged with the least possible delay. The features distinguishing the segments of *T. solium* and *T. saginata* (which is at least 50 times the commoner worm) are illustrated in Figure 20.5. Tapeworms can readily be destroyed by a single dose of niclosamide (Yomesan) 2 g. The tablets should be chewed before swallowing. No starvation or purgation is necessary and there are no side-effects. Epilepsy due to cerebral cysticercosis is treated symptomatically.

Trematodes

PARAGONIMIASIS. Among more familiar causes of haemoptysis in the Chinese is the lung-fluke *Paragonimus.* Living in the terminal bronchi it causes what is in effect a parasitic bronchiectasis. The symptoms are a chronic cough, worst in the mornings, productive of brownish sputum with occasional moderate haemoptysis. The diagnosis is easily made by microscopical examination of the sputum for ova. Successful treatment of paragonimiasis has been achieved with two drugs, hexachloroparaxylene (Chloxyle) 250 mg per kg body weight twice daily for 10 days or bithionol (Actamer) 50 mg per kg on alternate days for three weeks.

SCHISTOSOMIASIS. Vesical schistosomiasis should always be considered as a likely cause of painless haematuria in patients from Africa. The diagnosis is readily established by finding the characteristic terminally spined eggs in the urinary deposit. The infection can usually be cured quite easily by a single i m injection of hyacanthone (Etrenol) 3 mg per kg body weight (maximum dose 3 g). An alternative drug is niridazole (Ambilhar) 25 mg per kg body weight daily for seven days. It is given by mouth and the maximum dose should not exceed 500 mg three times daily. The drug colours the urine dark brown. It is usually well tolerated but may cause headache, mental confusion and rarely convulsions, so should only be used under careful supervision.

Nematodes

ANKYLOSTOMIASIS. Hookworms are the usual cause of iron-deficiency anaemia in tropical and sub-tropical countries. The amount of blood lost is directly proportional to the number of worms, and if this is in excess of many hundreds the ensuing anaemia will be profound and may be fatal. Microscopical examination of the stools will reveal the hookworms eggs and from their number a rough assessment of the number of worms can be made. Effective anthelmintic drugs are bephenium (Alcopar) 5 g, thiabendazole (Mintezol) 3 g. and tetrachloroethylene 3 ml. A dose of one or other of these is usually sufficient to reduce the number of worms to an insignificant level. Thereafter it is necessary to give a course of oral iron to accelerate restoration of haemoglobin to normal levels.

FILARIASIS. Infections with the filarial worm *Loa loa* are readily acquired by residents in certain areas of the western half of tropical Africa. The adult worms are threadlike creatures from 2 to 7 cm long. They migrate about the body in the connective tissues and occasionally cross the eye subconjunctivally, when their movement is felt and seen. They more usually manifest themselves by provoking large painless oedematous swellings ('Calabar swellings') often on the back of the hand or forearm, lasting about three days. The infection is associated with an intense eosinophil leucocytosis. It can be cured by a three-week course of diethylcarbamazine (Hetrazan,

Banocide) increasing the dose gradually during the first week from 50 mg to 200 mg three times a day.

MISCELLANEOUS CONDITIONS

Sickle-cell anaemia

The crises of sickle-cell anaemia are responsible for a variety of acute symptoms in Negro children who are homozygous for the sickling gene. These include severe haemolytic anaemia, bone pains with associated soft tissue swelling, bone abscesses infected with *Salmonella* and abdominal pain, which may be so severe as to suggest a surgical emergency. The crises are often precipitated by bacterial or protozoal infections. Their frequency and duration can be reduced in malarial regions by regular anti-malarial prophylaxis and there and elsewhere by prompt long-term antibiotic therapy. The pains of the crises can often be relieved by analgesics, anti-coagulants or by the i v or i m injections of tolazoline (Priscol) 25 mg. Packed red cell transfusion is also frequently necessary. Iron is contraindicated.

Lassa fever (see p. 440).

Heatstroke

This is due to reduction or cessation of sweating and consequent rise of body temperature and may occur in persons engaged in physical effort in hot climates. In severe cases confusion, convulsions and coma ensue. The body temperature is in excess of 40·6°C. Treatment is directed to reducing the rectal temperature by any physical means that are available, such as covering the patient with wet towels under a fan. The rectal temperature is taken at five-minute intervals and when it has fallen to 38·9°C the patient is maintained in cool surroundings.

Dehydration (see also p. 602)

Conditions associated with severe loss of water and electrolytes from the bowel such as cholera, and occasionally bacillary dysentery, must be treated by i v infusions according to the needs of the case. In cholera, where vomiting and diarrhoea are usually profuse, rehydration of the patient should be rapid. The first litre of isosmotic sodium chloride solution should be given i v in 15 minutes, the second over 45 minutes; and thereafter 1 litre every two or three hours, so that between 5 and 10 litres are given during the first 24 hours, after which i v therapy can usually be discontinued.

D. R. SEATON

FOR FURTHER READING

ADAMS, A. R. D. & MAEGRAITH, B. G. *Clinical Tropical Diseases,* 5th ed. Oxford: Blackwell. 1971.

JOPLING, W. H. *The treatment of Tropical Diseases,* 2nd ed. Bristol: John Wright & Sons. 1968.

WILCOCKS, C. & MANSON-BAHR, P. E. C. *Manson's Tropical Diseases,* 17th ed. London: Ballière, Tindall and Cassell. 1972.

WILMOT, A. J. *Clinical Amoebiasis.* Oxford: Blackwell. 1962.

CHAPTER 21

Emergencies In Occupational Medicine

(For list of Industrial Diseases see p. 687)

THE doctor practising in industry needs two complementary sides to his medical expertise: he must be prepared to deal with any emergency and should know the local specific industrial hazards. Local practitioners also should be aware of occupational diseases likely to occur where they practise. As more and more new compounds are made and used industrial toxicology becomes more complicated and perhaps bewildering for the family doctor or the casualty officer faced with an acute condition requiring immediate action.

Many of the emergencies described in other chapters occur at work. Their management in occupational and general medicine has much in common. This chapter deals only with special problems arising at work and with the following four groups of special occupational hazards—gassings, chemical poisonings, physical injuries, zoonoses and infections.

The action to be taken depends on whether the patient is inside or outside the works.

Inside the workplace

If the condition is serious the doctor or nurse will have to go into the plant. Portable equipment is then essential including the standard bag with dressings and analgesics such as morphine or heroin for immediate first aid. Factories in Great Britain employing more than fifty persons are required by law to have on site at least one trained first-aider. Portable breathing apparatus (the Ambu bag, p. 731, and oxygen face masks, p. 740) will be useful. A portable electrocardiogram can help in deciding on the early management of severe myocardial infarction. Unless, however, the emergency occurs far from a hospital, rapid transfer by ambulance is preferable.

Full-time doctors who work for large industrial organisations have detailed plans for dealing with large-scale emergencies such as widespread gassing or for treating a worker taken ill in some inaccessible position. Rescue teams consisting of a doctor, nurse and first-aiders are trained to deal with these problems. Practice exercises keep the team in constant readiness. A useful additional person is someone who from intimate knowledge of the layout can lead the team quickly to the victims. When the doctor reaches the casualty the first measure to be taken will be the immediate treatment of coma, asphyxia or severe pulmonary irritation. The victims must be removed quickly and given oxygen by mask (p. 740). Most firms using or manufacturing hazardous agents issue written instructions on how to deal with poisoning by them. When the patient is transferred to hospital this information together with any other details should go with him. Emergencies in industry may be widespread; the escape of noxious fumes of liquids may as a result of fire or explosion affect many people. Major accident contingency plans should be drawn up in conjunction with the local emergency services, the fire brigade, police and the nearest hospital. A designated person should implement such plans. Management has ' third party ' responsibility to the community living near the plant as well as to its employees.

Outside the workplace

Not all industrial emergencies present immediately after exposure. Delayed symptoms may cause an acutely ill person to be seen by the family or hospital doctor. He should enquire in detail into the patient's occupation and if he is in any way suspicious of industrial poisoning or injury he should make direct enquiries at the place of work. In Great Britain the Employment Medical Adviser (EMA) for the area may be helpful (EMA Headquarters, Baynards House, 1 Chepstow Place, W2 4TY 01-229 3456). Help can also be obtained from the Poisons Information Centre (see Appendix 12, p. 813) and the Information and Advisory Service of the TUC Centenary Institute of Occupational Health, London School of Hygiene and Tropical Medicine, Keppel Street, London WC1E 7HT (01-580 2386 office hours).

Leakage of dangerous liquids and gases from large tankers may result from an accident in transit. Most manufacturers insist that clear instructions on what to do are written on the tankers and also any necessary telephone number.

General measures

Few occupational emergencies require specific antidotes; if the patient is unconscious a good airway and adequate ventilation must be maintained. Measures may be needed to correct specific dysfunction. Important points are the nature of the noxious agent, the length of and time since exposure and a knowledge of the methods of treatment.

GASSINGS

Types of gases

Simple asphyxiants: Nitrogen, Carbon dioxide, Hydrogen, Methane.

Chemical asphyxiants: Carbon monoxide (p. 28). Hydrogen cyanide.

Gases irritant to the upper respiratory tract: Sulphur dioxide, Ammonia.

Gases irritant to the lower respiratory tract: Nitrous fumes, Ozone, Phosgene.

Anaesthetic vapours. Carbon tetrachloride, Trichloroethylene.

Systemic poisons. Hydrogen sulphide, Arsine, Phosphine.

Asphyxia as an emergency at work is usually due to gassing and certain measures must be carried out rapidly.

Removal of the affected person to a safe place

The source of the leak must be found and the emission of gas stopped immediately. Approach should be from the windward side and rescuers should be attached by lifeline to others standing at a safe distance. Where the gas is known to be lighter than air (nitrogen, hydrogen, ammonia) then the rescue team should crawl into the danger area to extract the victim. Knowledge of gas density enables the rescuers to work where the concentration is lowest. Breathing apparatus should be worn if the gas is extensive and ventilation should be increased by opening windows and doors. Those linking with other rooms should be closed. Clothing contaminated with an asphyxiant such as hydrogen cyanide should be removed and the patient rinsed with water.

Treatment. Lay the patient flat and maintain an airway. Give oxygen and use resuscitation measures on the journey to hospital. The decision to abandon treatment should only be made after prolonged attempts to revive the victim (see p. 735). It cannot be stressed too much that prompt action is essential. Delay in commencing ventilation may be disastrous. Almost invariably there are advantages in taking oxygen to the patient in the rescue manoeuvre rather than waiting until he is removed to a safer place. The only exception is where oxygen may form an explosive mixture in the presence of the offending gas, for example, hydrogen.

Occupational asthma

Certain industrial exposures can cause severe asthma. The iso-cyanates, for example toluene di-isocyanate (TDI), can cause marked bronchoconstriction in the sensitised worker. TDI because of its higher volatility is more dangerous in this respect than di-isocyanate di-phenyl-methane (MDI). Platinum, osmium and iridium if inhaled as dusts can cause respiratory irritation. Some people are allergic to certain wood dusts such as redwood. Treatment is as for asthma of non-occupational origin (p. 194). Sensitisation from further exposure should be avoided.

SIMPLE ASPHYXIANTS

These act by simple substitution of oxygen and there is no direct chemical injury to any system. Treatment is to remove the victim from the source and give him oxygen. Carbon dioxide is a hazard of the fermentation rooms in breweries and can also be dangerous in ship holds, refrigeration plants and lime calcining works. As CO_2 is heavier than air, workers in immediate danger of gassing should leave the area by the most elevated route and never crawl out. The gas is odourless and colourless and if a CO_2-filled room is entered the victim is 'pole-axed' by asphyxia so suddenly that he cannot take evading action or warn others.

CHEMICAL ASPHYXIANTS

These act specifically on blood or tissue cells irrespective of oxygen concentration.

Carbon monoxide (CO) is the most important member of this group (see p. 28). It is explosive and results from incomplete combustion of carbonaceous products. Firemen, coalminers and blast furnace men are particularly at risk. Before methane gas was generally used for domestic purposes CO was one of the commonest poisons used by suicides. In 1971 it was responsible for a quarter of the gassing accidents reported in Great Britain and 40 per cent of gassing fatalities. Hyperbaric oxygen (p. 814) is particularly effective in lowering the carboxyhaemoglobin concentrations.

Hydrogen cyanide (HCN) is a highly dangerous gas which acts by interfering with oxygen transfer from haemoglobin to tissue cells. The cyanide radicle causes enzyme damage. Other cyanide compounds are also dangerous. As HCN is a volatile liquid it is more dangerous in practice than, say, sodium cyanide which is a solid. Cyanide salts are hazardous mainly because, in the presence of

16

acid (including gastric hydrochloric acid), HCN is released. In industry cyanides are encountered in the manufacture of plastics, in fumigation operations and in metal hardening. Careful precautions are necessary to avoid inhalation of gaseous cyanide, as its infamous ' bitter almonds ' smell is not always noted even in high concentrations. Skin absorption of liquid HCN is also possible. HCN poisoning is rapidly fatal, producing respiratory paralysis by ' tissue apnoea ' in a matter of seconds. Test papers similar to those described for hydrogen sulphide (p. 465) are available and the rescue methods outlined earlier must be implemented immediately a leakage occurs.

Poisoning causes a metallic taste in the mouth and mucous membrane irritation followed by dizziness, nausea and frontal headache. Rapidly progressive tissue anoxia leads to a feeling of chest constriction, hyperpnoea, weakness and finally to fits, coma and death. Cyanide poisoning is a medical emergency requiring the highest priority and the swiftest possible action. Apart from extracting the victim, removing contaminated clothing and starting artificial respiration immediately, the inhalation of amyl nitrite may help to revive a partially conscious victim. Cobalt EDTA (Kelocyanor Rona) should be given i v without delay by the first competent person to arrive. The dose is two ampoules (40 ml), i.e. 300 mg i v using a large needle to ensure rapid injection. Follow it immediately with 50 ml of Dextrose Injection Strong BPC (50 g/dl). A third ampoule (150 mg) may be given followed by dextrose if there is insufficient improvement as shown by a failure of blood pressure to rise. Blood for cyanide estimation should be taken through the same venepuncture *before* administration of Cobalt EDTA. Recovery is often rapid after one dose but it may cause retching, hypotension and tachycardia. Further doses should be given if no improvement occurs within a few minutes. One of the newer kits should be kept in all premises using cyanide compounds. The old method of giving sodium nitrite and sodium thiosulphate i v has been superseded as sodium nitrite is itself toxic. Hydroxocobalamine (aqua-cobalamine vitamin B_{12} a) (100 ml of 10 g/dl solution i v) has been used successfully, and may be preferable as it is non-toxic (K. D. Friedberg *et al.*, 1966).

IRRITANT GASES

The distinction between upper and lower respiratory tract irritants is not merely a convenient subdivision. It indicates the differing symptomatology of the two types and also the kind of medical equipment required. The danger is inversely proportional to the solubility of the gas in water, the less soluble being more insidious in its action as its irritant nature is less well recognised.

UPPER RESPIRATORY TRACT IRRITANTS

Ammonia, chlorine and **sulphur dioxide** are highly soluble and are absorbed on the mucous membranes closest to the outside atmosphere. This causes lacrimation, conjunctivitis, laryngitis and acute dyspnoea and may lead to pulmonary oedema. Most people are forced to leave an atmosphere of such gases before pulmonary oedema supervenes but if this is not possible death from respiratory failure will occur. Removal from the gas and the administration of oxygen are the first steps to take. Inhalation of Friars' Balsam (Compound Tincture of Benzoin BP) 10 ml in 1 litre of hot water often alleviates the symptoms but the painful cough may require antitussives (p. 210). Morphine or atropine are usually not very effective and may be dangerous.

LOWER RESPIRATORY TRACT IRRITANTS

Pulmonary oedema and respiratory failure are more insidious in this group, the warning signs of upper respiratory tract irritation often being absent. Nitrogen dioxide classically produces this syndrome and anyone known to have been exposed to it, e.g. burners of nitrated compounds, arc welders or silo-fillers, should be admitted to hospital and kept under close surveillance for 24 hours. The occasional and frequently mild cough or eye irritation passes off quickly and 2 to 20 hours later the severely exposed individual will rapidly develop pulmonary oedema with cyanosis, cough, haemoptysis and tachypnoea. The treatment is similar to that described for ammonia, chlorine and sulphur dioxide gassing but hyperbaric oxygen may be particularly efficacious (p. 814).

Phosgene ($COCl_2$) has effects similar to those of nitrogen dioxide. Its danger lies in the fact that the gas can be released when certain chlorinated hydrocarbons, such as carbon tetrachloride, trichloroethane and chloroform come into contact with an open flame or hot metal. Firemen are frequently at risk from such reactions.

Inhalation of **nickel carbonyl** (odourless) causes a dry cough, dyspnoea and retro-sternal pain coming on 24 to 36 hours after exposure. Close observation for this period is advised after a gassing accident. Treatment is by oxygen inhalation, bed rest and measures for pulmonary oedema (p. 229). The best chelating agent is sodium diethyldithiocarbamate trihydrate (Dithiocarb*) prepared by adding 10 ml of phosphate buffer (0·5 g NaH_2PO_4 per 100 ml) to 1.0 g powdered dithiocarb. The solution contains 100 mg of dithiocarb per ml. The suggested initial dose i m is 25 mg/kg BW (total in 24 hours limited to 100 mg/kg BW). Orally the dose is 30 mg/kg BW.

ANAESTHETIC VAPOURS

These include a number of chlorinated hydrocarbons in industry as well as benzene and toluene. These compounds are used mainly as degreasers and some, such as trichloroethylene, are used in anaesthesia. Apart from the risk of mental confusion or narcosis, hepatic damage is frequent, **carbon tetrachloride** being one of the most dangerous. Others cause blood dyscrasias and benzene, which can cause aplastic anaemia, is now banned from most uses as a solvent in industry. Efficient ventilation of degreasing tanks should prevent the danger of excessive inhalation but no naked flame should be allowed near the liquids. Not all these compounds are inflammable but may release phosgene when heated. Anyone suffering from even mild narcosis due to chlorinated hydrocarbons should rest and be kept under observation for 48 hours. Liver function should also be monitored though treatment remains symptomatic.

Addiction to some of these compounds is well recognised and a number of **trichloroethylene** 'sniffers' have died as a result of injudicious inhalation. **Carbon tetrachloride** as well as producing liver necrosis, can cause severe gastro-intestinal disturbances with diarrhoea, vomiting and abdominal pain which may confuse the clinical picture and suggest an abdominal emergency (p. 121).

SYSTEMIC POISONS

These include hydrogen sulphide, arsine and phosphine all of which are local irritants but this is not their main action. **Hydrogen sulphide** from the smelting of sulphurous ores is well known for its nauseating 'rotten eggs' smell but olfactory fatigue is not uncommon and workers who have tolerated low concentrations have become suddenly unconscious when the concentration has risen. Small amounts irritate the mucous membranes leading to sore throat, sneezing, conjunctivitis and even keratitis. Paralysis of the

* Obtainable from Sigma (London), Norbiton Station Yard, Kingston-upon-Thames, Surrey, KT2 7BH. Tel. 01-549 3171 (reversed charges) as product D 3506. It is only available in Britain as a laboratory chemical. This does not prevent a doctor from using it clinically if he sees fit and there is no statutory enactment to prevent him from so doing.

respiratory muscles can occur in higher concentrations. Lead acetate paper darkens in its presence and may therefore give some warning as the speed of darkening is directly proportional to the concentration. Treatment is the same as for simple asphyxiants. **Arsine** (AsH_3 arseniuretted hydrogen) is formed in smelting operations when nascent hydrogen reacts with trivalent arsenic in the ore. It is not produced intentionally and is of no commercial use. **Phosphine** (PH_3) is a by-product of acetylene when this is produced from crude carbide. Both are lower respiratory tract irritants but they also cause nausea, vomiting and abdominal pain. Convulsions and coma may supervene before pulmonary oedema starts. Arsine can also cause severe haemolytic anaemia and kidney damage. Neither is a common industrial hazard. Arsine poisoning is treated with British Anti-Lewisite (BAL, Dimercaprol) (see p. 35) and blood transfusion if haemolysis is severe. Peritoneal dialysis (p. 716) or haemodialysis (p. 805) has been shown to lower the mortality from severe arsine poisoning (*Lancet*, 1971). There is no antidote for phosphine.

CHEMICAL POISONING

The number of chemical poisons is enormous and here we concentrate on the more important ones. They enter by ingestion, skin absorption and inhalation.

INGESTION

This is uncommon unless the worker is immersed in the liquid or is manipulating it close to his mouth, e.g pipetting. It is more commonly a mode of suicide.

SKIN ABSORPTION

This occurs with water-soluble and fat-soluble compounds. The range is vast and includes aniline, pesticides such as DDT and organo-phosphorous compounds, cyanides, phenol (pp. 37, 473 and 559), tetra-ethyl lead and the chlorinated hydrocarbons. A knowledge of whether a given compound can be absorbed is essential as it is useless to treat the victim unless his contaminated clothes are removed and his skin cleaned. If such compounds are present in large quantities at the workplace an emergency shower bath should be provided close to the source of the material. The victim can then be washed immediately before he is removed for further treatment.

INHALATION

This is by far the most important route of entry in industrial practice. Dusts, gases and vapours all act by absorption through or by their effect on, the respiratory tract. Speed of action is the most important feature and allows the following somewhat artificial division to be made.

RAPID ONSET. Metal fume fever. Cyanides.

MEDIUM ONSET. Pesticides. Aniline compounds.

SLOW ONSET. Lead. Mercury. Benzene. Carbon disulphide. Beryllium.

Some poisons could be included in more than one category and some are only harmful in the gaseous phase, e.g. benzene. The examples given illustrate the range of problems that may face a doctor confronted with a poisoned patient and underline the importance of a detailed history of possible exposure to noxious materials when dealing with a seriously ill patient.

POISONING OF RAPID ONSET

Metal fume fever

This is rarely serious and occurs when there is exposure to molten metals, especially zinc, as at brass foundries and rolling mills and during welding operations.

Fever, chills and dry cough commence four to eight hours after exposure. Polyuria and diarrhoea may occur. The mechanism is presumably allergic and immunity can be acquired. The symptoms are worst on Monday mornings and after a prolonged absence from work. The diagnosis is made by taking the occupational history. Treatment is symptomatic. As welders can be affected it is important to distinguish this syndrome from ozone poisoning which tends to cause more severe upper respiratory tract irritation.

Ozone poisoning (O_3)

Electrical discharges produce ozone and welders therefore are at special risk. Water purification and bleaching operations sometimes use ozone. The acute effects are upper respiratory tract irritation (p. 463). Treatment is symptomatic. Oxygen is often essential. Chronic low dosage exposure can cause permanent lung damage.

Cyanides (see p. 461)

Fluorine and hydrofluoric acid

Fluorine gas is released in the smelting of fluoride (aluminium) ores. It is combined with various chemicals to produce refrigerants (Fluon) and ' non-stick' surfaces (PTFE). Hydrofluoric acid is used to etch glass and cloud electric light bulbs and to ' print' circuits in electronic factories. It is occasionally added to the water used by window cleaners to clear roof lights. Small amounts of fluorine and hydrofluoric acid can cause abdominal pain, salivation and pruritus. One gram by causing severe irritation to mucous membranes and pulmonary oedema is rapidly fatal. Skin burns are severe and need immediate treatment. The area should be flooded with water or preferably warm saturated sodium carbonate solution for at least 20 minutes. A quaternary ammonium derivative such as benzalkonium chloride (Roccal) in a 1 g/l solution should be applied as an ice cold soak for one to four hours. After the soak a paste made of two parts glycerine and one part magnesium oxide should be massaged into the burn and left as a dressing which is changed daily. Chronic low concentration exposure to fluorine leads to fluorosis with increased bone density, pitted teeth and backache.

POISONING OF MEDIUM ONSET

Pesticides. These cover a wide range of chemicals. Most of them enter the body by skin absorption and skin decontamination is therefore vital.

Dinitro compounds, e.g. Dinitro-orthocresol (DNOC).

These herbicides uncouple oxidative phosphorylation and stimulate metabolism by extrathyroid routes. The patient presents in a hyperexcitable state, sweating and thirsty. Tachycardia, insomnia and loss of weight may be the presenting symptoms depending on the duration and severity of exposure. The skin and hair may be stained yellow. Treatment depends on the DNOC concentrations but is largely symptomatic. Sedation, fluids, cooling and oxygen may be needed in severe cases.

Organochlorine compounds (DDT, BHC, Lindane, Eldrin).

These are 'persistent' pesticides and acute overdosage involves the central nervous system and causes excitement, muscle fibrillation, tremors and convulsions. Tachypnoea is eventually superseded by apnoea. Oral ingestion calls for gastric lavage. The effects on the central nervous system are best controlled with diazepam (Valium). Artificial ventilation may be required.

Organophosphorus compounds (Parathion, TEPP, Dimefox)

These compounds inhibit cholinesterase and their effect is to produce parasympathetic overstimulation with nausea, vomiting, abdominal cramps, salivation, sweating and pupillary constriction.

Generalised muscle twitching leading to convulsions and coma may follow. Apart from skin decontamination, atropine sulphate 2 mg should be given i m as soon as the diagnosis is established. This large dose should be repeated if symptoms are not relieved immediately. A total dosage of up to 100 mg has been recorded. After taking blood for cholinesterase estimation a cholinesterase reactivator such as pralidoxime (P_2S) should be given in a dose of 1·0 g in 2 to 3 ml of water i m or 1·0 g in 6 to 20 ml of water i v. Pralidoxime (p. 767) is complementary to atropine and both can be administered simultaneously. The maintenance of pulmonary ventilation is of prime importance throughout the treatment.

Bipyridilium compounds (Diquat, Paraquat)

Few cases of occupationally acquired poisoning by these contact herbicides are recorded but poisoning from accidental or suicidal ingestion is fairly common. Paraquat is supplied by registered horticultural merchants and pharmacists under the names Dextrone, Dexuron, Gramonol and Terraklene. Diquat is sold as Aquacide and Reglone. Pathclear and Weedol contain both Diquat and Paraquat (see p. 38).

Aniline and the nitro and amino benzene derivatives

These compounds cause methaemoglobinaemia and a grey-blue pallor of the lips and gums is characteristic. Skin absorption is an important mode of entry. The acute effects include cyanosis, dyspnoea, confusion and convulsions. Chronic low dose exposure causes anaemia, lethargy, headache and digestive disturbances in addition to cyanosis. Treatment consists of skin decontamination, oxygen and a reducing agent such as ascorbic acid or methylene blue (a slow i v injection of 2 mg per kg body weight as a 1·0 g/dl solution).

Phosphorus

The symptomatology of phosphorus poisoning can be very varied, depending on the chemical configuration:

Yellow phosphorus: Severe jaundice and ' Phossy jaw '.

Red phosphorus: Non-poisonous.

Tri-ortho-cresyl-phosphate (TOCP): Peripheral neuropathy (' Jake paralysis ').

Organo-phosphorus: Parasympathetic stimulation (p. 467).

The mandibular necrosis of yellow phosphorous poisoning is virtually unknown now as the substance is banned in the manufacture of matches. It was treated by antibiotics and surgery. TOCP is a plasticiser and is hazardous because it volatilises so readily. There are three stages of poisoning: the first occurs after a latent period of 3 to 21 days and is characterised by gastrointestinal upset. Then foot drop may supervene and by the end of four weeks the third stage of upper limb involvement begins. Treatment is largely symptomatic but cholinesterase reactivators (Pralidoxime, P_2S, see p. 468 and p. 767) may be helpful. There may be residual weakness or numbness.

Cadmium

This illustrates the difficulty in classifying toxic chemicals on the basis of speed of onset of symptoms. Cadmium fumes produced during welding or alloying can cause pulmonary oedema and act like a lower respiratory irritant gas. The symptoms commence 24 to 36 hours after exposure and if severe, death will supervene within a few days. Survival or chronic low concentration exposure may be followed by chronic pulmonary emphysema or acute renal tubular damage leading to proteinuria, aminoaciduria or glycosuria. Rhinitis, anosmia, testicular atrophy and yellow rings on the teeth have also been described. Acute inhalation is treated with Calcium EDTA i v in a concentration not to exceed 3 per cent. The maximal dose per course of treatment is 2·5 g per 4·5 kg body weight. The rate of infusion per 4·5 kg BW should not exceed 170 mg per hour; 330 mg/day or 1 670 mg/week. Chronic poisoning can be treated with i v calcium EDTA or by oral administration of 0·5 g calcium EDTA every two hours while awake for one to two weeks.

Arsenic

This is a common contaminant of metalliferous ores and is a hazard in smelting plants. Its use in insecticides, weed killers and as a glass opacifier extends the potential risk to other industries. Acute poisoning occurs within 12 to 24 hours of ingestion or inhalation and results in severe gastrointestinal disturbances and haemolysis leading to coma and death. Emergency measures are blood transfusion and renal dialysis. Chronic poisoning causes digestive upsets, peripheral neuritis, which is predominantly sensory, and jaundice. White striae on the nails, ' rain drop ' skin, depigmentation and the peripheral neuropathy are almost pathognomonic of chronic arsenical poisoning. Dimercaprol (BAL) is the treatment of choice (see p. 35).

Lead

Lead is one of the oldest known metals and is a major industrial hazard. The signs and symptoms of inorganic and organic lead intoxication differ and will be considered separately.

Inorganic lead. Poisoning can occur among those who are occupationally exposed to lead dust or fumes: smelters, ship builders and breakers, scrap yard workers, battery makers and plumbers, lead paint manufacturers, amateur potters, glass makers, chemical and plastic workers. Absorption is almost invariably by inhalation and the effects can be classified as early or late though in fact there is a continuum from normal blood levels through excessive absorption to frank poisoning. Early symptoms are fatigue, lassitude, anorexia, headache, arthralgia, facial pallor, dyspepsia, constipation or intermittent diarrhoea, and a metallic taste in the mouth. Late symptoms are abdominal discomfort, colic, vomiting, weakness of muscle groups leading to wrist drop, blue line on the gums and kidney damage with proteinuria and casts. The diagnosis depends on blood and urine lead estimation, coproporphyrinuria and the clinical findings.

Treatment is by symptomatic management and the use of chelating agents such as calcium sodium EDTA (3 g in 600 ml of dextrose 5 g/dl i v over two hours and repeated if necessary). Calcium gluconate 10 ml of 10 per cent solution i v and atropine subcutaneously are used for lead colic. D-Penicillamine 600 to 1 500 mg daily by mouth is an alternative to EDTA.

Organic lead. Tetraethyl and tetramethyl lead are antiknock agents in petrol. Both are lipid-soluble and readily absorbed from the lungs, skin and gastrointestinal tract. Although ethyl lead is more toxic, both cross the blood-brain barrier and it is the central nervous system signs which predominate in organic lead poisoning. The latent period is two to three hours between exposure and symptoms. Fatal cases develop severe delirium, alternating mania and depression, convulsions, hallucinations and coma. Less severe manifestations include anxiety states, nightmares and abdominal pains. The most useful investigations are the blood and urine lead levels. Treatment is by skin decontamination and D-Penicillamine or calcium EDTA in two to three repeated seven-day courses. Symptomatic treatment with diazepam (Valium) is helpful but morphine should not be given.

Mercury (see also p. 38)

Like lead this is a long-established hazard but it is even more insidious in its effects. Few people seem to realise that metallic mercury has a vapour pressure and that it can be absorbed from the skin as well as from the lungs and gut. (For method of sweeping up spilled mercury and risks in aircraft see p. 73). Inorganic mercury is used in making pharmaceuticals, paints, amalgams, instruments and neon signs and in dentistry. Organic mercury is used as a seed dressing and in the explosives industry. Acute poisoning is rarely a problem in industry but when it occurs it causes gastrointestinal disorders, convulsions and acute oliguric renal failure. The common more chronic mercurialism classically causes ' erethism ' which is a psychiatric syndrome of self-consciousness, paranoia, timidity, anxiety and headaches. Dermatographia, a fine intention tremor and slurred speech may also occur. Organic mercury does not cause erethism but spastic quadriparesis and ataxia with contraction of the visual fields is more frequently seen. A late manifestation of both types of compound may be the nephrotic syndrome. Penicillamine (p. 470) is the treatment of choice combined with symptomatic management of the renal and central nervous system disorders.

Benzene

This has acute narcotic effects with euphoria, giddiness and excitement. After recovery there should be continued surveillance as the long-term sequelae include aplastic anaemia, leukaemias of several varieties, a common one being the Di-Gugliemo syndrome (erythroleukaemia and hyperplasia or dysplasia of red cell precursors in the bone marrow and a peripheral blood picture showing normocytic and hypochromic anaemia, nucleated red cells, thrombocytopenia and a low or normal white cell count). Chromosomal aberrations have also been described. Benzene illustrates the importance of following up apparently successful recovery from industrial poisoning to try and prevent, or institute early treamtent of, more serious later effects.

Carbon disulphide

This highly volatile liquid is used in the viscose rayon industry, in cold vulcanisation of rubber, pesticide manufacture and as a solvent in other industries. Its acute effects are largely confined to the central nervous system and include mania, depression, amnesia, hallucinations, psychosis and dementia. Sensory and motor neuropathies and abdominal discomfort can also occur. The treatment is symptomatic. Long-term effects include Parkinsonism and an increased tendency to myocardial infarction.

Beryllium

This is used in fluorescent light manufacture and for various alloys and is hazardous when inhaled as a dust. Acute respiratory embarrassment with pneumonitis commences within hours of exposure and recovery takes one to four weeks. Chronic beryllium disease is a sarcoid-like granulomatous affection of the lungs and liver. Corticosteroids if used early may arrest the process.

This account of chemical poisonings is not exhaustive but it illustrates the wide range of symptoms and the need for the doctor to consider differential diagnoses of various syndromes. These include acute confusional states, convulsions, peripheral neuropathy and gastrointestinal disorders as well as the ubiquitous respiratory embarrassment. Toxicological investigations may reveal an occupational source for the poisoning but the doctor must always keep in the back of his mind the possibility of criminal intent however remote this may seem. One of us (J. M. H.) recently investigated an outbreak of peripheral neuropathy of the Guillain-Barré type associated with alopecia and severe gastroenteritis. The clinical diagnosis was thallium poisoning but this was not occupationally acquired, being due to deliberate poisoning of his colleagues by a fellow worker.

PHYSICAL INJURIES

In industry most serious or fatal physical injuries are caused by machinery or are the result of transport or handling procedures. The injuries are no different from similar accidents in the home or on the road but some specific physical hazards will be mentioned.

High temperatures

Burns and scalds in Great Britain in 1972 accounted for 3 per cent of industrial accidents reported to the Chief Inspector of Factories. Heat syncope may also occur particularly among furnace men and similar workers. The symptoms are dizziness, nausea and blurred vision. Treatment is by rest, cooling and salted drinks. In heat exhaustion the patient may be suffering from salt or water depletion (see p. 602).

Low temperatures (see also p. 489)

Work in cold storage rooms may cause hypothermia and peripheral vasoconstriction if exposure is lengthy or the protective clothing inadequate. Serious cardiac arrhythmias are common at body temperatures below 30°C. The management of acute hypothermia is rapid rewarming. If hypothermia has been prolonged fluid balance must be carefully monitored as peripheral vasodilatation in response to warming may lead to a further lowering of ' core ' temperature in the initial stage of treatment The ECG may be helpful (see p. 362).

Chemical burns

Strong acids, alkalis, phenol and hydrofluoric acid (p. 466) are the commonest agents causing skin damage. Particular attention should be paid to the eyes when treating chemical splashes. Appropriate eye wash bottles should be strategically sited in areas where the risk of chemical burns is high. Isosmotic sodium chloride solution is the best general purpose eye-wash. Boric acid 10 mg to 1 litre should be added to discourage fungus growth. Other solutions for various chemical eye burns are described on page 530. Unless the wash bottle is known to be clean and recently replenished, flushing the eyes with water will suffice until fresh saline arrives. All skin injuries should, in the first instance, be treated by copious washing with water. Skin damaged by corrosives such as caustic soda (NaOH) or hydrochloric acid (HCl) should be washed with isosmotic sodium chloride solution. Phenol burns require swabbing with glycerol, polyethylene glycol (PEG) or a 70/30 PEG methylated spirit solution for at least ten minutes. Phenolic eye burns should be flushed with large amounts of water followed by local anaesthetic and oily drops if necessary (see p. 559).

Lasers

The increasing use of laser beams in industry carries with it the risk of burning, particularly to the eye. Damage to the cornea, retina and lens may be severe and permanent leading to partial or total blindness. Apart from first-aid measures an ophthalmologist should be consulted as soon as possible.

Abnormal pressures

High and low environmental pressure can cause decompression sickness when the worker is returned to normal pressures. This is a hazard to caisson workers and high altitude fliers (p. 506) as well as to deep sea divers (p. 494).

Electric shock (see also p. 648)

Electricity was responsible for 5 per cent of all fatal industrial accidents reported to the Chief Inspector of Factories in 1972. Most electric shock injuries or deaths are due to contact with alternating currents, usually of 50 or 60 Hz (cycles per second). The severity of the effect is inversely proportional to the electrical resistance of the body, the latter being decreased by wet skin or clothing. The current pathway is also important. Most fatal shocks have a pathway across the heart and only 3 per cent of currents which cause death pass through the head. Currents crossing the chest in excess of 20-40 mA produce tetanic contractions of the chest muscles and apnoea. If the current is not interrupted within two to three minutes death ensues. Ventricular fibrillation is the most important cause of death, however, and normal rhythm rarely returns spontaneously. Current passing through the respiratory centre in the brain stem may cause persistent respiratory paralysis even when the current ceases to flow. Immediate resuscitation is essential and should be instituted as soon as the victim is disconnected. (For details see p. 724.)

Electrical burns are treated similarly to thermal burns (p. 554) except that severe burning may produce chromoproteinuria due to excess of myoglobin from the muscles damaged by severe contraction. Alkaline infusions may reduce the risk of renal damage. Various neurological sequelae have been described and may be due to injury to spinal nerves caused by the violent movement of vertebrae resulting from massive muscular contractions.

ZOONOSES AND INFECTIONS

Occupationally acquired infections from animals or from handling infected materials are uncommon but they are important because failure to diagnose them early can have serious consequences.

Anthrax (see p. 549).

Leptospirosis (see p. 441).

Brucellosis is common among farmworkers and veterinarians.

Tetanus (see p. 637) is more likely to occur in farming communities than urban ones.

Failure to make an early diagnosis in an occupational disease can have serious consequences in the community if the disease is highly contagious. 'Natural' smallpox, cholera, typhus and tuberculosis are all now rare in western countries but they pose a threat to medical laboratory workers. Most emergencies in occupational medicine are avoidable and every case should be investigated to find the cause. Cases of lead poisoning or anilism, for example, should be followed up to decide whether other people at work are similarly affected. Some of the industrial emergencies described here have to be reported either for the purpose of prevention (the Notifiable Diseases, see p. 687) or for compensation for the affected worker (the Prescribed Diseases). None of the wide variety of conditions mentioned is particularly difficult to diagnose so long as the doctor is aware of the possibility that the illness may have been occupationally acquired. This is usually revealed by asking the patient's occupation.

J. M. HARRINGTON

R. S. F. SCHILLING

FOR FURTHER READING

ANNUAL REPORT. HM Chief Inspector of Factories. Cmnd 5398. London: HMSO. 1973.

CHIEF EMPLOYMENT MEDICAL ADVISER'S NOTES OF GUIDANCE. EMAS Department of Employment. London: HMSO. 1973.

EDITORIAL (1971). The arsine hazard. *Lancet,* 1, 71.

FRIEDBERG, K. D., GRÜTZMACHER, J. & LENDLE, L. (1966). Die Bedeutung der Wirkungsgeschwendigkeit von Antidoten bei der Behandlung der Blausäyrevergiftung. *Archiv Für Toxikologie,* 22, 176-191.

OCCUPATIONAL HEALTH AND SAFETY (2 vols.). Geneva: International Labour Office. 1971.

TECHNICAL DATA NOTES 1-41. Department of Employment. London: HMSO. 1972.

TREVETHICK, R. A. *Environmental and Industrial Health Hazards.* London: Heinemann. 1973.

CHAPTER 22

Medical Emergencies at Sea

(For medical advice by radio to ships at sea see p. 694)
(For broadcasting SOS messages see p. 694)
(For removal of patients by helicopter see p. 825)

No matter what size his ship or how long his journey the doctor has the priceless advantage of being able to anticipate the demands which may be made on him while on passage. Time spent in thought in preparation for the voyage is seldom wasted and it is an advantage to join the ship early.

Medicine afloat has to be practised without the benefit of sophisticated aids. Judicious inquiries should be made about the particular skills of medical passengers. Many a ship's doctor has slept more soundly in the knowledge that there is a surgeon or gynaecologist sleeping on B deck. Beware however lest a man's doctorate is in law or economics.

Learning to find one's way about is essential. This includes finding out how to reach parts difficult of access without destroying the watertight integrity of the ship. Passenger ships registered in Britain permanently exhibit plans showing watertight doors, the position of their controls and other relevant details. Booklets giving similar information are available to ship's officers (1965. 1103). Get an engineer to take you round the ship and wander round yourself to see where drugs, dressings and stretchers could be obtained in an emergency. Consider also what routes you would use for removing a casualty. After such inquiries many ship's doctors decide never to turn in without a morphine syringe and shoes, clothes, jersey and torch ready at hand.

Ship's rounds with the master provide another way of learning one's way about. A ship is sometimes described as a floating warehouse with a hotel complex. However hygienically maintained it enters ports of varying standard and is frequently at risk of recontamination by insects and rats. *Aedes aegypti* readily breeds on ships where small pools of fresh water occur and is probably the only significant vector to breed aboard. Most other insects as well as rats and mice join the ship in cargo. Oil seeds, copra, bulk bones and bananas may carry flies. Cockroaches frequently contaminate flour and animals bring fleas. Only constant vigilance will ensure that such contamination is recognised early. Rats are the reservoirs of plague and, in tropical areas, of murine typhus. Many rodents excrete *Salmonella typhimurium* and other organisms, and may play a part in transmitting Q fever, lymphocytic choriomeningitis and trichinosis. International Health Regulations (1969) require every ship to be either periodically deratted or kept permanently so. The Port Health Authority will always give advice and a list of designated ports for certification of deratting or of exemption from it is published by WHO (1974).

The crew

In times past ships carried large crews of relatively unskilled men who could turn their hands to most things and absence among them was easily made up from the rest of the complement. Modern seamen are more skilled but often less able to do other men's jobs. In addition there are fewer of them so that absence throws a greater strain on others. They have to work in extremes of heat, cold and humidity (Oliver, 1973). Lastly, a ship is in some ways like a village whose efficient functioning depends on a disciplined hierarchical structure. At the head is the master, a professional seaman who combines with this role that of squire, Justice of the Peace and parson, supported by his officers who may be very jealous of their departments. This structure the doctor must support in the knowledge that, like all villages, a ship thrives on rumour and gossip. He can be hard put to it to preserve medical confidences, support his captain, allay anxiety and take appropriate medical action.

The passengers

British ships required to carry a doctor are foreign-going vessels with upwards of a hundred persons, including crew. They are largely restricted to cruise liners. Their environments are no place for the aged, the unsteady or the severely disabled. The decision whether a passenger embarks is generally taken by the passenger himself and his family doctor. Sometimes the ship's doctor may be consulted. Passengers who are taking drugs should carry a letter giving up-to-date information. At sea they are not covered by the National Health Service and medical stores are limited; they must therefore carry adequate supplies of their medicines. Crew and sometimes passengers are treated gratis at sea but on most ships the care of passengers is a private matter and so attracts a fee. As there is always a risk of litigation the doctor should be sure that his subscription to his protection society is not in arrears. Membership affords unlimited indemnity against claims of professional negligence and is open to medical practitioners holding a qualification registrable with the General Medical Council who are on the register of the country in which they practice (other than the USA and, in the case of the Medical and Dental Defence Union of Scotland, in Canada also). But cover is given to members sued in US (and Canadian) Courts in respect of claims arising from treatment given as ship's surgeons. Against the cost of personal illness the doctor would be wise to take out an insurance policy.

MEDICO-LEGAL MATTERS AT SEA

The master is in law totally responsible for the ship and the safety of its crew and passengers. His authority is absolute and the doctor being one of his officers must obey his orders. The master is most unlikely, however, to disregard medical advice without good reason. The doctor must comply with the order of the master but should state any objection in writing for resolution later of the legal aspect before the owners, agents and British Consul. He must keep the master informed of health matters affecting the safety of the ship and those on board.

At sea the doctor has three loyalties which may conflict.

1. To the ship's company as a whole. Here he is acting in the capacity of a community physician with the authority to devise detention of the ship in quarantine and the right to enter all cabins. On arrival in port the master is required to prepare the ' Maritime Declaration of Health '. This provides evidence about plague, cholera, yellow fever, smallpox, typhus or relapsing fever which occurred on board or was suspected on passage, details of any illness on board on arrival and of any death which was not due to accident. It also requires evidence of plague in rats on board. The granting of a ' free pratique ' depends on the declaration or in some ports on equivalent application by radio. A second opinion can usually be obtained from the Port Medical Officer. Although he has the authority to require the isolation of contacts with infective diseases during the incubation period in question this rarely happens. Passengers are generally permitted to disembark under ' surveillance '. Rarely disinfection may be insisted upon.

2. To the owners and Ministry of Transport. Records of illness particularly in the crew and third class passengers are required. Accidents on board sometimes involve litigation so full records must be kept.

3. To the patient. The same considerations of professional secrecy apply as when ashore.

Restraint or confinement may sometimes be necessary in the potentially hazardous environment of a ship. Any such action must be recorded in the ship's log. A written second opinion from a medically qualified passenger is valuable support. The landing of a patient because of illness must be recorded as it is an offence to put ashore a passenger at a wrong port without his consent.

ALCOHOLISM

Drunkenness is an offence under the Merchant Shipping Act and can be punished by the master. The doctor may be called upon to examine a person and to give a firm opinion 'drunk or sober' (p. 677). By implication he excludes other factors (drugs, head injuries and cerebral malaria). The alcoholic may be a nuisance to others and the onus of any action is on the master. Amongst the crew and particularly if it is an officer who is drinking to excess it is often expedient to persuade the person to 'go sick' when abstinence can be enforced for a time.

MEDICAL EQUIPMENT AT SEA

The scale of medical stores in ocean-going vessels registered in the UK are laid down in the Merchant Shipping (Medical Scales) Regulations 1974 and the doctor should examine the scale before sailing since he may wish to supplement it. While some ships have extensively equipped sick bays most doctors will add their own drugs. An emergency bag (p. 1) is valuable not only on the ship but when called to another vessel. It is advisable to ensure that first aid equipment is ready wherever accidents may occur.

SEASICKNESS

For this disorder there is as yet no panacea. Most people will be seasick in rough weather but most regain their 'sea legs' in 24 to 48 hours. The usual remedies are hyoscine 0·6 mg followed by 0·3 mg six-hourly; promethazine (Avomine) 25 mg; dimenhydrinate (Dramamine) 50 mg. These are given one or two hours before rough weather and continued for 48 hours. They cause dryness of the mouth and disturbance of near vision but have a useful sedative effect. If the victim can sleep he often wakes much eased. The hopes held out for metoclopramide (Maxolon) (McMurray, 1973) have not been fully realised. For those prostrated by the disorder promethazine 25 mg i m followed by sleep is probably the most effective. Certain factors seem to make seasickness more obtrusive, such as malaise from another cause, peptic ulcer and excessive intake of alcohol. Apart from babes in arms young children are very prone to seasickness and may become dizzy and fall unexpectedly. They should be sent below when the early signs of yawning, swallowing and nausea appear and before they fall down. Prolonged seasickness can cause dehydration but the need to give fluid other than orally is rare. Some blood-streaking of vomit from oesophageal tears is not uncommon (Mallory-Weiss syndrome, p. 157) and the associated oesophagitis may need Asilone or alkalis for symptomatic relief. Probably the most dangerous features are injuries from falls whilst moving about a vessel in turbulent motion when one's balance is disturbed. As serious underlying disease may be concealed all should be examined for evidence of an acute abdominal emergency, tonsillitis, meningitis or middle ear disease. Even pregnancy can present as *mal-de-mer*.

PLAGUE

Rat-infestation is now rare in ships but it is still possible for plague to arise unexpectedly. Infection of humans is always preceded by an epidemic amongst the rats so that the finding of dead rats aboard should be looked into with alacrity. Particular features which obtain at sea favour dissemination amongst crew and passengers. Asian and African people may conceal an infected person on board since they are aware of and recognise buboes. The ventilation system may transmit *Pasteurella pestis* readily, resulting in pneumonic plague passed from person to person by droplet infection.

Whether the disease is bubonic or septicaemic the following action is recommended:

1. Isolate the patient in a cabin liberally dusted with DDT powder or similar insecticide. This should be used on all rat holes and runs and on the bodies of rats before disposal in the furnace or over the side.

2. All those attending the patient should wear masks, gowns and seaboots and, if the disease is septicaemic or pneumonic, goggles also.

3. Streptomycin 1 g i m followed by 500 mg six-hourly until afebrile for 24 hours or tetracycline 1 g i v followed by 1 g six-hourly by mouth for 48 hours. In neither of these is available give full doses of sulphonamides (12 g daily for adults).

4. All contacts should take tetracycline 2 g daily or sulphadimidine 3 g daily for one week.

5. Notify the owners by radio. They will tell the Department of Health who will notify WHO. (This applies also to cholera, yellow fever and smallpox at sea.)

PULMONARY EMBOLIC DISEASE

Seafarers tend to lead sedentary lives and when on their feet they are often standing on hot decks in engine rooms. They may develop some dependent oedema by the end of a watch. In addition, fungus infections of the feet with secondary infection are common. All these factors contribute to the subjective impression that in relatively young men deep venous thrombosis of the calves and pulmonary embolic disease are more common at sea than ashore. Such patients present with episodes of minor pulmonary embolism shown by transient dyspnoea and chest pain or a small haemoptysis. These episodes may lead to chronic thrombo-embolic pulmonary hypertension which sometimes precedes massive pulmonary embolism (p. 241). It may be that cardiac ' massage ' (p. 725) can reduce the amount of lung affected by forcing emboli deeper into the pulmonary tree.

In both major and minor embolism an immediate i v injection of 15 000 units of heparin reduces serotonin release from platelets which may diminish secondary bronchial and pulmonary artery constriction. Heparin is the only anticoagulant that can be monitored at sea, by using the coagulation time alone (p. 943). It can therefore be used for a few days giving 5 000 to 10 000 units i v every six to eight hours or by adding 40 000 units to dextrose 5 g/dl and giving 1 000 units over 24 hours. One should aim at a clotting time of two to three times the normal control. Heparin activity can be rapidly reversed by protamine sulphate BP (p. 283).

PSYCHIATRIC EMERGENCIES AT SEA

A ship is perhaps the most dangerous of all environments for the disturbed patient. Opportunities for self injury abound and many a depressive has just slipped over the side at night. It is not only lovers who stand on the fan-tail observing the wake. An elderly and widely experienced doctor used to make it a habit to take a walk round the stern at night before he turned in. Not only are the depressed at risk for an excited or alcoholic person is liable to fall on ladders and moving decks.

The handling of such cases depends very much on one's past experience. It is strongly recommended that the doctor should ensure his ability to handle a small number of drugs with confidence. The most useful are Largactil (chlorpromazine), Serenace (haloperidol) and Valium (diazepam). As alcohol potentiates the effects of chlorpromazine and barbiturates their dose should be reduced accordingly. The side effects are uncommon and on the credit side the anti-emetic effect is valuable at sea. Delirium tremens can be handled with chlorpromazine (Largactil) but chlormethiazide (Heminevrin) is in my experience better in calming delirium when shadows and lights are constantly on the move. Serenace (haloperidol) is a valuable alternative for the manic, agitated or schizophrenic; control requiring 3 to 9 mg daily. In acute outbursts 3 to 5 mg i v or i m should suffice.

Depression

Depressive states at sea can be most difficult to handle because supervisory staff is insufficient. Antidepressive drugs take about a week to act and when they do agitation is sometimes increased. There is much to be said for relying on sedation with chlorpromazine, support from discussion and such close supervision and protection from self harm as can be devised. It often helps to talk out the question of suicide in the light of assured help on reaching port. With this approach the patient is possibly less likely to attempt it while he retains the faith that the doctor can offer treatment in the foreseeable future. The most dangerous times are the early stages of depression and when the mood begins to lift; should these be while still out at sea very close observation should somehow be maintained.

MALARIA IN SHIPS

The endemicity, susceptibility of parasites to drugs and resistance of patients are all variables in malaria. *Anopheles* does not usually breed aboard ship (though *Aedes* mosquitoes which carry yellow fever and Arbor virus infections do so readily). Despite this an offshore wind may carry *Anopheles* on board. Passengers and crew who go ashore in malarious areas should wear long sleeves and trousers, particularly in the evening and early morning. Details of the malarial status of ports can be obtained from the local Port Health Authority and forward planning can be based on the WHO Epidemiological Record published twice a year. Briefly, one must anticipate malaria anywhere in the tropical seaboards of the world. (Fig. 20.1, p. 449).

Prophylaxis

Prophylactic regimes must be started on entering a malarial endemic area. The choice is:

1. Proguanil (Paludrine) 100 or 200 mg daily. Resistance is not common and 200 mg daily is effective at present, particularly in falciparum infections.

2. Pyrimethamine (Daraprim) 25 or 50 mg once weekly.

3. Chloroquine (Avlochlor, Resochin, Nivaquine) or amodiaquine (Camoquin) 300 mg once weekly. Chloroquine 100 mg of the base daily on six days of the week may be preferred.

4. Pyrimethamine (Daraprim) 40 mg once weekly combined with an appropriate dose of long-acting sulphonamide such as Sulfadoxine (Fanasil) 1 g or Sulfalene 2 g.

Since these drugs do not act on the pre-erythrocytic schizont malaria may develop later. Passengers must therefore continue them for four weeks after leaving a malarious area and tell their doctors where they have been if they become ill at home. These regimes should completely prevent *P. falciparum* parasitaemia. They will not prevent recurrence due to *P. vivax, ovale* or *malariae*. To avoid this an eight-week course of 300 mg chloroquine base combined with primaquine 45 mg once a week will usually cure relapsing malaria.

Clinical malaria

Certain diagnosis depends on demonstrating the parasite in a blood film but as this may be impossible on passage the following advice is given: always suspect malaria in any feverish illness and do not wait for it to evolve into a textbook pattern. If you do, many of those with malignant malaria will die. Treat on suspicion but first make thick and thin blood films for expert examination. The more ill the patient the more likely he is to have malignant malaria and the more urgent is the need for treatment (see p. 449; also British National Formulary 1974-76, p. 116).

Chloroquine resistant malaria (see also p. 448)

The distribution of strains of *P. falciparum* resistant to chloroquine is likely to vary but the situation as it obtains today is that resistance of *P. falciparum* to chloroquine has been proved but resistance of *P. vivax* and *P. malariae* has not been observed. The present distribution of chloroquine resistant strains is:

S AND CENTRAL AMERICA: Columbia, Brazil, Guyana, Surinam, Venezuela, Bolivia, Panama.

SE ASIA: Burma, E Malaysia, Philippines, Borneo, Thailand, Khymer Republic (Cambodia), Laos, Vietnam.

There is no evidence of chloroquine resistance in Africa, in Asia west of Burma or in the Western Pacific but there is widespread resistance to proguanil and pyrimethamine. For treatment see p. 450. More detailed advice is given in Chemotherapy of Malaria and Resistance to Antimalarials, WHO Technical Report Series No. 529, Geneva 1973.

DIARRHOEA AT SEA

The closed environment of a ship is ideal for the development of food poisoning and bacillary dysentery in epidemic proportions. The doctor should keep an eye on food preparation and handling and remember that cargoes can introduce organisms such as salmonellae from animal foodstuffs. It is uncommon for an epidemic of diarrhoea to be due to a specific organism and there is little evidence to support the belief that outbreaks are due to virus infections. Most travellers abroad get diarrhoea but whether this is due to recolonisation of the gut, alteration of the diet or other factors remains *sub judice*. (For treatment see p. 136.)

True bacillary dysentery acquired ashore in foreign ports can be a problem since sensitivities to antibiotics cannot be determined. There is widespread resistance of Shigellae to sulphonamides and streptomycin, particularly in the Mediterranean area and the Far East. The simple approach at sea is to regard acute toxic diarrhoeas with blood and slime in the stool as potential bacillary dysentery and to give neomycin 1 g six-hourly for five days or tetracycline.

Another cause is the flagellate *Giardia lamblia*. Stools tend to be two or three a day, often pale and explosive and associated with abdominal distension. Only rarely is the infestation severe enough to cause dehydration and malabsorption. It responds rapidly to metroidazole (Flagyl) 200 mg three times a day for seven days. An additional advantage is that in double this dosage it is a very effective amoebicide and if microscopy of the stools is not possible two objectives may be achieved in a rather empirical manner.

Diarrhoea causes anxiety amongst passengers. It is therefore often advisable to issue a statement, preferably through the captain, to allay anxiety. It is also expedient to be seen to pay attention to the methods and personal hygiene of food handlers. One of them may be a carrier of a specific organism. The advice of the Port Health Authority is invaluable.

In an epidemic the supply or storage of drinking water should be suspect. The delivery hose from ashore may be dropped into contaminated harbour water and then infect the water tank. Chlorination is harmless and may do much good. Instructions are given in *The Ship's Captain's Medical Guide* and on the cans of chloride of lime. Each of these carries sufficient to chlorinate 900 litres of water.

DENTAL EMERGENCIES AT SEA
(See also p. 642)

The ship's doctor should prepare himself by instruction from a dental colleague or by seeing the two films *Treatment of Dental Emergencies by Medical Staff,* No. 2290, obtainable from the Director of Dental Training and Research, Institute of Naval Medicine, Alverstoke, Hants., and by reading the accompanying handbook. Occasionally an epidemic of Vincent's stomatitis (acute necrotising ulcerative gingivitis) may spread rapidly amongst passengers or crew. Metronidazole (Flagyl) 200 mg three times a day has proved highly effective.

ARTHROPOD-BORNE VIRUS INFECTIONS

These are acquired by those who go ashore and the unsalted visitor to the tropics is particularly at risk. The most serious, yellow fever, should not occur if the international regulations on vaccination are observed. Both dengue and sand fly fevers are common in the tourist areas of the Mediterranean and Far East. Dengue fever is transmitted by culicine mosquitoes, particularly *Aedes aegypti,* and sand-fly fever by the sand fly *Phlebotomus papatasii.* Because of strain differences a patient seldom shows all the features described in a standard textbook. These acute febrile illnesses tend to affect visitors who were ashore in the endemic areas, particularly in the evenings during the hot seasons, some three to five days before the sudden onset of pyrexia, severe headache, backache and muscle pain. Dengue fever lasts seven to eight days with a drop in temperature half way through. They may show a morbilliform rash starting on the hands or feet and sometimes mild lymphadenopathy. Sandfly fever lasts three days, is generally milder and shows no rash. Both may cause depression, fatigue and prostration. Malaria and meningitis must be considered in the differential diagnosis. Treatment is entirely symptomatic.

EVACUATION OF PATIENTS FROM SHIPS IN AN EMERGENCY

There should be good clinical reasons whenever one calls for the evacuation of a patient from the relative security of a bunk in a sound ship at sea. Transfer from ship to boat is essentially a matter of seamanship; preparations can be made at leisure with one's seamen colleagues. The journey to port in a small boat may be rough, wet, cold and slow. For these reasons helicopter evacuation is better, giving a smoother ride direct to a hospital. The main problems are the noise and lack of heating in a helicopter cabin.

When requesting transfer, whether by boat or helicopter, the doctor and the master should prepare their wireless communications together and include details of age, sex, diagnosis and special needs. By international agreement ship's radios stop transmission at 15 to 18 and 45 to 48 minutes past the hour (Zulu time*). Radio requests for aid should be made at these times and addressed as described on p. 695.

Before arrival of the helicopter the patient should be brought to a sheltered space with convenient access to the upper deck and enough room to allow transfer to the Stokes Litter or Neil Robertson stretcher brought by the aircraft. Explain to him what is going to happen and make a trial of ear protectors or plugs of cotton wool. These should be removed and reinserted at the last moment. The notes should be packed underneath the patient and adequate blankets will be required. These must be tucked round the patient with no flapping ends to be caught by the wind. If a drip is running make sure there are means of clipping it off at the last minute. If possible the patient should wear a life jacket. When this is impossible have two available to attach to the top and bottom of the stretcher to keep it afloat in case of ditching. The usual procedure is for the helicopter to land a crewman on the ship to prepare for the patient's lift, taking station on the port side until all is ready. The helicopter pilot must be in charge of the evacuation procedure. The crewman landed is his agent; he is an expert and has done it all before. So heed his instructions. Only if there is the possibility of real clinical harm should the doctor argue about the instructions given. Any escort is generally lifted after the patient. He should be warmly clad and wear a life jacket. On arrival ashore he must wait with the patient until told to get out of the aircraft; the rotors may be in motion.

* The world-wide communicator's descriptive phrase for Greenwich mean time.

GENERAL DONT'S FOR THOSE ON BOARD

Don't touch the lowered hook or cable until it has rested on deck and discharged its static electrical charge.

Don't clip, foul or otherwise attach the cable to any part of the ship.

Don't wear a peak or brimmed hat; it will only blow off and perhaps damage the rotors.

Don't approach a helicopter that has landed on deck unless summoned by the crewman. The tail and overhead rotors may be running and both are dangerous. When instructed to approach always do so at right angles to the pilot from his starboard (right) side and watch him or the crewman for instructions.

MANHANDLING PATIENTS BETWEEN DECKS

Although only made of bamboo sewn on to white canvas, the Neil Robertson stretcher remains one of the best means of carrying a patient through narrow tunnels and up ladders. It can also be passed between ships and used for a helicopter lift off. It effectively restrains a violent patient for short periods while waiting for drugs to act. When used thus an entry must be made in the ship's log. The patient must never be left. As the device facilitates handling there is a risk of holding a patient too long with the feet dependent and so accentuating cerebral hypoxia. A slightly head-down position is best. In the tropics overheating of the encased patient is a risk.

SHIPWRECK AND SURVIVAL ON ABANDONING SHIP

Survival equipment is the responsibility of the master but the doctor should maintain a tactful interest in its efficiency. He should take part in lifeboat practices and make a point of being about and wearing his own life jacket when passengers do lifeboat drill. The heavy casualties amongst those forced to take to the boats during the last war have made it clear that a simple commonsense approach to abandoning ship will not suffice. This is because drowning is only the first hazard and once surmounted hypothermia becomes the most lethal threat.

The difference between the specific heat of water and air combined with the thermal conductivity of water causes a very rapid loss of body heat which may be 25 times the loss in air at 20°C. Maximal shivering will generate just about enough heat to balance the loss at this temperature but below 33°C shivering is replaced by muscle stiffness inhibiting the generation of heat. In a person of average build even exercise has no effect as the body temperature continues to fall in water at 25°C and also the turbulence created by activity hastens body cooling. Somewhat above that temperature the increase in blood flow to the limbs increases the heat loss from the body core and it is the central core temperature that matters. Heat is conserved naturally by subcutaneous fat and by clothing. Keating (1972) has demonstrated that volunteers in underwear, sweater, trousers and socks cooled at a quarter the rate of those unclothed in water at 5°C. The immediate advice to those abandoning ship should be:

1. Put on warm clothes, including gloves and footwear.

2. Put the life preserver on correctly over your clothes.

3. Take a long drink of water but avoid alcohol because of its sedative and peripheral dilator effects.

4. Float as quietly as possible on your life preserver and do not attempt to swim more than a few yards. Wait to be picked up by the lifeboat.

The open lifeboat gives little protection against cold and allows exposure to the sun but the modern liferaft is both a boat and a floating tent. It generally carries 25 persons and even in freezing conditions maintains, when occupied, a temperature of 20°C. In the tropics it can be cooled by dashing sea water over the outer fabric which can also catch rain water or dew. If it is possible to enter a liferaft clothed and dry one is very fortunate, but even if wet heat losses are minimal once the openings are closed to exclude wind. A useful series of papers came from a symposium on Cold/Wet Survival at the Institute of Naval Medicine in 1971 and published in the Journal of the Royal Naval Medical Service in 1972. Guide lines based on the priorities for survival are shown in Table 22.1.

MANAGEMENT OF RESCUED HYPOTHERMIC PATIENTS

In the absence of a low reading thermometer (p. 362) action must be based on clinical parameters alone. Provided the patient has a clear airway it is almost always better to get him below as quickly as possible maintaining a head-down rather than a feet-down posture and ensuring that all movements are as gentle as possible. Control of body core temperature depends upon sweating, vasomotor adjustments and shivering. These begin to fail at 33°C and failure is complete at 30°C when consciousness is lost and tendon reflexes disappear. The degree of hypothermia can be judged clinically as shown below.

APPROXIMATE CORE TEMPERATURE	CLINICAL MANIFESTATIONS	TREATMENT
35°C	Confused and disorientated Skin feels cold to observer Shivering	Rapidly rewarm bath of stirred hot water at 40-42°C keeping arms and legs out if possible
33°C	Semiconscious Pupils dilated	
30°C	Cardiac arrhythmia Persistent muscle rigidity Shivering absent Unconscious Tendon reflexes absent	Minimum handling Rapidly rewarm in stirred hot water at 44-46°C. Give oxygen and warmed i v bicarbonate to combat metabolic acidosis. When subjectively warm move to warmed bed.
28°C	Ventricular fibrillation	
27°C	Loss of muscle rigidity Bradycardia Slowed respiration	
26-25°C	Death	

Opinion seems agreed that at sea the treatment of hypothermia is rapid rewarming. It should always be tried immediately unless drowning is the primary condition since the diagnosis of death in the severely hypothermic is very difficult unless the patient has failed to respond to rewarming. Recent work is summarised in two papers by Hervey (1973) and Golden (1973). The essential changes in hypothermia are:

CARDIAC. Progressive bradycardia with prolongation of systole and a parallel drop in blood pressure. Atrial fibrillation is followed by ventricular fibrillation. From 33°C downwards cardiac irritability increases.

METABOLIC. Severe hypothermia results in a metabolic acidosis.

RESPIRATORY. Though hyperventilation may occur immediately on immersion hypothermia rapidly causes slow breathing and a decline in tidal volume.

It is on these changes that the current advice rests to avoid extra-cardiac massage with its risk of ventricular fibrillation until the patient is rewarmed. Bicarbonate i v may be of value (pp. 11 and 727). Three particular complications may arise during rewarming one of which, the ' after drop ' of core temperature, may account for death in the post-rescue period. As the circulation, with rewarming, resumes its flow, cold blood from the periphery may cause a further drop in core temperature of up to 3°C. Hypotensive episodes may occur and finally the fibrillating ventricle remains unresponsive to drugs and to electrical defibrillation.

MANAGEMENT OF NEAR-DROWNING

If conscious or semi-conscious the priority is to treat the drowning since the patient will not be likely to die from hypothermia. If unconscious with dilated pupils, muscle rigidity favours hypothermia as the primary factor. The core temperature is likely to be around 30°C. Rewarming has priority because hypoxia consequent upon partial drowning is unlikely to do fundamental damage below 30°C. Once the temperature rises attention can be directed to drowning.

The doctor at sea has good facilities for first aid but must compromise about further techniques. The drowning process is variable. Immersion in cold water itself stimulates breathing: this is followed by breath holding and struggling. At some time water reaches the larynx and may initiate laryngospasm which persists until relaxation comes with death. Others inhale water directly, while all tend to swallow it in large amounts during the phase of breath holding. Cyanosis from breath holding or laryngospasm develops in about a minute; consciousness is lost in two or three minutes and cardiac arrest occurs in five to ten minutes. The need for immediate rescue is obvious. Thereafter the airway should be cleared and mouth-to-mouth respiration started (p. 732). Spontaneous breathing efforts should be watched for and if the femoral or carotid pulses are absent closed cardiac ' massage ' should be started (p. 725) and maintained for a prolonged period (p. 727). Intubation, oxygen administration and positive pressure ventilation should be used if available. Once the airway is established and cardiac activity confirmed empty the stomach with a Senorans's evacuator. In view of chemical and bacterial contaminants in the water inhaled start hydrocortisone 1 g six-hourly and ampicillin 250 mg six-hourly.

The pathophysiology of near drowning in fresh water and salt water show the following differences (Rivers, 1972) (see p. 491).

All resuscitated patients must be kept under close observation for at least 24 hours as certain effects of near-drowning may be delayed. These are:

Increasing respiratory distress. This may develop rapidly at any moment and demand intubation and oxygen. In sea water drowning the use of an i v diuretic should be considered even though electrolyte monitoring is impossible.

Hypotension. As soon as this is noted the feet should be raised and a plasma or Dextran infusion started.

Cardiac arrhythmia. Without monitoring facilities treatment is difficult but multiple extrasystoles are an indication for ' blind ' administration of lignocaine (see p. 225).

FRESH WATER	SALT WATER
Hypotonic fluid inhaled crosses the alveolar barrier entering the vascular compartment of the body	Hypertonic fluid inhaled extracts fluid from the vascular compartment into the alveoli
Consequences: Hypervolaemia Haemolysis Electrolyte disturbance	*Consequences:* Pulmonary oedema Hypovolaemia Vascular shock
Death from ventricular fibrillation	Death from cardiac standstill

UNDERWATER EMERGENCIES

(N.B. Industrial Compressed Air Illness is notifiable.)

Submarines

The advent of nuclear power without a need for air lines has led to the evolution of submarines that can remain submerged for long periods so that control of their atmosphere for months at a time is necessary. The production of oxygen by electrolysis of sea water and the removal of CO, CO_2, aerosols and toxic contaminants creates new problems of monitoring. Minor changes in the environment when they go on for weeks on end create changes in human biochemical status and these in turn alter physiological function (Davies, 1973). Further information is likely to emerge from studies in a controlled environment chamber recently opened in the Institute of Naval Medicine, Alverstoke.

Diving

Accidents are all too frequent amongst swimmers, scuba divers, underwater fishermen and others despite the efforts of bodies such as the British Sub-aqua Club. These problems may present to any doctor but for the medical officer going to sea with working divers special training is needed. Courses in underwater medicine for doctors are held at the Institue of Naval Medicine, Alverstoke, Gosport PO12 2DL. Inquiries should be sent to the Director of Studies.

Medical examination of candidates for training in leisure diving is often requested and is a trend to be encouraged. The following is a basis on which a doctor with little experience of underwater activities can give an opinion. Candidates should be considered unfit for diving:

1. If not physically fit in the usual sense for athletic activities up to local club standard.

2. If temporarily unwell for any reason, particularly if incubating coryza or other virus infection.

3. If there is nasal obstruction or sinusitis.

4. If the outer ear is not clear of wax.

5. If the eardrums are perforated or not clearly mobile on Valsalva's manoeuvre.

6. If there is recent pulmonary disease or old scarring.

Various terms have been used to express the increasing pressure to which a diver's body is subjected as he descends. Divers spoke in terms of water and atmospheres ('At 33 feet the pressure is 2 atmospheres') and engineers of pounds per square inch or p.s.i. Scientists in this field use the bar but eventually the derived SI unit for pressure or pascal will be used everywhere and the present confused state will disappear. The pascal is derived from the newton (the SI unit for force) and is one newton per square metre. One bar = 100 kilo newtons per square metre (kNm^2) and this is 100 kPa or in old terminology 14·5 p.s.i. One standard atmosphere is 101·325 kNm^2. One mm Hg = 0·133 kPa.

The diver's first concern is the relationship between pressure and the volume of gas. Boyle's law states that at constant pressure the volume of a gas is inversely proportional to its pressure. Thus if at the surface volume the pressure is one atmosphere (1 a.t.a.) or 14·7 p.s.i. (101·1 kPa) (100 per cent), at 33 feet or 2 atmospheres (2 a.t.a) or 29 p.s.i. (202·2 kPa) the volume is 50 per cent, and so on.

When the diver has gone down to 100 feet the air in his lungs is compressed to a quarter of its volume at the surface which is approximately that of the residual volume in the respiratory tree after maximal expiration. Further compression of the thorax to expire is impossible and the excess pressure results in what divers call a 'squeeze' leading to pulmonary oedema, bleeding and sub-conjunctival haemorrhage. This occurs in rapid descents at relatively low levels where gas volume changes are greatest. As the diver descends air in any body cavity (ear, sinuses and under dental fillings) undergoes similar changes. The diver equilibrates these pressures and volumes by swallowing during descent to open his

Eustachian tubes. Dental pain is not uncommon and here adjustment is impossible. On ascent similar adjustments are most needed near the surface and the free diver and schnorkeller may go through considerable pressure changes between the surface and 50 feet. Inability to achieve these adjustments results in ototic and sinus barotrauma and occasionally in interstitial pulmonary emphysema. The features of barotrauma are (Head, 1973):—

CAUSES	SIGNS AND SYMPTOMS	TREATMENT
Otitic barotrauma		
Occlusion of external meatus by wax etc.	Sensation of fullness Discomfort and deafness Pain	Look at meatus and clear it Equalise pressure
Occlusion of Eustachian tube		Use nasal decongestants
Infections Allergy Scarring New growths Fright ' locking ' Dental malocclusion	Rupture of drum and bloodstained discharge Drum looks congested and haemorrhagic. May show a fluid level	Myringotomy or Eustachian catheterisation unless compression-decompression facilities are available. If drum is ruptured give broad spectrum antibiotic for 5 days
Sinus barotrauma		
Old nasal injury or deviated septum	Pain over antra or frontal sinuses followed by sero-sanguineous discharge	
Acute or chronic disease of nose or sinuses	Toothache Sinus tenderness Fluid level on X ray	Nasal decongestant Ephedrine 0·5 g/dl or Adrenaline 1 in 80 000 to middle meatus

Behaviour of air in the lungs

Mucus plugs, bronchospasm, panic ascent with mouth and nose closed and deliberate breath-holding as in the schnorkeller will all trap air under increased pressure. It may break out into the peribronchial alveolar tissue and cause interstitial and mediastinal emphysema or air embolism. Or it may rupture into the pleura and cause a pneumothorax. Lung compliance is the critical factor and is the main reason for recommending those with even healed disease to eschew diving. Since pressure will reduce the volume of air

17

bubbles immediate recompression is the conventional treatment, the doctor accompanying the patient in the compression chamber.

Effects of gases breathed under pressure

Nitrogen and oxygen have significant pharmacological activities under pressure. Nitrogen narcosis ('rapture of the deep') is a subjective condition very akin to alcoholic intoxication. It begins to affect most people at somewhere round 100 feet. Beyond that the untrained become jovial, garrulous, clumsy and irresponsible. Recovery is rapid on return to the surface though there may be amnesia or sleepiness. Essentially it is the limitation imposed on man by the narcotic effect of nitrogen under pressure that determines the need for deep diving to be carried out with oxygen helium mixtures, the latter gas being virtually inert.

Nitrogen moves into solution in physiological fluids with ease and equally readily comes out again. Henry's law states that 'at constant temperature the amount of gas which dissolves in a liquid with which it is in contact is proportional to the partial pressure of that gas'. Since air is 79 per cent nitrogen and 21 per cent oxygen at 1 atmosphere pressure (101·1 kPa) 1·85 ml of nitrogen is dissolved in 100 ml of water and 1·03 ml of oxygen once equilibrium at the air/water interface is achieved. The partial pressure of nitrogen is then 600 mm Hg (79·8 kPa) and of oxygen 160 mm Hg (21·3 kPa). As the total pressure is increased to 2 atmospheres the partial pressure of nitrogen rises to 1 200 mm Hg (159·6 kPa) and at 4 atmospheres to 2 400 mm Hg (319·2 kPa) with a proportional increase in the volume of the gas dissolved. At normal atmospheric pressure 1 ml of nitrogen is dissolved in 100 ml of blood but 5 ml in a similar amount of fat. Diffusion through these two fluids occurs at different rates. The total amount of gas dissolved depends upon the pressure and time spent under it. Caisson workers can stay at 18 p.s.i. (1 atmosphere or 225 kPa) and divers at 30 feet (202·2 kPa) for indefinite periods but once the pressure is increased more than this they are at risk of developing decompression sickness if brought back to normal atmospheric pressure too quickly. This hazard is increased the longer they have been under pressure.

Rapid decompression results in nitrogen coming out of solution and forming bubbles which act as micro-emboli. Argument continues as to whether this simple explanation is sufficient but whether or not other mechanisms come into play there is no doubt that recompressing the patient immediately alleviates the symptoms. This, combined with slow decompression, is the essential measure to wash out dissolved nitrogen. (For more detailed discussion see

Elliot *et al.*, 1974). The severity of decompression sickness appears to depend upon the size of the bubbles and therefore of the micro-infarcts caused. Symptoms range from mild joint pains (' niggles '), itching and burning of the skin and ecchymoses to true ' bends ' when there is severe boring joint pain, unaffected by movement but alleviated by recompression. The more serious manifestations are caused by nitrogen bubble emboli in the central nervous system or in the pulmonary vessels causing dyspnoea, pain and tightness in the chest, tachyhypnoea, collapse and shock ('chokes '). In the brain all functions may be disturbed while in the spinal cord bubbles cause weakness, paralysis, retention of urine and sensory disturbances. These symptoms occur 6 to 24 hours after reaching the surface. Advice on the nearest recompression facilities can be obtained in England from Superintendent of Diving, HMS Vernon, Portsmouth 22351 (STD 0705 ext 87 2366) or out of working hours, Duty Lieutenant Commander, HMS Vernon, Portsmouth 22351 (STD 0705) ext 872413-415. Discussion continues as to the best schedule on which to work when treating decompression sickness. Recent work is summarised by Barnard (1972). The main point is to decompress to a level that alleviates symptoms and then to reconsider the appropriate rate of ascent at relative leisure. Supplementary measures should be considered, in particular plasma expanders when there is hypovolaemic shock, mannitol and dexamethasone to reduce oedema in cerebral and spinal bends, heparin and hypothermia. Controlled studies are difficult to find and one can only advise seeking help from HMS Vernon.

Pain is a useful marker for monitoring adequate recompression and though one may be forced to relieve it analgesics are probably best avoided.

PETER PRESTON

REFERENCES

Health of seafarers

Regulations

MERCHANT SHIPPING (PASSENGER SHIP CONSTRUCTION). HMSO. 1103. Rule 22 1965.

PORTS DESIGNATED IN APPLICATION OF THE INTERNATIONAL HEALTH REGULA-TIONS (1969). Situation Jan. 1974. Geneva: WHO. 1974.

THE MERCHANT SHIPPING (MEDICAL SCALES) REGULATIONS No. 1193. London: HMSO. 1974.

THE MERCHANT SHIPPING (MEDICAL SCALES) (FISHING VESSELS) REGULATIONS No. 1192. London: HMSO. 1974.

MCMURRAY, G. N. (1973). An evaluation of metoclopramide as an anti-emetic in seasickness. *Postgraduate Medical Journal.* July Suppl. 38-41.

OLIVER, P. O. (1973). Health problems of seafarers. *Practitioner* **211**, 202-208.

Shipwreck

COLD/WET SURVIVAL SYMPOSIUM (1972). *Journal of the Royal Naval Medical Service.* LVIII.

GOLDEN, F. STC. (1973). Recognition and treatment of immersion hypothermia. *Proceedings of the Royal Society of Medicine*, **66**, 1058-1061.

GOLDEN, F. STC. (1974). Shipwreck and survival. *Journal of the Royal Naval Medical Service*, **60**, 8-14.

HERVEY, G. R. (1973). Physiological changes encountered in hypothermia. *Proceedings of The Royal Society of Medicine*, **66**, 1053-1067.

KEATINGE, W. R. (1972). Cold immersion and swimming. *Journal of the Royal Naval Medical Service*. LVIII, 171.

THE MERCHANT SHIPPING (LIFE SAVING APPLIANCES) RULES No. 1105. London: HMSO, 1965.

RIVERS, J. F. (1972). Near drowning. *British Journal of Hospital Medicine*, **8**, 299-300.

Underwater medicine

BARNARD, E. E. P. (1972). Formula and fashion in the treatment of decompression sickness. *Journal of the Royal Naval Medical Service*. LVIII, 4-8.

DAVIES, D. M. (1973). Sixty days in a submarine. The pathophysiological and metabolic cost. *Journal of The Royal College of Physicians*, **7**, 2, 132-144.

ELLIOTT, D. H., HALLENBECK, J. M. & BOVE, A. A. (1974). Acute decompression sickness. *Lancet* **2**, 1193-1199.

HEAD, P. W. (1973). Otitic and sinus barotrauma. *Practitioner*, **211**, 738-744.

CHAPTER 23

Medical Emergencies in the Air

(For risks of mercury in aircraft see p. 73)
(For flying and alcohol see p. 681)
Note.—1 000 feet may be regarded as 300 metres (strictly 305).

A MODERN aircraft is an immensely complex collection of machinery, and the possibility of failure of one of its components is correspondingly high. The potential for disaster is also great, for in apparent defiance of the rules of gravity and commonsense an airliner carries a large number of people at high speed through an environment that is inimical to life. In spite of these obvious objections to the whole principle of travel by air, the safety of commercial aviation is the envy of most other forms of transport. (Space flight has a better record in terms of fatalities per passenger-kilometre, but it falls far short of conventional flight when the figures are related to the population at risk.)

Standards of design and construction are far better for aircraft than, say, for motor cars, and national and international regulations provide further safeguards against catastrophe. Failures do occur in flight, but few of them constitute emergencies. Those incidents that may be so classed do not, in most cases, even come to the notice of the passengers, and the number that result in discomfort, disorder or death is extremely small. The practitioner is rather unlikely ever to see a true medical emergency resulting from flight; he will be unusual indeed if he encounters a medical emergency in the air. However, he may sometimes be asked to advise his patients on their fitness for air travel, and it is well that he should know something of the stresses to which they will *not* be exposed.

EMERGENCIES DUE TO ALTITUDE

The adverse effects of high altitude arise, directly or indirectly, from the relationship between height and barometeric pressure. The rate at which the pressure falls decreases with altitude; at sea level the total barometric pressure is 760 mm Hg (1 atmosphere or 101·325 kilo Pascals), and it has fallen to half of this value at 18 000 feet. At 27 000 feet the pressure is one third, and at 40 000 feet one fifth, of the standard atmosphere. Decompression increases the volume assumed by a given mass of gas; if the pressure is halved, the volume will be doubled provided that the walls of the container are free to expand. (It is for this reason that balloonists leave the ground with the envelope only partially filled.) Changes of pressure also affect the solubility of gases in liquids, and this property is exploited by the aerated drink industry. The body contains both dissolved and confined gases, and problems can arise during ascent, sojourn at altitude, or descent.

At the altitudes reached by present-day aircraft the composition of the atmosphere is much the same as that at sea level, about 21 per cent of the total pressure being contributed by oxygen. The partial pressure exerted by this fraction, however, declines in parallel with the total pressure, from about 160 mm Hg (21·332 kPa) at ground level to 30 mm Hg (4·0 kPa) at 40 000 feet. Indeed, at the latter height the *total* barometric pressure is less than the tension of oxygen in air at sea level, so that there will be some deficiency even if the environment contains nothing but oxygen. This fact has considerable implications for flight at very great altitudes.

Table 23.1 lists the total and partial pressures associated with various heights, and gives some landmarks in the progress towards the ultimate emergencies of altitude. The ideal solution to the problem of a reducing barometric pressure is to maintain the environment artificially at the equivalent of ground level by a fully pressurised cabin. The engineering penalties of this approach would be prohibitive (although it has been consistently adopted by the Russians for their space vehicles) and from a physiological point of view it is unnecessary to insist on ground level conditions. The pressure in a passenger aircraft is usually never allowed to fall below about 570 mm Hg (25·994 kPa) (equivalent to a local altitude of 8 000 feet). In military aviation the use of lower cabin pressures, and higher equivalent altitudes, is often necessary, and personal oxygen equipment must be worn by the crew. A well designed system ensures that the inspired oxygen tension remains close to the normal value regardless of the effective altitude within the cabin.

OXYGEN LACK

The pressure of oxygen available for gas exchange in the lungs is lower than the examination of Table 23.1 would suggest. Alveolar gas is saturated with water vapour which exerts a partial pressure of 47 mm Hg (6·266 kPa) at body temperature, and it also contains carbon dioxide at a pressure of about 40 mm Hg (5·333 kPa). At sea level, these components reduce the oxygen tension from 160 mm Hg (21·332 kPa) in the inspired air to around 100 mm Hg (13·332 kPa) in the lung. Their effect becomes even greater as the barometric pressure falls, for the contribution that they make remains relatively constant as altitude increases. At 18 000 feet the partial pressure of oxygen in the alveoli would be less than 30 mm Hg (4·0 kPa) unless compensatory mechanisms, in the form of increased rate and depth of respiration, helped to raise it. No generalisations can be made about either the extent or the effect of these mechanisms, and for this reason alveolar tensions are not quoted in the Table. It should be noted, however, that an increase in oxygen is not necessarily of benefit to the tissues if it is achieved at the expense of carbon dioxide in the alveoli and arterial blood.

The effect of small reductions in alveolar oxygen tension is minimised by the S-shape of the oxyhaemoglobin dissociation curve (see p. 29) which allows small reductions of oxygen pressure to occur, without greatly affecting the saturation of arterial blood. Once the partial pressure of oxygen reaches 60-65 mm Hg, the dissociation curve steepens, and thereafter small changes of oxygen produce large variations in arterial saturation. It is generally accepted that 10 000 feet is the critical level above which air-breathing will result in significant decrement, and at higher altitudes supplementary oxygen is necessary. For routine passenger flight, an even lower equivalent altitude is clearly desirable, for not all passengers can achieve the standard of fitness regarded as normal in military aviation. Although a pressure equivalent to 8 000 feet is regarded as the maximum acceptable, it is rare for even this height to be maintained in commercial operations, and 5 000 feet is a more usually-encountered value. At this height, even patients with a moderate reduction in respiratory reserve are unlikely to experience symptoms of hypoxia.

Signs and symptoms

Hypoxia is notoriously insidious in its effects, and the initial symptoms vary greatly, although they are usually constant in any one individual. This relative constancy makes it slightly more likely that a pilot will recognise that he is hypoxic if he has received previous training, but one of the most dangerous features of the condition is loss of insight so that the sufferer does not realise that he is affected.

The first symptom may be an apparent dimming and loss of contrast in vision, but this may only be realised in retrospect when

a return to full oxygenation restores lights to their normal bright-
ness. Listlessness and apathy commonly occur, and irritability or
light-headed irresponsibility may also be present. Hypoxia of this
degree is found at heights of about 12 000 to 15 000 feet, and it does

Table 23.1. *Characteristics of the Standard Atmosphere*
(1 Bar = 100 k Pascals, see p. 492)

ALTITUDE		BAROMETRIC PRESSURE		INSPIRED PO_2	REMARKS
FEET	METRES	MM HG	MBARS	MM HG	
0	0	760·0	1 013·3	159·6	
2 000	610	706·6	942·1	148·4	
4 000	1 219	656·4	875·1	137·8	Impaired night vision
6 000	1 829	609·1	812·0	127·9	
8 000	2 438	564·5	752·6	118·5	
10 000	3 048	522·7	696·8	109·8	Air-breathing limit
12 000	3 658	483·4	644·4	101·5	
14 000	4 267	446·5	595·3	93·8	
16 000	4 876	411·9	549·2	86·5	
18 000	5 486	379·5	506·0	80·0	Half sea-level pressure
20 000	6 096	349·3	465·7	73·4	
22 000	6 706	320·9	427·9	67·4	
24 000	7 315	294·6	392·7	61·9	Lower limit for decompres-
26 000	7 925	270·0	359·9	56·7	sion sickness
28 000	8 534	247·1	329·4	51·9	
30 000	9 144	225·7	300·9	47·4	
32 000	9 754	205·9	274·5	43·2	100 per cent oxygen required;
34 000	10 363	187·5	250·0	39·4	= sea-level, breathing air
36 000	10 973	170·5	227·4	35·8	
38 000	11 582	154·9	206·5	32·5	
40 000	12 192	140·7	187·5	29·5	100 per cent oxygen limit;
50 000	15 240	87·0	116·0	18·3	= 10,000 ft breathing air
60 000	18 288	53·7	71·6	11·2	
65 000	19 812	42·2	56·2	8·9	Cruising altitude; supersonic transport

not constitute an emergency in normal people. Cyanosis may be
detected at this stage, especially in the ears and the nail beds, but
it is only of use in diagnosis if the observer is not too affected by
hypoxia to recognise its significance. The degree of arterial saturation found at this altitude stimulates chemoreceptors in the aortic
and carotid regions, causing hyperventilation which rapidly becomes
more marked as the altitude is further increased.

At about 20 000 to 25 000 feet, the acuity of hearing is diminished, and the careless rapture of mild oxygen lack progresses to the ' drunkenness ' of serious hypoxia. The severity of the symptoms is likely to be increased by activity, and any exertion may result in unconsciousness. This may have far reaching consequences, for the would-be helper of a passenger smitten with hypoxia is liable to suffer the same fate unless oxygen equipment is used. A passenger unconscious in his seat is undesirable but a pile of comatose people on the floor would be a real emergency.

At altitudes greater than about 30 000 feet decompression results in rapid unconsciousness, jactitations, Cheyne-Stokes respiration and coma. Death may ensue unless the effective altitude is rapidly lowered. The time of ' useful ' consciousness, which represents the period in which purposeful action to correct hypoxia must be taken, varies considerably with altitude, as shown in Fig. 23.1. The administration of oxygen before the time of useful consciousness has elapsed will not necessarily prevent transient collapse some seconds later. Moreover, in some people the phenomenon of ' oxygen paradox' may appear. This is temporary worsening of symptoms manifested, in extreme cases, by loss of consciousness and convulsions. A rapid return to normal is the rule.

Extreme degrees of oxygen lack are very rarely seen in normal air passengers, but even mild hypoxia may constitute a medical emergency in the aged or infirm. Little is known of the effects of oxygen deprivation on the elderly, but those with circulatory or respiratory disease tolerate it badly. Persons with coronary insufficiency, for example, are poor candidates for high altitude flight, since even in normal subjects the uptake of oxygen by the myocardium is almost complete. The normal response to hypoxia is coronary vasodilation to maintain full oxygenation of the cardiac muscle, but patients with relative myocardial ischemia are unable to achieve this. Similarly, cardiac or pulmonary disease which involves arterial desaturation at rest or on moderate exercise will be adversely affected by oxygen lack. Exact limits cannot be stated, but patients with a greatly reduced vital capacity and maximum breathing capacity may become severely hypoxic even at 8 000 feet. Any condition in which the tidal volume is an appreciable proportion of the vital capacity is hazardous. For the same reason, anaemia reduces tolerance for hypoxia. It is unlikely that any patient fit to travel at all will be made unconscious by oxygen lack at altitudes usually encountered in airliners, but the symptoms of altitude will undoubtedly be more severe in those whose haemoglobin is less than about 8 g/dl.

Diagnosis

In severe cases, the diagnosis should be in little doubt. The history, the symptoms, and the presence of cyanosis will usually be conclusive. Diagnosis in-flight is, however, rendered more difficult by

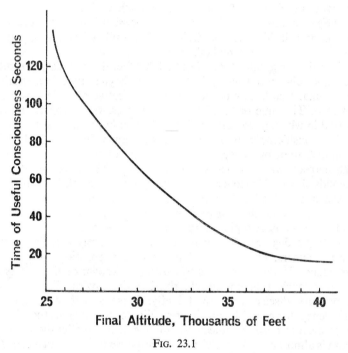

FIG. 23.1

The duration of useful consciousness when hypoxia is induced by rapid decompression from 10 000 feet, breathing air.

impairment of judgement, and for the same reason any mechanical altitude indicator in the cabin may be ignored. Breathlessness, or cardiac pain occurring in ill patients during flight should arouse the suspicion of hypoxia, but it must be emphasised that these symptoms are more likely to have a clinical origin than to be due to a failure of cabin pressurisation.

Treatment. The only treatment required in most instances is a speedy restoration to the normal oxygen tension. This can be achieved by descent to a lower altitude, by increasing the cabin pressure with respect ot the outside environment, or by the administration of supplementary oxygen.

Descent alone is a sufficient remedy if the cruising height of the aircraft is less than 25 000 feet, but jet airliners flying at 40 000 feet or above may not be able, for structural reasons, to descend very rapidly to a safe height of below 10 000 feet. If the defect in the cabin is small, and the rate of depressurisation is low, profound hypoxia may be prevented by increasing the flow of air via the normal pressurisation controls. In a more serious emergency, descent must be supplemented by the administration of oxygen to all occupants (including, of course, the crew). The latter have equipment immediately to hand, and are trained in its use, but passenger systems must be as foolproof as possible. It is usual to provide a simple face mask and re-breathing bag in a compartment above each passenger seat, and to arrange that the stowage doors are opened and the oxygen is turned on should the cabin pressure fail. The mask falls into a position from which it can easily be applied to the face. A simple demonstration of the use of this equipment is usually given to travellers before high altitude flights.

In addition, oxygen supplies sufficient for about 10 per cent of the passengers are normally carried as part of the medical stores. A flow rate of about 3 litres/min (0·05 l/sec) is adequate for most cases, but if the cabin altitude rises to 20 000 feet or more, the high setting of the regulator should be used, giving a flow of approximately 10 litres/min (0·167 l/sec. Cardiac patients may also require supportive treatment.

Sequelae

Mild hypoxia of short duration is usually followed by fatigue and headache, which are self-limiting and can be treated symptomatically. If the oxygen lack is severe and prolonged, cerebral dysfunction may appear and last for hours or days. The pattern and course depend upon individual susceptibility, but full recovery is the rule. Deaths from hypoxia are very rare, and treatment with oxygen, artificial respiration, heat, and stimulants should be continued even when the possibility of resuscitation seems very remote.

EFFECTS OF PRESSURE CHANGE

The inverse relationship between barometric pressure and the volume of a given mass of gas has already been mentioned. The two extreme cases are that of a perfectly elastic container which will double its volume as the ambient pressure is halved, and a rigid system in which decompression causes an increase in the differential pressure between inside and outside without change of volume.

The gas-containing organs of the body are neither perfectly elastic nor completely rigid, and they are not usually entirely closed. The physical effects of decompression and recompression are accordingly mixed. The gas will expand until it is constrained by the tension built up in the stretched wall, or until its pressure is high enough to overcome any obstruction to its egress. For cavities having some communication with the outside air the results will depend in part upon the rate of decompression. For example, most changes of barometric pressure encountered in practice are sufficiently slow to allow the free escape of air from the lungs, but very rapid or ' explosive ' decompression may produce damage because the rate of expansion of the gas may exceed the rate at which the excess can be voided from the lung, and very high intrathoracic pressures may temporarily develop. Similarly, gas in the middle ear will expand until its pressure is high enough to force open the flap valve at the lower end of the Eustachian tube, although here the results of decompression are rarely significant. (Recompression may, however, cause problems, and these are discussed later.)

One curious consequence of the gas laws appears at 63 000 feet, where the total barometric pressure is 47 mm Hg (6·266 kPa). This is equal to the vapour pressure of water at body temperature, with the result that water will ' boil ' at 37°C. All the available ' gas space ' in the lungs will therefore be filled with ' steam ' at this height. At still greater altitudes the water in the tissues may boil, and the circulation will then become gas-locked with water vapour. This hardly constitutes an emergency likely to be met with in everyday medical practice!

Intestinal pain

The average gastrointestinal tract contains between a half and one litre of gas at sea level pressures, and it generates about an equal volume each day. Most of the gas is in the large intestine, although in some people the stomach is a sizeable reservoir. Decompression to the 8 000 foot equivalent of a pressure cabin involves a theoretical increase in volume of approximately 25 per cent, although in fact the expansion is to some extent reduced by a small increase of intraluminal pressure. These changes can easily be accommodated without discomfort, but exposure to altitudes above 20 000 feet may give rise to feelings of distension or pain. A sudden loss of cabin pressure, during a rapid decompression to, say, 30 000 feet, will produce a sudden and large increase in the volume of intestinal gas. Severe colic, sometimes with shortness of breath, may result, and in some subjects this may be followed by syncopal collapse. There is some evidence that a heavy meal predisposes to this condition, and although the stigma commonly attached to baked beans in this connection is probably unjustified, a diet of gas-forming foods is not to be recommended to high fliers.

In most cases the abdominal distension is self-limiting, and the passage of the excess gas in either direction rapidly brings relief. There are some unfortunates whose physiological or social inhibitions will not allow them to void the gas; for these, only descent will bring a cure.

The diagnosis is usually obvious, but the symptoms may be overlaid by those of hypoxia. Rapid decompression is so uncommon in civilian aircraft that the effects of sudden abdominal distension upon ill or feeble passengers cannot be fully documented.

Toothache

A badly filled dental cavity may sometimes contain a bubble of gas beneath the stopping. Decompression can then lead to considerable tension within the cavity, resulting in pain so excruciating as to necessitate descent. Immediate relief may occur spontaneously at altitude if the defective filling is forced out by the high pressure behind it.

Ear and sinus pain

During ascent, the gas in these semi-closed cavities expands and bubbles harmlessly to the outside. The only symptoms during this phase of flight are a feeling of fullness, and slight deafness as the pressure in the middle ear increases. When the atmospheric pressure increases again during descent, the lower end of the Eustachiain tube closes, trapping gas within the middle ear. The progressive contraction of this gas builds up a pressure differential between mouth and ear, causing pain and deafness. At normal rates of descent, plenty of time is available for equilibration of this pressure, aided by yawning, swallowing, or moving the jaws. During an emergency descent from high altitude, however, the overall pressure change may be both high and rapid, and in these circumstances many passengers will experience severe pain. Rupture of the drum may also occur.

Frequent travellers soon learn the trick of clearing their ears during descent. Some airlines assist them by providing boiled sweets, which give a pleasant inducement to movements of the jaws. If other measures fail, swallowing while performing a mild Valsalva manoeuvre is usually effective. The old recommendation to stop the external auditory meatus with cotton wool has, mercifully, been generally abandoned.

The paranasal sinuses generally give no trouble unless the mucous membrane at their ostia is swollen. Such swelling may produce a flap valve, or even a closed cavity. For this reason, passengers with Eustachian catarrh or with blocked sinuses should be discouraged from travelling by air until the infection has subsided. If it is essential that they should fly, they should use a decongestant spray. Very occasionally, severe pain in the ear or sinuses may not regress spontaneously, and re-ascent, followed by a slower recompression, may be required.

'Explosive' decompression

The large volume of a passenger cabin ensures that even after the loss of a door or window the rate of change of pressure is comparatively low. Very rapid decompressions, occurring in one-fiftieth of a second or less, will only result from a catastrophic break-up of the aircraft structure. The problem of explosive decompression is therefore confined to military aircraft, and even in these, serious consequences are rare. The predominant features of the few reported cases have been pneumothorax, mediastinal and subcutaneous emphysema, and air embolism.

DECOMPRESSION SICKNESS

Acute exposures to the low barometric pressures associated with great heights can also result in symptoms which in some respects at least resemble those of the aquanaut. The omnibus term 'decompression sickness' is applied to both groups of conditions, but it comprises a variety of syndromes which have only their aetiology in common.

The body is normally in an uneasy equilibrium with the gases of the atmosphere, and if the total barometric pressure is changed this balance is disturbed. Oxygen and carbon dioxide pose no problem, because their interchange between tissues and blood and between blood and lungs is rapid and direct. Nitrogen is a different matter, for it has a poor coefficient of diffusion, and is preferentially held in some tissues. Equilibrium between the gas in the blood and that in the lung is rapidly restored, but the tissues may become supersaturated with nitrogen, which may then be released from solution in the form of bubbles. The equations governing bubble formation are complex, but they depend partly upon the blood supply and partly upon the solubility of the gas. Adipose tissue, for example, combines a relatively poor perfusion with a high affinity for nitrogen, and fat is the probable source of many gas foci.

If the bubbles were released directly into the venous blood and carried to the catchment area of the lungs, little harm would ensue, but this is not the case in practice. Relatively large collections of gas may accumulate locally, and bubbles may be carried through the arterial tree to lodge in the peripheral vascular beds. In some cases the relationship between bubbles and symptoms is obvious enough, and X rays may reveal free gas in joints which are the seat of pain, but in many instances the cause cannot be so easily identified. Not all frank bubbles produce pain, and not all pains are associated with demonstrable bubbles.

As the theory of its causation would suggest, the incidence of decompression sickness is strongly correlated with the altitude to which the aviator is exposed. The condition is extremely uncommon below 25 000 feet, although cases have been reported at 18 000 feet or even lower. At greater heights the risk rises rapidly, and at altitudes above 35 000 feet about half of the population will suffer symptoms if the time of exposure is sufficiently long. Decompression sickness is a disease of high altitude, and the most likely candidate for it is the ageing, short, broad chested aviator well endowed with adipose tissue. Thus, its primary target is the man who suffers both the environment of military aircrew and the physique of an airline passenger. Two other external circumstances affect susceptibility. The first is cold, which is a not uncommon accompaniment of exposure to a low cabin pressure, and the second is previous exposure to pressures greater than atmospheric, by indulgence in scuba diving. In both cases the additional stress may result in the appearance of symptoms at relatively low altitude.

Most cases of decompression sickness are cured by descent, and result in no sequelae. However, an occasional sufferer will develop delayed symptoms, and it is necessary that the practitioner should consider decompression sickness as a possible diagnosis in all cases exhibiting bizarre symptoms after flight.

Signs and symptoms

The two major syndromes of decompression sickness, known as ' bends ' and ' chokes ', are similar to those seen in deep sea divers. The ' bends ' usually starts as a dull poorly localised pain in the region of a large joint, and it is often compared to muscular cramp. Temporary relief can sometimes be obtained by movement or by rubbing of the affected part, but the pain soon returns with increased severity. The knee and shoulder are most commonly affected, followed by the elbow, wrist, hand, ankle and foot; for some un-known reason the hip is rarely involved. More than one joint may be painful at any one time, and there is some evidence that symptoms appear first at the site of an old injury. The pain may be associated with skin reactions, such as itching or tingling, or formication; urticarial rashes sometimes also occur. All these signs usually regress spontaneously upon return to ground level, and the joint pains may also disappear without further treat-ment. If the altitude is maintained, the discomfort usually spreads to involve muscle groups, and it can become so agonising that collapse occurs. Sometimes the condition presents as a painless swelling of the joints accompanied by crepitus from the presence of gas in joint spaces and tendon sheaths.

The ' chokes ' differs in some important respects from the condi-tion given that name by divers. It usually begins with tightness of the chest, accompanied by burning retrosternal pain which is aggra-vated by deep breathing. A hard paroxysmal unproductive cough develops, and the sufferer may become cyanosed and collapse. The occurrence of the ' chokes ' is of much more serious import than the complaint of uncomplicated ' bends '.

Neurological signs and symptoms may accompany either ' bends ' or ' chokes ' but they may more rarely occur independently. The pain that heralds the onset of ' the bends ' may be confined to the distribution of one peripheral nerve, and paralysis of one or more limbs may supervene. Generalised convulsions may occa-sionally appear, but more commonly the neurological picture is that of a migraine attack. This may follow the classical course from fortification spectra to vomiting, or it may be arrested at an earlier stage. Unlike other symptoms of decompression sickness, neuro-logical manifestations are not usually cured immediately by a descent to lower altitude.

Malaise, with nausea, pallor, and sweating, but without pain, may be the presenting symptoms. Vasomotor collapse soon follows, with bradycardia, low blood pressure, and loss of consciousness. In such cases the diagnosis of hypoxia may be difficult to exclude, but the return to normality is usually more protracted in the case of decompression collapse. Doubt should not delay the administra-tion of oxygen, which is an appropriate treatment for both con-ditions.

Post-decompression shock

A patient who has apparently shown a full and complete recovery from any of the manifestations of decompression sickness may be taken ill again minutes or hours after his return to ground level. Nausea, headache, and mild neurological disturbance can progress rapidly to acute secondary shock, with haemoconcentration, hypotension, and coma. Pulmonary oedema or pleural effusion may also appear, and unless the appropriate treatment is rapidly initiated death may occur. Post-decompression shock is a real medical emergency, and any unusual symptoms appearing in patients who have been exposed to altitudes in excess of 18 000 feet in the preceding 24 hours should be regarded as possible indications of this condition, until an alternative diagnosis is established.

Persistent neurological signs are of less serious import. Migrainous headaches, and perhaps vomiting, may fail to resolve after return to a normal barometric pressure, but more severe motor signs such as local paresis or aphasia may also remain for as long as 48 hours. Unless new signs appear, full recovery may confidently be predicted.

Diagnosis

The nature of the signs and symptoms is usually sufficient to establish a diagnosis of decompression sickness, but if the episode follows a loss of cabin pressure, hypoxia or hyperventilation may be suspected. Although the range of variation is great, decompression sickness does not usually appear for at least 30 minutes after exposure to the reduced barometric pressure, while hypoxia produces ill-effects within a matter of seconds. In nearly every case, the differentiation is academic, for the immediate treatment must consist of a return to ground level.

Treatment

PROPHYLACTIC. In some rare instances, prolonged exposure to extreme altitudes is a calculated risk. (Balloonists in quest of records provide one example.) In these circumstances, susceptible individuals can be protected by pre-oxygenation, which consists of breathing pure oxygen at sea level before the flight. It acts by establishing a gradient for nitrogen between the tissues and the lungs, resulting in the washing out of inert gas, and its replacement by oxygen. Unfortunately, the rate of clearance is very different for different tissues, and denitrogenation must be very prolonged if the stores in adipose tissue are to be adequately depleted. Three hours of oxygen breathing will remove about 80 per cent of the nitrogen from the body, but the remaining 20 per cent is contained largely in tissues where bubbles form most readily. The ' half-life ' of inert gas in these regions is exceedingly long. Oxygen breathing must, of course, continue during the preparation for flight, and throughout the ascent itself.

THERAPEUTIC. Uncomplicated decompression sickness is almost invariably cured by reducing the effective altitude to less than 18 000 feet, and a return to ground level is all that is usually required for a complete cure. Further exposure to altitude should be forbidden for at least 48 hours after an attack.

All cases that do not immediately resolve should be regarded as potential victims of post-decompression shock. Strict observation in hospital should be instituted, and if possible serial estimations of packed cell volume should be carried out. (Measurements of the haemoglobin concentration are less valuable, but they are better than nothing.) Haemoconcentration should be treated promptly by the i v infusion of fluid, preferably dextran or plasma. Cyanosis is an indication for the administration of oxygen, and paraldehyde (p. 755) is the best sedative drug if restlessness proves a problem. If i v fluids are administered, a watch should be maintained on the electrolyte balance. The role of cortisone derivatives is as much the subject of dispute as it is in other varieties of shock.

In any case showing deterioration, compression to a high pressure should be instituted at the earliest possible moment. A hyperbaric environment should be maintained until symptoms have completely disappeared, when a very slow staged decompression to sea level may be started. Both the Royal Air Force and the Royal Navy operate compression chambers as an emergency service, and will give advice and assistance when required. The current interest in hyperbaric oxygen therapy makes it likely that a single-patient chamber capable of compression to 2 or 3 atmospheres (202·650 kPa to 303·975 kPa) absolute pressure will be available at a not-too-distant hospital (see p. 814). Exposure should be to the highest pressure compatible with the administration of 100 per cent oxygen.

EFFECTS OF ACCELERATION

The human body relies for its appreciation of speed upon visual cues which may themselves be misleading. Alterations in either speed or in the direction of travel constitute accelerations, and to these the body is very sensitive. In physical terms, accelerations are measured as the forces which result when they act upon a mass; these forces give an object its weight. Resting weight results from the action of the earth's gravity, which is defined as an acceleration of 32 ft/sec per second (0·981 m/sec). It is convenient to specify other accelerative forces in terms of this standard, denoted by the letter G. Thus at an acceleration of 10 G an average man will weigh about three quarters of a ton, and he will need to exert ten times as much effort as usual to raise his arm. (Ten G is about the maximum acceleration to which astronauts are subjected during the re-entry of their space vehicle.)

The effects of acceleration depend upon a number of factors, of which duration and direction of action are the most important. Forces lasting for less than one second are usually associated with crashes and forced landings or, in military aircraft, with escape by ejection seat. The word acceleration implies an increase in speed, and the examples given constitute decelerations. However, it is the *change* in velocity that produces the force, and the physiological effects of acceleration and deceleration are the same. The former term is established by long usage.)

Forces of long duration (greater than one second) result from aircraft manoeuvres, such as turns, rolls, or loops. A fighter aircraft flying at 500 mph (223·5 m/sec) may execute a turn with a radius of about one mile, and take 35 seconds to complete a full circle. The force applied to the machine and to its occupant will be approximately 5 G. An airliner travelling at a similar speed may take $2\frac{1}{2}$ minutes to complete a full circuit. Its radius of turn will be nearly four miles, and the accelerative force applied to the passengers will not exceed 1·2 G. The crash landing of either aircraft may produce forces as high as 30 G, lasting for up to half a second.

Accelerations of short duration usually act predominantly in the transverse direction; that is, from front to back or from back to front. In general, tolerance for transverse forces is higher than for those in the head to foot direction, and these in turn have less serious effects than accelerations directed towards the head. Even in the vertical axis, tolerance is high if the duration of the applied force is brief. An ejection seat, for example, may subject the pilot to a force of 20 G, aligned parallel to his spine, for about 0·15 seconds.

Accelerations of long duration

The effects of prolonged acceleration in the long axis of the body and directed from head to foot (the so-called ' positive ' acceleration) are most apparent in the circulatory system. Even in normal circumstances, the blood pressure at head level is lower than that at the heart, and unless the body takes some compensating action, this pressure difference will be exaggerated in direct proportion to the applied acceleration. Thus, at 5 G, the pressure in the aorta must exceed 250 mm Hg if arterial blood pressure at the eye is to be maintained. Compensation of this degree is never achieved, and the retinal and cerebral circulations suffer accordingly. At the same time, and for the same reason, arterial and venous pressures in the lower part of the body increase, and venous return to the heart is impaired.

The pulmonary circulation is also disturbed, and at accelerations in excess of about 3 G only the lower lobes of the lung receive an adequate blood supply. Ventilation is relatively unaffected, but the gas reaching the upper zones of the lungs never comes into contact with blood, and merely adds to the respiratory dead space. In some circumstances, minor air ducts at the bases of the lung may be occluded, and perfusion then continues without adequate ventilation. If the alveoli in these regions contain only oxygen, that gas will rapidly be absorbed, leading to patchy collapse of lung tissue.

Symptoms

The initial symptoms of acceleration are those of increased weight in the direction of the applied force. A feeling of being squashed into the seat is accompanied by difficulty in moving the limbs and head. The soft tissues of the face sag, and heaviness of the lower jaw may produce some difficulty in speaking. As the G is increased, these initial symptoms are followed by a progressive failure of vision. Generalised misting or veiling of objects is associated with an apparent loss of contrast, and a reduction of the peripheral visual fields soon follows. As the applied force rises, the restriction of vision spreads inwards until central vision also disappears. The subject is then ' blacked-out '. The retinal arterial pressure is normally lower than that of the cerebral circulation, because the inflow of blood to the eye is opposed by a positive intraocular pressure. Black-out therefore precedes unconsciousness, but the margin between the two conditions is small.

The loss of consciousness is quite unlike the vasovagal syncope that sometimes results from mild hypoxia. It is a sudden event, unaccompanied by pallor, nausea or sweating. Bradycardia is also usually absent. When the stress is removed, recovery is rapid, although confusion and amnesia may occur, and violent jactitations frequently accompany the return to consciousness. Very prolonged exposures to lower accelerations may result in circulatory collapse, and here the mechanism is similar to that seen in other forms of blood loss. The continued pooling of blood in the lower limbs, and the filtration of fluid into the tissues, results in a critical reduction in the effective blood volume, and the sufferer faints. This syndrome is entirely analogous to that of the guardsman who faints on parade. Premonitory symptoms are the rule, and the collapse can be delayed by voluntary measures to promote venous return from the periphery.

The symptoms of impaired pulmonary function do not usually arise until the removal of the accelerative force. It is then found that a deep breath causes pain, and often provokes a fit of coughing. This helps to re-expand the collapsed lung, but discomfort and soreness in the chest may persist for up to 24 hours after flights in which exposure to centrifugal accelerations and to pure oxygen have been combined.

The effects of forces acting from foot to head (so-called ' negative ' acceleration) are more serious. They result from manoeuvres which are usually prohibited in Service aircraft, but which may inadvertently be encountered during loss of control or structural failure, or which may be deliberately performed by intrepid aerobatic pilots of light aircraft. The most common manoeuvres of this kind are inverted spins and outside loops. The symptoms are similar to those of standing on one's head, but the greater forces involved lead to the rupture of blood vessels in the face and the conjunctiva. The high arterial blood pressure in the head and neck stimulates the carotid sinus, causing bradycardia, cardiac arrhythmias and even asystole. It is probable that the latter is responsible for the unconsciousness that sometimes supervenes. Cerebral haemorrhage does not occur, because the brain is protected by a high pressure in the cerebrospinal fluid.

Diagnosis

The diagnosis is usually obvious from the history of the flight, and from the progress of the symptoms. Centrifugal force is one factor which must always be considered when the causes of unconsciousness or impaired performance in-flight are reviewed, but it is likely to be low on the list of possibilities. Complicating factors should be suspected if the collapse apparently results from acceleration of 3 G or less. Such secondary conditions are not uncommon, and heat, hypoxia, hypoglycaemia and particularly hyperventilation can greatly reduce the tolerance for quite small accelerative forces.

Chest pain after flight must be distinguished from ' chokes '. The diagnosis rests upon a history of exposure to centrifugal force while breathing oxygen, and the absence of a decompression to more than 25 000 feet. Confirmation is provided by the re-expansion of the collapsed lung when deep breaths are taken, but if any doubt remains, a chest X-ray will serve to distinguish the two conditions.

A diagnosis of symptoms caused by negative G cannot be missed. Petechial hemorrhages confined to the face, head and neck, with gross bleeding into the conjunctivae, are pathognomonic.

Treatment

Therapy for long duration accelerations should be entirely preventative. Voluntary tensing of the muscles, straining, or shouting will minimise or delay the symptoms, and many pilots have tricks of their own. Military aircrew constantly exposed to risk are equipped with anti-G suits which, by means of inflated bladders, apply counter-pressure to the abdomen and legs to prevent the pooling of blood and to limit the descent of the diaphragm.

Accelerations of short duration

Tolerance for brief acceleration depends upon the structural strength of the body, because there is no time for major haemodynamic effects to occur. Large forces applied to the chest or abdomen can produce a transient rise in cardiovascular pressures sufficient to cause conjunctival hemorrhages and petechiae in the soft tissues, but the significance of these is small compared with the major injuries likely also to be present.

Accelerations of short duration are usually encountered in aircraft crashes, and they act primarily in the front to back direction. As the aircraft stops abruptly, there is a tendency for the body to be thrown forward from its seat unless adequate restraint is provided, but the initial impact may be followed by break-up of the cabin or by slewing or rolling which may lead to secondary forces applied in other axes. Research using rocket sleds has shown that human tolerance for abrupt deceleration is greater than the strength of standard aircraft seats, provided that the body is adequately supported in all planes. Harness restraint systems developed for military aircraft provide such full protection, but the same is not true of civil practice.

Ordinary aircraft seats face forwards, and have only a simple lap strap for restraint. A crash can result in extreme flexion about the hips with the harness as a pivot. The distance between the seats is such that impact of the head with the back of the seat is certain, and fracture of the skull is a common cause of death in such accidents. Injury to viscera and rupture of blood vessels may result from the snubbing action of the safety belt, and the likelihood of such lesions is increased if disruption of the seat from the floor allows space for flexion of the body to be complete. In many instances, some warning of an impeding crash can be given to passengers, and some protective measures can be taken. Recommendations vary somewhat between different airlines, but the general principle is that the sudden flexion of the head and torso should be prevented. The head may be protected by the arms, and the trunk flexed forward so that both head and arms rest on the back of the seat in front. It can be argued that greater benefit would be obtained by reclining the seat fully and bracing the feet against the most solid structure within reach. The danger of this method is that extra loads would be progressively applied along the line of seats and the failure of one would cause the entire line to collapse like a house of cards.

Because injury is caused by differential movement of the body relative to the seat, the greatest protection will be afforded by a form of restraint which is applied over a large area of the body and which supports the head. Rearward-facing seats provide just such protection. There has been much controversy over the feasibility, or even the desirability, of incorporating backward-facing seats into civilian airliners. Passenger resistance is an oft-quoted argument against this scheme, but there is no evidence that the railways suffer a loss of revenue simply because only half their seats face in the direction of travel. The Royal Air Force has, for many years, used rearward-facing seats exclusively in its transport aircraft, and although the statistics are mercifully few, the risk of death or serious injury in a crash is thereby greatly reduced. There can be no doubt that if this principle were universally adopted by the provision of adequately stressed backward-facing seats the number of medical emergencies occurring in aircraft would be significantly fewer.

AIR SICKNESS

Air sickness results, in part at least, from the action upon the vestibular labyrinth of the repeated small accelerations encountered in every flight. Individuals vary widely in their susceptibility, and although a poor traveller is likely to be made sick by any form of transport, there are some who are unduly sensitive to the random multi-directional motion encountered in aircraft. As in other forms of motion sickness, psychological factors and previous unhappy experience of air travel greatly increase the probability of an attack.

Air sickness may be violent and disabling, but it can only be regarded as a true emergency in casualties and invalids. The danger to patients with head injuries, heart disease, peptic ulcers or recent abdominal operations, or advanced pregnancy, is obvious. Repeated vomiting may also have serious metabolic consequences in severe diabetics.

Although almost all normal people can be nauseated by stimuli of significant magnitude, incapacitating motion sickness in-flight is confined to passengers. Crew members who are subject to the affliction are detected and eliminated at an early stage of training.

Treatment

Air sickness is not basically different from other forms of motion sickness, and treatment should follow similar lines (see p. 479). In the air little can be done to help the sufferer, and prevention is the most important consideration. Prostrated passengers should lie flat as close to the centre of gravity of the aircraft as possible, and head movement should be avoided. Symptoms usually abate rapidly after landing, but the traditional use of hot sweet tea as a restorative for shattered nerves has much to recommend it. It should be liberally prescribed, both to the patient and to those who have nursed him through his difficult hours in-flight.

FITNESS FOR AIR TRAVEL

The hospitable environment of modern airliners enables most of the population to travel without risk, and patients to fly without detriment to their clinical conditions. Indeed, travel by air is often the method of choice for the elderly and infirm, for in speed and comfort it usually heavily outweighs other forms of transport. In most instances medical commonsense is enough to decide whether or not a patient is fit to travel by air, but it is impossible to lay down hard and fast rules for every case. Most major airlines retain specialist medical staff who can advise the practitioner concerning difficult cases, and make special medical arrangements for the carriage of individuals if necessary. In this country, enquiries may be addressed to ' The Medical Officer (Passenger Services), British Airways Medical Service, Central Area Medical Unit, London (Heathrow) Airport, Hounslow, Middlesex (Telephone 01-759 5511 Extension 2378) '. The Medical Service also issues a useful booklet entitled ' Carriage of Invalids by Air ', and it is from this that much of the following information is derived.

In 1961 a Joint Committee of the Aerospace Medical Association and the American Medical Association published a comprehensive report on ' Medical Criteria for Passengers Flying on Scheduled Commercial Fights ', and although the recommendations made there are not mandatory, they are almost universally accepted. A good general rule is that a person who looks normal, feels normal, smells normal, and can walk (or be assisted) up the steps of an aircraft can fly without the likelihood of difficulty. It does not necessarily follow that a patient failing to meet one or more or these criteria should not be allowed to travel by air.

CONTRA-INDICATIONS TO AIR TRAVEL

Patients in the following categories will not be welcomed by any airline.

1. **Infectious diseases.** An airline cannot accept infectious or contagious cases until the risk to other passengers has passed. This embargo is, of course, shared with other forms of public transport.

2. **Advanced pregnancy.** Women are not usually accepted on international journeys after the end of the 35th week of pregnancy, but an extra week's grace may be granted for short domestic flights. Even with these restrictions, premature labour may sometimes be induced by the physiological and psychological excitements of air travel, but to an efficient cabin staff even an in-flight delivery can hardly be counted as a medical emergency.

Some precautions can ease the lot of the heavily pregnant. It may be desirable to prescribe a suitable drug to reduce the risk of motion sickness (see p. 479). If possible, a rearward facing seat should be selected, so that the seat belt need not be uncomfortably tight. Passengers near to term should be warned that false labour pains sometimes occur for a day or two after flight, and given the necessary reassurance.

3. **Offensive passengers.** Patients whose appearance, behaviour, or medical condition may offend other passengers cannot be carried, but they may sometimes be accepted as stretcher cases in a specially screened compartment.

Potentially violent, disturbed, or suicidal patients must be adequately sedated and accompanied by trained staff. Even the ' harmless ' psychotic may present a problem, for he may be incapable of conducting his journey to a successful conclusion, especially if this involves a change of aircraft. Airlines insist that such passengers shall be accompanied by a responsible person, if only to ensure that the patient does not get lost en route.

4. **Terminal cases.** Gravely ill patients who are likely to die before their journey is completed pose special problems, because of the great administrative difficulties resulting from an in-flight death. Nevertheless, many terminal cases *are* carried when there are strong compassionate grounds, and special arrangements can often be made by discussion with the Medical Service of the airline concerned.

OTHER MEDICAL CONDITIONS

Cardiovascular disease

Although the effective cabin altitude of an airliner rarely exceeds 6 000 feet, even mild hypoxia may cause adverse reactions in patients with severe heart disease. For this reason, severe uncompensated heart failure and recent myocardial infarction should be considered as contra-indications to flight. Passengers with angina, and those recovered from a coronary attack (last episode at least 6-8 weeks ago, and with no residual symptoms and signs) may safely be carried, but advance warning should be given to the airline, and the need for extra oxygen should be indicated.

Uncomplicated hypertension is an acceptable condition, especially if the patient has had previous experience of air travel. An emotional rise of blood pressure is not uncommon in those who fly for the first time, and this may present some difficulties if there is concomitant cerebrovascular disease. A sedative should be given to such patients before flight. If the resting blood pressure exceeds 200/100, or if cardiac arrhythmias, marked albuminuria, or retinitis complicate the hypertension, an alternative means of transport should be considered.

Passengers prone to thrombotic conditions may be in some jeopardy on prolonged journeys from the enforced immobility and consequent venous stasis. The hazard can be minimised by frequent movements of the legs, and an occasional walk along the aisle of the aircraft.

Anaemic patients may fly in pressurised aircraft, unless their haemoglobin level is unduly low. A red cell count lower than about $2\frac{1}{2}$ million cells/mm^3 ($2 \cdot 5 \times 10^{12}$/l) is probably an indication for a 'top-up' transfusion. The aim should be to raise the haemoglobin level to at least 9 g/dl. Mild hypoxia may cause sickling in patients with this trait. Individual susceptibility varies widely, but cases known to suffer from this disorder should be discussed with the airline Medical Authorities before flight is contemplated.

Respiratory disease

Hypoxia is again the major problem, and the criteria used for judging cardiac conditions may also be applied to cases of respiratory disease. If doubt exists as to the adequacy of pulmonary function, supplementary oxygen should be available.

The maxim that sufferers from upper respiratory infections should not fly until the cold has cured itself cannot always be observed, but the chance of a blocked ear or sinus can be reduced by the judicious use of decongestants before and during flight. Similar advice should be given to sufferers from hayfever and allergic rhinitis.

Patients with asthma, bronchiectasis and emphysema sometimes find that breathing is easier in the slightly rarified atmosphere of a pressure cabin, but this improvement may be offset by the apprehension associated with a first flight. Moreover, aircraft cabins usually have a low humidity, and this may have an adverse effect. Cases of active pulmonary tuberculosis are excluded because of their infectious nature, but healed or quiescent lesions do not constitute a bar to flying.

Gastrointestinal disease

The primary consideration must be the possible effects of gas expansion. Haemorrhage or perforation may be precipitated in cases of acute peptic ulceration; colic can affect the martyr to a spastic colon; a large unsupported hernia may strangulate. If travel by air is essential, medication and mechanical support should be prescribed as appropriate. Patients who have had abdominal surgery should not fly for at least 10 days, even if the operation was a simple appendicectomy or laparotomy. In cases of peptic ulcer, at least three weeks should be allowed to elapse if major bleeding has been a problem.

A well behaved colostomy or ileostomy is acceptable on most airlines. The patient should be warned in advance of the probable results of exposure to a reduced barometric pressure, and advised to carry extra dressings so as to avoid embarrassing himself and others during flight. Babies are the only incontinent travellers welcomed in an aircraft.

Central nervous system diseases

Well controlled epileptics may travel by air, but they may be more liable than usual to seizures during a long journey; it is therefore desirable that they should be accompanied by an informed and understanding companion. Extra anticonvulsant medication may be required, and a mild sedative taken shortly before take-off will, by allaying some anxiety, make overbreathing less likely and thus decrease the risk of an attack. The airline should always be informed when an epileptic intends to fly, and the information should also be passed quietly to the cabin staff where possible.

In some unusual cases epilepsy may be triggered by travel in helicopters. The precipitating factor is the visual stimulus produced by blade flicker at the critical frequency of 8-12 cycles/second (8-12 Hz).

Degenerative cerebral disease, particularly if it is of vascular origin, may be made worse by the mild hypoxia of flight. Such patients become confused especially on a long journey and this possibility must be considered when long distance flights involving several changes of aircraft are contemplated.

Diabetes

Diabetic passengers should not fly unless their condition is fully stabilised by diet, drugs, or insulin. Most airlines will provide special diets on request, but require that the travellers shall manage their own medication. Severe complications may make the diabetic an unacceptable risk. Sufferers should be aware of the problems caused by time zone changes and by motion sickness. They are best advised to ignore local times during their flight and to remain on the schedule to which they are accustomed. Readjustment to local conditions may safely be undertaken upon arrival at the destination.

Age

There are no age limits for air travel, but it is advisable for prospective passengers over the age of 65 who are to make a long air journey for the first time to submit to a routine medical examination to exclude serious organic disease. (Old people are usually enthusiastic about their first flight.)

Infants also travel very well, and will often sleep throughout the flight with an equanimity that is the envy of their more senior companions. The short Eustachian tubes of the baby protect him against blocked ears during the descent. Any discomfort results in crying, and this has the effect of ventilating the middle ear. A bottle feed is an effective substitute for wailing, and may cause less disturbance to other passengers than the more natural source of infant nutrition.

Summary of contra-indications to air travel

The following list of general contra-indications may be useful. It is reprinted from the British Airlines Medical Service booklet mentioned earlier.

1. Anaemia of severe degree.
2. Severe cases of otitis media and sinusitis.
3. Acute contagious or communicable disease.
4. Myocardial infarction within six weeks of onset.
5. Uncontrolled cardiac failure.
6. Peptic ulceration with recent haemorrhages (i.e. within three weeks).

8. Post-operative cases:
   (1) Within 10 days of simple abdominal operation.
   (2) Within 21 days of major chest surgery.
9. Skin diseases which are contagious or repulsive in appearance.
10. Fractures of the mandible with fixed wiring of the jaw. (Because of the risk of vomiting with disastrous consequences.)
11. Mental illness without escort and sedation.
12. Pregnancies beyond the 35th week for long international journeys and beyond 36th week for short journeys.
13. Introduction of air to body cavities for diagnostic or therapeutic purposes within 7-10 days.

SUPERSONIC FLIGHT

Despite alarmist statements in some popular periodicals, supersonic flight is not an unexplored and hazardous domain. The problems that it poses are little different from those encountered in other aircraft, and there is no reason to suppose that medical emergencies will be more common in Concorde and its successors than in present day machines. Indeed, they may well be less so, because improvements in technology lead not only to greater speeds but also to greater safety and reliability.

Supersonic travel of itself produces no physiological effects, and passengers will be unaware that they have penetrated the mythical ' sound barrier '. However, the shorter time required to cover large distances will exacerbate an existing problem of intercontinental flights; that of crossing time zones. For example, a departure at 11 a.m. followed by a four-hour flight from West to East in a supersonic airliner may result in arrival at the destination at midnight. The physiological clock of the unfortunate passenger reads only 3 p.m., and he must adjust his metabolism to the loss of nine hours if he is to conform to local habits. Even experienced travellers may take some days to compensate fully for time changes of this extent, and the problem becomes more pressing if several such journeys are made over a short period of time. The ' desynchronosis ' or ' jet lag ' is more of an annoyance than an emergency, but diabetics and others requiring regular meals or medication must be advised of the potential problem.

The economical cruising altitude of a supersonic airliner is 65 000 feet or more, but this simply means that a higher pressure differential must exist between the cabin and the atmosphere so that a habitable environment can be maintained within. The passenger oxygen systems of current airliners are effective only up to a cabin altitude of about 35 000 feet, and they would be of little value at the cruising height of commercial supersonic airliners. Full protection against these altitudes demands the use of pressure suits, which obviously cannot be provided for passengers. The only practicable alternative is to ensure that in the event of a decompression the cabin altitude does not exceed the capability of the standard oxygen equipment. By careful design and engineering it has been possible to limit the depressurisation following an emergency such as the loss of a door or a window to the equivalent of no more than 25 000 feet. A more serious but most unlikely defect in the cabin could involve exposure to altitudes of more than 36 000 feet, with a reduction to 10 000 feet or less in 5-8 minutes. In such an event cases of unconsciousness would be expected, but it has been shown that decompression profiles of this kind do not result in permanent neurological damage, even when oxygen is not available.

The height at which supersonic aircraft fly introduces two potential hazards that are not found at lower altitude. The concentration of ozone in the atmosphere increases steadily, to reach a maximum at about 90 000 feet, and at the cruising altitude of Concorde up to 10 parts/million may be present in the ambient air. The requirement that the concentration of ozone within the cabin shall be less than 0·1 parts/million is easily met. Most of the gas is broken down to oxygen by the heat associated with the cabin pressurisation equipment, and a catalytic filter is fitted as a second line of defence.

Much has been made of the potential danger from cosmic radiation, the flux of which increases at high altitude because the attenuation provided by the atmosphere is smaller. It is estimated that the total dose received by a passenger in a transatlantic crossing will, in normal circumstances, amount to only about 4 per cent of that experienced during a chest X-ray. The dose rate depends in part upon the activity of the sun, and large solar flares can produce intense bursts of radiation. Monitoring equipment in the aircraft and on the ground can give warning of an increase in the radiation hazard, and if abnormal conditions are encountered it may be necessary for the flight to be conducted at a lower altitude.

Envoi

An aircraft is not a sanctuary from the medical problems of everyday life, and an airline ticket is not a talisman against appendicitis. Emergencies in the air are much more likely to have familiar clinical causes than to result from the environment of flight. In aviation, as in other fields of medical practice, the mundane conditions are the ones that are most frequently encountered.

PETER HOWARD.

FOR FURTHER READING

General

GILLIES, J. A. *A Textbook of Aviation Physiology.* London: Pergamon Press. 1965. (A comprehensive and authoritative account of the whole of aviation medicine, as practised and preached by the Royal Air Force.)

RANDEL, H. W. (ed.). *Aerospace Medicine.* Baltimore: The Williams and Wilkins Company. 1971. (A slimmer and less ambitious work, based on American principles.)

Passenger Flying

AEROSPACE MEDICINE ASSOCIATION AND THE AMERICAN MEDICAL ASSOCIATION (1961). Medical criteria for passenger flying on scheduled commercial flights. Joint committee report. *Archives of Environmental Health,* **2,** 136. (The report states both physiological and clinical principles.)

Supersonic Flight

BENNETT, G. (1965). Human factors in the Concorde SST. *Aerospace Medicine,* **36,** 1094.

STRUHRING, D. H. (1963). The medical aspects of supersonic flight. *Journal of the American Medical Association,* **185,** 94.

Aircraft Accidents

MASON, J. K. *Aviation Accident Pathology.* London: Butterworth. 1962.

CHAPTER 24

Ophthalmic Emergencies

FOREIGN BODY IN THE EYE

THIS rather commonplace injury has several diagnostic pitfalls to trap the unwary and care in history taking and examination is essential. The mode of entry should be particularly noted. Some particles are simply carried in by a current of air and these are usually lightly adherent to the conjunctiva or cornea. Others enter with force as in hammering or grinding; these are often firmly embedded and may actually penetrate the globe.

The cornea and conjunctival sac must be carefully explored. If photophobia makes examination difficult, instil a drop of 1 per cent amethocaine hydrochloride (there is no contraindication to this in any type of painful eye). Illumination is best provided by a strong spotlight directed obliquely.

1. Inspect the corneal surface carefully, sector by sector, remembering to direct attention to the transparent dome and not to the deeper and more obvious iris markings.

2. Examine the bulbar conjunctiva and lower fornix.

3. Evert the upper lid (Fig. 24.1). A foreign body is frequently lodged in the tarsal sulcus which runs some 2 to 3 mm from the free margin of the lid.

If no foreign body is found, suspect:

1. Spontaneous exit leaving a small corneal abrasion. The site of this can be found by ' staining '. An area denuded of epithelium shows up as a green spot after staining with fluorescein impregnated filter paper and washing out with isosmotic sodium chloride solution. (Fluorescein eyedrops can be dangerous, p. 86).

2. An in-turning eyelash.

3. Penetration of the globe. The entry must be forcible for this to occur but the possibility is frequently forgotten.

Removal of foreign body

A foreign body under the upper lid is best removed by everting the lid and wiping it off with a damp cottonwool stick or corner of a clean handkerchief (Fig. 24.1). Occasionally a particle lodges right up in the upper fornix. It can be removed by everting the lid and sweeping the upper conjunctival fold with a cottonwool stick.

A corneal foreign body is dealt with as shown in Fig. 24.2. As fainting is an occasional complication during removal, the patient should lie on a couch. If this is not possible, the head must be kept back and rested firmly on a support. Three drops of 1 per cent amethocaine are instilled at minute intervals. It is important to gain the patient's confidence before starting the removal by demonstrating that the procedure will be painless. This is best done by first testing the relatively insensitive bulbar conjunctiva before touching the cornea.

The gaze is then directed upward to some suitably placed spot and an assistant focuses a spotlight obliquely on the cornea. Figure 24.2 shows the method of holding the lids to prevent blinking and also how the hand holding the instrument is steadied by resting it on the patient's cheek. If the operator is right-handed, he should stand on the patient's right side for either right or left eye.

The choice of instrument used depends on the degree of adherence of the foreign body and the experience of the operator. Removal can frequently be effected with a damp cottonwool wick, but the spud will be necessary for more firmly embedded particles. The least traumatising procedure is to use a pointed instrument such as a Bowman's needle or a large straight triangular surgical needle (these may with advantage be used in conjunction with a magnifying loupe). The point is introduced under the foreign body which is then lifted off the cornea.

After removal instil one drop of 0·5 per cent Chloramphenicol Eye-Drops. Keep the eye padded until healing is complete—this normally takes 24 to 48 hours. A sensation as though the particle is still present indicates that the area has not yet been covered by epithelium and that padding for a further period is required.

COMPLICATIONS OF REMOVAL OF A FOREIGN BODY. There are three main complications of this procedure:

1. *Extensive corneal abrasions.* These usually result from repeated unsuccessful attempts to dislodge a particle which may have penetrated deeply. The use of a slit lamp may be required to gauge the depth of a deeply embedded particle. The removal of this type of foreign body is a matter for the expert.

2. *Perforation of the cornea.* This complication usually occurs during the removal of a large deeply situated foreign body. A gush of aqueous and a shallow anterior chamber indicate this complication which fortunately is not usually so serious as might be expected. The attempt at removal is, of course, abandoned. Several drops of 0·5 per cent Chloramphenicol Eye-Drops are instilled and one of 1 per cent atropine. The eye is lightly bandaged and the patient treated as for penetrating injury (p. 527).

3. *Corneal ulceration.* This is a later complication caused by infection of the traumatised area. It is most likely to occur if the eye is left unbandaged before the wound has become properly healed.

SPECIAL TYPES OF FOREIGN BODY

Rust ring

A ring of very adherent brown stain often occurs around a steel or emery wheel particle. The parent foreign body is often quite easy to deal with, but the eye usually remains irritable until the rust ring has been removed. The cornea softens around the ring and it is usually quite easy to scrape the whole area away with a sharp needle or small dental burr.

Sparks from contacts between electrically driven bumper-cars and the wire mesh carrying the current release showers of tiny molten metallic particles. These may penetrate the cornea but symptoms are often delayed for up to 48 hours. They may leave a rust ring.

Glass

Glass particles are difficult to see although they may glint in a bright light. Even quite small particles may, however, be discovered by instilling 1 per cent amethocaine and then running the ball of the little finger along the lower fornix and over the surface of the everted upper lid. A moistened cottonwool wick is then gently passed around the upper fornix.

Lime (p. 530).

Indelible pencil

Chips of indelible pencil or aniline dye in any form set up an intense conjunctivitis. Remove any visible particles with cottonwool wick or fine forceps and instil pure glycerine at 10-minute intervals for two hours.

Multiple particles

Sand, dust and other particles are best removed by liberal irrigations of the eye with a stream of isosmotic sodium chloride solution.

Chewing gum (p. 642).

INJURIES TO THE GLOBE

These injuries fall into two groups :

1. Those perforating or rupturing the globe. Penetration is commonly caused by pointed instruments or missiles. Intraocular foreign bodies also come into this category.

2. Those causing contusion of the globe. Injuries of all grades of severity may be caused by rounded objects such as knuckles, tennis balls, and projections on furniture.

A sharp instrument may damage the eye without entering it and a blunt instrument may cause rupture of the globe. Hence the history may be misleading. A careful examinatiaon is essential.

Method of examination

1. Estimate the vision of the injured eye. Even when the lids are severely bruised they can be gently separated and the test applied. Vision is conveniently assessed by finding what size newsprint can be read or at what distance fingers can be counted. If good vision has been retained, many serious possibilities are excluded.

2. Examine the lids, cornea and sclera for evidence of puncture wounds.

3. Stain the cornea with fluorescein (pp. 524 and 86) for evidence of abrasion (a common injury).

4. Examine the anterior chamber, noting the depth and the presence or absence of blood.

5. Examine the iris, noting any displacement or distortion of the pupil and compare direct and consensual light reflex with the uninjured eye.

6. Dilate the pupil with 1 per cent homatropine and examine the lens, vitreous and fundus with the ophthalmoscope.

7. X ray the orbit if an intraocular foreign body is suspected. *On no account should an attempt be made to test the ocular tension.* Little information would be gained thereby and prolapse of intraocular contents may be caused if perforation has occurred.

PENETRATING INJURIES

Signs of penetration of the globe

1. If the wound is in the cornea or corneo-scleral junction, the pupil is drawn up towards the wound and there is likely to be a prolapse of iris through it. This will appear as a small brown or black bead on the surface, often with a thread of fibrin or mucus attached. The anterior chamber may be shallow or absent.

2. If the wound is in the sclera, it is more difficult to decide whether penetration has occurred as subconjunctival bleeding usually obscures the wound area. The appearance of brown uveal tissue or the presence of vitreous will clinch the diagnosis.

Complications

Apart from damage to the transparent media and nervous tissues there is risk of intraocular infection and sympathetic ophthalmia.

Emergency treatment of penetrating injuries

Pending removal to hospital, emergency treatment consists in combating possible infection by instillation of 0·5 per cent Chloramphenicol Eye-Drops and applying a light pad and bandage.

General treatment consists in preventing further prolapse or intraocular haemorrhage by keeping the head still and the body relaxed. Valium 5 mg is a useful sedative but morphine must be avoided as it may provoke vomiting. The patient should be taken to hospital in the prone position or, if this is not possible, sitting back comfortably with the head supported.

NON-PENETRATING INJURIES

The possible effects of a non-penetrating injury are:

1. *Bruising of the lids.* This may make examination of the globe difficult although the visual acuity can usually be assessed.

2. *Fracture of orbital bones.* The orbit may suffer a ' blow out ' fracture with herniation of its contents through the floor. This causes enophthalmos and limitation of upward movement of the eye. Fractures of the zygoma and inferior orbital margin may also occur. Always X ray the orbit if there is extensive bruising.

3. *Corneal abrasion.* This is a common injury. The extent can be ascertained by fluorescein staining (pp. 86 and 524).

4. *Intraocular haemorrhage.* In the anterior chamber blood may be seen by the naked eye. In the vitreous it often obscures the red fundus reflex. Retinal haemorrhages and also white patches of oedema (commotio retinae) in the fundus are seen by ophthalmoscopy.

5. *Injury to iris and pupil.* The pupil may suffer traumatic mydriasis and the iris show tears at the pupil margin or at its peripheral attachment.

6. *Injury to lens.* A displaced lens may give rise to a tremulous iris and its rounded edge may be observed through the pupil on ophthalmoscopy. Cataract formation may occur in the ensuing weeks.

7. *Retinal detachment.* This important complication, with its characteristic symptom of loss of part of the visual field, may not be apparent for some days or weeks after the injury.

8. *Secondary glaucoma.* Severe pain in the eye, forehead or temple should arouse suspicion of increased intra-ocular tension. It is most likely to occur after intraocular haemorrhage.

Treatment of non-penetrating injuries

The swelling of even severely bruised lids soon resolves with a cold saline compress and firm bandage. Corneal abrasions are treated by 1 per cent Homatropine Eye-Drops twice daily and padding the eye until healed. If any intraocular damage is suspected, the patient should be kept quietly in bed with the head supported on two pillows and the advice of an ophthalmologist obtained. Intraocular haemorrhage usually means hospitalisation as recurrent haemorrhage and secondary glaucoma are ever-present dangers. These cases need constant expert surveillance.

PHYSICAL INJURIES

Burns of the lids

These usually occur from accidents such as ' blow-backs ' from gas stoves, petrol explosions and the like (p. 558). The skin of the lids and face may suffer any degree of burn. The eyes suffer corneal abrasions and may receive multiple foreign bodies which are either the products of the explosion or fragments of the patient's charred lashes.

Treatment. Gently cleanse the lids with warm isosmotic sodium chloride solution and remove dead skin with scissors. Clip the lashes almost to the roots; scissors smeared with petroleum jelly will be found helpful as the cut lashes adhere to the blades instead of dropping into the eye. Irrigate with warm saline to remove foreign particles and examine the cornea for abrasions after fluorescein staining. Instil 0·5 per cent Chloramphenicol Eye-Drops and cover the closed lids with tulle gras dressings. Apply a light pad and bandage.

Exposure to ultraviolet light

This occurs in arc-welders working with their eyes inadequately protected by goggles, and in electricians from short circuit flashes. It is common as snow-blindness in alpinists and skiers and sometimes follows exposure to mercury vapour lamps. The symptoms start after a latent interval of some hours. There is intense pain, lachrymation, photophobia and oedema of the lids.

Treatment is simple as the condition is self-limiting. Reassure the patient that the symptoms will pass off in a matter of hours and that the sight will not be affected. Apply hydrocortisone ointment to the conjunctival sac, cover the eyes with cold saline compresses and put the patient to bed. Pethidine should be given if the pain is severe.

CHEMICAL INJURIES

In general, chemical injuries are confined to the cornea and the conjunctiva, particularly of the lower fornix. The cornea is frequently abraded and if the erosion penetrates deeper than the epithelium a permanent scar will result. The conjunctiva is intensely injected and there is usually some discharge. Loss of epithelium in the fornices may result in symblepharon, a disabling adhesion of the inner side of the lid of the globe. It must not be forgotten that chemical injuries may involve other parts also, e.g. the glottis where oedema coming on later, particularly after an ammonia attack, may necessitate urgent treatment (p. 225).

Treatment

In any type of chemical injury immediate douching will dilute the irritant and prevent further tissue injury. A tap-water douche at once is better than the theoretical antidote administered with complete asepsis an hour later so hold the victim's head under the cold water tap (clothes regardless). Speed is the only thing that counts.

Unless there is actual tissue destruction by strong acids, ammonia, caustic soda or lime (see below) isosmotic sodium chloride solution is the most effective and least irritating solution to wash out irritants including liquid fuels, spirits, cleaning agents and antiseptics. Certain chemicals which cause actual tissue destruction are with advantage washed out with neutralising solutions as follows:

For strong acids. Irrigate freely with sodium bicarbonate 2·5 g/dl.

For caustic soda. Irrigate freely with ammonium chloride solution 5 g/dl.

For lime or plaster-lime. As this causes severe pain a preliminary instillation of 1 per cent amethocaine is advisable. All solid particles are first removed using a cottonwool stick moistened with sodium edathamil (EDTA) 0·4 g/dl, the best neutralising agent. Some of the more adherent particles may have to be scraped off with a spud. The upper lid must be everted and cleaned for quite large plaques frequently adhere there. Finally give a copious irrigation with sodium edathamil (EDTA) 0·4 g/dl.

(For eye injuries from spitting snakes see p. 632, from indelible pencil see p. 826, and from phenol see p. 37).

After removal of the irritant ascertain the extent of the tissue damage by staining with fluorescein (p. 524). A corneal abrasion

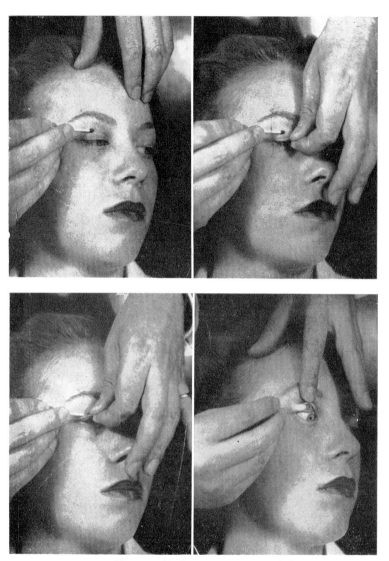

(*Photographic Department, St. Bartholomew's Hospital.*)

FIG. 24.1. Eversion of the upper lid.

Facing page 530

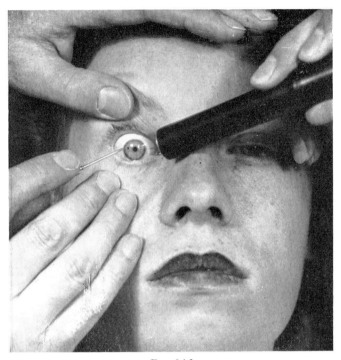

FIG. 24.2
Removal of corneal foreign body.

The patient is directed to fix the gaze on some distant object. The left thumb retracts the upper lid to prevent closure during the operation. The hand holding the spud is steadied by resting the lower three fingers on the patient's cheek.

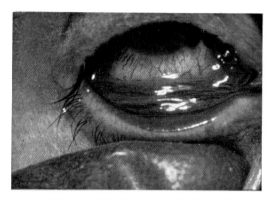

(*Photographic Department, St Bartholomew's
Hospital.*)

Fig. 24.3
Acute conjunctivitis showing the superficial type of
congestion most marked in the fornices and brick red
in colour.

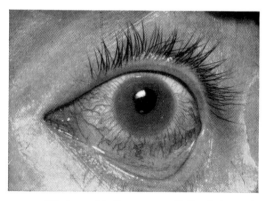

(*Photographic Department, St Bartholomew's
Hospital.*)

Fig. 24.4
Acute iritis showing the deep or ciliary type of
congestion most marked in the peri-corneal zone
and purplish in hue. The patient is under treatment
with atropine which has caused the pupil to be
dilated and irregular.

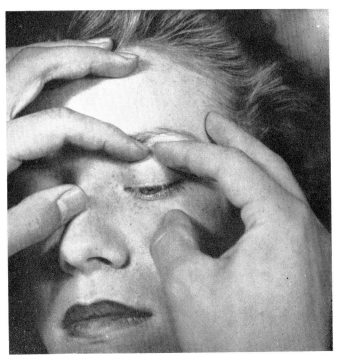

(*Photographic Department, St. Bartholomew's Hospital.*)

Fig. 24.5

Estimation of intraocular tension.

The patient is directed to look right down. The forefingers are placed on the lid above the tarsal plate. The left forefinger steadies the globe while the right gently palpates. The resistance offered to the palpating finger gives an estimation of the tension.

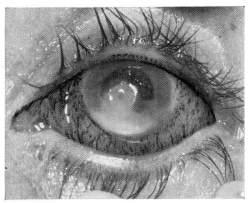

(*Photographic Department, St. Bartholomew's Hospital.*)

Fig. 24.6

Large corneal ulcer, stained with fluorescein. Note the presence of hypopyon.

will stain green and a loss of conjunctival epithelium a greenish-yellow. An ointment containing chloramphenicol 1 per cent and hydrocortisone acetate 0·5 per cent is helpful in reducing the inflammation and preventing secondary infection. If a corneal abrasion is found insert in addition some Eye Ointment of Atropine BP 1 per cent and apply a pad and bandage. If the conjunctival epithelium in the fornices is damaged symblepharon can be prevented by instilling 1 per cent amethocaine and gently drawing a glass rod smeared with Chloramphenicol Eye Ointment 1 per cent around upper and lower fornix thereby breaking down any adhesions which may be forming. This procedure is repeated every day for a week.

Unless mild it is always safest to refer actual burns for specialist treatment since severe tissue loss in the fornices is best treated by mucous membrane graft within the first few hours.

INFLAMMATIONS OF THE GLOBE

DIFFERENTIAL DIAGNOSIS OF AN INFLAMED EYE

Four groups of ocular lesions give rise to general congestion of the globe:

1. Acute conjunctivitis (Fig. 24.3).

2. Acute keratitis. The most usual type of keratitis is the single corneal ulcer. The presence of pus in the anterior chamber (hypopyon) is a sign of especial gravity (Fig. 24.6). The herpetic (dendritic) type often coincides with the onset of a febrile illness. Multiple punctate erosions, a corneal foreign body and the deep or interstitial type of corneal inflammation are also included in the term keratitis.

3. Acute iritis or iridio-cyclitis (Fig. 24.4).

4. Acute glaucoma.

These four groups are differentiated by a careful history and examination of *both* eyes (Table 24.1).

Episcleritis is diagnosed by congestion of *a sector* of the sclera. It is unlikely to be confused with the four conditions mentioned above because it is localised. It is not associated with loss of vision or discharge and responds dramatically to local steroids.

Further diagnostic points

1. *Discharge.* Conjunctivitis is the only one of the four conditions with discharge which varies in amount from a slight crusting of the lids on waking to an intense purulent exudate.

2. *Pain.* Conjunctivitis gives discomfort only, not pain. The pain of acute glaucoma may be sufficiently severe to cause vomiting.

3. *Vision.* Vision in glaucoma is greatly reduced. The patient may give a history of coloured haloes around lights.

4. *Types of congestion* (Figs 24.3 and 24.4). In the conjunctival or superficial type of congestion the redness is maximal at the fornices and the colour a brick red. In the ciliary or deep type the congestion is circumcorneal and has a violet hue. It is of the utmost importance to recognise this type of congestion (even though in some cases there is a super-added conjunctival congestion) as keratitis, iridocyclitis and glaucoma are all serious conditions.

5. *Corneal transparency.* Compare the transparency of the two corneae and note if any opacity is localised (keratitis) or generalised. Always stain with fluorescein (pp. 86 and 524) as an active ulcer, especially a small one, can only be seen by this means (Fig. 24.6).

6. *Anterior chamber.* Compare the depth on the two sides. Inspect the lower parts carefully for evidence of hypopyon.

7. *Iris and pupil.* These differ in iritis and glaucoma. The pupil in iritis is small and the margin may be bound down or seen to be filled with exudate. The iris shows a ' muddy ' discoloration. The pupil in acute glaucoma is dilated, often oval with the long axis vertical. Reaction to light is absent or poor in both conditions.

8. *Tension* (Fig. 24.5). Compare the resistance of the globe on the two sides.

9. *Examination of the other eye.* Never omit this, as it often provides important diagnostic clues.

Common diagnostic difficulties

A small corneal foreign body is easily missed as is an inturning eyelash. Small ulcers, especially those near the corneal margin, are common, and will escape notice unless looked for carefully after staining. Sometimes a conjunctivitis and a keratitis (in the form of a corneal ulcer) may exist together. Further, an acute iritis may give rise to a secondary glaucoma.

EMERGENCY TREATMENT OF THE RED EYE

Congestion apart from that of simple conjunctivitis and small ulcers, should be treated at hospital as diagnosis may necessitate the use of special instruments. If this is not possible the following measures should be carried out.

Conjunctivitis

Take a conjunctival swab (for direct smear, culture and sensitivity to antibiotics) before any treatment is started. Cleanse any discharge

Table 24.1. *Differential diagnosis of the red eye.*

	CONJUNCTIVITIS	KERATITIS	IRITIS	GLAUCOMA
1. Discharge	Present			
2. Pain	Discomfort only	Watering only Pain	Watering only Pain + or + +	Watering only Pain + + or + + + may cause vomiting
3. Vision	Normal	Depends on area of opacity covering the pupil	Reduced	Much reduced
4. Type of congestion	Conjunctival	Ciliary	Ciliary	Ciliary
5. Corneal transparency	Cornea normal	Opacity is localised	General haze	General clouding
6. Anterior chamber	Normal depth	Normal depth	Normal or deep	Shallow
7. Iris and pupil	Normal size Normal reactions	May be small; reacts to light	Pupil small and often bound Reflexes poor or absent. Iris discoloured	Pupil dilated No reaction to light
8. Tension	Normal	Normal	May be somewhat increased	Greatly increased
9. Examination of other eye	Condition often bilateral	May be old scars of previous ulcers	Pupil may be bound from past iritis	Disc may be cupped. May be evidence of previous glaucoma operation

from the lids with saline swabs. Apply 0·5 per cent Chloramphenicol
Eye-Drops every two hours. If the inflammation has not considerably improved in 36 hours the organism is almost certainly resistant
and treatment should be changed to weak Eye-Drops of Sulphacet-
amide BPC (10 per cent) four-hourly. Order dark glasses. (Never
use a pad.) Where there is severe purulent discharge either in the
adult or the newborn, suspect a gonococcal infection and give the
following: 0·5 per cent chloramphenicol eye-drops every minute
for 30 minutes, then every 15 minutes for the next two hours and
finally every two hours until the inflammation has subsided. In
addition give full doses of sulphadimidine (Sulphamezathine) orally.

Corneal ulcer

Apply 1 per cent atropine ointment and Chloramphenicol Eye-
Drops 0·5 per cent three times a day followed by a hot steaming
pad and bandage. Local steroids should not be used. If hypopyon
is present (Fig. 24.6), anaesthetise the conjunctiva with a drop of 1
per cent amethocaine and inject 100 mg of Soframycin in 0·5 ml
distilled water beneath the lower bulbar conjunctiva.

Iritis

Apply 1 per cent atropine ointment three times a day, followed
by hot steamings. Order dark glasses. If atropine fails to dilate the
pupil inject 0·3 ml of Mydricaine beneath the lower bulbar conjunctiva.

Mydricaine is obtainable from Macarthy's Laboratories Ltd.,
Chesham House, Chesham Close, Romford, RM1 4JX (Romford
46033 STD).

It is made in two strengths. The dose of each must not exceed
0·3 ml.

	Mydricaine No. 1	Mydricaine No. 2
Atropine sulphate	0·5 mg	1·0 mg
Procaine hydrochloride	3·0 mg	6·0 mg
Adrenaline solution BP	0·06 mg	0·12 ml
Boric acid	5·0 mg	5·0 mg
Sodium metabisulphite	0·3 mg	0·3 mg
Water for injection	0·3 mg	0·3 mg

Acute glaucoma

Instil 4 per cent pilocarpine into the affected eye two-hourly
and 1 per cent pilocarpine into the opposite eye twice daily since
it is also liable to an acute attack. In addition give acetazolamide

(Diamox) 500 mg by mouth and further doses of 250 mg at six-hourly intervals. Pethidine should be given if pain is severe. Following resolution of acute glaucoma a peripheral iridectomy is always necessary and is advisable in the other eye as this also is liable to develop an acute attack.

PAIN IN AND AROUND THE EYE

When eye pain is a presenting symptom the following conditions should be considered.

1. Acute glaucoma (p. 534, Fig. 24.5).
2. Iritis (p. 534, Fig. 24.4).
3. Keratitis (Table 24.1, p. 533).
4. Herpes zoster ophthalmics (p. 552).
5. Trigeminal neuralgia (p. 325). Here the pain occurs in paroxysms and is sharp or burning and around rather than in the eye. The globe is normal and vision unimpaired.
6. Frontal sinusitis. Here as well as pain there is tenderness over the affected sinus.
7. Retro-bulbar neuritis (see below)

SUDDEN BLINDNESS
(For Amblyopia in Renal Disease see p. 383)

Blindness in one eye

When of rapid onset this is usually caused by one of the following vascular accidents:

1. Thrombosis of the central vein. The disc is swollen, the veins engorged and there are multiple haemorrhages and exudates along their course.

2. Thrombosis, spasm or embolism of the central artery (sometimes associated with temporal arteritis). The disc and retina are pale while the macula shows up as a ' cherry spot '. The arteries are thread-like. Unless the circulation is restored in three hours loss of vision will probably be permanent. Dilatation of vessels may be effected by an inhalation of amyl nitrite or (a measure well worth trying) by massaging the globe with the finger tips through the closed lids and using moderately firm pressure for 10 minutes. Further treatment (in hospital) is by paracentesis of the anterior chamber or by stellate ganglion block (p. 711). If temporal (giant cell) arteritis is diagnosed prompt treatment with steroids is indicated because of the high risk of blindness from involvement of ophthalmic vessels. When one eye is affected steroids may prevent blindness in the other eye.

3. Intraocular haemorrhage. The lesion may be of any size from a small haemorrhage at the macula to a vitreous full of blood. It may complicate any conditions of which bleeding is a feature (p. 275). Among these are proliferative diabetic retinopathy, Eales' disease (periphlebitis of retinal veins), sickle cell disease and new vessel formation after a branch vein thrombosis.

Conditions causing less sudden blindness in one eye are :

1. Retro-bulbar neuritis. Here there may be pain on movement of the globe and a central scotoma. The pupil reacts sluggishly to light, but the consensual reaction is normal. Treatment is that of the causal condition.

2. Detachment of the retina. This is characterised by progressive loss of the visual field and needs immediate treatment in hospital for reattachment.

3. Central choroiditis. A patch of choroiditis near the macula or disc may cause a loss of vision which increases over a period of days.

4. Hysteria. Hysterical blindness may be partial or complete and is occasionally bilateral. The patient avoids obstacles in his path and shows the blink reaction to menace. The pupils and fundi are normal.

Blindness affecting both eyes.

This is almost always due to general causes such as :

1. Toxic substances: methyl alcohol (p. 34), quinine, and (rarely) lead, arsenic, carbon disulphide, ergot, and filix mas. Chloroquine and allied drugs may cause all degrees of loss of vision.

2. Severe haemorrhage particularly from the gastrointestinal tract p. 164). uterus and lungs. The blindness comes on several days after the main loss.

3. Hypertensive states and toxaemia of pregnancy.

4. Renal disease (p. 383).

5. Diabetes.

6. Diseases of the central nervous system including vascular lesions involving the visual pathways (usually causing a hemianopic field loss), haemorrhage into a pituitary tumour, gross papilloedema and acute encephalo-myelitis.

J. H. DOBREE

CHAPTER 25

Emergencies in Skin Diseases

SKIN diseases though rarely fatal in themselves may be of urgent importance. Systemic visceral disease may coexist as in lupus erythematosus, polyarteritis nodosa, dermatomyositis, reticulosis, epithelioma, melanoma and toxic and allergic dermatoses, as well as with widespread pruritus. Secondary infection may develop when there is exudation, erosion, fissuring, ulceration or any break in the epidermis. Lymphangitis, lymphadenitis and even septicaemia can result. Loss of protein may occur in exfoliative dermatitis and of fluid, protein and electrolytes also in pemphigus. Cardiac failure may result from the greatly increased blood flow through the skin. Patients with erythroderma may suffer excessive heat loss, causing hypothermia. A skin condition may cause great anxiety or be the outward sign of a psychoneurosis or psychosis. The differentiation of some non-infectious skin conditions from infectious exanthemata may demand instant decisions. Lastly, itching may become intolerable and distressingly urgent.

THE DIAGNOSIS OF ACUTE ERUPTIONS

A discussion on the finer points of differential diagnosis cannot be made in a book of this nature; but a list of the more likely causes for various types of eruption may prove of value in an emergency. An eruption for which immediate treatment is expected may be widespread (one of the specific fevers, a toxic erythema, a specific skin disease or a generalised eczema) or it may be local (of bacterial, viral or fungal origin, or eczematous in nature).

WIDESPREAD ERUPTIONS

Erythematous

Scarlatina; morbilli; rubella; other virus infections, drug exanthems and erythemata of undetermined causes; urticaria, purpura, erythema multiforme, erythema nodosum; and the roseolar syphilide (palms involved).

Scaly erythematous

Pityriasis rosea and its mimicry by drug eruptions and scaly syphilides; scaly seborrhoeides (sweat grooves); guttate psoriasis (silvery scaling may only be revealed by rubbing with a spatula); peeling scarlatina (coarse and glove-like on hands and feet).

Papular and papulo-vesicular

Lichen planus (flat-topped polygonal violaceous papules with a 'waxy glance'), widespread eczemas from internal or external causes, including eruptions secondary to hypostatic eczema (eczematides) often arising from secondary infection or from the use of sensitising or occlusive applications; dermatophytides; varicella (polymorphic lesions especially affecting covered areas, e.g., axillae); variola (single or multiple, monomorphic, favouring exposed areas); papular urticaria (extensor aspects of limbs, also trunk and often grouped), (examine pets and the chairs and rugs on which they lie for parasites and ova); halogen eruptions; papular syphilides, pityriasis lichenoides et varioliformis (scabbed and necrotising papules and small ulcers).

Bullous

Insect bites (mostly on the legs; examine pets for infestations and surroundings for bugs, fleas and other biting arthropods); urticaria (lesions fade rapidly without trace); erythema multiforme (persistent, often with iris lesions, distally distributed and with oral, ocular and genital lesions in the severe Stevens-Johnson form); varicella, variola, vaccinia, Kaposi's varicelliform eruption (generalised herpes simplex or generalised vaccinia); drug eruptions; plant dermatitis; juvenile dermatitis herpetiformis (mostly around the mouth and genitalia); toxic epidermal necrolysis (extensive scald-like blistering, p. 546).

LOCALISED ERUPTIONS

Infective dermatoses are, as a rule, crusted or exudative and patchy in distribution tending to affect flexures and follicles and with peripheral 'satellites'. Localised virus infections such as vaccinia, herpes simplex, orf and milker's nodes are tense, oedematous, sometimes necrotising lesions. Eczematous dermatoses are usually papulo-vesicular or erythemato-squamous, and are more diffuse and ill-defined, with the exception of discoid eczema of the extremities in which de-fatting of the skin and sensitisation to skin organisms seem to play a part. Mixed eczematous and infective conditions are not uncommon. With annular lesions, likely diagnoses include tinea, impetigo, pityriasis rosea, syphilis, psoriasis, lichen planus, erythema multiforme, lupus erythematosus, and granuloma annulare. The differential diagnosis of these eruptions depends on a careful history and on their distribution and detailed morphology. In the diagnosis of fungal infections physical signs alone cannot be relied upon and it is necessary to examine a scraping microscopically in liquor potassae after applying gentle heat. The septate branching mycelium can be seen with the 16 mm objective with the diaphragm stopped down and confirmed under the 4 mm objective. Fungal infections are often markedly atypical after topical corticosteroids have been applied. A fixed or recurrent localised erythema may be caused by phenolphthalein, iodides, sulphonamides, barbiturates, oxyphenbutazone, tetracyclines, chlordiazepoxide, acetylsalicylic acid and quinine.

DRUG ERUPTIONS

Drug eruptions are usually mild and transient but may be severe and even fatal if a vital organ or tissue is also affected, particularly the bone marrow, vessel walls, kidneys, liver, or the heat-regulating centre. Drugs particularly liable to cause eruptions include allopurinol, amidopyrine, amiphenazole, ampicillin and other antibiotics, arsenic, barbiturates, carbromal, oral contraceptives, gold, phenolphthalein, phenothiazines, phenylbutazone, quinine and sulphonamides. The list continually changes with the introduction of new drugs and the abandonment of old ones.

Arsenic, carbromal, amiphenazole and the halogens cause characteristic eruptions, but with most other drugs the eruptions are non-specific and to identify the cause reliance must be placed on the history, perhaps followed by a sub-therapeutic (one-tenth) test dose at a later date.

A possible drug causation should be considered in erythematous eruptions, whether morbilliform, scarlatiniform, urticarial, purpuric, or erythema multiforme-like; in stomatitis; in eruptions resembling pityriasis rosea, ' seborrhoeic dermatitis,' psoriasis, or lichen planus; in exfoliative dermatitis, eczematoid, furuncular, acneiform or rosacea-like conditions when there is light-sensitivity or vasculitis, and in granulomatous lesions. Acne vulgaris and rosacea may be aggravated by halogens. Pruritus may be caused by opiates, including codeine; also by belladonna and cocaine. Sometimes it precedes a drug eruption.

Before giving treatment, an attempt should be made to decide whether a drug eruption is due to direct action on the skin or to indirect effects resulting from the action of the drug on other organs.

Direct toxic action on the epidermis may cause exfoliative, dyskeratotic, necrolytic or pigmentary changes. Allergic hypersensitivity causes eczematous changes in the epidermis and erythema, urticaria or purpura in the dermis.

Drug action on the bone marrow may cause purpura and cutaneous or oral ulceration. Action on the liver may cause infective, exfoliative or phrynodermatous eruptions or photosensitivity. Oedema and haematuria may result from renal involvement. Myxoedema may appear if the thyroid gland is damaged and unexplained pyrexia may occur if the heat-regulating centre is involved. Oral antibiotics, especially the tetracyclines and chloramphenicol, may disturb the bacterial flora of the gut and cause anogenital pruritus and *Candida albicans* infection (angular stomatitis, intertriginous dermatitis, paronychia, balanitis or vulvitis).

Treatment. In severe cases the patient should be confined to bed and given ample fluids and a light diet. All suspected drugs should be withheld. Local treatment consists of bland, non-sensitising applications. The specific antidote should be used if there is one, for example, dimercaprol (BAL) (p. 35). Antihistamine drugs are helpful for urticarial eruptions. Cyanocobalamin injections 1 000 μg daily, and vitamin supplements by mouth are indicated when a drug-induced nutritional deficiency is likely. Blood transfusion and vitamins C and K may be helpful if there is evidence of damage to the bone marrow (p. 275). Prednisone is indicated in severe erythema multiforme and prednisolone 20 to 40 mg in severe acute conditions, e.g. anaphylactic shock.

When the patient develops sensitivity to a drug the administration of which is very important for his welfare, e.g. PAS, an attempt may be made to desensitise, giving a short course of corticotrophin by i m injection in daily doses of 60, 40, 20, and 10 units on successive days. It may thus only be necessary to interrupt the drug for two days after which it may be possible to continue without ill effect.

THE RELIEF OF ITCHING

The patient should be kept at rest in cool surroundings. A cradle should be placed over the legs, and smooth bedwear should be worn. In acute vesicular eczema wet dressings and lotions are best, such as isosmotic sodium chloride solution; or oily lotion of calamine, BPC.

A diluted steroid application (betamethasone valerate 0·01 per cent, fluocinolone acetonide 0·0025 per cent or triamcinolone acetonide 0·01 per cent) helps to minimise the inflammatory process and relieves smarting, discomfort and itching.

Adequate sedation should be given with phenobarbitone 30 to 60 mg or promethazine hydrochloride (Phenergan) 10 to 25 mg twice a day, and sometimes an additional 50 mg at night.

In itching of dermal or of combined dermal and epidermal origin (urticaria, erythema multiforme, prurigo), Calamine Lotion BP is useful. Topical steroids may relieve prurigo but are relatively ineffective in urticaria and in erythema multiforme. Internally, antihistamine drugs should be given in a dosage just sufficient to control the symptoms, with gradual reduction as these are relieved. In pruritus without obvious skin abnormality relief mainly depends on adequate sedation by mouth. Defatting of the skin is a factor in the elderly especially in winter and when hot baths and bath salts are used excessively. Aqueous cream may be helpful and emulsifying ointment as a substitute for soap in the bath. In severe prurigo with intolerable itching it is justifiable to give prednisone 10 mg twice a day and to reduce the dose slowly.

SOME CONTRAINDICATIONS IN THE TREATMENT OF ACUTE SKIN CONDITIONS

Local applications

1. Ointments which are immiscible with water should not be used in acute cases. They prevent evaporation and macerate the skin, increase itching and encourage the spread of infection. Lotions or powders should be used in acute cases and emulsions or creams in subacute cases.

2. Antiseptic or antibiotic applications should not be used unless infection is clearly present but in discoid eczema clioquinol is often helpful especially when combined with a steroid. Antibiotics should preferably only be used topically under bacteriological guidance but in acute conditions e.g. impetigo or infected dermatitis chlortetracycline ointment is the safest application. For mixed bacterial and *Candida albicans* infections a combination of neomycin, gramicidin and nystatin is useful.

3. It is risky to use sulphonamides and penicillin topically because of the risk of sensitisation.

4. Benzocaine antipruritic applications are very liable to sensitise the skin. The topical use of antihistamine drugs is also fraught with this risk.

5. For secondarily infected fungal infections of the feet soaks of potassium permanganate 1 in 7 500 are useful (4 ml of a 4 per cent solution in 1 200 ml of boiled water. A saturated solution, deep purple in colour, is 5 g/dl. If there is no secondary bacterial

infection, the application of magenta paint at night and 3·0 per cent salicylic acid compound powder in the morning is often effective.

6. Emulsifying ointment is the best base for use in hairy areas, where shake lotions or pastes cause unpleasant matting and are difficult to remove.

7. The use of 'blunderbuss' prescriptions should be avoided. They increase the risk of sensitisation and if this occurs it is difficult to find which ingredient is responsible.

8. Mercurials or dithranol should not be used in subacute or extensive psoriasis or on flexural lesions as exfoliative dermatitis may follow. When using dithranol care should be taken to ensure that it does not get into the eyes.

9. Ulcers should not be treated with topical corticosteroids as these may extend and deepen them.

A few examples of eczematisation commonly resulting from faulty and perhaps over-vigorous treatment may be helpful:

Cuts and abrasions dressed with acriflavine or parachlormetaxylenol may develop spreading eczema in the vicinity and if the cause is not soon recognised this may become widespread.

The herald spot of pityriasis rosea is sometimes diagnosed as ringworm and treated with a fungicide. If the eruption that follows is interpreted as a spread of an infection and similarly treated, an obstinate eczema may be superimposed on this relatively trivial, self-limited skin disorder.

If hypostatic ulcers are treated with antiseptic or antibiotic applications a localised spread of eczema may suddenly develop and become generalised.

Systemic treatment

1. Unless their use is essential, sulphonamides should not be used systemically if sensitisation has occurred from their previous topical application.

2. Drugs (except antihistamines) should not be given in urticaria and other eruptions suspected of being toxic or allergic in origin.

3. Sufferers from acute dermatoses should be protected from sunlight, heat, humidity, exertion and excitement.

4. Steroid hormones should only be prescribed for systemic use after careful consideration of the contraindications (dyspepsia, peptic ulceration, infections, hypertension and mental instability). In dermatological practice they should be used in acute conditions only when life or vital organs are threatened as in pemphigus, lupus erythematosus, severe erythema multiforme, severe drug reactions,

herpes gestationis and Behçet's syndrome. In the worst forms of prurigo a systemic steroid may have to be used but its withdrawal may subsequently prove difficult. Systemic steroids should not be given in the milder cases.

ACUTE SUNBURN
(For effects on the eyes see p. 458)

This may result from over exposure of a normal person, especially if fair-skinned, or from moderate exposure of someone who has been sensitised to ultraviolet light. This sensitisation may be by various drugs, chloroquine, barbiturates, dipheniramine, gold, chlordiazepoxide, antibiotics and phenothiazines and by surface contact with many substances such as certain plant juices, citrus fruits, dyes (acriflavine and fluorescein), halogenated salicylanilides, bithional or hexachlorophane in soaps or cosmetics, local anaesthetics, phenothiazines, sulphonamides, quinine and Jadit (buclosamide).

Prevention. The emergency of acute sunburn can be prevented by applying substances which protect against ultra-violet light. All are effective for two to four hours but not all are aesthetically acceptable. Substances used are tannic acid, quinine hydrochloride and pyribenzamine, all 5 per cent, and salol 10 per cent in a vanishing cream base. Esters of para-aminobenzoic acid are used as in Spectraban Stiefel which contains 2·5 per cent of isoamyl-p-N dimethylaminobenzoate in lotion form. In Uvistat cream (W. B. Pharmaceuticals) 4 per cent mexenone, a benzophenone derivative is used. Para-Amino benzoic acid, although a sun screen, can cause photosensitivity in some people.

Treatment

Severe sunburn with circulatory collapse calls for treatment as for thermal burns (p. 554). Systemic corticosteroids are needed in severe burns and topical applications or oily calamine lotion in milder ones. The oedema of acute sunburn can be suppressed by Chymoral two tablets every four hours for three doses and then two tablets every six hours. (Each enteric-coated tablet contains 50 000 units of trypsin Armour with Chymotrypsin in the ratio of 6 to 1.) (Burke, 1969.)

Blisters should be opened under aseptic conditions and the raw areas covered with oily calamine lotion. Sedatives may be needed to ensure sleep.

PRICKLY HEAT (Miliaria Rubra)

This disorder is common in the tropics and is sometimes seen in temperate climates as a complication of dermatitis. The onset may be sudden. Relief may be obtained and sweating occur following the inunction of lanolin, ointment of wool alcohols, or Oily Cream BP (Hydrous Ointment). The underclothing should be light and pervious; excessive washing should be avoided, and lotions containing spirit, antiseptics and powders should not be used. Ascorbic acid, up to 1 g daily is reported to bring brisk relief.

CHILBLAINS (Erythema Pernio)

Chilblains are caused by cold and damp acting on those predisposed to them by poor peripheral circulation and insufficient exercise. As a first-aid remedy the affected parts should be cleaned and massaged gently from the periphery with olive oil or Oily Lotion of Calamine, BPC.

ACUTE CONTACT DERMATITIS

From a carefully taken history and the distribution of the eruption, it may be possible to determine the cause and prevent further exposure. Acute dermatitis of the scalp and neck may be caused by the dye paraphenylenediamine used on the hair, in hair nets or in furs. It may also arise from permanent-wave solutions. Acute dermatitis mainly involving the face and neck may be due to air-borne agents, some plants (most commonly *Primula obconica* and chrysanthemum), occupational and other dusts, formalin vapour, and insecticides. It may also arise from hand-transferred substances including nail varnish, hair lacquer, and other cosmetics, medicated soaps, and many substances handled in work and hobbies, including alkalis, glues, photographic chemicals, and procaine. Dermatitis around the eyes may result from the use of eye lotions containing sulphonamides, antibiotics, silver, mercury or atropine. Nurses sensitive to streptomycin usually present with conjunctivitis or dermatitis of the eyelids. Nickel dermatitis often affects the eyelids as well as sites of direct contact with the metal. Lichen simplex also occurs on the eyelids, closely mimicking contact dermatitis. Acute dermatitis of the face and other exposed areas, with light sensitivity, may arise from the topical use of acriflavine, Jadit (buclosamide) p-aminobenzoic acid derivatives, penicillin, phenothiazines, quinine, sulphonamides or tar. Many internally administered drugs may also cause light sensitivity: they include sulphonamides, antibiotics, barbiturates, gold, phenothiazines, chloroquine and diphenhydramine. Some drugs including griseofulvin, streptomycin, sulphonamides, tetracycline and thiouracil have been reported to cause lupus erythematosus-like conditions. Barbiturates, griseofulvin, sulphonamides and phenothiazines may activate or exacerbate porphyria. Dermatitis of the hands and forearms arises from innumerable occupational irritants and sensitisers. Dermatitis from rubber gloves and rubber in garments is common. Dermatitis elsewhere on the body may follow the use or abuse of antiseptics and parasiticides in soaps, lotions and ointments, and counter-irritants. Dermatitis from a heavy irritant dust such as cement may particularly affect the collar line, the waist and the legs at the sock level. Genital dermatitis sometimes arises from quinine or mercurial contraceptives, rubber condoms or from antiseptics. Dermatitis of the feet sometimes develops from dyes, glues or leather in footwear or from antifungal remedies. Some of the commoner outwardly applied remedies causing eczematous reactions are antihistamines, local anaesthetics of the benzocaine group, antibiotics (particularly neomycin, soframycin, bacitracin, penicillin and streptomycin), antiseptics of the hydroxyquinoline group and also parabens and lanolin in vehicles.

Treatment. After removing the cause, one of the applications for the relief of itching (p. 540) should be employed. For cleaning the skin olive oil should replace soap and water during the acute phase. When the condition is resolving a non-scented superfatted soap should be used with tepid water. The patient should rest and avoid exposure to sunlight, cold winds and the warmth of fires.

A steroid ointment or lotion is indicated for acute eczematous dermatitis but not for application to skin damaged by a primary irritant, for example, an alkali. In primary irritant dermatitis oily calamine lotion or Lassar's paste is useful and in defatting eczema aqueous cream or emulsifying ointment. If secondary infection is present, the appropriate antibiotic should be applied according to the bacteriological findings. It is justifiable in infected eczematous conditions to apply a steroid-antibiotic or steroid-clioquinol mixture.

Adequate sedation is usually obtained with promethazine hydrochloride (Phenergan) 25 mg twice a day.

ACUTE WIDESPREAD SENSITISATION DERMATITIS

This condition, fortunately becoming rarer, may occur after the topical use of some antibiotics, antihistamines, benzocaine local anaesthetics, parachlormetaxylenol in Dettol or even from lanolin. Paraphenylenediamine in hair dye may cause it. In the past topically applied sulphonamides, penicillin, ammoniated mercury and flavine were often responsible.

Generalised eczema may also originate from secondarily infected or over-treated hypostatic ulcers and eczema, or from the use of occlusive dressings, e.g. paraffin ointment (autolytic eczema).

The same local principles apply as for treatment of acute contact dermatitis. A diluted steroid cream (e.g. one part of betamethasone valerate cream with nine parts of aqueous cream) should be applied.

Severe Erythema Multiforme
(Stevens-Johnson syndrome)

This severe and febrile form of erythema multiforme affects the skin, eyes, mouth and ano-genital region causing bullae and haemorrhagic crusts. Corneal ulceration, anterior uveitis or panophthalmitis may occur and also bronchitis, pneumonia, otitis media, polyarthritis and renal involvement with haematuria. Untreated, the mortality is 5 to 25 per cent. Treatment consists of bed rest with good nursing; prednisone 30 to 60 mg daily reducing gradually over two to four weeks and a systematic antibiotic to control any secondary infection.

TOXIC EPIDERMAL NECROLYSIS

This condition, sometimes called Lyell's or the ' scalded skin ' syndrome develops as an extensive erythema proceeding to the formation of flaccid bullae and sodden epidermal necrosis which strips off in sheets and so resembles extensive scalding. Only the hair-bearing areas escape. Healing occurs within two weeks without scarring but there may be recurrence. There is a 25 per cent mortality rate and the condition is particularly serious in infants. Cases have followed infections such as measles or even impetigo and drugs such as phenytoin sodium, sulphonamides, penicillin, phenylbutazone, phenolphthalein and hydantoin. It has followed radiotherapy. Sometimes no cause can be found. Birke et al. (1971) recommend plasma, Ringer-lactate and dextrose 5 g/dl, five to six litres daily for an adult and cortisone and ACTH by infusion: no local treatment is indicated for the exposed skin lesions but the provision on a specially designed bed of warm, dry air at 40°C with relative humidity of 20 per cent at a flow rate of about two litres per minute.

ACUTE URTICARIA

Acute urticaria most commonly arises from gastrointestinal allergens: food (especially shell-fish, strawberries, wheat, eggs, milk, chocolate), drugs and sera, or from insect bites. Inhaled allergens sometimes cause it. The cause may be obvious and easily removed. An emotional upset can lower the threshold of response to an allergen. If a gastro-intestinal cause is suspected, a dose of 30 ml of Mixture of Magnesium Sulphate BPC may help.

The choice of an antihistamine drug depends to some extent on the preferences of the prescriber. Individual patients may respond better to one than to another and so it is well to have choices in mind. Chlorpheniramine maleate (Piriton) is useful in a dose of 4 mg three times a day, raised if necessary to 8 mg three times a day. Promethazine hydrochloride (Phenergan) 25 to 50 mg or triprolidine hydrochloride (Actidil) 5 mg at night usually ensures adequate sleep. Individual reactions are marked and patients should be warned that their faculties may not be fully alert while under the influence of the drug. It should not be taken before driving a motor vehicle and no alcohol should be taken concurrently. Any other drugs which the patient is taking by mouth, injection or inhalation should be stopped unless essential.

Locally Calamine Lotion BP is suitable. If the lesions are very extensive, or involve the mouth, tongue or throat, 0·1 to 0·5 ml of Adrenaline Injection BP should be given subcutaneously, in a single dose; or by repeated injections of 0·06 ml every minute until the lesions are controlled.

ANGIO-OEDEMA

(Quincke's oedema; Giant urticaria)

Angio-oedema is a form of urticaria in which the lesions are mostly or entirely subcutaneous. There are two varieties: a relatively common allergic form and a rare, very serious, non-allergic, hereditary form. In the allergic form the eyelids, lips and external genitalia are often affected and the tongue, oropharynx or larynx may also be involved. The non-itchy swellings appear suddenly, distorting the features.

Treatment. This is as described above for urticaria. If the larynx is affected adrenaline is the drug of choice, usually given subcutaneously or, if there is circulatory collapse from shock, i m or i v, in which case noradrenaline is preferable as it avoids dangerous side effects on the heart. For recurrent attacks the patient may either be taught to inject adrenaline or instructed to use isoprenaline or ephedrine sublingually at the same time taking a large dose of a rapidly absorbed antihistamine orally (chlorpheniramine 8-12 mg). Occasionally a permanent tracheostomy is needed to make the patient safe.

In the **non-allergic hereditary form** (called hereditary angio-edema (HAE) in USA), which is very serious but, fortunately rare, the inheritance is as an autosomal dominant. It is not caused by the release of histamine but by a deficiency of the serum inhibitor (C/I esterase) of the first component of complement (complement being involved in the production of the oedema). It often starts in childhood. There is nausea, vomiting or diarrhoea and colicky abdominal pain but no accompanying urticaria. Lesions may be caused by local trauma such as dental extractions and also by pressure, physical or psychological stress or infections. In the past 20 per cent of patients have died from it before reaching middle age.

Treatment. In attacks tranfusion of fresh-frozen normal plasma (from Regional Blood Transfusion Centres, p. 802) is indicated but carries with it the danger of causing serum hepatitis or of bringing about temporary exacerbation before improvement occurs by supplying more substrate for the C/I esterase to work upon. Prophylaxis is by the administration of the anti-fibrinolytic agent E-amino caproic acid (EACA) 0·1 g per Kg body weight daily (Champion and Lachmann, 1969). This substance reduces the incidence and severity of attacks by reducing the drain on the already short supply of C/I esterase (see p. 285).

ACUTE INFECTIONS

Bullous Impetigo of the Newborn

(*Pemphigus neonatorum*)

This *staphylococcus pyogenes* infection of the skin of the newborn is usually acquired from a medical, nursing or other nasal carrier of pathogenic staphylococci. It is one of the most dreaded infections in nurseries, the mortality being as high as 10 per cent depending on the virulence of the strain of organisms. The skin of the newborn is highly susceptible to superficial invasion by staphylococci. Large bullae on the face, body and limbs contain clear or purulent fluid. It is probable that transmission from one infant to another is by the hands of attendants more often than by the airborne route. Virulent strains may cause lung abscesses, pneumonia or osteomyelitis. Premature and undernourished infants are particularly susceptible and especially males.

Treatment. A systemic antibiotic in full dosage is advisable in addition to a topical antibiotic, the choice depending on culture and sensitivity of the organisms. If it is considered too urgent to await bacteriological findings a tetracycline is probably the best choice.

Echthyma gangrenosum of the newborn

This presents as a spreading erythema from the umbilicus with an offensive bluish green discharge caused by infection with *Pseudomonas aeruginosa*. Scattered pustules may also develop proceeding to necrosis and ulceration. Treatment is by gentamicin or polymyxin topically and, if there is no rapid response by oral demethylchlortetracycline (Ledermycin) and colistin by injection.

Infected pompholyx and infected epidermophytosis

Vesicular eruptions about the hands and feet often become secondarily infected, causing local pyoderma, lymphangitis, lymphadenitis, abscess or cellulitis (erysipelas). The patient should rest, with the affected part elevated. If the infection is superficial, purulent bullae should be incised and drained, and the affected part soaked for 10 minutes twice a day in a solution of potassium permanganate 1 in 7 500 (p. 541) and then dressed with the most suitable antibiotic, depending on the bacteriological findings. In the presence of lymphangitis and lymphadenitis, the affected part should be elevated, and the patient should receive either i m injections of procaine penicillin 300 000 units daily until the condition has subsided, or a course of sulphadimidine (Sulphamezathine) or tetracycline.

Boils on the nose and lip

Boils about the nose need special care, owing to the danger of spread of infection through the superficial and deep venous anastomoses. All boils in this area should be treated with the utmost respect and the sufferer kept in bed and strongly warned against the risk of manipulation. Pledgets of wool soaked in hot saline may be gently applied. The area should be immobilised as far as possible, talking minimised, and the patient fed with liquids. All general measures must be employed to encourage resolution, including penicillin, tetracycline, or some other suitable antibiotic. When the boil starts to discharge, frequent applications of warm hypertonic saline should be made without squeezing or pressure.

Anthrax (N.B. Notifiable)

Being rare this disease may be easily missed but it should be thought of if a worker in the bone and hide trade develops a skin lesion. (Some Regional Health Authorities keep a register of industrial premises in which there is an anthrax risk.) Laboratory workers are occasionally infected and should remember that staining does not kill anthrax spores. Exposed areas are affected and lesions are more often single than multiple. An irritable papule rapidly becomes bullous and possibly haemorrhagic with, later, a black crust (malignant pustule.) Around the crust there is erythema and oedema, sometimes with small vesicles. There is relatively slight regional adenitis. Constitutional symptoms may be slight or grave with severe prostration and a mortality risk of 20 per cent. Material from a vesicle or slough should be sent for examination preferably to a designated hospital (p. 812) but treatment should not await the result. Penicillin G should be given i v in a daily dose of 300 000 to 600 000 units for 10 days. The second choice is tetracycline 500 mg every four hours. The part should be immobilised and chlortetracycline ointment applied to the lesion. Anthrax anti-serum is held at certain hospitals (p. 767) but as it causes severe reactions it is doubtful whether it should ever be used in view of the effectiveness of antibiotics. It might be considered for pulmonary anthrax (wool-sorter's disease).

Purpura-fulminans (see pp. 276 and 432) and **Waterhouse-Friderichsen syndrome** (see pp 355 and 438).

Cutaneous diphtheria.

Cutaneous diphtheria is most commonly a complication of nasal diphtheria or of a nasal carrier state, though it may occur by itself. The lesions may be ulcerative, impetiginous, or eczematoid. There is often a blood-stained nasal discharge. Culture and animal virulence tests are necessary but treatment (p. 433) should be started on clinical evidence alone. Locally, the most suitable antibiotic should be applied to clear the associated coccal infection. Three or more consecutive negative skin and nasal swabs should be obtained before the patient is discharged.

ERYSIPELAS

(Streptococcal cellulitis)

This infection of the dermis with virulent strains of *Streptococcus pyogenes* was once more serious than it is today; nevertheless it remains a threat to life particularly in the newborn and the aged. Susceptibility to it is increased by malnutrition, alcoholism, recent infections and dysgammaglobulinaemia. In recurrent attacks the presence of impaired lymphatic drainage is likely or there may be oedema of renal origin. The affected skin is red, swollen and tense, with a well defined spreading edge where some vesicles may be visible. In infants the abdominal skin is mostly affected; in older children the face, scalp or a limb; and in adults a leg is more often affected than the face or an ear. Nephritis, abscesses or septicaemia may develop and, without effective treatment, the mortality in infants is 40 per cent. Treatment is by penicillin for a week and, in recurrent cases, with a smaller maintenance dose, Tetracycline is the second choice of antibiotic.

Erysipeloid

This is usually an occupational disease of food handlers and is caused by the introduction, through a prick or abrasion, of the organism of swine erysipelas (*Erysipelothrix rhusiopathiae*). A finger or thumb, a hand or a forearm is usually affected. Three days after the prick a hot dusky red swelling develops around the site of injury. The well demarcated border may be vesicular. Fever and malaise are unusual but there is a rare form in which systemic erysipeloid develops soon after the primary lesion with widespread bullae and red plaques. Treatment is with penicillin or tetracycline systemically.

HERPES SIMPLEX

A 5 per cent solution of idoxuridine in dimethyl sulphoxide (DMSO) (Herpid, WB Pharmaceuticals) penetrates the skin deeply within minutes of application and is effective in the early stages of herpes simplex. It should be applied to the lesions with a soft brush four times a day for up to four days. More prolonged use may macerate the skin. Rapid regression usually follows. DMSO should never be applied to the conjunctiva as it is toxic to the lens. Idoxuridine eye drops (100 mg/dl aqueous solution) should be used if need be.

For genital herpes simplex and herpetic whitlows greater concentrations are needed as the virus is more resistant in these situations. For herpetic whitlow the digit should be splinted and the arm slung in an elevated position. The use of corticosteroids both topically and systemically is strongly contra-indicated in herpes simplex.

ECZEMA HERPETICUM: ECZEMA VACCINATUM

Special hazards face the eczema-prurigo patient. Infants suffering from eczema are specially susceptible to viral infections and sudden death may occur, apparently from overwhelming general infection. the skin being the portal of entry. After exposure to herpes simplex an eczematous infant may develop a generalised form of herpes with a considerable death rate. Vaccination of an eczematous person may be followed by generalised vaccinia. Both these conditions are included in the term Kaposi's varicelliform eruption. Because of these risks it is inadvisable to admit to hospital children who are suffering from eczema, particularly if under one year of age. The contact of eczematous children with recently vaccinated individuals or with those suffering from herpes simplex, zoster or varicella should be avoided. Vaccination of such children should be deferred until the skin has been clear for at least a year. Any superimposed infection in an eczematous child should be treated topically with the appropriate antibiotic. Cubicle nursing is desirable. Cytarabine (Cytosar, Upjohn) may be used in eczema herpeticum giving by rapid i v injection a single daily dose of 2 mg/kg for up to 5 days. Cytarabine is a desperate remedy and potentially very toxic. So it should only be used when life is threatened and preferably on the advice of a physician experienced in cancer chemotherapy.

Herpes Zoster

Zoster lesions of the skin, if treated early, respond well to Herpid (see Herpes simplex) which shortens the duration of an attack and lessens post-herpetic pain and scarring and also the risk of secondary infection. It is a major advance in therapy. Cytarabine (see above) is indicated in generalised zoster, zoster encephalitis and zoster involving the naso-ciliary branch of the ophthalmic nerve.

Gasserian herpes zoster when it affects the first branch of the trigeminal nerve is often of the severe gangrenous type. The *side* of the nose is supplied by the naso-ciliary nerve after the branches to the globe have been given off and if the ala nasi is involved then the risk of corneal zoster is greater. The common eye lesions are keratitis and iritis but episcleritis, paralysis of the external ocular muscles and retro-bulbar neuritis may also occur (herpes zoster opthalmicus). The first sign of inflammation of the globe (usually within a week of the onset of skin lesions) is ciliary congestion.

Atropine Sulphate Eye-drops BPC 1 per cent should be instilled twice daily and Predsol Eye-drops (prednisolone sodium phosphate 0·5 per cent) hourly, preferably in hospital. The skin of the forehead and lids should be treated by application of gauze soaked in 5 per cent idoxuridine in dimethyl sulphoxide (DMSO) (Herpid). This should be resoaked frequently but not removed for up to a week. DMSO must never be used in the eye as it is toxic to the lens. Failing Herpid, idoxuridine eye-drops and wet dressings such as slightly hypertonic saline or potassium permanganate solution 1 in 7 500 (p. 541) are best. The sloughs take several days to separate and care must be taken to prevent any superimposed infection or retention of discharges under occlusive dressings.

For the non-gangrenous areas, Calamine Lotion BP is suitable. Collodion should only be used on unbroken lesions in mild cases. When the sloughs have separated a sterile yellow soft paraffin 2 mm mesh Tulle-gras dressing will be found most comfortable. Chlortetracycline ointment, 3 per cent, is useful for preventing or controlling secondary infection. For the relief of pain paracetamol with codeine may be adequate. Promazine (Sparine) 25 mg three times a day is also useful but in severe cases it is sometimes necessary to give heroin (diamorphine) 10 mg sublingually or even morphine parenterally in order to obtain a night's rest.

URGENT SKIN DISEASES ASSOCIATED WITH PREGNANCY

Herpes gestationis

Herpes gestationis usually appears in the third trimester but it may start earlier or may only develop in the puerperium. It is an intensely, itchy, polycyclic, erythematous eruption with bullae. The distal parts of the limbs may be especially affected, or the eruption may be widespread on the trunk and limbs. It is not thought to be a virus infection but is more akin to dermatitis herpetiformis.

Sufficient prednisone should be taken to give 75 per cent relief; this may be up to 30 mg a day. It is advisable to tail off this dosage before delivery. Good results have also been reported from progesterone up to 100 mg daily, later reduced to a maintenance dose of between 25 to 50 mg daily. The patient should not take iodides or bromides in any form. Oestrogens may cause an exacerbation. Local treatment consists of the application of Calamine Lotion BP.

Impetigo herpetiformis (Hebra)

This is a very rare condition usually occurring during the last trimester of pregnancy. Irregular polycyclic clusters of small pustules are present mostly in the flexures, each lesion being surrounded by an inflammatory halo. Ulcers may appear in the mouth. The lesions are sterile. There is grave constitutional disturbance with fever, vomiting, diarrhoea, nephritis and splenomegaly. Hypoparathyroidism is often present. Tetany may develop. The condition is sometimes fatal.

Calcium in large doses and dihydrotachysterol 1.25 mg (1 ml) (p. 369) daily are said to help the condition. An antibiotic, e.g. tetracycline, should be given by mouth and applied topically for any secondary infection. Corticosteroids are also justified. Gonadotropic hormone may prevent or lessen the severity of a recurrence.

Induction of labour may be necessary. Therapeutic abortion in any future pregnancy should be considered.

BRIAN RUSSELL

REFERENCES

BIRKE, G., LILJEDAHL, S-O., RAJKA, G. (1971). Lyell's syndrome. Metabolic and clinical results of a new form of treatment. *Acta-Dermato-Venereologica*, **51**, 199.
BURKE, D. T. (1969). On sunburn: an orally effective cure. *Medical Journal of Australia*, **1**, 1186.
CHAMPION, R. H. & LACHMANN, P. J. (1969). Hereditary angioedema treated with E-amino caproic acid. *British Journal of Dermatology*, **81**, 763.
JUEL-JENSEN, B. E. (1973). Herpes simplex and zoster. *British Medical Journal*, **1**, 406.
PICKERING, R. J., GOOD, R. A., KELLY, J. R. & GEWURZ, H. (1969). Replacement therapy in hereditary angioedema. Successful treatment of two patients with fresh frozen plasma. *Lancet*, **1**, 326.

BURNS

The emergency treatment of burns consists of the prevention of shock, the prevention of infection and damage by mechanical and chemical trauma, and the replacement of areas of full thickness skin destruction at the earliest moment. (For eyelid burns see p. 529.)

Shock

This is the commonest cause of death in untreated large burns and the first complication to be prevented. For first aid treatment the extensively burned patient should be wrapped in a clean sheet, kept warm with blankets if necessary, and taken to hospital immediately. Victims overcome by smoke, particularly black smoke, may also have CO poisoning. An HbCO estimation may indicate oxygen therapy (see p. 740). The supreme need is early and adequate transfusion, and local treatment takes second place. One effective dose of morphine may be given i v if the patient complains of pain but extensive deep burns are not usually painful. Oral fluids may be given to relieve thirst but should be limited to about 50 ml an hour for children and 100 ml an hour for adults to discourage vomiting. Chilled isotonic saline-bicarbonate solution should be the principal one given by mouth once the patient reaches hospital. This may be made by adding 5 g (1 level teaspoon) NaCl and 4 g (1 level teaspoon) $NaHCO_3$ to one litre of cold water.

The treatment of patients who will become shocked if not given i v fluid is made easier by the rough relationship which exists between the area burned and the amount of plasma lost. A child with more than 10 per cent of the body surface burned, or an adult with more than 15 per cent, excluding erythema, will lose sufficient plasma to require resuscitation if clinical shock is to be prevented. The estimation of these areas is made easier by using the 'rule of nines' method (Fig. 25.1) and by using for measurement the area of the patient's outstretched palm and fingers, which is about 1 per cent of his body surface.

Orthodox methods of resuscitation employ plasma or dextran

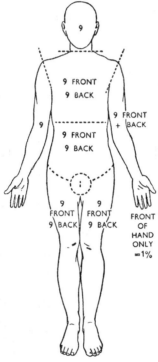

FIG. 25.1

The Rule of Nines

Correction for head and neck and legs in children:
Subtract age in years from 12.
For head and neck *add* result to the head and neck
  figure of 9 per cent.
For legs *subtract* the result from the adult figure of
  36 per cent for the legs.

in saline and sometimes blood, to restore the blood volume to near normal. Increasingly plasma is combined with equal volumes or more of electrolyte solution (Hartmann's solution described in the British Pharmacopoeia 1968 under the title Compound Sodium

Lactate Injection but better known as Ringer-lactate solution). A similar proprietary solution is Plasma-lyte 148 (Baxter). The body is well able to compensate for some degree of oligaemia but without treatment this may become extreme in two or three hours and be a factor in causing fatal renal damage.

Transfusion should start promptly and not later than 15 minutes after admission to hospital. This means that transfusion equipment

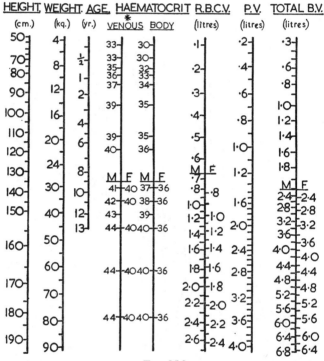

Fig. 25.2

Average normal values for plasma volume, red cell volume, and blood volume for different ages, weights, and heights. * The figures for venous haematocrit have been corrected for trapped plasma. The samples were centrifuged for 55 minutes at 3 000 r.p.m.

By courtesy of Dr E. Topley and the Editor of the Journal of Clinical Pathology.

must be ready and sterile wherever burns may be admitted. The transfusion should continue as long as there is appreciable loss of plasma, which is usually 24 to 48 hours.

The rate and amount of transfusion should be controlled by the trend of all available information studied as a whole. Outside burns units this means in practice a combination of (1) a surface area formula, (2) changes in haematocrit and (3) certain physical signs.

1. Surface area formula. Adults require 1 to 1·5 litres of colloid or equal volumes of colloid and Ringer-lactate for every 10 per cent of the body surface burned, excluding erythema. Children up to 12 years need a similar infusion equal to the patient's plasma volume (Fig. 25.2) for every 15 per cent burned. These are the amounts for the first 24 hours and half of this should be given in the first eight hours. Burns of more than 25 to 30 per cent of the body surface usually require continuation of the infusion into the second day. The amount for this 24 hour period may have to be about half of that given on the first day.

2. Average normal venous haematocrit figures (corrected for trapped plasma) are available, and vary from 0·36 at 1 year to 0·44 for adult males (Fig. 25.3). Serial haematocrit readings may be obtained every one or two hours using capillary blood from any warm area of skin. It is desirable to return the haematocrit to about the average normal initially, and then perhaps even below

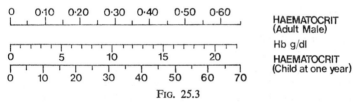

FIG. 25.3

Average normal values for venous haematocrit corrected for trapped plasma. (Modified from Veall and Mollison, 1950. *Lancet* 2, 792.)

normal if this seems necessary to correct clinical shock or to obtain an adequate urine output. A rising haematocrit indicates a falling blood volume, but a normal haematocrit does not mean a normal blood volume as losses up to 40 per cent of the red cell volume occur in 20 to 50 per cent burns in the shock period.

3. Pallor, thirst, a cold nose and forehead and apathy often indicate inadequate colloid replacement. Restlessness is a sign of hypoxia which may be due to inhaled smoke or carboxyhaemo-globinaemia sometimes superimposed on a pre-existent anaemia. Oliguria is commonly found, but the hourly urine output should be kept at over 30 ml for adults and 20 ml for children by adequate transfusion. Greater outputs than 75 ml in an adult and 50 ml in a child indicate overtransfusion. It should be stressed that it is the *trend* of these guides that should be followed.

In addition to i v therapy to prevent shock about three quarters of the patient's normal fluid intake should be given by mouth as chilled isosmotic saline-bicarbonate solution (Na 133 m mol/l; Cl 85 mmol/l; HCO_3 48 mmol/l). This amount (about 60 ml for a child and 120 ml for an adult) is taken quite well by burned patients but if vomiting occurs it should be added to the infusion as Ringer-lactate or Plasma-lyte 148 (Baxter).

Infection

Ninety per cent of recently burned patients arriving at a burn unit had no pathogenic organisms on the burned surface. In other words, *a new burn is a clean wound,* but one which is especially liable to infection because of its large area. Bacterial contamination may result from direct contact with hands and clothes, or by airborne spread from mouths and noses.

To prevent this complication, first aid treatment should afford immediate cover for the burn with a sterile or freshly laundered cloth until the lesion can be examined by the surgeon to determine its depth. It should then be properly dressed or grafted. Prophylactic systemic antibiotic cover for one week to prevent tetanus and colonisation with Group A haemolytic streptococci is advisable (e.g. oral erythromycin or flucloxacillin six-hourly).

There are at present two principal local treatments, the *closed* and the *exposure* methods. Choice should be made between these two by considering which method can be carried out most efficiently for the particular burn, patient, and environment. The *closed* method aims at covering the clean wound with an efficient antibacterial barrier and renewing it every day or two. This may be a cream or tulle gras impregnated with antibiotic or chemotherapeutic agent e.g. silver nitrate 0·5 per cent and chlorhexidine 0·2 per cent in cream, or one per cent silver sulphadiazine cream. The *exposure* method is based on the principle that since it is difficult to prevent bacterial colonisation completely with a dressing, an alternative is to secure drying of the burned surface by exposure. Bacterial growth will then be limited by the dry and cool environment and exposure to light. Success with the *closed* method depends largely on sufficient dry wool to prevent the exudate soaking through; the *exposure* method depends partly on adequate immobilisation to prevent cracking of the eschar. The closed method is of universal application except for burns of the face, buttocks and genitalia, and in hot climates; the *exposure* method is an in-patient treatment especially valuable where closed dressings are difficult and for burns of one side of the trunk only. Neither method requires an anaesthetic. It is important to keep the exposed patient warm, preferably in an environment of 32° C and 20 to 30 per cent humidity.

Recently there has been a return to treatment with silver nitrate compresses (0·5 per cent in distilled water) (Moyer *et al.,* 1965). The compress should consist of about 10 layers of sterile gauze soaked in silver nitrate and it should be resoaked every two hours by pouring on more warmed silver nitrate solution to keep it wet. The dressings should be changed daily. Severe staining of bed-clothes and furniture is inevitable, but the treatment is most effective in preventing colonisation of the burns with *Ps. aeruginosa* and, to a lesser extent, *Proteus* species. Patients treated in this way require a daily electrolyte supplement by mouth related to the size of the burn and body weight, and the following guide is suggested: sodium chloride (10 to 30 g), calcium lactate (4 to 8 g), and potassium glutamate (15 to 22 g). If more than 15 g of salt is given daily in the diet, 30 to 80 ml of molar sodium lactate should also be given by mouth to prevent acidosis. Sulfamylon (Winthrop) (Maphenide) 10 per cent in a water-soluble cream is an alternative application which can be smeared over the burn after a daily bath and left exposed. It stings on application and causes skin sensitivity in 10 per cent of patients but it has prophylactic and therapeutic effect against *Ps. aeruginosa.* Silver sulphadiazine cream 1 per cent offers equal protection against Gram negative infection without staining, stinging or likely skin sensitivity.

Since the presence of dead tissue encourages the growth of organisms, whenever possible a deep burn should be excised and grafted at once as the best method of preventing infection.

Chemical burns

Immediate vigorous washing with water is the emergency treatment for acid and alkali burns. This should be followed by a compress of buffer phosphate solution for 20 minutes. This solution is non-irritant and can be used in the eyes. (Composition: KH_2PO_4, 30 g; Na_2HPO_4 $12H_2O$, 220 g; in 850 ml of water; this makes 1 000 ml of solution.) Failing this the caustic may be neutralised with sodium bicarbonate or vinegar. Further treatment is the same as for thermal burns. Burns by phenol and its derivatives are particularly dangerous; for example, a 7 per cent cresylic acid burn absorbed sufficient chemical to cause fatal renal failure although it was only a red partial skin loss burn. Phenol should only be washed off the skin with water as a last resort because phenol is absorbed more easily when diluted. It should be wiped off the skin with gauze or cotton wool soaked in glycerine, methylated spirit or polyethylene glycol. Emergency surgical excision may be life saving by reducing absorption. For hydrofluoric acid burns see p. 466.

Skin grafting

The modern classification of burns is into two categories, partial thickness skin loss which generally heals without scarring from remaining epithelial elements in the burned skin, and full thickness skin loss which heals slowly by contraction of the wound and epithelial cell migration from the edge.

Full thickness burns which are analgesic to pin prick should be grafted as soon as possible to limit infection, fibrosis and scarring, and this can often be started by the end of the third week after removing residual slough. In about a quarter of these deep burns, however, it is possible to shorten the healing time by excision of the burn on the day of injury or soon after with immediate closure of the wound by skin grafting. This procedure is advised for burns of up to 5 per cent of the body surface, provided one can be *certain* that the burn has caused full thickness skin loss.

Some analgesic deep dermal burns which would perhaps heal spontaneously in four to eight weeks with bad scarring can be tangentially excised and grafted three or four days after injury. This gives quicker healing and a better cosmetic appearance and is one of the few important recent advances in burns management. It is important for even small analgesic burns to be assessed by a burns surgeon in the first three days. Blood loss may be considerable with excision unless a tourniquet is used but with adequate blood replacement excisions of 15 to 20 per cent of the body surface are regularly performed in some centres.

The only grafts which take permanently are autografts or homografts from an identical twin. However, some benefit may be obtained by using living skin grafts from human donors or cadavers less than 24 hours old. These homografts are often stored in a refrigerator at 4°C or over liquid nitrogen (minus 196°C). Skin grafts from pigs or dogs (xenografts), usually collected and freeze-dried commercially, are an alternative. Both may be used to limit fluid, protein and evaporative heat loss and to reduce temporarily the size of the open wound and the risk of bacterial invasion.

D. MacG. Jackson

REFERENCES

Artz, C. P. & Moncrief, J. A. *The Treatment of Burns*. Philadelphia : Saunders. 1969.

JACKSON, D. The management of the burned patient. Chapter 31, pp. 676-687, in *A Practical Guide to the Care of the Injured*, by London, P. S. Edinburgh: E. & S. Livingstone. 1967.

MOYER, C. A.. BRENTANO, L., GRAVENS. D. L., MARGRAF, H. W. & MONAFO, W. W. (1965). Treatment of large human burns with 0·5% silver nitrate solution. *Archives of Surgery*, **90**, 812-867.

MUIR, I. F. K. & BARCLAY, T. L. *Burns and their Treatment*. 2nd ed. London: Lloyd-Luke. 1974.

SEVITT, S. *Burns : Pathology and Therapeutic Applications*. London : Butterworth: 1957.

CHAPTER 26

Emergencies during Anaesthesia

MANY emergencies during anaesthesia are preventable being due to failure to appreciate such factors as pre-existing disease, preoperative medication, overdosage of drugs and departure from accepted techniques. Preoperative assessment is, therefore, important. Careful scrutiny of the history may disclose, for example, that the patient is taking a tranquilliser potentially capable of modifying the action of drugs used in anaesthesia. During operation and in the postoperative period, observation of the pulse rate, blood pressure, respiration rate and tidal volume are essential, though more intricate observations such as venous pressure, ECG, arterial pH, $PaCO_2$ and PaO_2 might be required.

EMERGENCIES CONSEQUENT ON A PRE-EXISTING DISEASE

DIABETES

(See also Diabetic Acute Abdomen, pp. 118 and 340. Surgical Operations in Diabetics, p. 349.)

The commonest emergency in diabetics during operation is hypoglycaemia. This may result from long-acting insulin and oral hypoglycaemic agents, especially chlorpropamide whose effect lasts 36 hours (see p. 348). The preoperative management of diabetics is described on p. 348. Hypoglycaemia is recognised by tachycardia, sweating and dilated pupils. Ganglion blocking drugs and high spinal and epidural anaesthesia mask these signs by preventing the outpouring of adrenaline which raises the blood sugar. For this reason, hypotensive techniques are contraindicated in diabetes. The treatment of hypoglycaemia is to give 50 to 100 ml 25 per cent dextrose 25 g/dl i v. Diabetics are prone to vascular degenerative changes and so are liable to myocardial infarction.

CONDITIONS REQUIRING STEROID THERAPY

Patients with Addison's disease, those who have had bilateral adrenalectomy and those who are taking, or who have taken steroids within the last two months (Plumpton *et al.*, 1969) may all respond to the stress of operation by developing adrenal failure with profound hypotension.

Treatment. This is on the lines laid down on p. 354.

PATIENTS WITH CARDIOVASCULAR DISEASE

Prevention of emergencies in these patients calls for careful preoperative assessment of the heart and consideration of any drugs being taken. Operation should be delayed, if possible, for at least three months after a cardiac infarct. Patients who need special care are those with pulmonary hypertension (they are difficult to resuscitate after cardiac arrest), those with heart block and those whose cardiac output is fixed from constrictive pericarditis or aortic stenosis.

Oxygen administration for two minutes should precede the induction of anaesthesia and all anaesthetic agents should be given slowly and in reduced amounts. Thiopentone should not be used in those with a fixed cardiac output. Hypoxia and CO_2 retention should be avoided at all costs for hypoxia causes further damage to a diseased myocardium. They can also, by causing pulmonary hypertension, lead to a reversal of shunts in congenital heart disease. Drugs for hypertension should be continued except propranolol which should be stopped 48 hours before operation. Diuretics should be reduced since by lowering the body potassium they accentuate digoxin arrhythmias and by lowering the plasma volume they decrease the response to vasopressor drugs. The venous, as well as the arterial, pressure should be monitored along with the ECG in patients with cardiovascular disease who undergo surgery. Monitoring should be continued into the post-operative phase and oxygen should be given. (As this may induce respiratory failure in the respiratory cripple (see p. 197) it is safer then to use oxygen in a known percentage, e.g. 28 per cent by a Ventimask (p. 740, Fig. 32.20).

PATIENTS WITH RESPIRATORY DISEASE

Patients with pre-existing disease of the respiratory tract are prone to become emergencies from respiratory obstruction, respiratory depression and prolonged apnoea when submitted to anaesthesia.

Conditions which should be recognised before operation include retrosternal goitre, scars on the neck from burns and malignant disease of the mouth and pharynx. All these are potential causes of respiratory obstruction. In small children, under-development of the lower jaw (micrognathia) can lead to obstruction with the additional hazard of a cleft palate which is often present.

The normal dose of anaesthetic agent becomes an overdose and leads to respiratory depression in the elderly and debilitated and in those suffering from muscular dystrophy, myasthenia gravis, kyphoscoliosis and ankylosing spondylitis, certain neurological diseases, abdominal distension and lung disease (bronchitis, asthma and emphysema). If there is a weakness of the laryngeal muscles (bulbar paralysis) inhalation of secretions and vomit may occur.

The risks are assessed by clinical and radiological investigation, blood gas analysis and respiratory function tests (p. 195). If the forced expiratory volume over one second (FEV 1) divided by the forced vital capacity (FVC) is less than 65 per cent there is significant bronchial obstruction. If the maximum expiratory pressure (MEP) is reduced from the normal 80 mm Hg to 20 mm Hg there is extensive muscle weakness (see Table 8.1, p. 195). Observation of the patient during normal sleep may be helpful; respiratory obstruction may be noted while shallow respiration and a tracheal tug may indicate respiratory depression. Treatment is described on p. 198.

HEPATIC DISEASE

Anaesthetics after hepatitis may cause liver necrosis and so should be avoided if possible for three months after the attack and until liver function tests have been done. There is less risk in cirrhosis and here halothane may be used. Repeated halothane anaesthesia may cause hepatitis and an interval of one month should elapse before it is given again. Hypersensitivity, unexplained fever, eosinophilia and jaundice 5 to 14 days after giving halothane are all contraindications to its further use. Tubarine is bound to globulin and as this is increased in patients with liver disease they may be resistant to this muscle relaxant. Promethazine can safely be used for premedication but morphine and pethidine should be avoided and thiopentone only used in small amounts. As the pseudocholinesterase level may be depressed, the use of suxamethonium may result in prolonged apnoea (p. 569). (Send clotted blood for serum estimation.) Detoxication of local anaesthetic agents may be similarly impaired. The prothrombin level may be low and so techniques likely to cause even minimal trauma, e.g. nasal intubation and nerve blocks are not recommended.

RENAL DISEASE

If renal disease is severe, drugs which are excreted in the urine unchanged, such as gallamine (Flaxedil), decamethonium (Eulissin) and hexamethonium give rise to prolonged paralysis or hypotension.

HAEMORRHAGIC CONDITIONS

When there are defects in the clotting mechanism or when anti-coagulants have been given, subcutaneous and i m injections may produce extensive haematomas. Premedication should be given orally or i v, either directly or into the i v infusion. Nerve blocks and epidural anaesthesia are contraindicated and nasal intubation should be avoided. Patients with sickle cell anaemia or a sickle cell trait may have a crisis if there is hypoxia or hypothermia or if a tourniquet is used.

THE POOR RISK PATIENT

Under this heading we place patients who have myocardial ischaemia and severe sepsis or who have had repeated or extensive operations. We also include those who have suffered blood loss or who have a reduced blood volume from prolonged intestinal obstruction.

A close watch is necessary on blood pressure, pulse rate, venous pressure and ECG, even prior to operation. The central venous pressure (p. 751) is relatively easy to measure by means of a catheter inserted into the external jugular vein (Sykes, 1963). The tubing and manometer are readily available in presterilised disposable packs. The normal pressure range is 6 to 14 cm of water. A pressure less than 6 cm with a falling blood pressure indicates a low circulatory blood volume. Blood should be transfused. If rapid massive transfusion (more than 3 litres an hour) is necessary the blood should be warmed to body temperature to avoid cardiac arrhythmia or arrest. Calcium chloride 0·5 g with each unit (568 ml) of blood is recommended. Bicarbonate may also be necessary to combat the metabolic acidosis (p. 194) which results from inadequate tissue perfusion and the use of stored blood. A rising venous pressure (above 14 cm) and a falling blood pressure indicate cardiac failure. Treatment is to give digoxin, to improve ventilation and to control the resulting metabolic acidosis.

Lillehei *et al.*, (1964) have drawn up a programme of treatment for irreversible shock using vasodilator drugs (see p. 240).

Emergencies consequent on previous medication

The monoamine oxidase inhibitors (MAOI) are the main source of trouble under this heading (see also p. 88). They include iproniazid (Marsalid), isocarboxazid (Marplan), nialamide (Niamid), pargyline (Eutonyl), phenelzine (Nardil), tranylcypromine (Parnate), tranylcypromine with trifluoperazine (Parstelin). These drugs may enhance or potentiate the actions of other drugs such as:

1. Morphine and pethidine causing hypotension and coma.
2. General and local anaesthetic agents.
3. Pressor amines e.g. methylamphetamine (Methedrine) causing hypertension and excitement.
4. Imipramine (Tofranil) causing circulatory collapse.
5. Ganglion blocking drugs and diuretics. They reverse the action of some hypertensive drugs.

All monoamine oxidase inhibitors should be avoided in pregnancy, for at least two weeks prior to surgery and when there is liver disease. If operation becomes necessary in a patient taking a monoamine oxidase inhibitor, the following regime is advisable.

1. Avoid morphine and pethidine for premedication and use instead promethazine 25 mg and atropine 0·4 mg for the average adult.
2. Give thiopentone very slowly and in reduced dosage.
3. Measure the blood pressure frequently.
4. Use one tenth of the usual dose of analgesics for post-operative pain.
5. Avoid the use of vasopressors.

If, despite precautions, hypertension occurs. it should be treated with phentolamine 5 mg i v. Should coma result from morphine or pethidine, give nalorphine 5 to 10 mg i v or naloxone (Narcan) (p. 37). Acidification of the urine increases the excretion of pethidine and is best achieved giving 10 to 20 g of arginine hydrochloride dissolved in 500 ml of dextrose 5 g/dl as an i v drip over three to four hours. Afterwards, acidification can be maintained by giving ammonium chloride 2 g two hourly by mouth. If coma is accompanied by hypotension, then hydrocortisone and a reduced dose of vasopressor should be given.

The tricyclic anti-depressant drugs imipramine (Tofranil), nortriptyline (Aventyl) and amitriptyline (Laroxyl) should not be used with MAOI and pressor amines (Boakes et al., 1973). They have a strong atropine-like action and may precipitate glaucoma.

EMERGENCIES DUE TO PREMEDICATION

The important emergencies caused by premedication are respiratory depression, hypotension and restlessness.

For respiratory depression, inflate the patient's lungs by mouth-to-mouth ventilation (p. 732) or give oxygen by mask and reservoir bag. Nalorphine 5 to 10 mg or preferably naloxone (Narcan) (p. 570) may be needed. Hypotension occurs after morphine, pethidine and phenothiazine derivatives (chlorpromazine—Largactil), and is usually postural. Lay the patient flat and, if necessary, give 5 to 10 mg methylamphetamine (Methedrine) i v. Restlessness with disorientation and hallucinations occurs in the young and the elderly after hyoscine. Sedation or the induction of anaesthesia may be necessary to abolish it.

RESPIRATORY OBSTRUCTION

Respiratory obstruction is recognised by inadequate tidal exchange, excessive abdominal movement, retraction of the chest wall and finally cessation of respiration. Respiration may be noisy (crowsaturation had fallen below 75 per cent. Cyanosis (see p. 192) depends on the presence of not less than 0·7 g/dl of reduced haemoglobin and hence may not be present if the patient is also severely anaemic.

Causes

The commonest cause is falling back of the tongue on the posterior pharyngeal wall. Treatment is to extend the head and to insert a pharyngeal airway. The jaw should be pushed well forward by pressing behind its angle. Excessive and prolonged pressure may damage the facial nerves so that intubation of the trachea may be preferable to maintain a clear airway. To avoid respiratory obstruction in the post-operative period, the patient should be placed on his side so that the tongue does not fall back.

Another cause is laryngeal spasm. This may be due to direct stimulation of the vocal cords by anaesthetic agents such as ether, by foreign material such as saliva, blood and vomit or attempting to intubate under light anaesthesia. Indirect stimulation may result from the painful stimuli of anal and cervical dilatation.

Treatment

This depends on the cause. Debris should be removed from the pharynx, surgical stimuli halted and irritant anaesthetic gases avoided. Oxygen should be administered, the level of anaesthesia deepened and the patient intubated, if necessary, with the aid of a muscle relaxant.

Bronchospasm

Bronchospasm means obstruction in the lower respiratory tract. This may be due to surgical stimulation under light anaesthesia, an asthmatic attack, inhalation of foreign material and an irritable tracheo-bronchial tree, such as is often seen after influenza, morphine and thiopentone.

Bronchospasm may be simulated by obstruction and distortion of the endotracheal tube if it becomes kinked or if its bevel becomes compressed against the tracheal wall or its cuff overdistended so that it overrides the bevel or becomes compressed during surgical manipulation of the neck. The endotracheal tube may enter a bronchus and provoke an attack of wheezing.

Treatment. Bronchospasm is treated by the i v administration of hydrocortisone 100 mg or aminophylline 0·25 to 0·5 g (see p. 196). Faults in the endotracheal tube are corrected by deflating the cuff, altering the position of the tube, or, if necessary, replacing it. Compression of the tube may be avoided by using an armoured one. After intubation, air entry over both lungs should be checked with a stethoscope.

Pre-existing respiratory obstruction

On no account must any patient with respiratory obstruction be given respiratory depressant drugs. If obstruction is severe, a preliminary tracheostomy under local anaesthesia is advisable. If this is impracticable, as in severe throat inflammation, a nasotracheal tube should be passed under local anaesthesia, using cocaine in a dose of 3 mg/kg with a maximum of 200 mg for a 70 kg adult (see p. 61). With the tube *in situ,* anaesthesia is maintained with nitrous oxide, oxygen and halothane. The tube is left in position until recovery from the anaesthetic is complete and the patient wide awake. Children with micrognathia should be anaesthetised by an inhalational technique, avoiding relaxants for intubation.

Note. Oral intubation is normally preferred to nasal intubation except in operations in the mouth. However, in patients with short necks, nasal intubation by the ' blind ' method may be the only technique possible.

RESPIRATORY DEPRESSION

Some degree of respiratory depression is often present under general anaesthesia with the patient breathing spontaneously. It is accentuated by pre-existing respiratory disease and by surgical procedures which interfere with ventilation.

Recognition of the condition may be hampered by the absence of cyanosis because the patient is breathing an oxygen-enriched mixture or by relying on the excursions of the reservoir bag, as an indication of the depth of respiration. It may be detected with a Wright respirometer which measures tidal volume.

Treatment

(For use of drugs for IPPV see p. 17.)

If the patient is still in the theatre, assisted or controlled ventilation via an endotracheal tube should be used. In the postoperative period respiratory depression may occur when the patient is still in the recovery bay or ward. It may be unnoticed until it becomes very marked. Emergency treatment will then call for mouth-to-mouth respiration (p. 732) until a mask, reservoir bag and supply of oxygen can be obtained. The jaw should be held well forward and ventilation continued at the rate of 14 to 20 per minute. The carotid pulse should be felt to confirm that circulation is intact. Endotracheal intubation may become necessary. Treatment must be immediate and only when it is under way should the causes of profound respiratory depression be reviewed. These are considered in the next section on apnoea.

APNOEA

The cause of apnoea is either central (depression of the respiratory centre) or peripheral (from the effects of muscle relaxants). They may be differentiated by stimulation of the ulnar nerve at the elbow; if the muscles of the hand do not contract, the cause is peripheral. Respiration is not a good index of the state of the neuromuscular blockade. The commonest cause of apnoea at the end of an operation is the combined effect of premedication, thiopentone and suxamethonium together with local anaesthesia of the trachea followed by hyperventilation with halothane. Hypocapnia and apnoea readily ensue and may last throughout the operation. This type is amenable to simple measures like moving the endotracheal tube, deflating the cuff, lightening the anaesthesia and even allowing the accumulation of CO_2.

Many other factors contribute to apnoea and they may be grouped as follows:

Pre-existing disease

This includes disease in most systems of the body and especially liver disease (causing low pseudocholinesterase levels and poor detoxication of drugs), kidney disease (impairing excretion of drugs), neuromuscular disorders such as myasthenia gravis (causing excessive response to relaxants and sedatives), endocrine disorders, severe anaemia, electrolyte imbalance, dehydration and metabolic acidosis.

Pre-existing medication with mecamylamine (but not other anti-hypertensive drugs), chlorpromazine (Largactil) and streptomycin also plays a part. Neomycin instilled into the peritoneal cavity has a neuromuscular blocking effect and can cause apnoea. Kanamycin may also potentiate muscle relaxant drugs.

Surgical causes

Under this heading are operations on the posterior fossa of the skull, abdominal operations which lower the vital capacity, pulmonary collapse and blood loss.

Anaesthetic causes

These are chiefly the respiratory depressants (morphine, thiopentone and cyclopropane). On controlled respiration, apnoea may be due to CO_2 lack and spontaneous respiration will not start again until CO_2 is added. Tubocurarine and gallamine must be mentioned specially since their effects may be prolonged in a patient with myasthenia gravis or electrolyte imbalance as well as excessive dosage or impaired excretion. Hypotension may contribute to apnoea. Hypothermia prolongs the action of depolarising relaxants (suxamethonium). Decamethonium and gallamine which are excreted by the kidneys will have an enhanced effect if there is kidney disease. Pseudocholinesterase is low in liver diseases and so this will enhance the effect of suxamethonium as also will local anaesthetics and trimetaphan (Arfonad).

MANAGEMENT OF APNOEA

1. Maintain adequate ventilation.
2. Diagnose the cause—using the nerve stimulator to decide whether it is central or peripheral. Do not give any drugs until the cause is known.
3. If metabolic or respiratory acidosis is suspected, measure the arterial pH, $PaCO_2$, bicarbonate and serum potassium.
4. If apnoea results from an overdose of thiopentone give doxapram (Dopram) $1 \cdot 0$ to $1 \cdot 5$ mg/kg; if morphine or pethidine is the cause give nalorphine (Lethidrone) 5 to 10 mg (nalorphine can itself cause respiratory depression). Naloxone (Narcan) antagonises pentazocine (Fortral) as well as morphine and pethidine but has no effect on non-opioid drugs. Naloxone should be given in a dose of $0 \cdot 1$ to $0 \cdot 2$ mg i v aiming to achieve adequate respiration without loss of analgesia. It acts within five minutes and its effects last for one hour; this dose may be repeated i v or i m.

5. Take the temperature.

6. If the cause is peripheral (due to non-polarising muscle relaxants such as Tubarine or Gallamine), give atropine 1 mg followed by 2·5 to 5·0 mg neostigmine after an interval of five minutes. These drugs should not be used if apnoea results after depolarising relaxants such as suxamethonium. Spontaneous respiration need not be awaited as it will be inadequate and the accompanying CO_2 retention will, in the presence of neostigmine, lead to cardiac arrhythmias.

If apnoea lasting an hour occurs after a 50 mg dose of suxamethonium then low pseudocholinesterase should be suspected. The serum level should be estimated and the *dibucaine number* (DN), the percentage inhibition of pseudocholinesterase by dibucaine (Nupercaine), should be measured. This will show whether the cause is liver damage or an inherited atypical enzyme, resistant to inhibition so that the DN is low. When prolonged, intermittent dosage of suxamethonium is followed by apnoea, it is the breakdown products which are responsible. Suxamethonium apnoea is treated by adequate ventilation and not by drugs.

The cause of apnoea is usually easily determined from the clinical condition of the patient and the course of the anaesthesia. Metabolic and electrolyte disturbances are rare. Metabolic acidosis is rectified by bicarbonate solution (pp. 11 and 727). Correction of a low serum potassium may be hazardous without ECG control (see p. 602), especially in patients who are digitalised. Not more than 20 mmol should be given in an hour.

To avoid the risk of inhaling secretions, no patient even though apparently breathing adequately, should leave the care of the anaesthetist with any signs of paralysis of the laryngeal or pharyngeal muscles.

ASPIRATION OF FOREIGN MATERIAL INTO THE TRACHEO-BRONCHIAL TRACT

(See also p. 601.)

This can occur during induction of anaesthesia, during operation and in the post-operative period. In debilitated and heavily sedated patients it can occur even without anaesthesia. Aspirated material may come from the mouth, tonsils, sinuses and from the stomach and intestinal tract. Food may be vomited, despite adequate precautions, for its passage from the stomach may be retarded by pain and emotion, especially in children. The inhaled material can lead to laryngeal spasm, pulmonary collapse, bronchopneumonia and 'peptic aspiration pneumonia' (Mendelson's syndrome p. 601), lung abscess and reflex cardiac arrest.

Prevention

If there is any doubt about the stomach being empty, intubation with a cuffed endotracheal tube should be performed under local anaesthesia. Measure the amount of local anaesthetic to be used and do not exceed it (4 ml of 2 per cent lignocaine is enough for the average adult) (see p. 62). Anaesthetise the internal laryngeal nerve by using Krause's laryngeal forceps to apply dental mops soaked in anaesthetic solution to the piriform fossae, then spray the tongue and pharynx with the remainder of the solution. Insert the laryngoscope, pass the tube and blow up its cuff. Continue anaesthesia with nitrous oxide, oxygen, halothane and relaxants if necessary.

Under general anaesthesia, two techniques are possible but in each it is imperative to empty the stomach first by oesophageal tube (size 12).

1. After preoxygenation induce anaesthesia by thiopentone and suxamethonium with the patient in the steep head-up position. This may cause hypotension so, in the elderly, substitute cyclopropane for thiopentone. Another danger is that the stomach contents may flood the pharynx before the tube is inserted. Pressure on the cricoid by an assistant may prevent this.

2. Induce by inhalational methods only. Place the patient in the Trendelenburg position and on his side and intubate.

A reliable suction apparatus should always be running during induction of anaesthesia.

Treatment

If aspiration has occurred, place the patient in a head-down position and turn him to one side. Clear obvious debris by hand and the rest by suction. Give oxygen by mask. Intubate when possible continuing with oxygen by endotracheal tube and control ventilation as necessary. Give hydrocortisone hemisuccinate 100 mg i v and repeat if necessary. Some may be given down the endotracheal tube. Give aminophylline 0·25 to 0·5 g i v, and repeat if necessary. Bronchial lavage should be limited to four washings as repeated lavage removes 'surfactant'. Antibiotic cover is advisable. The chest should be X rayed and physiotherapy started.

This account deals mainly with aspiration during induction of anaesthesia. If it occurs after operation and coughing is ineffectual, a nasotracheal tube should be inserted under local anaesthesia by the blind technique and a similar regime carried out.

CARDIOVASCULAR EMERGENCIES
(For cardiac arrest see pp. 724 to 730.)

BRADYCARDIA

Causes and treatment

1. Pulling on abdominal viscera when it is accompanied by hypotension. If it persists after cessation of stimulus give methylamphetamine 5 mg.

2. Halothane, especially if hyoscine has been used for premedication instead of atropine. Reduce the concentration of halothane and give atropine 0·5 to 1·0 mg i v.

3. Repeated doses of suxamethonium. These can also cause arrhythmias and cardiac arrest due to the release of potassium. Give atropine i v.

Patients with muscle disease, recent hemiplegia and burns are specially liable to bradycardia and cardiac arrest after suxamethonium.

TACHYCARDIA

Causes and treatment

1. Blood loss.

2. Atropine, gallamine and ganglion-blocking drugs, e.g. hexamethonium.

3. Adrenaline in the local anaesthetic. The strength, for this purpose, should not exceed 1 in 200 000.

Excess of adrenaline may be secreted during light anaesthesia or if there is CO_2 retention or hypoglycaemia. Treatment is to deepen the level of anaesthesia and ensure adequate ventilation. If tachycardia is very troublesome, the heart may be slowed by propranolol (Inderal) 0·5 to 1·0 mg.

HYPERTENSION

Causes and treatment

Inadequate ventilation or defective absorption of carbon dioxide can cause hypertension. (In the post-operative period hypotension may result.) Pressor amines, if injected, in pre-eclamptics and in patients who have had ergometrine will cause hypertension. Endogenous secretion may arise from a phaeochromocytoma. It will respond to phentolamine 2·5 to 5·0 mg i v. The accompanying tachycardia will respond to propranolol (Inderal) (p. 253).

HYPOTENSION

This results from reduced cardiac output, vasodilatation and diminished blood volume.

Causes and treatment

1. Halothane. This depresses cardiac output and causes peripheral vasodilatation especially in the presence of tubarine (d-tubo-curarine chloride). The concentration of halothane should be reduced and a vasopressor such as metaraminol (Aramine) 0·5 to 2·0 mg given i v.

2. Chlorpromazine (Largactil) and reserpine cause hypotension by depleting the body's stores of noradrenaline.

3. Morphine, pethidine and the rapid injection of thiopentone. Treatment is to give a vasopressor drug.

4. Interference with venous return. This may be by pressure on the inferior vena cava by retractors and packs. The gravid uterus compresses the vena cava when the patient lies flat (supine hypotensive syndrome) even before anaesthesia is induced. Treatment is to place the patient on her side.

5. Removal of a phaeochromocytoma. A noradrenaline drip (see p. 85) should be set up in a concentration of 8 μg per ml.

6. Traction on abdominal viscera.

7. Removal of leg tourniquets. Treatment is to raise the legs.

8. Removal of clamps from major vessels, after resection of the aorta. Treatment is rapid transfusion of warmed blood and the use of bicarbonate (p. 616) and even calcium chloride.

9. Inadequate tissue perfusion with resulting metabolic acidosis (p. 194). Treatment is rapid transfusion and the use of bicarbonate (pp. 616 and 727).

10. Adrenocortical failure (p. 353).

11. Patients with neurological disease (tabes or peripheral neuropathies) have poor circulatory reflexes and develop profound hypotension during anaesthesia. Treatment is to use reduced amounts of anaesthetic agents and to support the circulation with vasopressors.

12. Hypotension may be deliberately induced during anaesthesia by ganglion-blocking drugs. In these patients blood loss must rapidly be replaced as otherwise profound hypotension and cardiac arrest may ensue.

13. Local anaesthesia used for nerve blocks or infiltration or if it is excessive or given inadvertently into a vein. Hypotension, cardiac arrest and convulsions may ensue. Extensive sympathetic paralysis may result if the subarachnoid space is entered unintentionally during epidural anaesthesia—the result being total spinal

anaesthesia, apnoea and coma with dilated pupils. Treatment is to put the patient in the head down position, ventilate him and give vasopressors.

CARDIAC ARRHYTHMIAS

The cardiac arrhythmias of great concern during anaesthesia are ventricular in origin. To detect them, the heart should be monitored continuously by ECG in patients with cardiac disease who undergo anaesthesia. The cause is adrenaline, either secreted in excess under the stimulus of CO_2 retention or light anaesthesia or injected in local anaesthetic. Halothane, trichloroethylene and cyclopropane also play a part since the myocardium is specially sensitive to them in the presence of adrenaline (p. 89). Adrenaline solution should not be used for infiltration in vascular areas when halogen anaesthetics are used.

Treatment

Ventricular arrhythmias may disappear with adequate ventilation to decrease the arterial $PaCO_2$. The arterial PaO_2 should be increased by raising the percentage of oxygen in the inhaled gases to even 100 per cent. Painful stimuli should be avoided. Lignocaine i v up to 50 mg should be tried and if unsuccessful practolol (Eraldin) 5 to 20 mg may be given very slowly. Propranolol is dangerous during a sudden haemorrhage and in asthmatics and in those in cardiac failure and metabolic acidosis. If ventricular fibrillation ensues, external cardiac massage must be started at once as for circulatory arrest (p. 724).

CONVULSIONS

Convulsions during anaesthesia are usually due to an overdose of local anaesthetic. They should be quickly controlled by diazepam (Valium) 5 to 20 mg i v. Alternatively, suxamethonium 50 mg i v should be given and followed by intubation and controlled ventilation. An i v barbiturate should be avoided lest it damage the heart already depressed by anaesthetic. If the patient has been prepared only for local anaesthesia a further emergency may arise from inhalation of gastric contents.

MALIGNANT HYPERPYREXIA

This rare condition may occur during and after operation. It is characterised by severe sustained generalised contraction of the skeletal muscles and may be triggered off by atropine, suxamethonium and halothane. The body temperature rises by $2°C$ per hour. Muscular rigidity may not be present in every case. An effective method of diagnosis is the routine monitoring of body temperature. Death occurs from respiratory and cardiovascular collapse with a high incidence of metabolic acidosis. A careful family history should be taken. Patients with musculo-skeletal abnormalities should be treated with great care. A rise in the level of serum creatine phosphokinase (CPK or CK2.7.3.1.) (Reference value ('Normal' range) 30-170 u/l) may indicate patients liable to develop this condition. Treatment must be rapid by surface or gastric cooling (p. 723). Dehydration and metabolic acidosis must be corrected. Oxygen should be given and CO_2 removed by hyperventilation. Measures may be needed to prevent cerebral oedema (p. 301). Procaine 30 to 40 mg per kg followed by 0·2 per kg per minute and hydrocortisone have been recommended.

ANAESTHESIA IN OBSTETRICS

Regurgitation and vomiting occur readily during labour and if the acid gastric contents are inhaled fatal pulmonary oedema can result (Mendelson's syndrome, p. 601). The general management should be as for anaesthesia in intestinal obstruction. Profound hypotension can complicate anaesthesia late in pregnancy when the uterus presses on the inferior vena cava. Treatment is to try to displace the uterus laterally, to turn the patient on to her side and to give up to 30 mg of ephedrine i v. Allergic responses have been reported with repeated Althesin anaesthesia.

DENTAL ANAESTHESIA

Postural hypotension and syncope may occur with both general and local anaesthesia in the sitting posture. Management is largely by prevention. Many extractions under local anaesthesia should be performed with the patient flat. If general anaesthesia is proposed for a long procedure an endotracheal technique with the patient recumbent is advisable and is possible even for out-patients if there are recovery facilities. Valium (diazepam) up to 20 mg in 2·5 increments i v is a valuable drug for use in difficult extractions. It must be combined with good local anaesthesia. For shorter procedures using i v drugs such as thiopentone, methohexitone (Brietal) or propanidid (Epontal) or inhalational anaesthesia using halothane, the patient should be recumbent with some degree of head-down tilt. The pharynx must be meticulously packed off otherwise blood, pus or a tooth may be inhaled. Should fainting occur in the sitting position let down the back of the chair to lower the head. For cardiac arrest see p. 724.

Entonox

Emergency analgesia is sometimes called for after an accident or to cover a painful procedure. I v opiates all constrict the pupils—a disadvantage in head injury cases. Injected drugs often cause vomiting. Inhalation of a mixture of equal parts of nitrous oxide and oxygen (Entonox, Fig. 4.6) avoids these disadvantages. It is rapid in action and somewhat euphoric in its effects. Provided one is aware of the risk of gas-induced drowsiness passing into unconsciousness from other causes it is a safe emergency analgesic. Repeated administration as for painful dressings is not recommended as it may cause leucopenia. A storage hazard is that low temperature causes separation of the gases which could result in anoxia. Inverting the cylinder a few times avoids this risk.

NEW INTRAVENOUS INDUCTION AGENTS

These are propanidid (Epontal), ketamine (Ketalar) and alphoxalone (Althesin). Propanidid is very short acting as it is destroyed by pseudocholinesterase. Episodes of hypersensitivity have been recorded requiring treatment with i v hydrocortisone. The drug is viscous and has to be given into a large vein but it may be diluted with saline. Ketamine has been recommended for short operations and for procedures such as frequent change of dressings as in burns. It frequently causes unpleasant dreams and recall phenomena which can be lessened by diazepam (Valium) 5 to 10 mg i v. Althesin is a mixture of steroids with anaesthetic properties. Recovery is rapid. Tachycardia may be caused and there has been one report of a convulsion (Uppington, 1973). Allergic responses have been reported with repeated Althesin anaesthesia.

ANAESTHETIC ACCIDENTS

Eyes

The conjunctiva and the cornea may be abraded if the face is covered during operation. The eyes should be kept closed by ' clear tape ' (Johnson) and protected with paraffin gauze. Abrasions should be treated with 0·5 per cent Chloramphenicol Eye-Drops instilled at hourly intervals. Pressure on the eye during hypotensive anaesthesia is thought to be the cause of central retinal thrombosis. Hypotension may also damage the occipital cortex and cause blindness.

Mouth

The mucosa of the gums may be abraded during intubation or the insertion of an airway. Treatment is to apply 5 per cent lignocaine ointment to the affected area. Care should be taken that a dislodged tooth is not inhaled. If it is a permanent tooth in a child, it should be replaced, splinted and the child referred to a dentist for immediate attention.

Accidents from apparatus

Trichloroethylene may come into contact with soda lime in the closed circuit so that dichloracetylene is formed and this can cause cranial nerve damage. Hypoxia can result from oxygen failure. A warning device such as the ' Bosun ' may lead to a false sense of security since it depends on the nitrous oxide which may also become exhausted. The battery used to operate the Bosun light may run down or fail to operate when used with certain ventilators for controlled respiration. An overdose of halothane may be given with vaporisers and even with the supposedly safe Fluotec vaporiser if controlled ventilation is used with low flow rates. Mediastinal emphysema (p. 599) may occur with over-distension of alveoli during positive pressure anaesthesia and also from perforation of the trachea or a bronchus and from brachial plexus block. Thiopentone is dangerous if given into an artery (p. 52) or extravenously when the median nerve may be damaged. (For N_2O frostbite see p. 654).

Pollution in the operating theatre

Halothane vapour inhaled by the theatre staff has been suspected as a cause of abortions, genetic defects and jaundice. This is difficult to prove but it would be wise to see that air changes in operating theatres are not less than 20 per hour. If possible all gases including nitrous oxide should be vented to the outside atmosphere using the Penlon or Enderby valve.

NEONATAL RESUSCITATION
(See also p. 396)

Respiratory depression in the newborn may have many causes for all of which resuscitation must be quick, adequate and atraumatic.

1. Aspirate secretions from the pharynx with a mucus catheter (beware of blowing down it to clear it). This may stimulate respiration.

2. Using a small rubber funnel, insufflate the baby's mouth with oxygen at 2 litres per minute.

3. If there is no response after one minute and especially if the heart is slowing, intubate the infant. The laryngoscope should have the infant Magill blade except in micrognathia when the Seward blade is preferable. The tube (diameter is 3 mm; size 00) is available

presterilised (the Portsmouth Riplex tube size 14 F.G.) is joined by a light weight connection (Rendell Baker) to the Jackson Rees modification of the Ayre's T piece. Insufflation by mask is not recommended as this distends the stomach.

4. Ventilate with oxygen at the rate of 40 per minute and an oxygen flow rate of 3 litres per minute.

5. Aspirate secretions with a sterile plastic catheter (Riplex Portsmouth pattern size 3) down the endotracheal tube. Aspiration should not be too vigorous or prolonged lest air is sucked from the lungs with resulting hypoxia.

6. Aspirate the stomach.

7. If cardiac arrest or bradycardia does not respond to one minute of positive pressure ventilation, perform external cardiac massage, compressing the lower third of the sternum with the index and middle fingers at the rate of 100 to 200 per minute. Interrupt every five seconds to inflate the lungs (p. 732).

8. Correct metabolic acidosis by i v injections of 4 mmol of sodium bicarbonate (p. 727).

9. Prescribe an antibiotic.

If the mother has received large doses of analgesics during labour, she should be given nalorphine 5 to 10 mg or naloxone (Narcan) (p. 570) before delivery. Otherwise it should be withheld and only given if the infant shows respiratory depression. The dose is 0·2 mg into the umbilical vein or i m.

POST-OPERATIVE RESTLESSNESS AND COMA

Restlessness may be caused by inadequate analgesia and by hypoxia of which it may be the only sign. Differentiation is important —for example an analgesic given to a child who is restless from hypoxia after a cleft palate repair might prove fatal. If the cause is clearly pain, an analgesic should be given i m or even i v. Restlessness after halothane may be accompanied by shivering and a fall of body temperature. For confusion in the elderly after operation, use promazine (Sparine) 25 mg by mouth, diazepam (Valium) 10 to 20 mg i m or 5 to 10 mg i v into a large vein or paraldehyde 5 to 10 ml i m from an all glass syringe (p. 755).

The causes of coma and delay in the recovery of consciousness after anaesthesia are many. These may be previous illness: cardiovascular, cerebrovascular, metabolic or failure of renal, hepatic and adrenocortical function. Electrolyte imbalance, especially hypokalaemia, may play a part. Causes closely connected with anaesthesia are hypothermia, hypotensive technique, prolonged anaesthesia, CO_2 retention and a hypoxic episode. Prior administration of drugs, e.g. monoamine oxidase inhibitors (p. 565), must be remembered. The previous history, the course of anaesthesia and a full clinical examination will reveal which of these causes is responsible. At all times during assessment of the cause, care should be taken to see that ventilation and circulation are well maintained.

LEON KAUFMAN

REFERENCES

BOAKES, A. J., LAURENCE, D. R., TEOH, P. C., BARAR, F. S. U., BENEDIKTER, L. T. & PRICHARD, B. N. C. (1973). Interactions between sympathomimetic amines and antidepressant agents in man. *British Medical Journal,* **1,** 311.

ELLIS, F. R. (1973). Malignant hyperpyrexia. *Anaesthesia,* **28,** 245.

ISAACS, H. & BARLOW, M. B. (1973). Malignant hyperpyrexia. *Journal of Neurology, Neurosurgery and Psychiatry,* **36,** 228-243.

LILLEHEI, R. C., LONGERBEAM, J. K., BLOCH, J. H. & MANAX, W. G. (1964). The nature of irreversible shock: experimental and clinical observations. *Annals of Surgery,* **160,** 682.

PLUMPTON, F. S., BESSER, G. M. & COLE, P. V. (1969). Corticosteroid treatment and surgery. *Anaesthesia,* **24,** 3 and 12.

SYKES, M. K. (1963). Venous pressure as a clinical indication of adequacy of transfusion. *Annals of the Royal College of Surgeons,* **38,** 185.

UPPINGTON, J. (1973). Epileptiform convulsion with Althesin. *Anaesthesia,* **28,** 546.

CHAPTER 27

Emergencies Resulting from Ionising Radiations

(Notifiable if of industrial origin, see p. 687.)

Ionising radiations used in medicine

ALL the treatment of any effects of ionising radiations on the body is best carried out in the specialised centres where these radiations are used in the investigation and treatment of disease. The use of these rays in medicine and industry is now so extensive that all medical practitioners should know something of their action and of the hazards associated with their use.

X RAYS. These are electro-magnetic waves similar to wireless, heat, light and ultraviolet waves but of much shorter wavelength. They are produced at potentials of thousands or millions of volts—the higher the energy the more penetrating the rays and the greater the quantity of energy absorbed by the body. Linear accelerators now installed in many radiotherapy centres are examples of ' super· voltage ' X ray machines with energies of 4 to 45 million volts.

GAMMA RAYS. These are similar to X rays and are produced during the disintegration of radioactive elements such as radium which occurs naturally and $cobalt_{60}$, $iodine_{131}$, $caesium_{137}$, $gold_{198}$ and $iridium_{192}$ which are produced artificially in an atomic pile.

NUCLEAR PARTICLES. These are minute particles which may bear an electric charge. They are expelled from the nuclei of atoms during disintegration and are found in the emissions of many radio-active isotopes as well as in cosmic rays and atmospheric radiation.

Sealed and unsealed sources

Alpha particles are identical with the nucleus of helium. Neutrons are nuclear particles without electrical charge and beta particles are negatively charged electrons. All ionising radiations cause injury to living cells by physical ionisation of the molecules in the nucleus —the degree of damage depending upon the quantity of energy absorbed from the beam. Beams of electrons and neutrons are used in radiotherapy while workers in atomic power installations may be exposed accidentally to highly ionising neutron irradiation.

Cells vary in their sensitivity to irradiation—tissues such as the marrow, lymph nodes and gonads are very sensitive while differentiated adult tissues such as muscle and brain are insensitive.

Dividing cells are very sensitive and therefore the basal cells of the skin and mucosae and intestinal epithelium are more sensitive than are the superficial layers of the skin or differentiated adenomas of the bowel. The action of all the rays described is similar but their penetration below the surface of the body depends on their nature and energy. The radiotherapist chooses that agent which will best deliver the correct quantity of radiation to the chosen volume in the chosen time.

While most patients are treated by X or gamma rays applied externally, others may have encapsulated sources of radium, cobalt, caesium or iridium inserted into hollow organs or into the tissues in order to irradiate a small volume to a high dose. When by accident or for therapy or investigation an unsealed isotope is ingested its chemical composition determines the site at which it is concentrated and there it continues to emit radiation for the terms of its physical activity. Radium, for instance, is deposited like calcium in bone and will decay only to half its activity in over 1 600 years during which time it emits highly ionising alpha particles and has long been known to result ultimately in aplasia of the marrow and bone sarcoma. Iodine 131 used in the investigation and treatment of disease of the thyroid and concentrated in that organ has a half-life of only 8-14 days. Extreme care is therefore necessary in the custody of radium and its gaseous derivative radon. These elements are being replaced in clinical use by the physically more stable nucleides already mentioned.

Plutonium is a radioactive element extensively used in the nuclear fuel industry. If particles are ingested, inhaled or absorbed through lacerations they become localised in the lungs, reticulo-endothelial system and bone and remain for years, during which time, as with radium, alpha particles are produced. It should be noted that the tissues of a patient treated by any form of external irradiation, excepting high energy neutrons, are not radioactive but a patient who has absorbed an unsealed radioactive isotope is so since rays from the absorbed isotope in the tissues pass out through the surface of the body. Any object touched may also become temporarily radioactive from contamination with sweat, saliva or excretions, all of which contain the isotope and so may contaminate others by skin contact and subsequent ingestion or inhalation.

GENERAL CONSIDERATIONS

External irradiation

Everything on the earth's surface is continually subjected to a small amount of radiation. This comes from cosmic sources, from the atmosphere and from radioactive rocks. In recent years the quantity of radiation received by man has risen because of its steadily increasing use in medicine and industry. Compared with this, the increased atmospheric pollution and fall out from nuclear tests is slight but it is important since fission products may be inhaled or ingested by man often after incorporation in plants or animals.

Internal irradiation

All animals and plants are subjected to continuous internal irradiation from the radioactive atoms of carbon and other elements of which they are composed. The content of radioactive elements is increased by any factors which increase the quantity present in the atmosphere or on the surface of the earth. In medicine, radioactive isotopes of many different elements are administered in small ' tracer ' quantities in the investigations, or in larger quantities in the treatment, of disease. In addition, minute quantities of unsealed radioactive isotopes are increasingly used in hospital laboratories, research departments and in industry.

Medical use of ionising radiation

The main cause of extra irradiation during recent years is the steadily increasing use of diagnostic radiology. While only a very small dose is received in any one investigation, the effects are cumulative and become important when repeated investigations are made. Larger doses can also be received in the prolonged screening of the patient made possible by modern techniques. The need to restrict these investigations and to confine the radiation to as small a part of the body as possible is now universally accepted. Even small doses are of real importance when repeated investigations are made, even over a number of years, or when the gonads are irradiated or a fetus is exposed *in utero*.

The increasing practice of nuclear medicine and the use of very small quantities of unsealed radioactive isotopes in the investigation of disease also adds to the quantity of radiation to which the population as a whole as well as the patient and personnel are exposed. Here also an unnecessary exposure even to such a small dose should be avoided.

In radiotherapy a much heavier dose of radiation is delivered but the effects on the population as a whole are of much less importance since the patients, because of their age or disease, are usually past child-bearing. While the risk to the patient is slight in comparison with that of the disease to be treated, radiotherapy should still not be used where any equally effective alternative exists.

REACTIONS TO WHOLE BODY IRRADIATION

Single large dose

The dose of irradiation received is measured in rads which are units of energy absorbed. The quantity tolerated by any individual is inversely proportional to the volume irradiated and increases with the length of time over which it is received. For instance, a tumour may be given a dose of 6 000 rads over a period of several weeks with little upset but few would survive 800 rads given to the whole body in a short time. Where a huge dose has been received in a short time, the first effects appear within a few hours and are caused by irradiation of the central nervous system. There is nausea and vomiting with profound mental depression, prostration and sometimes dehydration caused by sweating, diarrhoea and increased urinary output.

Digestive tract injuries

The endothelium of the digestive tract is extremely sensitive to radiation and its injury or destruction results in pain, and diarrhoea causing fluid loss and diminished absorption. Infection from local organisms increases the damage and ulceration may cause the patient's death. Where the patient survives heavy irradiation, severe bowel injury may still result in late obstruction and perforation.

Marrow injury and damage to the reticuloendothelial system

The stem cells are the most radiosensitive and the effect of the irradiation becomes obvious only after the more radioresistant adult cells in the circulating blood have disappeared. After some days, there is a fall in the platelet count with perhaps petechiae and bleeding from lungs or intestine which may prove fatal. There is leucopenia and the resistance to intercurrent infection is diminished as the immune response may be abolished for weeks or months. (This effect is deliberately produced prior to organ transplantation.) Anaemia may be profound, due partly to bleeding and partly to diminished red cell formation. Even after the patient has survived the initial bowel and blood changes, death may occur from marrow failure about a month after irradiation.

Other less serious reactions are:

SKIN EFFECTS. Where a dose of several hundred rads has been received epilation may occur after a few weeks but no very severe reaction is to be expected where a sublethal dose has been received by the whole body.

GONADS. There is a temporary loss of spermatozoa or some interruption of menstruation. Where sterility is not produced there is an increased risk of genetic changes in the next generation.

Prophylaxis

Much radiobiological research is at present directed towards the development of substances which will modify the effects of radiation. No antidote is known which is usefully effective in man against irradiation although certain substances have been found to have some protective action when given *before* irradiation. Because of this inability to counteract the effect of radiation, *prophylaxis is of the greatest importance* and all *unnecessary* radiation, however slight, should be avoided. The *Code of Practice* (p. 594) gives guidance on the dosage of radiation permissible for those regularly exposed and also on the protection of the patient and public from unnecessary irradiation. An EEC directive is also expected.

Treatment

This consists in relieving symptoms, avoiding complications and maintaining life until the natural recovery processes have taken place. Where a large dose has been received, patients should be treated in special centres where they are isolated and protected from infection. This is of greatest importance and they are nursed from the first with reversed barrier nursing precautions. Exertion is avoided and mental rest promoted by sedatives. A light diet is sufficient with copious fluids to correct dehydration. I v fluids may be necessary and steroids are sometimes of value for prostration or shock. No other treatment is necessary at this stage apart from antibiotics for any infection. Byron and Lajtha (1966). have shown in monkeys that the mortality rate can be diminished and intestinal ulceration avoided by sterilising the intestinal tract by antibiotics. In borderline cases, platelet, whole blood or marrow transfusions may tide the patient over until his own marrow function returns, (300 to 40 ml of fresh marrow from a person whose blood characteristics are as similar as possible to those of the patient being injected i v).

LATE RESULT OF A SINGLE LARGE DOSE
OR REPEATED SMALL DOSES

These may be considered as *somatic,* which affect the patient but are not transmitted to the next generation, and *genetic,* where the germ cell is altered and the effect seen only if fertilisation occurs.

Somatic changes

Where the whole body is heavily irradiated shortening of the life span is to be expected in man as in experimental animals. Most changes caused by irradiation neither affect the patient's life span nor are transmitted to children, e.g. the cataract which may result from small doses of irradiation or the skin changes common after radiotherapy. Children's tissues are more sensitive to irradiation than those of adults.

LATE MALIGNANT CHANGES. Malignant change may occur in irradiated tissues—well-known examples being the epithelioma on the hands of many early radiologists after years of exposure to frequent small doses, and the cases of leukaemia and other malignant diseases reported after a single large dose received at Hiroshima and Nagasaki. The incidence of leukaemia also shows a small but significant rise in patients with spondylitis treated by radiotherapy where the risk appears to be directly related to the volume irradiated and dose given. Such dangers, although too slight to contraindicate *necessary* irradiation in the diagnosis or treatment of disease, provide additional reasons for avoiding any unnecessary exposure.

Genetic changes

A very small dose of irradiation, such as may be received during a routine chest X-ray, may, unless special precautions are taken, be sufficient to cause important changes in the germ cells of the ovary or testis. Alteration in the chromosomes in these cells result in genetic mutations which could be transmitted to future generations. Although special precautions are now routinely taken in diagnostic departments to reduce irradiation of the gonads to the minimum, a responsibility rests on both practitioners and specialists to avoid any unnecessary investigation involving irradiation of the abdomen in children or women of child-bearing age.

EFFECTS OF IRRADIATION ON PREGNANT WOMEN AND CHILDREN. The growing cells of the embryo are especially sensitive to radiation and there is danger during the first three months of intrauterine life when malformations are most easily produced, many making the fetus unviable. Although these changes are less common in later pregnancy, the tissues of the fetus and young child are more sensitive to irradiation than are those of adults and there is evidence for the belief that very small doses received in diagnostic procedures when *in utero* or in early childhood is responsible for an increased incidence of leukaemia and other malignant disease. Irradiation of the germ cells in the gonads of the fetus or child can also cause genetic changes affecting the next generation.

Prophylaxis. While the risks are statistically small avoidance of unnecessary irradiation is of the utmost importance as, once received, its effects cannot be prevented. Much can be done to reduce unnecessary irradiation of patients in diagnostic radiological procedures and it is of the utmost importance that practitioners and specialists should cooperate in this with the radiologists since it is they who initiate the investigation involving the patient's exposure to ionising radiation. Special care must be taken when requesting an investigation involving irradiation of the abdomen in children or in young adults and, since the embryo is at its most sensitive before the pregnancy is usually diagnosed, this possibility must be considered in all women of child-bearing age. The Code of Practice lays down that the date of the last menstrual period should be entered on the request form and that it is the responsibility of the clinician to ascertain this. The Code advises that examinations involving radiation of the lower abdomen should be carried out within ten days following the first day of the menstrual period. Only absolutely essential examinations should be made during pregnancy. Mass miniature techniques should not be requested for chest examinations of pregnant women. Ultrasonic methods are replacing diagnostic radiology in the localisation of the placenta.

X ray investigations should never be needlessly repeated and clinicians and radiologists should consult before extensive or repeated investigations are performed in children or young adults. It should be remembered that *any* irradiation of the abdomen will involve the gonads to some extent.

A report on the hazards associated with diagnostic radiological procedures with special reference to their genetic significance to the population as a whole was published by the Adrian Committee (1966) and in this are found numerous technical and clinical recommendations aimed at reducing the dosage received during these procedures. A useful memorandum on the implementation of those recommendations which apply especially to clinicians was drawn up by the Radiation Protection Committee of the British Institute of Radiology (Memorandum, 1964). The Royal College of Radiologists suggests that, when appropriate, pregnancy tests should be carried out before the commencement of a course of radiotherapy or chemotherapy. The principles to be observed in avoiding unnecessary irradiation of any patient during the investigation of disease by diagnostic radiology or by unsealed radioactive isotopes are included in the Code of Practice.

TERMINATION OF PREGNANCY. The question of termination sometimes arises on the grounds of possible fetal malformation when a
patient (usually the mother) has received irradiation to the gonads.
The dose may be a few hundred rads received over a period of a
few weeks during a course of radiotherapy. While such patients
are usually advised not to have children because of the increased
risk of abnormality *there is no absolute indication for termination*
and many normal children have been born to patients whose germ
cells have been irradiated. Expert advice should be sought in every
case. The natural incidence of visible genetic abnormalities is about
15 000 per million live births and a dose of 1 rad might produce
visible genetic defects in another 20 cases per million live births.

LOCALISED HEAVY IRRADIATION

Reactions caused by radiotherapy should be treated primarily
by the radiotherapy department and when they do not appear to
be clearing up satisfactorily, the patient should be referred back
for advice. It must always be remembered, however, that reactions
ascribed to radiotherapy may, in fact, be due to the disease itself
or to such complications as intestinal obstruction etc., which
require further urgent treatment.

In those cases where a small part of the body only is irradiated,
symptoms are due partly to the general reaction and partly to
intense local reactions caused by the high dose of radiation given
to the tumour and surrounding tissues.

GENERAL REACTIONS TO LOCAL IRRADIATION

Fatigue, anorexia, depression, nausea and vomiting are all
common. The severity of the symptoms is greatest when the trunk
is irradiated or when large volumes of tissue are treated. It is
increased by fear and anxiety and poor general condition.

Treatment. General care is of prime importance. *Repeated* reassurance is of great value and, when anxiety is an important
factor, suitable sedatives and tranquillisers are useful. Hypnotics should be given at night to ensure sufficient sleep. An
adequate diet is important and, where there is difficulty in swallowing, a special fluid or soft diet must be provided. Vitamins and iron
are added as required. A fluid intake of 3 litres should be maintained except in those patients where this is contraindicated by
cardiac insufficiency or cerebral oedema. Regular bowel action is
important. Infections should receive appropriate treatment.

Persistent pain may contribute to the general reaction. The *regular* administration of mild analgesics often reduces or makes unnecessary the need for stronger drugs. Nepenthe 1 to 2 ml combined with Disprin 300 to 600 mg is invaluable in many cases with severe pain. Dipipanone (Diconal), physeptone and pethidine and pentazocine (Fortral) are all useful at times. Regular administration of adequate doses of a variety of analgesics at decreasing intervals should be tried before resorting to morphine or heroin in the treatment of advanced disease.

TRUE RADIATION SICKNESS

Some patients are extremely sensitive to radiation and may vomit throughout the treatment, especially in the early part of the day. Pyridoxine 50 to 100 mg is often effective and should be given three times a day, the first tablet being taken in bed before rising. Phenergan, Avomine and other antihistamines and sedatives all have their place, as also does metoclopramide (Maxolon). The choice of drug depends on the nature of the symptoms in each patient. Steroids may be useful in controlling nausea and in producing a feeling of well-being but are best avoided unless indicated by marrow depression.

LOCAL REACTIONS

Skin

Supervoltage therapy. Most treatments by external irradiation are now given with gamma rays from radiocobalt or radiocaesium units or from linear accelerators working at energies of 5 to 35 million volts. Deep X rays produced at much lower energies are, however, still used. In supervoltage treatment, there is little apparent effect on the skin but a marked effect on the subcutaneous tissues and a severe reaction in the region of the tumour where a very high dose is achieved. Dryness and pigmentation of the skin is followed after a few months by pronounced subcutaneous fibrosis. In obese patients, fat necrosis may occur some months after treatment when the whole area may temporarily become red and tender. The healing power is reduced and *surgical incisions through the irradiated area should be avoided.*

Superficial and deep X rays. When these are used, the skin reaction is much more severe and destruction of the epidermis may occur. Erythema develops during the first two weeks and is followed by first dry and then moist desquamation when areas of the dermis are exposed. Treatment is usually discontinued at this point and healing occurs within two or three weeks. Where a larger dose has

20

been given or the tissues are, for some reason, devitalised, delayed healing or even necrosis persisting for months may occur. Bone or cartilage necrosis is much more common with deep X rays than with supervoltage techniques.

Treatment. Throughout treatment the skin is protected from mechanical or chemical trauma. Tight clothing is avoided, no soap is allowed, the area is bathed and dried gently, treated with spirit and dusted with a non-irirtating baby powder. If erythema develops and the spirit stings, the area is bathed in sodium bicarbonate solution (the contents of a 5 ml teaspoonful to 500 ml of boiled water). For dry desquamation, the same treatment is continued or, if the area becomes painful, it is painted with 1 per cent aqueous solution of gentian violet.

In the later stages and after deep X-ray treatments, painting with gentian violet continues until the treatment is completed. Until then any ointment or lotion containing metal should be avoided, since this makes the reaction more severe. Once the irradiation has been completed, the gentian violet dressing may be continued or a bland ointment may be used, applied to the smooth side of a lint dressing. Lanoline, Tulle gras, Carbonet and Melolin non-stick dressings (T. J. Smith and Nephew) are all suitable and if there is infection, penicillin, Achromycin or Betnovate N cream may be useful. Ultralanum (Schering) is useful in tender areas such as the vulva or axilla and Nestosyl of value when there is ulceration and a combination of fungation and reaction. An ointment used in many centres consists of bismuth subnitrate 10 per cent, with 30 per cent each of arachis oil, lanoline and yellow soft paraffin.

Mucous membranes

Changes in the mouth and throat are similar to those occurring in skin with the addition of a yellow fibrinous exudate which covers the denuded surface when desquamation occurs. Such reactions may be very painful especially when they are associated with swelling of the tissues due to growth or infection, with possible obstruction of food or air passages.

Treatment. For pain use Disprin solution as a mouth wash or gargle, viscous lignocaine to swallow and appropriate analgesics and sedatives.

For infection and oedema use appropriate antibiotics with steroids (p. 756). Nystatin is extremely effective where there is infection with monilia.

Inevitable irradiation of the salivary glands makes the saliva thick and sticky while irradiation of the mouth and throat causes dryness, loss of taste and dysphagia. These effects are at best extremely unpleasant and encouragement is needed if an adequate fluid and calorie intake is to continue throughout the treatment. Sleep may be disturbed by discomfort or coughing. Some relief is obtained from mouth washes and sips of sodium bicarbonate (one teaspoonful to a cup of warm water), water and fruit juice. Although taste usually returns within a few months, some dryness of the throat may persist. Where the reaction is severe and the patient's condition does not improve quickly, admission to hospital is necessary. Extreme oedema will sometimes respond to steroids, combined with antibiotics, but in other cases, a tracheostomy is necessary for respiratory obstruction or passage of a Ryle's tube for dysphagia. Nutrition must be maintained by a soft or liquid diet. Complan and Carnation Milk Breakfast Food are useful additions to the diet.

Bowel

External irradiation. The use of modern supervoltage techniques in the treatment of extensive abdominal disease such as uterine or ovarian carcinoma necessarily involves the irradiation of a considerable length of small intestine as well as the pelvic colon and rectum. Erythema and loss of epithelium is caused similar to that occurring in squamous epithelium and late fibrosis diminishes the blood supply and may produce scarring, subacute obstruction or even necrosis of the bowel. Some degree of colic and diarrhoea is inevitable during the second half of these treatments and for a time afterwards and the patient should be kept on a bland, low residue diet with copious fluids until all reaction has subsided. Codeine phosphate 30 to 60 mg up to three times a day, Chalk and Opium Mixture BPC and Kaolin and Morphine Mixture BPC are all useful. Care must be taken to distinguish the condition from subacute or total obstruction.

Intracavitary irradiation. Where radium or other sources have been placed in the uterus or vagina a small area on the anterior rectal wall may receive very heavy irradiation. Local pain is associated with tenesmus, diarrhoea and the passage of mucus and blood. In rare cases ulceration may follow. Treatment is by rest, diet and medication as before with the addition of Predsol retention enemas (Glaxo) once or twice daily. Healing is usually rapid. Where symptoms persist, the patient should be referred back at once to the radiotherapy centre. Again, care must be taken to distinguish the condition from recurrence of the tumour.

Bone marrow

The modern treatment of Hodgkin's disease and other reticuloses may involve the heavy irradiation of the lymphatic glands as well as the liver and spleen. Investigations before treatment include examination of the bone marrow to exclude aplasia or infiltration by disease. The inevitable irradiation of the haemopoietic tissues causes depression of the marrow and a drop in the leucocyte or platelet count calling for suspension of treatment. With previously healthy marrow recovery is rapid and may be accelerated by prednisone 5 to 15 mg or betamethasone 1 to 2 mg three times a day (enteric coated if there is dyspepsia).

Diagnosis must be made between aplasia induced by therapy and that due to marrow infiltration and also from increased destruction of red cells caused by hypersplenism (see p. 721). The first dealt with by suspension of treatment, steroids and the correction of anaemia; the second by a combination of chemotherapy, steroids and blood transfusion. Hypersplenism is treated by splenectomy.

The reactions of haemopoietic tissues to irradiation are similar to those resulting from chemotherapy. Similar bone marrow depression may occur from irradiation of a large volume of tissue in other forms of malignant disease and in ankylosing spondylitis. Severe aplasia or even malignant change (leukaemia) may result in rare cases.

The immunological response is impaired in any patient treated by extensive irradiation or chemotherapy. This effect (deliberately produced in patients receiving organ transplants) renders those suffering from conditions often treated by multiple courses of irradiation or chemotherapy, very susceptible to infection. After this has been controlled by antibiotics on a number of occasions a respiratory fungoid infection becomes not uncommonly a final complication.

LATE RESULTS OF LOCALISED HEAVY IRRADIATION

Changes include permanent epilation, loss of sebaceous and sweat glands, changes in pigmentation, loss of subcutaneous fat, fibrosis in the subcutaneous tissues and telangiectasia. As the power of recovery of the scarred tissues is diminished, slight trauma or infection may later lead to necrosis of bone or cartilage or ulceration of skin and mucous membrane and, in a very small proportion of cases, malignant disease may, after many years, develop in the irradiated tissues. In most cases, post-radiation changes cause no trouble, but in those few where trauma results in necrosis or the appearance of the skin suggests the possibility of later malignant change, the affected area should be widely excised and grafted. When treatment has been by a cobalt unit or by X-rays from a high energy linear accelerator there may be no superficial evidence of irradiation but massive localised fibrosis may develop at depths of two or more centimetres and may simulate tumour formation.

Reactions of malignant disease to chemotherapy

Chemotherapy in malignant disease has progressed from a palliative and controlling role to become curative. At first single agents were used but now pulsed multi-agent therapy has been developed in which several drugs are used simultaneously over a few days. This is followed by an interval of two or three weeks without treatment during which the normal tissues (and to a lesser extent the tumour cells) recover from irradiation. The effect on the normal cells and especially the bone marrow controls the dosage. This is so calculated that its effect is the maximal possible to allow recovery. The drugs are chosen to act at different times in the mitotic cycle. This intensive intermittent treatment injures the neoplastic cells and also the sensitive normal marrow cells. The patient's immunological reaction is also depressed so that he becomes abnormally susceptible to infection just as he would from the same reaction to radiotherapy and chemotherapy before organ transplants.

Intensive chemotherapy has been shown to cure Hodgkin's disease and other reticuloses. It also cures such highly malignant tumours as chorion carcinoma. It is adjuvant to surgery and radiotherapy in the treatment of the malignant diseases which are resistant to combined surgery and radiotherapy and is increasingly used in the treatment of advanced ' solid ' tumours such as carcinoma of the breast, ovary and bronchus and of osteogenic sarcoma and as prophylactic therapy in early breast cancer.

Alternation between the injury produced by chemotherapy and the recovery interval maintains the general and immunological state of the patient who remains, however, on the border of marrow failure with impaired immunological response. The doctor must expect to find his patient responding poorly to any bacterial or fungoid infection and should start appropriate antibiotics and steroids. Admission to hospital for isolation in a reversed barrier nursing unit for treatment for haematopoietic and immunological failure should be considered.

ACCIDENTS INVOLVING RADIOACTIVE SOURCES

The NAIR scheme (National Arrangement for dealing with Incidents involving Radiation) produced by the National Radiation Protection Board covers the procedures for dealing with such accidents. The police, ambulance and fire services personnel are trained to deal with these problems and certain hospitals have been approved for the decontamination of skin and wounds and other treatment of irradiated persons.

Any such accidents in hospitals and industrial premises are controlled by Radiological Protection Advisers (RPA) who should also be called on if isotopes are mislaid or stolen. If necessary, they can be contacted through the police. No action should be taken before the RPA arrives but it is useful to remember that the risk from sealed sources is from external radiation only but from unsealed sources it is from ingestion, inhalation and skin contamination also. Care must be taken, therefore, not to spread the radioactive substances on shoes or clothing. Contaminated clothing, hair and eyes should be washed copiously with water and this should be tested for radioactivity before disposal. All these procedures should be directed by the Radiological Protection Adviser.

PERMISSIBLE EXPOSURE

A *Code of Practice* for the protection of persons against ionising radiations arising from medical and dental use has been issued by the Department of Health and Social Security. It lays down permissible dosage levels and gives guidance on procedures used in diagnostic and therapeutic radiology and on the treatment and management of patients investigated or treated by radioactive isotopes. Similar codes have been devised covering the use of ionising radiation in research and teaching.

The carrying out of the principles laid down in the *Code of Practice* is the responsibility of the governing bodies. These bodies appoint Regional Safety Committees whose constitution is laid down in the code and also a Radiological Protection Adviser who visits the hospitals and reviews the protection measures laid down in consultation with the heads of the departments. Radiological Safety Officers in each department ensure that the safety measures are carried out.

SPECIAL HAZARDS IN THE TREATMENT OF PATIENTS

With unsealed sources

Patients who have received a significant dose of any radioisotope are isolated in hospital until their radioactivity has dropped to a 'safe' level. All levels are laid down in the *Code of Practice* which also details the precautions to be observed including the nursing of the patient and the disposal of the radioactive excretions. Reversed barrier nursing is used and the radioactivity of the patient and surroundings estimated with Geiger counter daily. Excretions and contaminated sheets, dressings, etc., are stored until their radioactivity drops to such a level that they can safely be cleaned or disposed of with other refuse.

Patients whose bodies contain radioactive materials are allowed to return home when the activity has dropped to a certain level—the actual level depends both on the type of transport used (private or public) and the radioactive isotope employed, which may be $Iodine_{131}$, $Yttrium_{90}$, $Gold_{198}$ or $Phosphorus_{32}$. These amounts are based on the consideration of the maximum permissible doses for members of the public. It is the duty of the hospital to inform the family doctor of the dosage level and of the precautions to be observed and the date when they may be discontinued.

Patients are instructed before leaving hospital that they should not play with or nurse young children or share the same bed with a spouse of reproductive age until the activity has fallen to one quarter of the values at the time of discharge. Similarly, patients should not return to work or visit places of entertainment until the activity has fallen to one quarter. With normal standards of hygiene, there is no risk of any serious contaminations of bed linen and the excreta from such patients may be disposed of via the normal drains.

Post-mortems, embalming and cremations

The Code of Practice states that no special precautions are needed for post-mortem examinations outside treatment centres or for the embalming of corpses containing not more than five millicuries of colloidal $Yttrium_{90}$ or $Gold_{198}$; 10 millicuries of $Phosphorus_{32}$ of 15 millicuries of $Iodine_{131}$ or sealed $Yttrium_{90}$ or $Gold_{198}$. Corpses containing greater activities than these should not normally be embalmed or, if there are special reasons for doing so, embalmers should first consult the hospital where the treatment was given (see p. 762). No special precautions are necessary in the direct burial of deceased persons who have received therapeutic or diagnostic doses of isotopes, nor are they necessary for the cremation of corpses containing up to 30 millicuries of $Yttrium_{90}$, $Iodine_{131}$, $Gold_{198}$ or 10 millicuries of $Phosphorus_{32}$. Again, the family doctor will have been informed at the patient's discharge if special precautions are to be observed. If the patient dies before the date when precautions were to be lifted, the doctor should ask advice of the consultant in charge.

MARGARET D. SNELLING.

FOR FURTHER READING

Effects of irradiation

ADRIAN REPORT (1966). *Radiological Hazards to Patients.* London: H.M.S.O.

ALEXANDER, P. (1965). *Atomic Radiation and Life.* Revised ed. London: Penguin.

BACQ, Z. M. & ALEXANDER, P. (1961). *Fundamentals of Radiobiology.* London: Pergamon Press.

BYRON, J. W. & LAJTHA, L. G. (1966). Radio protection in total body irradiated primates. *Br. J. Radiol.* **39**, 382.

MEMORANDUM (1964). On implementation of the second report of the Adrian Committee on radiological hazards to patients. *British Journal of Radiology,* **37**, 485.

Incidence of genetic abnormalities

MEDICAL RESEARCH COUNCIL (1966). *The Assessment of the Possible Radiation Risks to the Population from Environmental Contamination.* London: H.M.S.O.

Permissible exposure and protection to be observed

MINISTRY OF LABOUR (1964). *Code of Practice for the Protection of Persons Exposed to Ionising Radiations in Research and Teaching.* London: H.M.S.O.

The Safe Use of Ionising Radiations. A Handbook for Nurses. London: H.M.S.O. 1965.

Code of Practice for the Protection of Persons Against Ionising Radiations Arising from Medical and Dental Use. London: H.M.S.O. 1972.

Radiological Protection in Universities (1966). The Association of Commonwealth Universities. 36 Gordon Square, London, W.C.1.

MINISTRY OF LABOUR (1961). *Factories (Ionising Radiations) Special Regulations.* London: H.M.S.O.

MINISTRY OF LABOUR (1961). *Factories, The Ionising Radiations (Sealed Sources) Regulations.* London: H.M.S.O.

Recommendations of the International Committee for Radiological Protection

ICRP PUBLICATION 2 (1960). *Permissible Doses of Internal Radiation.*

ICRP PUBLICATION 3 (1960). *Protection against X-rays up to Energies of 3 MeV and Beta- and Gamma-rays from Sealed Sources.*

ICRP PUBLICATION 5 (1965). *Handling and Disposal of Radioactive Materials in Hospitals and Medical Research Establishments.*

ICRP PUBLICATION 8 (1966). *The Evaluation of Risks from Radiation.*

CHAPTER 28

Post-operative Medical Emergencies

THE clinical problem presented by the patient who, within a few hours or days of an operation, becomes acutely ill is often difficult to solve. Correct management can only be learned by experience and here all that is attempted is to collect together the possibilities and to indicate the broad lines of management and treatment. More than one pathological process may be threatening life. The patient is the entity and not the disease and sometimes an intangible factor, his will to recover, will enable him to surmount the crisis. Many postoperative emergencies are within the province of the surgeon and anaesthetist and the physician is only called when something is thought to be wrong ' medically '. The emergency may be directly caused by the operation or the anaesthetic and if it arises within 48 hours of the operation it is wise to discuss it with the anaesthetist and surgeon in order to learn details of what was done and of the anaesthetic technique used. It is important to find out what the patient was like before operation and to make a note of all drugs which were being taken.

The following urgent postoperative complications will be considered.

Chest pain
        Myocardial infarction
        Pulmonary embolism
        Pneumothorax
        Mediastinal emphysema
        Diaphragmatic irritation

Dyspnoea
        Collapse of the lung
        Pulmonary aspiration
        Pleural effusion
        Fat embolism
        Left ventricular failure

Postoperative fluid and electrolyte disturbance
        Potassium depletion
        Potassium excess

Sodium depletion
Water depletion
Hypomagnesaemia

Abdominal pain and back pain

Acute porphyria
Addisonian crisis
Pancreatitis
Pyelonephritis
Diabetic ketosis
Acute dilatation of the stomach
Paralytic ileus

Hypotension and shock

Hypovolaemia
Hyponatraemia
Cardiogenic shock
Septicaemia
Endocrine failure
Postoperative bleeding
Collapse in a patient having corticosteroid therapy

Hypertension

Phaeochromocytoma
Thyrotoxicosis
Fluid overload
Pre-eclampsia

Coma

Diabetic ketosis. Hypoglycaemia
Hypothyroidism
Hepatocellular failure
Electrolyte imbalance

Convulsions

Paresis and Tetany

Hypothermia and pyrexia

Venous thrombosis

CHEST PAIN

Myocardial infarction

Patients with ischaemic heart disease are particularly prone to myocardial infarction either during the operation or immediately afterwards. Predisposing factors include hypotension, hypoxia and the onset of a dysrhythmia during the operation. For management see p. 233.

Pulmonary embolism

This generally occurs three to fourteen days after operation. Other predisposing factors are pregnancy, a low cardiac output state, mitral stenosis and prolonged bed rest. Chest pain may be central or lateral (pleuritic). For further details see p. 241.

Pneumothorax. See also p. 202.

Operations most commonly complicated by pneumothorax are those on the chest or close to the diaphragm, i.e. on the kidneys, spleen or liver. Predisposing factors are the insertion of a central venous pressure line via the subclavian vein (p. 751) and post-operative coughing in a patient with emphysema or a lung cyst. A pneumothorax developing after operation in a patient on a volume-cycled ventilator is a true emergency since tension in it develops very rapidly. The first indication is a rise of airway pressure shown on the pressure gauge of the ventilator followed by tachycardia and cyanosis.

Mediastinal emphysema

Air may enter the mediastinum following thyroidectomy, tonsillectomy and perforation of the oesophagus, stomach or intestine. It may complicate retroperitoneal insufflation of air. There is often a history of coughing or vomiting followed by severe retrosternal pain and dyspnoea. It is generally a benign condition which subsides spontaneously. Occasionally increased mediastinal pressure causes a shocked state with dyspnoea, cyanosis, engorged (often non-pulsatile) neck veins, low volume pulse and low blood pressure. Emphysema may be felt as crepitus in the neck. The apex beat may be impalpable and the area of cardiac dullness absent or diminished. The heart sounds are feeble. Hamman's sign (crunching sounds at the left sternal border synchronous with systole) is present in 60 per cent of cases and is diagnostic as is a chest radiograph (Fig. 28.1). This, because of gas between the diaphragm and the heart shadow, sometimes delineates the upper surface of the central part of the diaphragm (normally not seen). When there is sufficient gas to cause cardiovascular collapse its removal is called for by insertion of a needle through the third or fourth right intercostal space parallel to the deep surface of the sternum. Sometimes there is also a pneumothorax.

Diaphragmatic irritation

One of the difficult postoperative diagnostic problems is that of irritation of the diaphragm causing chest pain referred to the shoulder tip, the upper abdominal wall or the loins. This may be due to infection following renal surgery or leakage (of bile after cholecystectomy or of intestinal contents after operations on the bowel). It is often complicated by lower lobe collapse. A state of shock does not arise when the collapse is segmental. Pulmonary embolism and septicaemia should always be suspected when, in the absence of massive lung collapse, a shocked patient complains of lower pleuritic chest pain.

DYSPNOEA

Collapse of the lung (p. 205)

Atelectasis or partial collapse of the lung usually occurs within the first 24 hours after operation. Contributory factors are pain on coughing and depression of the cough reflex by drugs. There is a sudden rise of temperature and respiratory rate. The patient becomes cyanosed and restless. An increased pulse rate is usual. Localising signs are absent unless the area of collapse is large when there is tracheal deviation towards the side of the lesion associated with diminished chest expansion. Breath sounds are bronchial or absent. X-ray examination of the chest should always be made. A triangular shadow at one base is the collapsed and usually infected lobe. In the early stages vascular markings may be seen crowded together in it. The heart and mediastinum, diaphragm and lung fissures are all pulled toward the collapsed lobe. These traction effects distinguish collapse from consolidation. The narrowed intercostal spaces produce a ' roof tile ' appearance; the rest of the lung is radiolucent from compensatory emphysema.

Treatment. This is with antibiotics and vigorous physiotherapy. Multiple areas of atelectasis in an exhausted patient may call for endotracheal intubation under local anaesthesia. Following intubation the airways can be cleared by bronchial suction and the alveoli expanded by hand ventilation. Should breathing and the blood gases remain unsatisfactory a period of artificial ventilation may be

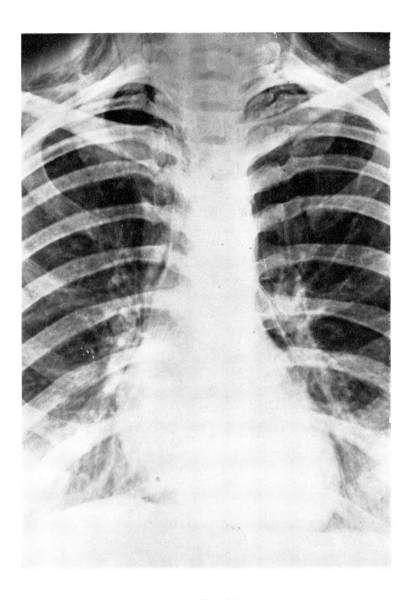

Fig. 28.1
Mediastinal Emphysema.
Note the outline of the mediastinal pleura and the subcutaneous air above
the clavicles. (Courtesy of Dr Cyril Barnes and Blackwell Scientific
Publications Ltd., Oxford.)

Facing p. 600

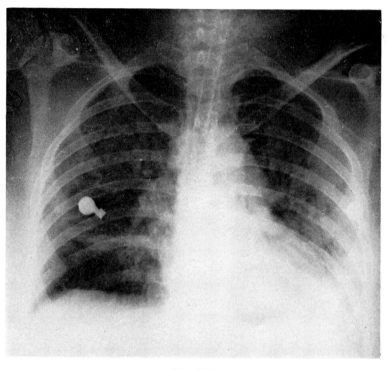

FIG. 28.2
Pulmonary aspiration complicating Caesarean section.
(Mendelson's syndrome.)

necessary. Accumulation of pulmonary secretions is particularly common following chest trauma or surgery. When there is massive collapse bronchoscopy is indicated followed by endotracheal intubation and IPPV. Occasionally collapse of the left lung may follow intubation. It is therefore most important when called to see a cyanosed distressed patient who has been recently intubated, to exclude intubation of the right main bronchus complicated by non-aeration of the left lung.

Pulmonary aspiration

Inhalation of vomit may occur in any debilitated patient whose cough reflex is diminished. It happens most commonly during the induction of anaesthesia in a patient with a full stomach. When it complicates an obstetric procedure it is termed Mendelson's syndrome (p. 571). The anaesthetist generally suspects aspiration but it may be overlooked when the amount aspirated is slight. Following the operation there is an interval of two to five hours when the patient's condition is satisfactory and this is followed by cyanosis, tachypnoea and tachycardia. On examination extensive crepitations (frequently restricted to the right lung) are heard and bronchospasm is common. The blood pressure is often low. X-rays show patchy consolidation (Fig. 28.2). When aspiration seems likely to occur, e.g. when the stomach is not emptied before anaesthesia, a pre-operative dose of antacid is wise. Further measures should be on the lines suggested on p. 572. Intermittent Positive Pressure Ventilation (IPPV) may be needed. A higher concentration than 60 per cent of oxygen should not be used since, assuming no leakage, it would carry the risk of oxygen toxicity. Should the PaO_2 be less than 70 mm Hg (9·3 kPa) using 60 per cent inspired oxygen in a patient with previously normal lungs then the use of Positive End Expiratory Pressure (PEEP) should be considered. This prevents the intra-alveolar pressure from dropping to zero at the end of inspiration and so alveolar collapse is prevented. The amount of PEEP needed varies from 5 to 15 cm of water and depends on the level of PaO_2. The CVP should be monitored since it is important that the dynamic blood volume should be normal before commencing PEEP.

LUNG ABSCESS. An aspiration or obstructive lung abscess sometimes arises in patients with infected gums and after tonsillectomy. An inhaled fragment reaches the most dependent part of the lung in the lying position, i.e. via the posterior branch of the right upper lobe bronchus, and causes an area of atelectasis with subsequent necrosis. Inhaled particles are more likely to reach the right lung because the right main bronchus is more in line with the trachea than the left. Radiographs, including a lateral view, initially show an area of consolidation followed by a rounded shadow with a fluid level in it. Treatment includes postural drainage and antibiotics. Surgery may have to be considered.

Pleural effusion

Postoperative accumulation of fluid in the pleural space may be sufficiently rapid to cause urgent dyspnoea and cyanosis. It usually arises after thoracic surgery but on rare occasions it complicates such procedures as the incorrect insertion of a central venous catheter via the subclavian vein (p. 747). Sometimes following oesophageal resection the anastomosis leaks and fluid may be regurgitated from the stomach through the anastomotic line into the pleural space. Shock may accompany the rapid accumulation of fluid in the pleural cavity. The erect position is best to show the effusion by X rays.

Treatment is by aspiration of the fluid and insertion of a drain. Thoracotomy may be indicated.

Pulmonary embolism. See p. 241.

Fat embolism. See p. 653.

Left ventricular failure

This can sometimes be diagnosed by the anaesthetist during the operation or it may show as dyspnoea and cyanosis several hours later. Precipitating factors are over-zealous infusion of fluids, the onset of dysrrhythmia or the development of myocardial infarction. Diagnosis and treatment are discussed on p. 229.

POSTOPERATIVE FLUID AND ELECTROLYTE DISTURBANCE

A normal adult needs 25 to 35 ml of water per kg body weight and 1·2 to 2·0 mmol per kg body weight of sodium ions. Less is needed for several days after operation because the endocrine response to stress causes water and salt retention so that the output of urine and its salt content are low. This might wrongly suggest that extra salt is needed when it is not.

Potassium depletion

This is a fairly common postoperative emergency. The patient may have been hypokalaemic before operation and this may show as inadequate breathing following anaesthesia. Hypokalaemia may follow massive intestinal resection, intestinal fistula formation, the aspiration of large volumes of gastro-intestinal fluid, the relief of obstructive uropathy and the pseudo-membranous colitis which sometimes complicates operations on the upper gastro-intestinal tract.

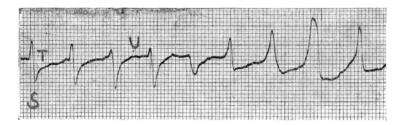

FIG. 28.3

A

A. Potassium deficit. (Serum level 1·5 mmol.) Low voltage, flattening of T waves. ST segment depression. Prominent U wave. Last four complexes show probable Left BBB pattern due to defective conduction. (Apparent widening of T wave sometimes seen is due to merging a low T wave with a U wave.)

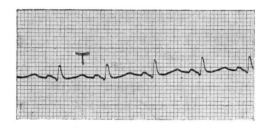

B

B. Same patient, Lead III, 48 hours after infusion of 300 mmol potassium ions. Serum level 4·0 mmol.

Potassium is predominantly an intracellular ion and so it is important to know the various factors which cause shifts of potassium between the intracellular and intravascular spaces. These are summarised in Table 28.1. A metabolic or respiratory acidosis causes a shift of potassium from the cells into the vascular compartment thereby giving the impression that the total body potassium is normal. The infusion of dextrose in a patient who is already hypokalaemic may precipitate hypokalaemic paresis because of shift of potassium into the cells.

The symptoms of hypokalaemia may come on insidiously and are muscular weakness, abdominal distension and mental confusion. Any patient with these symptoms who has lost potassium-containing fluids should have his plasma potassium measured. A 10 per cent depletion of total body potassium causes symptoms and a 30 per cent depletion is fatal. A normal ECG does not exclude a potassium deficit but changes are invariably present when the serum potassium is 2·8 mmol or less. The ECG changes are shown in Fig. 28.3A.

Treatment. In most patients with postoperative hypokalaemia the potassium has to be replaced i v. The amount to be given depends

Table 28.1. *Factors affecting plasma potassium*

CHANGES IN EXTERNAL BALANCE	
Sodium excess	Increase in extracellular fluid volume Replacement of cellular K^+ by Na^+
Acidosis	Replacement of cellular K^+ by Na^+ Increase in plasma K^+
Alkalosis	Replacement of cellular Na^+ by K^+ Decrease in plasma K^+
CHANGES IN CELL METABOLISM	
Cellular uptake of glucose	Uptake of K^+ by the cells Decreased secretion of K^+ Fall in plasma K^+
Protein Catabolism	Breakdown of cells Rise in plasma K^+
MISCELLANEOUS FACTORS	
Insulin	Uptake of K^+ by the cell
Adrenaline Steroids	Fall in plasma K^+ Increase in K^+ secretion by renal tubular cells Fall in plasma K^+

upon the probable rate of future loss and the total present potassium deficit. Sufficient potassium should be given to keep up with the losses expected over the next four hours. An attempt should be made to replace half to one third of the assessed potassium deficit over the ensuing 24 hours (but see p. 607). When replacing potassium to counter severe deficiency it is essential to use ECG monitoring control and serial potassium and electrolyte estimations. When there is also a metabolic acidosis it is essential to replace the potassium as potassium chloride in saline before correcting the acidosis with bicarbonate. To use sodium bicarbonate first might precipitate hypokalaemic paresis. The number of potassium ions required to correct severe hypokalaemia may be large. When faced with severe hypokalaemia and continuing potassium losses the advice of a metabolic physician should be sought. (For risks of i v potassium see pp. 89 and 105.)

Potassium excess (see also p. 379)

Hyperkalaemia may arise postoperatively when there is acute intravascular haemolysis (p. 271) or when the operation has been performed in the presence of acute renal failure. Serious hyperkalaemia may be precipitated by a respiratory or metabolic acidosis in a moderately hyperkalaemic patient. The clinical manifestations are listlessness, mental confusion, weakness and tingling of the extremities. The ECG changes are characteristic (Fig. 28.4) and the serum potassium is raised.

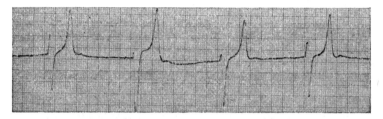

FIG. 28.4
Hyperkalaemia. Lead II. Increase of QRS interval. Tall peaked T. waves. No evidence of atrial activity. Serum level 9·2 mmol.

Treatment. In the postoperative hypercatabolic patient this depends upon renal function. Immediate interim treatment consists in the i v infusion over 30 minutes of 80 g glucose with soluble insulin 20 units. Potassium ions shift into the cells thereby lowering the serum potassium. In the presence of acute renal failure renal dialysis should be established as soon as possible, but where renal function is good, the excess potassium may be cleared by a thiazide diuretic.

Sodium depletion

Sodium depletion leads to a diminution in the intravascular volume and hence apathy, weakness and postural hypotension. This syndrome may come on after operation in patients who were depleted of sodium before operation and then lose large volumes of fluid from or into the gastro-intestinal tract during and following operation. Sodium depletion associated with a hypokalaemic metabolic alkalosis is common in patients who have prolonged gastric aspiration in the presence of inadequate saline and potassium replacement. Such patients become steadily hypovolaemic and if the metabolic deficit is not corrected before operation they collapse after it from hyponatraemia. The diagnosis is confirmed biochemically.

Treatment. Insert a central venous pressure line (p. 751) and rapidly infuse isosmotic sodium chloride solution until the central venous pressure is within normal limits. In the presence of oliguria and extreme hyponatraemia it may, on rare occasions, be necessary to use twice isosmolar sodium chloride solution (Na 300 mmol/litre). More than one litre of such a solution should not be given. CVP monitoring and frequent electrolyte estimations are essential.

The total quantity of sodium ions lost by a patient can frequently be assessed by estimating the concentration of sodium ions in the gastric aspirate and the volume of fluid lost over the previous few days. The quantity of sodium ions to be lost over the subsequent 24 hours can be assessed and to this should be added approximately half of the estimated sodium and chloride ions previously lost. A rough idea of the number of sodium ions required can be obtained by the following calculation.

Deficit of Na=(normal level−patient's level)× *volume* of extracellular fluid (volume of ECF=15 per cent BW in kilograms)

$$=(142-\text{patient's sodium level in mmol})\times\frac{15}{100}\text{ BW in Kg.}$$

For a 70 kg man with a plasma sodium of 118 mmol/litre deficit

$$=142-118\times\frac{15}{100}\times70=24\times10.5=252\text{ mmol.}$$

One litre of isosmotic sodium chloride solution = 154 mmol Na (approx.).

The required replacement is

$$\frac{\text{Deficit}}{154}\text{ litres of isosmotic sodium chloride solution}$$

=approx. 1·6 litres.

Such a calculation is only a rough guide for it is fallacious to suppose that, knowing the body weight and the plasma electrolyte levels, it is possible to calculate exactly how much salt is needed to bring the plasma level back to normal. Calculations cannot allow for the state of the intracellular fluid or the efficiency of the kidneys and they ignore the adjustments which are continually taking place between the intracellular and extracellular fluid compartments.

We should judge the patient's state by considering all the evidence; the history of fluid loss by vomiting, diarrhoea or through a gastric suction tube or a fistula; the presence or absence of thirst; the clinical signs of dehydration (slack skin, dry tongue and collapsed veins); the urinary volume, osmolality and chloride content and the serum sodium and potassium levels. It must be remembered too that in addition to replacement of deficits the patient must receive also his basic need of fluid (approximately 1·5 litres daily). The basic sodium requirements should be adjusted individually and approximated to the number of sodium ions lost in the urine. The number of sodium ions lost in sweat should also be considered.

Water depletion

Fluid lost from the lower intestinal tract as diarrhoea or from fistulas is generally of lower sodium content than that of gastric juice. Water depletion therefore becomes the more important feature of intestinal loss. Depletion of water (and, to a lesser extent, sodium) may arise when fluid replacement after operation is inadequate. The patient becomes weak and apathetic and complains of severe thirst. The hypotension and low tissue turgor of sodium depletion are not seen. The urine volume is small and the urine and plasma osmolality high.

Treatment. Give dextrose 5 g/dl (isotonic) i v until the serum osmolality and serum sodium reach normal levels (i.e. 285-300 m osmol/litre and 135-145 m mol/litre respectively). Approximately half the estimated previous loss plus the loss likely to occur over the subsequent 24 hours should be infused over the next 24 hours. The concentration of ions to be infused can frequently be assessed by biochemical analysis of the fluid lost. In clinical practice predominant water depletion is generally associated with mild sodium and moderate potassium depletion. Small quantities of sodium ions can be given as glucose (Na^+ 30 mmol/litre). Pure water depletion is treated with dextrose 5 g/dl.

Hypomagnesaemia

While a deficit is a reliable index of magnesium deficiency it is possible to have a normal plasma concentration with a generalised body depletion of the element. Like calcium the magnesium ion exists in the plasma in both the ionised and protein bound state. The serum concentration is 0·6 to 1·0 mmol (1·5 to 2·5 mEq/litre) of which approximately 35 per cent is protein bound. Many of the basic energy processes of the cell are mediated by enzymes activated by magnesium. Magnesium also affects neuromuscular function. Deficiency is frequently associated with calcium deficiency and may arise from excessive gastrointestinal fluid loss or follow parenteral administration of magnesium-free fluid. The symptoms and signs consist of disorientation, tremor and a positive Chvostek's sign. With increasing depletion the patient may develop convulsions and tetany.

Treatment. This is by the administration of 4 ml of a 50 g per dl solution of magnesium sulphate, i.e. 2·0 mmol Mg^{++}/ml given i m (preferably in equal doses given into two separate sites) or i v in 1 litre of dextrose saline over two to four hours.

ABDOMINAL PAIN AND BACK PAIN

Acute porphyria

Colicky abdominal pain following a negative laparotomy is the picture when the diagnosis has been missed. Any operation may precipitate an attack in a patient with porphyria (see p. 123).

Addisonian crisis

A patient with undiagnosed Addison's disease (p. 301) may present after operation with severe pain in the epigastrium and vomiting. A similar syndrome may occur in patients on long-term steroids if they are not prepared adequately before operation (see p. 354).

Pancreatitis

This may complicate operative procedures on the biliary tract and the upper gastrointestinal tract. The onset is dramatic with epigastric and back pain. Shock may be severe (see p. 113).

Pyelonephritis

Operations on the genito-urinary tract may be complicated by acute pyelonephritis. Patients particularly at risk are those who have infected urine not adequately controlled by antibiotics. The onset can be dramatic. Because of a septicaemic spread the patient becomes suddenly shocked. He has severe back pain and perhaps a rigor. There is tenderness over the affected kidney. Treatment should be with heavy doses of the appropriate antibiotic (see pp. 383 and 387) preferably i v. In order to ensure an adequate intake fluids should be given i v. It is essential to measure the output of urine since there is a risk of acute renal failure.

Diabetic ketosis

An undiagnosed diabetic may present after operation with acute epigastric pain and vomiting. The abdomen may appear distended and the clinical findings suggest a gastro-intestinal perforation. A known but inadequately prepared diabetic may develop severe ketosis with epigastric pain and vomiting following operation (see p. 349).

PARALYTIC ILEUS

This is a common finding after any abdominal operation and following generalised peritonitis. It may, however, occur in the absence of intra-abdominal pathology or operation, e.g. in uraemia, chest trauma, retroperitoneal haemorrhage, renal pathology and hypokalaemia.

Ileus for periods up to 48 hours is not serious and does not usually cause symptoms. Prolonged beyond this it may lead to severe vomiting, abdominal distension, absolute constipation and discomfort (though not colicky pain). On examination the abdomen is tympanitic all over and silent on auscultation. The diagnosis is confirmed by seeing gas and fluid levels in both small and large bowel on X-ray films taken in the erect position. Untreated, dehydration and electrolyte problems together with respiratory embarrassment will follow. Adequate fluid and electrolyte replacement by i v infusion and intestinal decompression by a nasogastric tube are the two mainstays of treatment. Sedation, antibiotic therapy in peritonitis and the use of a flatus tube may be helpful. Bowel stimulants (Carbachol and neostigmine) have no place in treatment and are dangerous.

ACUTE DILATATION OF THE STOMACH

The cause of this peculiar condition remains obscure. It is now a rare complication of abdominal or pelvic surgery but may occasionally be seen after spinal trauma or damage to retroperitoneal tissues. It is characterised by effortless vomiting of copious brown or black fluid. Before vomiting the patient may have hiccup and complain of nausea and abdominal discomfort. The pulse rate is increased, fulness may be noticed in the epigastrium and a loud sucussion splash can be detected. Whenever acute dilatation is suspected a nasogastric tube should be passed at once and the stomach kept empty by continuous drainage. This is the most important measure in preventing a fatal outcome. The fluid removed must be measured and an i v infusion of isosmotic sodium chloride solution started. Subsequent management will depend on the volume aspirated and the serum electrolytes. Hypokalaemia is a likely complication and should be treated as described on pp. 8 and 21.

HYPOTENSION AND SHOCK

Postoperative hypotension may be secondary to hypovolaemia, intrinsic myocardial failure and a multiplicity of factors such as septicaemia and endocrine failure.

Hypovolaemia

This may develop in patients who have bled during the operation and who have continued to bleed slowly afterwards. Hidden sources of bleeding must be sought. Bleeding into the abdominal or thoracic space can cause profound shock in the absence of overt bleeding. Haemorrhage into the thoracic space can generally be detected clinically. Severe intraperitoneal bleeding can be demonstrated by a four quadrant peritoneal tap. Retroperitoneal haemorrhage may complicate back injuries and should be suspected when the shocked patient who has signs of internal bleeding also complains of back pain. The management of haemorrhagic shock is discussed on p. 8.

Hyponatraemia

Sodium depletion diminishes the intravascular fluid volume and causes apathy, weakness and postural hypotension. This may develop after operation in patients whose salt intake was low before operation and who lose large volumes of fluid from or into the gastro-intestinal tract following operation. For treatment see p. 18.

Mixed sodium and water depletion may lead to a fall in intra-vascular volume and associated hypotension. This calls for appropriate fluid replacement with dextrose 5 g/l of isosmotic sodium chloride solution.

Cardiogenic shock

This is fully discussed on p. 238.

Septicaemia

Postoperative shock due to septicaemia is relatively common and should always be considered when patients, operated on for sepsis, particularly of the biliary and genito-urinary tracts, develop shock. The early signs are pyrexia (occasionally absent), sweating, restlessness, confusion and tachypnoea. There is a steady fall in blood pressure and a rise in pulse rate. Mild jaundice is common. The patient may deteriorate during the operation or fail to recover from the anaesthetic. Alternative diagnoses to be considered are myocardial failure, pulmonary embolism (p. 241), amniotic fluid embolism (p. 185), and an adverse drug reaction, incompatible blood transfusion (p. 103), transfusion of out-dated blood (p. 105) and loss of blood volume in the absence of septicaemia. As the condition deteriorates the patient becomes comatose, hypotensive and cyanosed and his skin cold and clammy and increasingly jaundiced. Acute renal failure and coagulation abnormalities are common. The differential diagnosis of the late picture includes a cerebral catastrophe, myocardial failure, pulmonary aspiration, thrombotic and amniotic fluid embolism, hepatocellular failure and blood loss.

Treatment. Close cooperation with the microbiologist is necessary in order to decide the best antibiotic to use (see p. 429). Shock should be treated on the lines described on pp. 8 and 238, except that the use of phenoxybenzamine (Dibenyline) (for reference see Lillehei, p. 240) is not advised since it can cause gross peripheral vasodilatation which, in spite of volume replacement, can be irreversible. Similarly the use of pressor agents is of doubtful value (p. 239). Adrenaline and noradrenaline are not advised and if an adrenergic drug is to be used isoprenaline is probably best because of its inotropic effect on the myocardium and its peripheral vasodilatory effect. For further discussion see bacteraemic shock, p. 428.

Endocrine failure

Hypotension may develop after operation in a patient with known endocrine failure who has been inadequately prepared. Alternatively hypotension may be precipitated in a patient whose endocrine failure (from Addison's disease, panhypopituitarism or hypothyroidism) has not yet been diagnosed.

POSTOPERATIVE BLEEDING

A mechanical factor, e.g. a slipped ligature, should always be looked for first. Once this has been excluded haemostatic failure should be considered. The commonest cause is loss of labile coagulation factors following massive blood transfusion (see p. 277). This can be prevented by infusing three packets of fresh frozen plasma after every five litres of blood. Haemorrhage due to a hereditary coagulation defect is generally seen during operation as a continuous ooze. Rarer causes of haemorrhage following operation are primary activation of the intrinsic coagulation system or of the fibrinolytic system or both, especially in obstetric practice following retention of a dead fetus, amniotic fluid embolism (p. 185) and septic abortion.

Operations involving handling of the lung may be followed by a haemorrhagic tendency. Generalised bleeding may occasionally develop following prostatectomy and is thought to be due to local fibrinolysis activated by the normal urinary constituent urokinase. Provided there is no evidence of activation of the intrinsic coagulation system the bleeding is strikingly diminished by giving the anti-fibrinolytic drug E-amino-caproic acid (p. 285).

The treatment of the emergency of intractable postoperative haemorrhage may be summarised as follows:

1. Exclude a source of bleeding.
2. Replace lost red blood cells.
3. Give vitamin K_1 if any suggestion of deficiency.
4. Exclude any drug anticoagulant effect.
5. Deficiency of coagulation factors in old blood: Give Fresh Frozen Plasma.
6. Hypofibrinogenaemia. Give FFP. Check fibrinogen level immediately and 30 minutes after infusion. If level has fallen suspect disseminated intravascular coagulation (DIC) or fibrinolysis.
7. DIC. Give FFP. Should clotting factors repeatedly fall and haemorrhage continue consult the haematologist. Consider heparin.
8. Platelet deficiency. Platelet count 100 000 cu. mm or less and clotting factors normal: give platelets. Platelet count 100 000 in the presence of DIC: replace clotting factors. Should bleeding continue give 4 to 6 packets of platelets or platelet-enriched plasma.
9. Fibrinolysis in isolation is rare. Do not give anti-fibrinolytic drugs without previous heparin therapy.

Postoperative collapse in a patient having corticosteroid therapy
(see p. 354)

Corticosteroids and corticotrophin will suppress the normal responsiveness of the pituitary-adrenal system to stress. The duration of this suppression depends partly on the dose but it is now thought that adrenal supression will have ceased when the patient has been off corticosteroids for two weeks. Any patient who has had steroid therapy should carry a steroid card showing his dose or a Medic-Alert bracelet or pendant (p. 822). The subject is fully dealt with on p. 354.

HYPERTENSION

Postoperative hypertension is unusual. It may arise from an endocrine crisis or from fluid overload or simply because the patient's hypotensive drugs were omitted before the operation. It can occur when the effect of these drugs, e.g. bethanidine (Esbatal), is posturally dependent.

Phaeochromocytoma

Patients who have any operative procedure and coincidentally have a phaeochromocytoma may present with tachycardia associated with severe diastolic hypertension. The crisis is generally associated with sweating and peripheral vasoconstriction producing a shocked appearance. Diagnosis and treatment is discussed on p. 357.

Thyrotoxicosis

Whether diagnosed or undiagnosed this may be precipitated into a crisis by an operation. It used to be a severe hazard following thyroidectomy in inadequately prepared patients with thyrotoxicosis. The syndrome may be suspected postoperatively if a patient who is hyperactive in spite of adequate sedation and with no evidence of hypovolaemia, has a tachycardia and hot moist hands. The temperature may be high and there is often a high pulse pressure. More careful examination in an undiagnosed patient may elicit thyroid enlargement and a thyroid bruit. The past history may be of help. The metabolic demands of a thyrotoxic crisis superimposed upon a recent operative procedure frequently necessitate sedation with chlorpromazine (Largactil) or diazepam (Valium) analgesia and IPPV. A muscle relaxant may be required to institute ventilation. β-adrenergic blockade with i v propranolol is essential in the presence of a pulse rate of greater than 140 per minute and is preferably given as a continuous infusion. For further treatment see p. 359.

Fluid overload

Shock during or after operation may be followed by acute renal failure. Excess fluid infused during the phase of oliguria may cause hypertension and acute left ventricular failure. Such a complication will require dialysis in order to remove the excess fluid (see p. 106).

Pre-eclampsia (See also p. 178.)

A rapid rise of blood pressure during the last ten weeks of pregnancy or within 48 hours of delivery may herald the onset of eclampsia. A rise of diastolic pressure about 110 must be treated as a matter of urgency. Blood pressure can be lowered most effectively by diazoxide (Eudemine) given i v rapidly (within 30 seconds) and undiluted. 300 mg usually lowers the blood pressure within five minutes.

COMA

(See also p. 579.)

Diabetic ketosis may follow operation in a known but inadequately controlled diabetic or it may be found in a previously unknown diabetic when an emergency operation has been done without a preoperative urine test. Poor renal perfusion may prevent glycosuria even though the blood sugar is high. For the first 24 hours after operation all insulin-dependent diabetics should have serial estimations of blood glucose. The management of diabetic ketosis is discussed in p. 341.

Hypoglycaemic coma classically follows the inappropriate administration of insulin to a diabetic. It may, however, be a feature of hepatocellular failure and one of the major features of adrenal failure. In hypoglycaemia there is generally sweating and restlessness. The condition is rapidly reversed by i v dextrose. Diabetics with an associated endocrinopathy are very susceptible to insulin hypoglycaemia. The dose of insulin following thyroidectomy in a diabetic should be reduced. Following delivery of a pregnant diabetic the dose of insulin should be half of that needed before pregnancy. There is a marked tendency to insulin-induced hypoglycaemia following Caesarean section in a known diabetic.

Hypothyroidism

A hypothyroid crisis may be precipitated by operative stress and show postoperatively as coma with hypothermia (p. 361) and bradycardia (p. 573). Coma may be the presenting feature of adrenal or pituitary failure (pp. 365 and 366).

Hepatocellular failure (p. 145)

This may develop after operation in any patient with liver cell disease. It is precipitated by blood transfusion, hypokalaemia and metabolic imbalance. Acute hepatocellular necrosis may complicate any operation on a shocked or hypoxic patient. After the operation he becomes jaundiced and comatose. There is frequently a haemorrhagic tendency associated with acute renal failure. In severe cases deterioration is rapid and the patient dies of hepatic failure within a few days of operation. Treatment is the same as that for any form of hepatocellular failure (pp. 151 and 155).

Electrolyte imbalance

Coma may develop following various electrolyte disturbances and is most often seen in hyper- and hyponatraemia, metabolic and respiratory acidosis and the hyperosmolality syndrome. Hyperosmolar coma may appear after operation as a consequence of sodium overload in the presence of relative water deficiency. It may also complicate the over-enthusiastic use of sodium bicarbonate to correct a metabolic acidosis. Electrolyte examination shows a raised serum sodium and often a raised blood sugar. The serum osmolality is high (normal 285-300 m osmol/kg) and a high blood urea may contribute to this. Treatment after operation is complicated by the tendency to retain sodium.

Treatment. Give hypotonic solutions either orally or i v to correct the hyperosmolality gradually over a period of 24 to 48 hours. Hyperglycaemia should be corrected by insulin and hypernatraemia by large volumes of hypotonic solution either as water via a Ryle's tube or i v as dextrose 5 g/dl. Severe hyperosmolality is frequently associated with impaired renal function or acute renal failure. In such cases a CVP line is essential since many of these patients have considerable expansion of the intravascular volume and are in danger of developing acute left ventricular failure. A hyperosmolar state associated with renal failure will necessitate peritoneal or haemodialysis using a hypotonic solution with a sodium concentration of no more than 135 mmol of sodium ions per litre of solution and a blood dextrose concentration of approximately 90 mg per 100 ml (4·95 mmol/l). Hyponatraemia when extreme may be associated with coma. Its diagnosis and treatment has already been discussed (p. 17).

Metabolic acidosis of sufficient severity to cause coma is rare after operations. It may follow severe shock and poor peripheral perfusion or it can develop more insidiously following the loss of base as from a fistula. The patient is confused and hyperventilating. Metabolic acidosis secondary to poor peripheral perfusion should be corrected by rewarming and volume replacement. When poor peripheral perfusion is associated with myocardial failure an inotropic agent such as isoprenaline with mild peripheral vasodilatory properties may be used. Sodium bicarbonate should be given if the base deficit is greater than 8. Base deficit and excess is defined under abnormalities of acid-base balance on p. 19. Correction of hypoxia and improvement in perfusion will lower base deficit and so we must avoid the over-correction and sodium overload which working to a base deficit of zero might bring. The approximate number of bicarbonate ions required to correct the patient deficit to 8 is given by the formula on p. 11. It is well to give the amount in two separate doses with an Astrup check in between.

CONVULSIONS

The stress of operation may precipitate a convulsion in a known epileptic. Such a patient must have his usual anticonvulsant drugs before and after operation by the i m route. Pyrexia and hypoxia may be precipitating factors. Postoperative cerebral embolism may present with a convulsion. Heparin should be given (see pp. 236 and 283). Hyperosmolality may first show as a convulsion. Convulsions may follow brain surgery. Pyrexia, extensive burns and injection of foreign protein may all precipitate a convulsion particularly in a child. While the underlying cause of a convulsion should be treated as soon as possible symptomatic treatment by diazepam (Valium) i v may be needed. Particular attention should be paid to the airway since these patients are very susceptible to hypoxia and pulmonary aspiration.

PARESIS AND TETANY

Muscle weakness and paresis are sometimes the dominant features of a postoperative electrolyte and metabolic disturbance (see sodium depletion p. 605, hypokalaemia p. 602, hyperkalaemia p. 605, metabolic alkalosis pp. 194 and 615, hypomagnesaemia p. 607).

Tetany

This may be mild (as in carpopedal spasm) or severe (with convulsions, coma and death). It can follow intestinal fluid loss but the commonest cause is inadvertent removal of or temporary damage to the parathyroid glands during thyroidectomy (see p. 368).

HYPOTHERMIA AND PYREXIA
(See Taking the temperature, p. 69.)

Hypothermia is a complication of any operative procedure in which the body is exposed for prolonged periods. Infants and hypothyroid patients are particularly susceptible. Acute hypothermia may develop as a result of rapid i v infusion of cold fluids, especially blood (see p. 13).

Moderate postoperative pyrexia only becomes an emergency when there are also other features such as rigor or convulsion or evidence of a septicaemia. Blood transfusion sometimes causes a pyrexial reaction (p. 102). When drugs are the cause there is usually a rash. Dextran can cause pyrexia with bronchospasm, generalised wheals and collapse due to histamine release. The infusion must be replaced at once by one of isosmotic sodium chloride solution and the drugs on the anaphylaxis tray (p. 745) used. For malignant hyperpyrexia see p. 575.

VENOUS THROMBOSIS

This is a dangerous, if initially silent, complication which should be looked for after any operation which keeps the patient in bed for more than a few days. The postoperative incidence is about 20 to 30 per cent. It may be symptomless and yet be complicated by pulmonary embolism. There is usually mild pyrexia. Early signs are slight oedema of the foot which masks the extensor tendons and slight fulness of the foot veins. Dorsiflexion of the ankle causes pain in the calf (Homan's sign), which is also tender on pressure. The diagnosis should be confirmed by venography. Anticoagulant therapy should be started at once as a continuous heparin infusion. An extensive thrombosis may be an indication for streptokinase therapy (p. 243) preceded by a venogram. If anticoagulant therapy is adequate it is rare for surgery to be required. There is evidence to suggest that heparin subcutaneously before and after operation may reduce the incidence of postoperative venous thrombosis (see pp. 242 and 283). (An occasional pitfall in diagnosis is rupture of a Baker's cyst with extravasation into the calf causing tenderness and Homan's sign. Knee arthrography with Hypaque will show the leak.)

GILLIAN C. HANSON

C. ALLAN BIRCH

CHAPTER 29

Geriatric Emergencies

CERTAIN peculiarities of old age alter the picture of common illnesses. Pain sense is diminished so that cardiac infarction, for example, may present with little or no pain and make the patient gravely ill before his plight is recognised. Homeostatic mechanisms are impaired, temperature regulation is poor and drugs are only slowly metabolised and excreted. Dehydration with raised blood urea is common to many illnesses in the elderly. Many old folk are socially disadvantaged and are living alone or are supported at great emotional cost by relatives. In such circumstances the help of the social worker is essential.

Many of the conditions presenting as emergencies in old age have been described in other chapters for they are not peculiar to the elderly. The urgent aspects of geriatric illness which warrant special consideration are: confusion, coma (including hypothermia) and disturbances of behaviour, mobility and continence.

CONFUSION

This is a characteristic of any physical illness in old age and corresponds to delirium in the young. It is commoner and occurs from lesser causes in those who have shown earlier mental impairment than in those previously normal. There may be a single incident or recurrent attacks, often at night. Unfamiliar surroundings play a part but physical illness is the main factor particularly when, as in respiratory infection, cardiac failure and anaemia, there is hypoxia. Dehydration, renal failure, diabetes, hypoglycaemia (often iatrogenic) and trauma, including operations (especially for fractured neck of femur), may all be complicated by confusion. Drugs causing confusion include barbiturates, atropine and atropine-like substances, anticholinergics, tricyclics, antispasmodics and digitalis. Simple discomfort from a distended bowel or an overfull or infected bladder sometimes provokes confusion.

The acutely confused old person is restless and uneasy. He cannot remember where he is. He has lost track of time. He fails to recognise his friends and relations and may resist their attentions. His perception is distorted and he misinterprets and is frightened by what he sees. His speech is rambling and incoherent. He may shout noisily for help. He is very likely to want to get out of bed.

Management. This is difficult in the acutely confused patient at home, especially at night. Sometimes a night light may restore normality. Admission to hospital (preferably a side ward) is often necessary and there the patient should not be left in the dark. The staff should help him to keep in touch with reality by talking to him. His attempts to get out of bed should not be resisted and he should be helped into a chair. It will take some time to diagnose the cause for a thorough examination of an acutely confused person is difficult. However, relief may come quickly if retention of urine or impaction of faeces are detected and dealt with. These conditions should always be in mind before drugs are considered. Of the tranquillisers it is doubtful if any are better than chlorpromazine (Largactil) 50 mg i m. Paraldehyde is best avoided. It gives the breath an unpleasant smell and may cause a sterile abscess (see p. 85). Recovery from its effects may be marked by noisiness and confusion so that it may create as many problems as it solves.

Coma
(See also p. 290.)

The commonest cause of coma in the elderly is a stroke. Usually there is evidence of hemiparesis which, even in the comatose patient, shows in that the paralysed arm when lifted falls back more heavily than does the normal one. There may be conjugate deviation of the eyes. The presence of other conditions may be over-shadowed by the stroke. Sometimes a fit marks the onset of stroke illness. Epilepsy may be the cause of unconsciousness but whereas this rarely lasts over half an hour in the young it may continue all day in the elderly.

Metabolic causes of coma are common in the old. A fall of 50 per cent in cerebral blood flow, or a drop of PaO_2 to 40 mm Hg (5·32 kPa) or of blood sugar to 40 mg/100 ml (2·2 mmol) will cause coma. Other commonly seen causes are acute cardiac dysrrhythmias, respiratory and renal failure, hypothyroidism and drug overdosage. While diabetic coma with ketosis is uncommon in old age hyperosmolar non-ketotic diabetic coma is more often seen (see p. 345). Hypoglycaemic coma in the elderly is usually due to oral hypoglycaemic agents, especially chlorpropamide (Diabinese). Tolbutamide (Rastinon) is safer but three daily doses are a disadvantage. A convenient once a day sulphonylurea preparation is glymidine (Gondafon) 0·5 to 1·0 g with breakfast. Diabetics on diguanidies are not in danger of hypoglycaemia but may become comatose from lactic acidosis. The serum lactate level (normal 3·6 to 13·5 mg/100 ml; 0·4 to 1·5 mmol/l) should be estimated if an elderly diabetic on diguanides shows any disturbance of consciousness.

Hypothermia

In addition to what is said about it on p. 361, hypothermia deserves special mention as a cause of coma in geriatric practice for it may occur in well heated surroundings. The abdomen and axillae, normally always warm, are cold to the touch. The risk of using an ordinary thermometer is mentioned on p. 69. Confirmation of hypothermia should be made rectally by a low-reading thermometer. Hypothyroidism is an associated condition in only a minority of cases and can be suspected if when the ankle jerk is present its relaxation phase is greatly prolonged. A recorder is needed to show that prolongation is more than it would be from hypothermia alone but clinical evidence such as a thyroid scar and *erythema ab igne* may point to the diagnosis. When this is definite triiodothyronine in low dosage (10 μg every 12 hours) should be given i v. Apart from this no drugs other than a broad spectrum antibiotic are needed. Simple nursing measures in a temperature of 27° to 30° C suffice but procedures like catheterisation and intubation should be avoided as they may provoke fatal ventricular fibrillation. The mortality is high from pneumonia and other associated illness.

DISTURBANCES OF BEHAVIOUR

Much peculiar behaviour in the old is tolerated until a crisis occurs which provokes a demand that 'Something must be done'. The causes are sometimes emotional and there is often organic mental disease also. In many cases there is underlying physical illness whose nature is not obvious at first. Often the necessary admission to hospital is refused. If a domiciliary consultation with the geriatric physician will not cause a change of mind compulsory admission under Section 47 of the National Assistance Act 1948 must be used because the patient is a danger to himself and to others. It is always wise to make sure first that a hospital bed will be available.

Depressive illness is sometimes the cause of the crisis. It is suggested by apathy, decreased activity, anorexia, carelessness about dress and estrangement from friends. The patient may complain of various pains and may be preoccupied with his bowels. He seeks constant reassurance. A diurnal swing of mood is suggestive. This picture is often resolved by tricyclic antidepressants (dothiepin (Prothiaden) 25 mg three times a day being the safest). When the depression lifts underlying disease may become apparent.

Dementia is often superimposed on a life-long personality trait such as irritability, greed, suspicion and eccentricity and some degree of mental impairment is found in 20 per cent of people over the age of 80. It is primarily dependent on memory defects but it results in disturbances of behaviour, social adjustment, emotional control and the ability to perform skilled tasks. Memory failure in later life is always greatest for recent events while those of early life are well remembered. There is often also disorientation in time and space. An old lady may, for example, get up in the middle of the night to see her husband off to work. Such happenings may lead to a crisis. Table manners, dressing habits and personal cleanliness are all impaired. As inhibitions are lost an old person may become aggressive when irritated and may lash out and injure others. Negativistic behaviour such as refusal to dress, faecal smearing and incontinence are sometimes a protest against an upsetting situation and may respond to understanding, affection and a more secure environment.

Loss of domestic skills may cause fear in the relatives that the house will be set alight. A patient of suspicious temperament may, when she loses, for example, her handbag, assume that it has been stolen and react angrily. In these situations the help of a psychogeriatric day hospital may keep the domestic tension bearable.

DISTURBANCE OF MOBILITY

Immobility is a great threat to a patient's independence and calls for urgent attention. Falls whether accidental or symptomatic (p. 290) cause loss of confidence and this *timor decadendi* restricts activity. Domestic circumstances such as poor lighting and loose rugs must be corrected and efforts made to restore confidence. Loss of ability to walk is often the result of a stroke (mortality 1 in 3) or acute joint pain. Urgent admission after a stroke depends on the balance between the social circumstances and the degree of disability.

Paraplegia is a rare type of paralysis in old age but the diagnosis is often delayed because the backache and walking difficulty are attributed to cervical and lumbar spondylosis—almost a physiological process. Although this causes symptoms it does not preclude more sinister pathology such as secondary deposits. The distinction is not merely academic for hormonal and deep X-ray therapy may bring relief.

21

An acute flare-up of arthritis bad enough to cause immobility is rare unless due to trauma and must be distinguished from such conditions as gout, septic arthritis and a stress fracture. For the minor exacerbations of osteoarthritis of the knee intra-articular hydrocortisone will bring dramatic relief (p. 644).

When an old person is sent to hospital it is most important to stress that this is not for terminal care when it is simply that he has temporarily lost his ability to move. Outdoor clothes should go with him and he should know that a retaining fee for the accommodation he has temporarily left has been paid.

Disturbance of Continence

Unless they cause retention of urine, sphincter disturbances seldom present as emergencies but urinary incontinence and more commonly faecal incontinence is often the last straw which upsets a precarious balance and makes admission to hospital necessary. Incontinence of urine is an almost universal complaint of acutely ill old people and is due to immobility and the effect of diuretics. Urinary tract infections rarely cause it. Catheterisation (p. 720) for less than a week carries only a negligible risk of ascending infection. Faecal incontinence is very distressing. It is rarely due to true diarrhoea and more often results from faecal retention. Disposable enemas usually suffice to cure it, but when there is impaction manual evacuation of the rectum is necessary.

The Relatives

Many crises in geriatrics are produced by collapse of morale among the relatives and friends. It is easy for a doctor to feel critical of them and his life would be simpler if only they would go on carrying the burden. So it is worth reflecting that the relatives of the elderly are often past middle age and when the patient is in his nineties his children may be past retirement. Advancing age brings increased incidence of illness and the relatives may be victims also. The demands of the old may provoke acute conflicts of loyalty particularly in the middle aged woman who finds herself torn between the needs of her parent and those of her husband and children. The situation is more difficult if she has had to give up work to care for the old person whose presence is resented also by the children. Those with more experience, however, are constantly impressed by what the family will endure to support the aged rather than by the readiness with which they will reject them.

In old age it is always vital to assess quickly the total problem and not to be content with the mere mechanical management of the predominant emergency. These criteria should be borne in mind when prescribing and the drugs used must not, as a side effect, deprive him of his mental integrity, his mobility or the control of his bladder and bowels.

R. E. IRVINE

THEODORE M. STROUTHIDIS

FOR FURTHER READING

AGATE, J. The Practice of Geriatrics. 2nd edition. London: Heinemann. 1970.

BERGMAN, K. The Aged—Their Understanding and Care. London: Wolfe Publishing Ltd. 1972.

BROCKLEHURST, J. C. Textbook of Geriatric Medicine and Gerontology. Edinburgh and London: Churchill Livingstone. 1973.

GARDINER-HILL, H. (Editor). Compendium of Emergencies. Chapter 23 by A. N. Exton-Smith. 3rd edition. London: Butterworths. 1971.

HARRISON, M. J. G. (1974). The diagnosis of coma. British Journal of Hospital Medicine 11, 783-791.

HODKINSON, M. H. An Outline of Geriatrics. London: Academic Press. 1975.

IRVINE, R. E. (1973). Hypothermia. Modern Geriatrics, 3, 464-470.

IRVINE, R. E., BAGNALL, M. K. & SMITH, B. J. (1974). The Older Patient. 3rd edition. London: English Universities Press. 1976.

ISAACS, B., LIVINGSTONE, M. & NEVILLE, Y. Survival of the Unfittest. London: Routledge & Kegan Paul. 1972.

STEVENS, R. S. (1966). Geriatric emergencies. Practitioner, 196, 539-545.

CHAPTER 30

Bites and Stings and Miscellaneous Emergencies

BITES AND STINGS
BEES AND WASPS

Prevention

THE chances of being stung by a honeybee are reduced by wearing clean, smooth-textured, light-coloured clothing and by avoiding sudden movements and sweating. Repellants smeared or sprayed on the hands are helpful. A few puffs from the beekeeper's smoker on the part stung will mask the sting odour and so discourage more stings. A visitor to an apiary should be careful not to cross the flight path of the bees or to place himself directly in front of a hive. He should wear a veil. It is best to open up a hive in warm sunny conditions.

A beekeeper who reacts badly to stings may prevent serious symptoms by taking ephedrine 15 mg or an antihistamine tablet before handling his bees. Aqueous desensitising vaccines made from extracts of whole bees (Bencard) can be used each year and are helpful if the reaction is of the anaphylactoid type. Venom itself would probably be more effective but is harder to prepare.

Reaction to stings

Most people have pain and local swelling only but a few react badly. Occasionally coma and death have followed within 20 minutes. In the ten years 1962-71 eleven people in England and Wales died from bee stings and 33 from wasp stings. Since in some of these cases no local reaction has occurred and the site has been on thin vascular skin it is thought that the venom entered a venule by chance. It is said that bee stings on the back of the neck are liable to cause fainting from reflex vagal inhibition. Status asthmaticus has followed a sting. Wasp stings can be equally serious but an individual generally receives fewer wasp than bee stings. Some antigens are common to bees, wasps and most members of the hymenoptera group but that of the wasp includes a polypeptide, kinin, whose effects are specially persistent.

A rare but picturesque beekeeping emergency is the occasion when a swarm settles on one's head. Don't panic or hit out. Sit tight in the hope that the scout bees will soon call the swarm to the new home they have chosen. Should a fellow apiarist spot the queen—an unlikely event—she should be put on a frame in a nearby empty hive. The workers will follow. Otherwise the beekeeper should move slowly to a place where the bees can be brushed off his head into a box or preferably an empty hive.

Treatment. A honeybee's sting is barbed so she leaves it behind in the skin together with its poison sac the muscles of which go on pumping in poison for several seconds. Hence it is best not to try to pick out the sting lest the fingers squeeze out more venom. The sting should be scraped out with a finger nail or wiped out with a handkerchief. A steroid cream is the best application to use but it would have to be applied very promptly. Putting on alkali (' blue bag ') for bee stings and vinegar for wasp stings is outmoded but any application can help by suggestion. As self-injection of adrenaline is usually impracticable isoprenaline 10 mg sublingually may be used for a bad reaction. Failing this, a Medihaler Iso Forte (Riker) (20 mg per ml) may be carried.

Anaphylactic shock following bee stings is a serious emergency. Adrenaline Injection BP 1 ml should be given i m followed by 50 mg of prednisolone 21 phosphate. Then 10 ml of 10 per cent calcium gluconate should be given slowly into a vein and chlorpheniramine (Piriton) 4 mg continued three times a day by mouth. It should be noted that the insulin requirements of a diabetic will be increased by a severe reaction to a bee sting.

The serum of some beekeepers who do not react badly to stings has a high level of protective antibody which might be used to treat severe reaction in others. It would be wise to follow this by a course of immunising injections of bee venom.

MOSQUITO AND HORSE FLY (CLEG) BITES

These are best treated by a dab of spirit or other antiseptic. If there is a severe reaction give ephedrine 30 mg by mouth and repeat if necessary.

BLISTERING BEETLES

These cause skin lesions requiring local treatment by alkaline solutions. If fluid from crushed beetles reaches the eyes it causes an acute conjunctivitis. The hairs of certain catterpillars act in the same way. Treatment is on general lines.

FISH STINGS

Weever fish (called Bishop fish in Cornwall) are found round the sandy Mediterranean coasts and those of the Eastern Atlantic including Britain. They are 15 to 40 cm long and have six large dorsal spines which are generally removed before sale for food. As the fish lies partially buried in the sand stings usually occur on the feet of bathers and those who go shrimping barefoot. It is wise to wear rubber slippers when paddling. Stings can cause pain which is often described in the strongest terms and accompanied by prostration. This may explain some otherwise unaccountable bathing fatalities. The site of the sting may show haemolytic staining of the skin and a kidney-shaped puncture wound corresponding to the shape of the first spine. The sting ray has a sharp spine which usually breaks off in the wound where it can by shown by X-rays. In tropical seas fish stings are a commoner hazard than jelly-fish stings and the bites of sea snakes (which incidentally are painless).

Treatment. The patient should be reassured in the strongest terms. Meddlesome measures at the site of the sting should be avoided. Weever fish stings are rare. Zammit* (1973) saw 10 cases between 1969 and 1973 in Malta and found the best treatment was the injection of 2 ml of 2 per cent lignocaine near the entry wound so that some of it oozed out of the puncture tract. This brought prompt relief. As the venom is deactivated by heat repeated momentary immersion of the foot in water as hot as the victim can bear has been advised but it is doubtful whether he would allow this.

JELLY FISH STINGS

Most jelly fish on British shores are fairly harmless but occasionally there is an invasion of the more sinister *Physalia* or Portuguese Man-of-War. It is very common on eastern Australian beaches, especially those of Sydney where it is called the bluebottle. It looks rather like a pale blue Cornish pastie with a dark line down its back. It is not just one animal but a colony of up to 1 000 separate organisms with different functions banded together and behaving as one unit. It cannot swim and simply drifts with the wind and probably gets its name from its resemblance to the lumbering galleons of the time when Portugal was a naval power. Tentacles trail up to 20 metres below the floating part and are beaded with myriads of swellings (nematocysts) which contain batteries of

---

* ZAMMIT, L. (1973). Weever fish stings. *The St Luke's Hospital Gazette,* Vol. VIII, No. 2, pp. 77-81. (Malta.)

stinging cells. These stinging elements retain their potency long after the rest of the body has withered in the sand so don't pick up a ' dead ' one. Stinging causes very painful urticarial wheals and only rarely is there a systemic reaction other than cramps. Cutaneous vasodilation from sunburn probably increases the absorption of toxin. Much more dangerous is the sea wasp or box jelly fish (*Cubomedusa*) of the Indo-pacific and North Australian waters— the world's most venomous creature. Found close inshore, its tentacles have millions of microscopic venom cells. Hence the total amount of toxin injected is large (see p. 777). Stings can be rapidly fatal. It has been found that the stinging cells of the sea anemone will not discharge in olive oil and this raises the possibility of protecting fishermen and swimmers by grease on the skin.

Treatment. Remove the tentacle having made a ' glove ' of wet sand on your hand first or apply cellophane tape to it. Methylated spirit or petrol will inactivate the nematocysts. Failing this rub the part with a towel. Measures for severe symptoms are Adrenaline Injection BP 1 ml subcutaneously or an antihistamine subcutaneously or by mouth. For very serious cases (sea wasp stings) a slow i v injection of 10 ml of calcium gluconate 10 g/dl and prednisolone 20 mg i v is advised. There is a potent sea wasp antivenom made by using the venom of *Chironex fleckeri* as antigen (for supplier see p. 777) but there is as yet no antivenom for the serious blue-ringed octopus of Australian waters. If transport to hospital is undertaken, avoidance of cerebral hypoxia on the journey is important.

SHARKS

Sharks are not a hazard to bathers in Britain but are a danger in some waters, e.g. in South Africa and Australia. So a brief note is made about them chiefly to help in avoiding an emergency. Warning notices about sharks should always be taken seriously. The barracuda or ' tiger fish ' and the blue fish are more dangerous than sharks.

Sharks are deep-water fish but some (baskers and loafers) live inshore and attack bathers. They do this purely by chance and, apart from the occasional man-eating rogue shark, they do not hunt or stalk human prey. In murky water the shark cannot see and avoid a swimmer and when he bumps against something soft he tries to eat it. The rough skin and sharp fins can cause severe abrasions. When blood flows there is danger for the shark is very sensitive to it and even a trace stimulates him to feed. Nothing will then stop him and a limb may soon be lost. Splashing water will not frighten him and the old explosive 'bang stick' was dangerous in that disruption of one shark only attracted more. There are chemical repellants such as copper acetate ('Shark Chaser') and the secretion of the Red Sea 'Moses' sole. Women should never bathe during menstruation if sharks are about.

POISONING FROM SPIDER BITES (ARACHNIDISM)

The bite of the 'Black Widow' spider of America (*Latrodectus*) (called Kapito in New Zealand and the red-back spider in Australia) and related species in the Mediterranean zone, South Africa, India and Russia is capable of causing severe symptoms. The male is less venomous than the female. As the spider often spins webs across latrine seats, a common site for the bite is the perineum or genitalia. The bite may not be felt but two small red spots are to be seen—the marks of the horny fangs through which the poison is injected. This, a non-haemolytic neurotoxin, causes cramping pain all over the body, often within 15 minutes of the bite; the muscles become rigid, and an 'acute abdomen' may be simulated (p. 121), but there is no tenderness or rise of pulse rate. Other features are pyrexia, leucocytosis and a macular rash. A burning sensation in the soles of the feet is said to be pathognomonic. Spider bites cause a high death rate in infants but are less serious in adults.

No British spiders inflict severe bites but a very aggresive one (*Phoneutria fera*) which strikes on the slightest provocation survives refrigeration on bananas. Only local symptoms result.

Treatment. Morphine may be required. Probably the best remedy is the one nearly always to hand, namely atropine 0·3 mg. Specific anti-venine should be used if available (Mulford Laboratories, Philadelphia). The dose is 2·5 ml and may be repeated. It is supplied dry and should be mixed with warm water. Avoid shaking as this causes troublesome foam. Failing this, a slow iv injection of calcium gluconate 10 to 20 ml of 10 g/dl solution is very effective. Antibacterial measures should be used. Corticotrophin (ACTH) has been recommended. For serum for Red Back Spider bite in Victoria, Australia, see p. 777. There is no antivenom for the dangerous funnel web spider in the Sydney area.

Scorpion Stings

Scorpions are arachnids of which some 650 species are known. Only a few, unrelated in size, are dangerous to man. A bulbous enlargement of the telson or last segment of the tail bears two poison glands and a terminal sting. The scorpion is a nocturnal creature and most stings occur at night. The effects vary from local pain to fatal collapse. The venom consists of many complex proteins. These cause a ' sympathetic storm ' similar to that caused by a phaeochromocytoma.

Treatment. A tourniquet should be applied if possible and suction started. Ammonia or rectified spirit in which scorpions have been killed should be applied. Atropine and calcium gluconate should be given as for spider bites. Lignocaine 2 g/dl, by injection, will relieve the pain but the best remedy is said to be an injection of emetine hydrochloride 30 mg into the site of the bite. Specific anti-venine is available in 1·0 ml doses (The Lister Institute, Elstree, Herts. WD6 3AX. 01-953 6191).

SNAKEBITE AND SNAKEBITE POISONING
IN BRITAIN

The only poisonous indigenous snake in Britain is the adder or Northern viper (*Vipera berus*) which is found chiefly in Scotland, the New Forest and on Dartmoor. It may be recognised from its general shape and appearance (Fig. 30.2) being stumpier than a grass snake and with a flatter and V-shaped head. The markings are variable and may be indistinct. They do not always conform to the book description—zigzag with a black V for viper on the head. Young males have a light grey body colour with black markings. These spread until the adult male is uniformly black. The female is more olive than grey. Colour changes with age and in the third year it may appear rusty. A melanistic variety devoid of markings and of a uniform grey colour is rare (Fig. 30.2). The eye is orange coloured with a vertical pupil. Adders rarely exceed 50 cm and a large snake over 75 cm long in Britain is almost certainly a harmless grass snake. An alleged snakebite in Ireland, the Isle of Man or the Channel Islands is probably a sting by an unnoticed insect as snakes are unknown in these parts (except perhaps in zoos). Adders rarely bite except when disturbed on coming out of hibernation in dry areas in the Spring. They migrate to damp places for the summer breeding season and so holiday makers on heaths and moors are rarely bitten. The ' deaf adder' is not deaf. It is warned of one's approach by scent and perhaps by vibration rather than sound. Most bites are on the fingers or hands because the adder is picked up. Expectant methods and reassurance are usually enough, particularly if there is no local swelling after 10 minutes. Kill and identify the snake if possible. Confirm the diagnosis of adder bite by finding the two punctures 1 cm apart (sometimes only one fang penetrates) (Figs. 30.1 and

30.3). Symptoms may be slight as when little poison enters because the adder has recently emptied its poison sacs. Wash the wound with water but do not incise it or apply a tourniquet. (The effects of any absorption of adder venom are slight compared with those of local swelling which a tourniquet would only aggravate.) Suction if used very promptly would seem reasonable but should be avoided

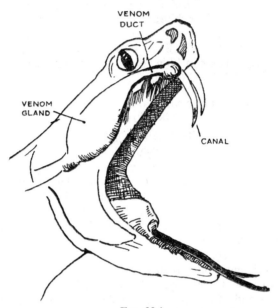

FIG. 30.1
Partly dissected head of adder (*Vipera berus*) *with* venom gland and duct displayed.
(*American Museum of Natural History.*)

if the lips are cracked. No drug other than an analgesic is usually indicated. If systemic effects suggest the need for anti-venom there is now one commercially available (p. 766). (The serum previously on sale was not prepared by using adder venom. Its use was discouraged by the Department of Health.)

A person bitten by a snake in a zoo may need specific anti-venom. At the London zoo each venomous snake's cage has a card attached giving a serum number and first aid procedure. Cases are treated at The Middlesex Hospital, Casualty Entrance, Nassau Street, London WIN 8AA (01.363 8333). A wide range of antivenoms is kept. A similar procedure is adopted at other zoos. There is no zoo in the Isle of Man (only a cattery).

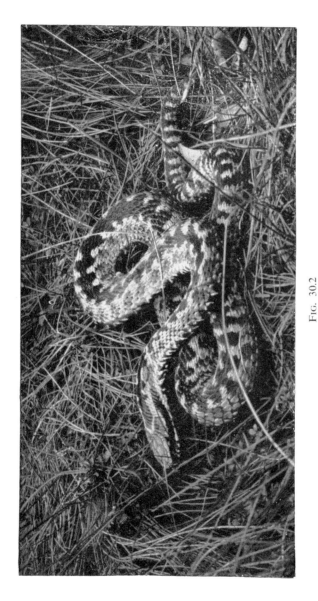

FIG. 30.2

A normal-coloured and a melanistic adder. The colouration of adders varies considerably with sex and age, though melanistic snakes are rare. Note the 'poison label'—the black zig-zag marking down the back of the normal-coloured adder.

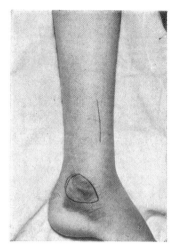

Fig. 30.3
Adder bite. Note within the red ringed area the two fang marks and the line of bruising. This case was fatal.
(*Dr James Macrae, Ham Green Hospital, Bristol.*)

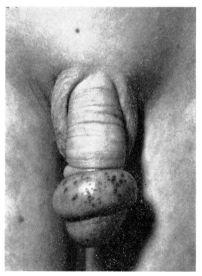

Fig. 30.4
Paraphimosis.

OUTSIDE BRITAIN

Poisonous snakes belong to three types: elapids (neurotoxic), sea-snakes (myotoxic) and vipers (vasculotoxic). The vipers are distinguished by having triangular heads and short bodies. Their fangs are erectile. Pit vipers, by virtue of a thermosensitive pit near the nose, can detect warm-blooded prey in the dark. Vipers are commoner than elapids in the tropics. They do not occur in the Pacific or Australian area.

Prevention

Although no snake will bite a human being unless provoked it is wise, in snake-infested country, never to reach up and put one hand on a rock or to step on a fallen log or approach a rough stone wall without testing-out first with a long stick. It is unwise to go into the jungle at night without boots, torch and stick. Beware of picking up a snake after ' killing ' it for it may only be stunned.

Diagnosis

Fang marks (Fig. 30.3) may be visible. As a snake only bites humans defensively a bite does not always mean poisoning. This only occurs in about one case in four and so it is important to decide whether it has taken place. If local signs are absent and the snake was recognised as a viper then poisoning can be excluded but generally identification of the snake is unimportant. The early signs of systemic poisoning are: viper—blood stained sputum and non-clotting blood (as tested in a capillary tube); elapid—ptosis and paralysis of swallowing; seasnake—myalgia and haemoglobinuria. Poisoning if it has occurred is usually evident by the time the doctor is seen.

Treatment

The victim may be seen in the latent period before symptoms begin and will be very frightened. Strong reassurance should be given and possibly a placebo injection (of tetanus toxoid). Local measures, beyond possibly immediate suction, are best avoided as they carry the risk of infection. Absorption of venom is very rapid but may be delayed by a promptly-applied tourniquet. This should be placed round the finger, arm or leg near to the bite and over the clothing if necessary. As venom is injected superficially and travels by lymphatics the tourniquet need not be very tight. Keep it on until other measures have been completed. If these last longer than an hour release it for a few seconds every half hour.

Antivenom (For sources of supply see p. 777.)

Although there is no antivenom for poisoning by coral snakes Australian tiger snake 'broad spectrum' antivenom is reported to be effective in sea-snake bite poisoning as well as in all types of neurotoxic poisoning. Haemolytic signs call for viperine antivenom. For neurotoxic signs without local swelling use mamba antivenom in Africa and krait antivenom in Asia. It may be easier to use a polyvalent serum. All antivenoms should be given by i v drip and the anaphylaxis tray (p. 745) should be ready. The response of the systemic effects to antivenom is prompt and dramatic even though it is not given until hours after the bite. For serious sea-snake bite poisoning up to 10 000 units of specific antivenom should be given i v.

General measures

Good nursing is of the greatest importance. The urine output must be carefully watched to detect acute renal failure. In elapid poisoning respiratory and circulatory failure (p. 6) may call for urgent measures. In severe viper poisoning blood transfusion can be life saving. As the victim often has ascorbic acid deficiency the effects of which are similar to those of venom it is reasonable (and harmless) to give vitamin C in large doses. Antihistamines are of no value and steroids have not been shown to help. Local necrosis may be extensive but it is nearly always confined to superficial tissues. Leaving the bitten area exposed without a dressing gives excellent results. If there is secondary infection antibiotics are indicated. Tetanus toxoid is recommended in all cases and has a reassuring effect if the victim does not know what was injected.

Spitting snakes

Certain kinds of cobra are able to eject their venom considerable distances and to aim it accurately. The patient usually sees the snake and almost immediately feels an intense burning in the eyes. Severe conjunctivitis results. Treatment consists in repeated irrigation with weak sodium bicarbonate solution or saline, and instillation of 4 per cent lignocaine eye-drops.

DOG AND CAT BITES
IN BRITAIN

The modern view is that a dog or cat bite should be treated like any other wound. It should be cleaned with soap and water but not scrubbed. Then it should be douched with hydrogen peroxide or cetrimide solution and covered with a dressing. It is advisable to give penicillin as bites are commonly infected by *Pasteurella septica*. Measures to prevent tetanus (p. 637) should be taken. For wound treatment to prevent rabies see p. 635.

OUTSIDE BRITAIN

Unfortunately rabies following a dog bite is still a possibility in many countries. Hence immediate treatment of the wound in an attempt to destroy the virus should be made. One per cent benzalkonium chloride (Roccal) is recommended and is better than fuming nitric acid which is very painful and may seal the virus deep in the wound. Injections of hyperimmune rabies serum (p. 767) round the bite are advised.

RABIES

Rabies is unlikely to be contracted at present in Britain but could occur from smuggled animals and from travellers who have been infected abroad. Workers in quarantine kennels and veterinary laboratories and those handling exotic animals are at risk and should receive rabies vaccine prophylactically. No one has died of rabies contracted in Britain since 1903 and all the ten fatal human cases in England since 1946 were infected abroad. Some 40 patients (and 12 000 dogs) die of it each year in U.S.A. where because of the ever increasing reservoir of infected wild animals (vampire bats, etc) it cannot be eradicated. Since the air of bat-infested caves may contain the virus the disease may be acquired without being bitten. Three foci of rabies exist on the Continent of Europe: (1) in the far north in silver foxes, (2) in Central Europe in the common fox (' wildfire rabies '), (3) in south-east Europe in wild and domestic animals (dogs) (' urban rabies ') but the disease is spreading nearer to the Channel Ports in wild animals. Cases may be expected in Britain when quarantine regulations are infringed or if the insectivorous bat now known to transmit rabies should cross the Channel. In 1974 213 animals were detected being illegally landed here. In these days of rapid travel persons infected when abroad may develop the disease here. Vaccination of animals against rabies is possible but is illegal in Britain.

Prevention of rabies in Britain depends on quarantine. Vaccination of animals may only be used on either an animal in quarantine to prevent cross infection or on an animal to be exported to meet the importing country's regulations. The sole distributors of rabies vaccine in Britain are Pharmaceutical Specialties (May & Baker) Ltd., Dagenham, Essex, RM10 7X2.

Treatment

Once symptoms have appeared rabies in man is almost invariably fatal. Symptomless or inapparent infections have been described in animals and there is some serological evidence that they may occasionally occur in man. Only one case, a boy aged 6, is known for certain to have survived rabies. He was found bitten by a bat which was captured. The wound was washed and vaccines started. Symptoms including coma developed but recovery was complete. The bat was proved to be rabid.

Prevention

It is a good rule for a traveller never to befriend any animal when abroad.

The bite of a possibly rabid animal always raises the urgent question of prophylaxis. In 95 per cent of human cases a dog bite is the cause but many other animals including cats, wolves, jackals and vampire bats may act as vectors of the virus. Saliva is the usual medium of infection and so this may result not only from biting but also when dogs lick fresh wounds, the abraded skin or mucosal surfaces. Attendants may be similarly affected by patients. Urine and CSF can also convey the virus. Rabies virus has been found in the milk and meat from a rabid animal.

Since specific treatment is not entirely innocuous (very rarely there are neurotoxic sequelae due not to the virus but to the animal tissue in which it is grown) the important question to answer is: ' Is the dog rabid?'

A rabid dog shows changes in disposition, becoming either morose or irritable. The bark changes. The dog is easily startled and appears ill. In this ' furious stage ' it will snap viciously at anything in its path. Later it has convulsions and paralysis. A rabid dog is infective for not more than four days before it develops symptoms after which it dies within six days. When possible, therefore, a suspected animal should be caged. If it survives 10 days it could not have been rabid at the time of biting. Modern fluorescent antibody techniques can show the virus even within 24 hours.

It is best not to kill a possibly rabid dog immediately but if circumstances demand it chloroform should be used and not violence. If a post-mortem has been made and rabies is suspected the head and neck should be wrapped in a cloth wrung out in 1 in 1 000 corrosive sublimate and sent to the Public Health Laboratory at

London, Newcastle, Liverpool or Cardiff (p. 776). Alternatively the whole body may be sent but in either case the regulations concerning sending pathological specimens by post (p. 698) must be strictly observed. Further advice can be obtained from the appropriate government health department (see Appendix 1, p. 764).

When any person is bitten by a dog or other animal *thought to be suffering from rabies* the wound should be washed at once with soap and water and a course of antirabies treatment started at the earliest possible moment without even waiting for confirmation of the diagnosis. The most important post-exposure treatment is to give human hyperimmune gamma globulin 15-40 i u/kg i v. This will ensure the production of antibody titres within 24 hours. If the animal is later found not to have rabies the full course of treatment need not be completed. This advice applies in particular to persons exposed to rabies abroad. In Britain the dog population is free from rabies at present so that vaccination is not ordinarily recommended.

The incubation period of rabies varies from two weeks to several months or even a year. It is usually 60 days, and depends on the virulence of the virus, and the site, severity and the amount of laceration caused by the bite. If a person is developing rabies this is shown by non-specific malaise. Pain and paraesthesia of the bitten area should make one suspicious. ' Furious ' rabies is shown by hydrophobia and ' dumb ' rabies by progressive flaccid paralysis. If seen within 24 hours of a bite the lesions should be thoroughly cleansed, preferably with soap solution or certrimide, each tooth wound being thoroughly flushed. Deep fang punctures should be irrigated and then probed with a swab dipped in Roccal (p. 633). The wound should not be sutured. Although of doubtful value the surrounding tissues may be infiltrated with antiserum. Tetanus prevention measures should be adopted (p. 637). When there is adequate reason to suspect a rabies infection vaccine treatment should be started without delay. Excess of antigen is needed to lessen any suppression of antibody production by the gamma globulin already given. The half life of this is 21 days and vaccine given early will produce an immune response about then. Hyperimmune serum when given together with a killed-type vaccine gives better results than vaccine treatment alone. Twelve to 21 daily subcutaneous injections of vaccine into the abdominal wall should be given together with antiserum on the first and second days. The serum should be used together with a vaccine in all cases of infection in the head region, and whenever there are extensive lacerated injuries. The serum given alone has an obvious potential value if the start of vaccine treatment has unavoidably to be delayed. Duck embryo vaccine is given and also serum concurrently during the first few days according to the probable intensity of the initial infection. Doses will be indicated on the material sent. Neurological complications of this vaccine are rare. The total dose should not be less than 40 international units per kg body weight. For sources of supply see p. 767. There is promise of an improved (two dose) regimen (Institut Merieux). Those nursing the patient with rabies must be free from minor cuts and abrasions and must take full precautions (rubber gloves and masks). The ' kiss of life ' must not be given to a patient moribund from rabies.

HUMAN BITES

These generally occur on the hands because the closed fist is hit against the teeth. The tendon carries infection upwards when the hand is opened if the sheath is lacerated. These bites should therefore be treated with great respect.

Measures to prevent tetanus (p. 637) should be taken. Suturing should be avoided and a surgeon's advice sought.

CAMEL BITES

These, though rare, are mentioned because of their special features. The supercilious, benign expression of the camel does not warn us against his bite. Because of his peculiar dentition (hook teeth) he can and does inflict severe crushing and avulsion injuries because the camel twists the arm just as he does the twigs of a tree. Prevention lies in avoiding a camel (male or female) at the rutting season especially if his nose is ringed. Treatment is on general (surgical) lines including tetanus prevention.

PARAPHIMOSIS

The normal prepuce reduces itself after retraction but if it is tight (phimosis) and not reduced it forms a constricting band with swelling of the glans beyond (paraphimosis) (Fig. 30.4). This is rare in children for the prepuce is not fully retractable before the age of two years. More often it follows sexual intercourse after a drinking bout for the patient forgets to pull the prepuce forwards. If seen early reduction is possible by simply squeezing the glans with one hand while the other eases the foreskin forwards. More severe cases are best dealt with by injecting the oedematous ring in four places with hyaluronidase 1 500 units in 4 ml of lignocaine 1 g/dl.

The penis is then wrapped in gauze wrung out in iced water and compressed by the hand for 10 minutes. Reduction is then usually easy but failure is an indication to try again. Sometimes a general anaesthetic is needed. If manual reduction is impossible the constricting band must be cut putting a grooved director under it first and avoiding the vessels in the midline. When the swelling has subsided a circumcision should be done.

TRISMUS

The urgency of trismus depends upon the fact that tetanus may be the cause, particularly if it is painless. If this is suspected treatment for tetanus must be started at once. Trismus of a few days' duration may set up an intense stomatitis. The danger then is that the trismus may be attributed to the foul mouth and not to tetanus and so urgent treatment may be delayed.

TETANUS

Probably between 150 and 200 cases of tetanus occur in England and Wales each year. They are medical emergencies with surgical aspects in that there is a wound, the commonest being a penetrating one of the hand. This may, however, be slight—a scratch or a small puncture from a nail (or needle in a drug addict) and can have healed by the time symptoms appear. Scab formation aids the development of tetanus. Hence tetanus may be unsuspected. Trismus ('lockjaw') and stiffness of the neck are usually the first symptoms followed by rigidity of the abdominal and thoracic muscles (a negative laparotomy is sometimes done) (p. 126). After an interval reflex spasms or convulsions may develop. Trismus or stiffness can have other causes and tetanus is unlikely if the patient has received active immunisation with tetanus toxoid within the previous five years. The likely severity can be gauged either from the incubation period, when known (under seven days it may be severe; over 14 days the prognosis is good); or from the period of onset, that is, the interval between the first symptoms and the first reflex spasm—the chances increase with each day that spasms are delayed after the first three days.

PREVENTION

Treament of wounds

Wounds and burns which call for tetanus prevention are: (1) those more than three or four hours old (especially if contaminated

22

by dirt), (2) penetrating wounds, (3) those which contain devitalised tissue or foreign bodies.

All contaminated wounds should be excised, however small. This applies particularly to penetrating wounds of the hands and feet. In all these cases order tetracycline 250 mg six-hourly for five days or crystalline penicillin (1 mega unit for adults) by i m injection daily for five days.

Immunological treatment

1. IMMUNE PERSONS. These are people who are definitely known to have received a full course of injections of tetanus vaccine (e.g. Service personnel). They require a booster dose of 0·5 ml tetanus vaccine (adsorbed) at once but they do not need tetanus antitoxin. They may be wearing a Medic-Alert bracelet or necklet (p. 822) saying ' Has had tetanus toxoid '.

2. NON-IMMUNE PERSONS. Those who are not known to have been given any tetanus vaccine previously are treated as non-immune. They should be given immediate protection by human antitetanus immunoglobulin (Humotet, Wellcome) 250 units (1 ml). Protection lasts four weeks as, unlike antitoxin of horse origin, Humotet is not rapidly metabolised. The warnings about the use of antitoxin of horse origin do not apply to Humotet. At the same time but in a different site the first dose (0·5 ml) of tetanus vaccine (adsorbed) should be given subcutaneously. (Intradermal injection does not provide an adequate stimulus and may cause a granuloma.) This course should be given to all non-immune persons irrespective of the assessment of the wound.

If only antitoxin of horse origin is available it must be avoided if there is a history of asthma, eczema or hay fever or if the patient has previously been given horse antitoxin. (In any case second and subsequent doses of horse antitoxin are ineffective as they are rapidly destroyed by the body.) If horse antitoxin has to be used then a test dose of 0·2 ml should be given subcutaneously. If sensitivity is shown it is wise to abandon the use of this antitoxin. Horse antitoxin should only be given after consultation with a senior colleague.

Full immunisation necessitates three doses of tetanus vaccine (adsorbed), the second and third doses being given after intervals of four to six weeks and six months. Every patient given a first dose of vaccine should receive a card indicating the dates on which subsequent doses are due.

DEGREES OF SEVERITY

Cole and Youngman* (1969) have shown the importance of assessing the severity of the illness and of placing the patient in one of three groups. It may be too late to save the patient once serious spasms begin. Their criteria are as follows:

Grade 1. Mild

Incubation period (injury to first symptom) over 14 days.
Period of onset (first symptoms to first spasm if any) over six days.
Trismus present but not severe.
Difficulty in eating and drinking—due to trismus not dysphagia.
Localised stiffness may occur (a) alone (b) preceding generalised rigidity by hours or days. This is ' local tetanus '.
Generalised spasms if present are short not violent, not interfering with breathing and slow to get worse.

Grade 2. Moderate

Incubation period 10 to 14 days.
Period of onset from over three to six days.
Trismus marked.
Dysphagia i.e. swallowing with choking or inability to swallow often present.
Rigidity generalised from the start. Vital capacity reduced.
Minute volume normal at rest.
Reflex spasms become more violent and frequent for several days but do not cause severe dyspnoea or cyanosis.

Grade 3. Severe

Incubation period under 10 days.
Period of onset three days or less.
Trismus and dysphagia severe, the latter causing aspiration of saliva and food or regurgitation early in the disease. It commonly occurs during the urgent inspiration at the end of a spasm. Rigidity may limit breathing and cause continuous asphyxia. Acute or chronic asphyxia is the commonest cause of death.
In severe tetanus there is over activity of the sympathetic nervous system with profuse sweating, salivation, hyperpyrexia, tachycardia, hypertension, arrhythmia and peripheral vasoconstriction.

Treatment (For special centres see p. 790.)

The severity of the illness must be decided early by using the above criteria. Detailed notes must be kept so that the grade of severity can be reassessed if need be. The patient must never be left alone.

All patients must be given antitoxin (up to 100 000 units for an adult) preferably as Humotet. The veto on antitoxin in persons who have received horse serum previously must be waived when it has to be used for the *treatment* of tetanus. (See p. 745 for precautions.)

---

* COLE, L. & YOUNGMAN, H. (1969). Treatment of tetanus. *Lancet,* **1,** 1017.

Grade 1. Mild

Treatment is by antitoxin and general nursing measures with sedation, feeding (by nasogastric tube if need be) and measures to prevent secondary infection. There may be the need for extensive surgical toilet of the wound. Elderly patients generally have dysphagia and so should be placed in Grade 2.

Grade 2. Moderate

Treatment is for a Grade 1 case plus tracheostomy by cuffed tube under general anaesthesia and feeding by nasogastric tube. The respiratory minute volume and blood pressure should be monitored every half hour at first.

Grade 3. Severe

Here rigidity and severe spasms call for curarisation (adult dose *d*-tubocurarine 15 to 20 mg) and artificial ventilation using preferably a positive pressure artificial ventilator and an air filter. Repeated doses of *d*-tubocurarine may be needed every 20 minutes if there is any sign of returning muscular activity. Emptying the bladder by catheter and the rectum by finger is necessary.

Sedation

Barbiturates, tranquillisers and opiates are all contraindicated because they may exaggerate respiratory embarrassment. The safest drug is paraldehyde (p. 755) up to 12 ml every four hours by stomach tube (diluted 1 in 10) or neat by i m injection (p. 54). Too heavy sedation carries the risk of making a severe case appear mild.

An attack of tetanus does not necessarily confer immunity and so survivors should be actively immunised with toxoid.

Lest anyone is tempted to give antitoxin intrathecally a warning is given that this route leads to complications in the central nervous system.

MISCELLANEOUS MISHAPS
THE FIXED WEDDING RING

A not uncommon emergency is caused by a wedding or other ring which cannot be removed and which causes swelling or even ulceration of the finger. Occasionally the real cause of trouble is a forgotten tight rubber band which has slipped under the ring. So look for this first. Division of the ring by cutters or a Gigli saw is often performed but most women have a sentimental objection to such methods which sacrifice the ring. The following simple method using a piece of string is very effective and should be tried first.

Beginning near the distal interphalangeal joint fine string is wound tightly round the finger up to the ring and the end hooked under it by a curved needle or pushed under by a match stick (Fig. 30.5). The end is then pulled towards the finger tip and as it unwinds the ring comes with it since the string provides a pull at an infinite number of points. Wedding rings come off well but rings with stones require patience and manipulation in the unwinding process.

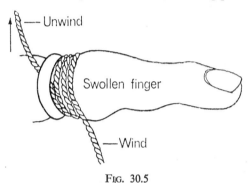

FIG. 30.5
How to remove a fixed wedding ring.

If this method fails 1 500 international units of hyaluronidase in 1 ml or procaine 1 g/dl should be injected into the finger and massaged a little. Then a length of thin rubber tubing should be wrapped round the finger from the tip up to and including the ring and left in place for five minutes. This will often reduce the swelling sufficiently to permit the ring to be drawn off or the string method to be used successfully.

FISHHOOK INJURIES

The treatment of these injuries may have to be undertaken by any doctor on a fishing holiday. To remove a fish hook there are two methods: pushing through and backing out. For each some local anaesthetic may be injected parallel to the shaft of the hook. If the hook has entered and come out again grasp the point and barb with a needle holder and withdraw the hook. It is often advisable to cut off the barb and also the eye first. If the hook has not quite emerged it can be pushed onwards and then dealt with as described. Backing out is best reserved for a hook which has come up under bone or a finger nail. The shaft should be moved up and down to disengage the barb. Then placing the shank parallel to the skin the fibres holding the barb can be cut and the hook extracted. Sometimes removal is easier if a small haemostat is pushed along the track and snapped on to the barb. If the hook impinges on cartilage as in the nose or ear it is best to push it through as backing out would be difficult. Similarly in the eyelid pushing through is best because backing out might tear the tissues badly. Backing out may be achieved rapidly by using a piece of string as shown in Fig. 30.6. Pass a loop of string over the hook and hold it close to the

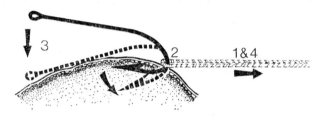

FIG. 30.6
Removal of fishhook.

skin with the index finger of the left hand (1 and 2). Depress the eye end of the hook (3) and hold it close to the skin with the middle finger and thumb of the left hand to disengage the hook. Take the string in the right hand and give it a sharp pull (4) to remove the hook through the entry point. Tetanus prophylaxis (p. 637) should be used.

CHEWING GUM ON THE EYELIDS

A minor emergency is caused when a playful child closes another's eyes with chewing gum. Removal pulls out eyelashes; most gum solvents injure the lids and cutting the eyelashes is mutilating and undesirable. Coconut oil is used to clean gum from machines in the chewing gum factory but as it is not usually at hand cocoa butter in the form of milk chocolate can be used instead. It will soften and plasticise chewing gum. So melt some in hot water and work it into the eyelids. The gum can then be washed off with soap and water. Several applications may be needed to get rid of all traces.

DENTAL EMERGENCIES*

The doctor may have to extract teeth and give other urgent dental treatment when a dentist is not at hand.

---

* SEWARD, G. R. (1966). Emergency dentistry for the general practitioner. 1. Pain from dental disease. 2. Treatment of the primary conditions causing pain. *British Medical Journal*, **2**, 509, 567.

TOOTHACHE

This has three main causes:

1. PULP INFECTION. This occurs secondarily to a cavity, and the tissues surrounding the tooth are normal. Gentle probing will usually elicit which tooth is affected.

Treatment. Unless the infection is gross, an attempt should be made to fill the cavity. Clean it out with a spoon excavator after an injection of 1 to 2 ml of procaine 2 g/dl round the tooth. Swab the cavity with oil of cloves and fill it with zinc oxide mixed with two or three drops of oil of cloves or Eugenol. This will relieve pain temporarily.

2. PERIODONTITIS. This occurs secondarily to pulpitis. The tooth is tender on pressure, raised in its socket, and pus may appear round it.

Treatment. Give very hot mouth washes, holding the liquid by the tongue around the tooth. Never apply hot fomentations to the cheek lest the abscess be caused to point externally. Extraction is often necessary when pus is present, and should always be done under general anaesthetic, injections into infected tissues being dangerous.

3. INFECTION ROUND ERUPTING LOWER WISDOM TEETH (pericoronitis). The patient complains of a dull pain, sometimes associated with trismus; there may be an inflamed gum flap over the tooth. Mouthwashes should be given and the flap painted with Weak Solution of Iodine BP.

ULCERATIVE GINGIVITIS (VINCENT'S ANGINA)

This is characterised by sore and bleeding gums, and sometimes tonsillitis is present also.

Treatment. In the acute phase stop brushing the teeth and discard the old toothbrush. Clean the teeth with cotton wool and wash the mouth out with Dettol or hydrogen peroxide thrice daily. Give penicillin i m or metronidazole (Flagyl) 200 mg three times a day by mouth for a week. A further measure is to apply chromic acid 10 g/dl carefully to the gums around the teeth on pledgets of cottonwool. Follow this with hydrogen peroxide similarly applied. Black chromic oxide is immediately produced and should be allowed to remain in the tissues for about a minute, following which a further peroxide mouthwash should be given.

THE BLEEDING TOOTH SOCKET

The bleeding tooth socket not infrequently causes the hospital resident to be summoned urgently. Sometimes a tendency to bleed because of treatment by anticoagulants, oestrogens and salicylates has been overlooked. More often there is a local cause. Removal of clot by excessive mouth washing is sometimes responsible. In the usual case the procedure is as follows. Reassure the patient and, if necessary, give him a sedative such as Valium 2 mg (diazepam). Sit him up and clear his mouth of loose clots, using cottonwool and isosmotic sodium chloride solution. Verify the site of bleeding. Make a roll of guaze like a cigar and put it across the socket. Tell the patient to bite on this. A bandage may be used to keep the jaws together. After 20 minutes remove the gauze gently. This is usually all that is necessary as the bleeding was capillary in origin. If bleeding continues the source is a lacerated gum or a vessel in the socket. If from the gum inject 2 g/dl procaine on each side and put in a horizontal suture of nylon or silk to draw the gum margins together. It is well to trim any sharp edges of bone first. If bleeding is from a vessel in the socket packing is necessary. Gauze soaked in Adrenaline Solution BP 1 in 1 000 may be used but absorbable hydrophilic dressing (Orahesive, Squibb) is better as it does not have to be removed. If oozing persists despite local measures and there is no blood dyscrasia a systemic haemostatic may be given; either Dicynene (ethamsylate) two tablets three or four times a day or Epsikapron (p. 285).

The approach should be rather different in a patient who is a known or suspected bleeder. Tight plugging and suturing should be avoided. A piece of Calgitex gauze soaked in thrombin solution should be put in the cavity and held in position by Orahesive. Anything more drastic should be avoided, but the patient may be transfused (see Haemophilia, p. 279).

ACUTE ARTHRITIS

This may present as an emergency when it strikes in circumstances which render the patient incapable of continuing to walk or use his arm or drive his car. The commonest examples of such urgent happenings are gout in the big toe (podagra) and an acute exacerbation of rheumatoid arthritis in the knees or elbows. Fortunately these large joints are the easiest to inject.

Acute rheumatoid arthritis of the knees and elbows

The best emergency measure for these joints is the intra-articular injection of 5 to 50 mg, according to the joint, of hydrocortisone acetate or up to 40 mg of a long-acting steroid methylprednisolone (Depo-Medrone), (40 mg/ml) using a 30 mm 63/100 needle. The injections can be given in any room provided a no-touch technique is used. A face mask should be worn and the hands scrubbed. The patient's skin should be swabbed with Hibitane (1 in 200 chlorhexidine in spirit 70 per cent v/v. An injection of lignocaine 2 g/dl may be given into the skin and subcutaneous tissues but this, in the case of the knee, is not always necessary. It is best to restrict movement of the joint for 24 hours after the injection. If fluid is encountered as much should be removed as comes easily but more should not be sought lest the cartilage be scratched.

The knee

With the joint relaxed and slightly flexed enter the needle 1 or 2 cm from the medial border of the patella and direct it outwards

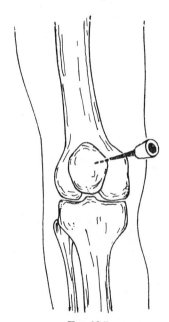

FIG. 30.7
The right knee extended. Antero-medial approach.

and backwards between the patella and medial femoral condyle (Fig. 30.7). It is not quite so easy from the lateral side. If osteophytes make this injection difficult then the knee should be flexed

to 90° and the needle inserted through the outer or inner part of
the tendon below the patella and directed backwards and slightly
upwards (Fig. 30.8). An alternative site for obtaining fluid (and
synovium for biopsy) is the supra-patellar pouch. The needle is
directed through the quadriceps muscle on either side of its insertion

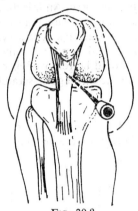

FIG. 30.8
The right knee flexed. Infra-patellar, antero-medial approach.

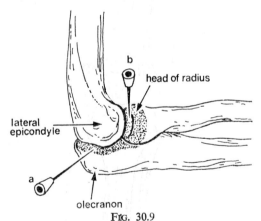

FIG. 30.9
The right elbow flexed. The stippled area shows the synovial membrane.

(Figs. 30.7, 30.8, 30.9 from Cawley, M. I. D. (1974) in *British Journal of
Hospital Medicine*, **3**, No. 5, p. 744. By courtesy of the author and editor.)

into the patella. Other bursae round the knee may call for injection.
The semi-membranosus bursa is not normally continuous with the
joint cavity and presents as a swelling in the popliteal fossa. After

its careful palpation on the postero-medial aspect of the knee joint a needle may be directed into it. Needling through the popliteal space should be avoided and is not needed for bursae which are continuous with the joint.

The elbow

Let the patient sit with his elbow resting on a table and flexed to 90°. Find the gap between the lower end of the lateral humeral condyle and the olecranon (Fig. 30.9). Insert the same needle as for the knee here and direct it anteromedially into the joint. Inject the steroid when the humero-ulnar joint space is entered. The humero-radial and superior radio-ulnar joint spaces are continuous with that of the humero-ulnar joint. If it is preferred to enter them separately the head of the radius is easy to feel and the joint is easily entered. When the olecranon bursa is involved it can be entered by a direct approach.

For help with other joints the reader is referred to an article on Arthrodesis in the *British Journal of Hospital Medicine* 1974, vol. II, page 74, by M. I. D. Cawley.

ACUTE GOUT

The pain of gout, commonly in the big toe, may be so severe as to occasion an emergency call. Colchicine, the traditional remedy, often caused diarrhoea and vomiting before pain was relieved. It has been replaced by indomethacin 50 mg immediately and 25 mg every two hours for four doses or until acute symptoms are relieved and then 100 to 150 mg a day. An alternative is phenylbutazone 200 mg a day for two days. This can be given i m if need be. Other measures are to spray the joint with a cooling spray of chloro-fluoromethane and to protect it from even trivial trauma by a cage. Corticotrophin (ACTH) may help but should be avoided during a remission as it may precipitate an acute attack. The metatarso-phalangeal joint of the big toe does not often call for treatment by injection of steroids but needling may be done to obtain material to confirm the diagnosis by finding crystals. It should be made on the dorsal surface on one or other side of the extensor tendon. Because of pain inhalation of Entonox (p. 577) may be necessary.

Pseudo-gout (synovitis and chondrocalcinosis caused by calcium pyro-phosphate) affects larger joints than true gout. It is best managed by joint aspiration and injection of prednisone. A common error is to diagnose septic arthritis in a case of pseudo-gout. Crystals should be looked for in the aspirated fluid.

ACUTE BERIBERI

Acute deficiency of vitamin B_1 causing beri beri rarely occurs in Britain but may be seen in the Far East where polished rice is the staple diet. The common manifestations of peripheral neuropathy and oedema do not cause urgent symptoms but the rarer cardiac and cerebral syndromes may present as emergencies either unheralded or in a patient known to have chronic beriberi.

ACUTE HEART FAILURE. The fulminating cardiac form of this deficiency disease is known by the Japanese term Shöshin beriberi (Sho = damage; shin = heart). Usually in a patient with chronic beriberi any cause for increased vitamin B_1 requirement such as fever and increased carbohydrate intake will precipitate acute cardiac failure. Sometimes muscular work in hot weather brings it on. The patient is very ill with a rapid regular enlarging heart, epigastric discomfort and great respiratory distress (see p. 229). Sometimes there is hoarseness caused by pressure on the recurrent laryngeal nerve by the dilated left auricle.

CEREBRAL SYMPTOMS. In addition to general symptoms such as loss of appetite, vomiting and insomnia the patient is confused and shows loss of memory for recent events with pseudo-reminiscences (Korsakow's syndrome). Mid-brain damage shows as oculomotor palsies and nystagmus (Wernicke's encephalopathy).

Treatment

Thiamine (vitamin B_1) 100 mg should be given i v at once either alone or with other B vitamins (Parentrovite, Bencard) and then 50 mg daily by mouth. The response of the heart is often dramatic but improvement in the cerebral signs is slow and may not be complete. The diet should contain 30 g of yeast each day.

ELECTROCUTION

The effects of an electric current on the body depend not only upon its amperage but also on the duration of the shock, the current pathway and the skin resistance. The most important effects from the emergency point of view are on the nervous system—coma and bulbar palsy. Burns and fractures may also occur. The patient may also be unconscious, pulseless, and apnoeic and appear to be dead.

About 100 persons lose their lives in England and Wales each year from electrocution. Many more receive non-fatal shocks from faulty wiring of domestic apparatus. Most fatal accidents occur in the voltage range 200 to 250. Water lowers skin resistance—hence the danger of electrocution in the bath. The doctor may be consulted after a minor shock and should be able to offer intelligent advice. The serious risk of electrocution and personal experience of cases prompts me to set out some elementary technical facts about electrical wiring, even in a book of this kind.

Many assume that because apparatus connected to a plug socket can be switched off at the socket it is therefore safe. It is only safe if there is a double pole switch on the lead to the apparatus or if the wall switch is wired in such a way that it breaks the live (brown) wire to the switch and not the neutral (blue) wire. The wiring can be easily tested by using a lamp in an insulated holder with a short

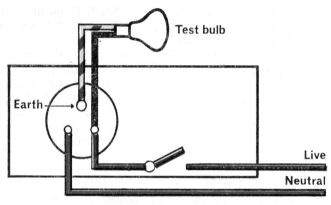

Fig. 30.10
Diagram showing electric lighting circuit being tested

length of flex connected to it. Not more than a quarter of an inch of wire should be bare at the end of each piece of flex. Push the test lamp leads into the 3-pin plug sockets as follows: one into the earth socket of a 3-pin plug and the other into one of the supply sockets. (If a 2-pin socket is being tested one lead from the test lamp must be connected to a convenient water pipe.) If the lamp does not light when switched on at the wall socket change the lead over to the other supply socket and try again. If the switch is correctly placed in the live wire (Fig. 30.10) the lamp will light when the switch is on and go out when the switch is off. If the lamp lights with the switch both on and off, then the supply socket is wrongly wired. Any apparatus connected to it will be ' live ' to earth even when switched off. In this dangerous condition the heating element of a fire, for example, would be alive at full mains voltage, even when switched off and cold. If touched, it could give a fatal shock. (If the lamp will not light at all when connected to earth and to either of the supply sockets and the switch is on, this is also a dangerous state, for it means that the earth socket is not connected to earth. If the apparatus developed an insulation fault the whole framework could become alive.) In testing, a small insulated screwdriver containing a neon bulb and a high-value resistor can be used instead of a lamp holder as it indicates a live point without the use of external wires.

Treatment

Switch off the current. If this would take too long pull the victim away or push him away with a broom-stick. Pad the hands with dry clothing or wear gloves while doing this. If found in contact with or near a high voltage cable or rail call the engineer; otherwise there may be two victims instead of one.

Carry out artificial respiration (for method and duration see page 732). Death is now known to occur in many cases from circulatory rather than respiratory arrest and so if the carotid pulse is absent proceed as indicated on p. 724. Give Nikethamide Injection BP 2 ml i m repeatedly, and apply warmth. If the patient remains comatose but is breathing, or if breathing does not establish itself, lumbar puncture, and removal of 5 to 10 ml cerebrospinal fluid is advisable.

Micro-ampère Electrocution

Faulty earthing of electrical apparatus can cause small leakage currents—180 μA—which if they pass through the heart can cause fatal ventricular fibrillation. As there is no objective evidence the death may be put down to natural causes.

LIGHTNING

During a thunderstorm it is best to stay inside with doors and windows closed. Keep away from the fireplace, the main electric switch and the wireless aerial. The telephone is safe to use being fitted with lightning arresters and fuses at both ends. If out of doors take refuge in a substantial building or closed (metal) car but keep away from crowds. Avoid solitary trees, walls, wire fences, ponds and river banks. Throw down your golf clubs. If in an open space it is best to keep moving. This is because a column of warm air rises from a stationary body and acts as a conductor. It is possible for a lightning stroke to kill several people or animals at a distance. The potential between two points is the product of the current times resistance (Ohm's Law) and conditions may be such that there is a considerable voltage drop between the legs of a man or animal.

This causes a current to flow between them which can be fatal. It is safer to be thoroughly soaked than to be dry since wet clothing may reduce the current which flows through the body sufficiently to prevent fatal injury. A person struck by lightning falls unconscious at once. He does not see the flash. No electric charge remains in his body and so he may be approached safely.

*Treatment**

In most cases apnoea and cardiac arrest are temporary but if the victim is not breathing spontaneously within a minute of the strike mouth-to-mouth artificial respiration (p. 732) and external cardiac massage (p. 725) must be started. Fixed dilated pupils and failure to hear heart sounds after a lightning strike do not indicate death. The heart can tick over inaudibly in these cases. As resuscitation may have to go on for several hours the patient should be moved to hospital. Blood gases should be measured and kept within normal limits. Temporary flaccid paralysis of the legs is common and requires no special treatment. Acute hysteria may demand emergency measures (p. 308).

HANGING

Death from hanging usually results from asphyxia. The heart continues to beat for some minutes after respiration ceases and it is wise to try artificial respiration, particularly if the person is found within five minutes of suspension. Recovery will be precluded if, as in judicial hanging, there has been a ' drop ', because this dislocates the cervical vertebrae.

DROWNING (see also p. 490)

Of the 1 327 deaths from drowning in the United Kingdom in 1971 290 were suicidal. One quarter of the rest occurred in the sea and three quarters in inland waters. About 20 per cent of deaths following immersion are due to asphyxia from glottic spasm (' dry drowning '). Fresh water entering the lungs is rapidly absorbed. Resulting haemolysis with potassium release causes ventricular fibrillation. Salt water is not absorbed but causes exudation of protein-rich fluid into the alveoli. These interesting differences are not of great practical importance in treatment. About one quarter of rescued victims die later from pneumonitis and metabolic acidosis (' secondary drowning '). A few deaths result from vagal inhibition

---

* For a review of management see HANSON, GILLIAN C. & MCILWRAITH, G. R. (1973). Lightning injury. *British Medical Journal*, **4**, 271.

caused by sudden impact with cold water (immersion syndrome). Death can follow the bad habit of hyperventilating before diving because it lowers $PaCO_2$ and constricts cerebral arterioles. Cerebral hypoxia follows when oxygen is used up before the $PaCO_2$ is sufficient to stimulate breathing. Fish stings, cramp and painful injuries such as a prolapsed intervertebral disc may all play a part in the causation of death from drowning.

Treatment

Artificial respiration by the mouth-to-mouth method (p. 732) must be started in the boat or as soon as the victim is landed. *Literally not one second must be wasted.* It must go on without interruption for at least 15 minutes and only then should any attention be paid (preferably by another person) to such measures as loosening clothes, listening to the heart and so on. A few breaths in the first few seconds will do more than pure oxygen through a perfect airway could do 10 seconds later. It is not possible to drain water from the lungs so time should not be wasted in attempting to do this. If the heart has stopped measures for circulatory arrest must be started (pp. 724 and 730).

When recovery is occurring the movements of artificial respiration must be timed to coincide with the patient's breathing. Watch must be kept for recurrence of respiratory failure. Excessive stimulation may be dangerous. Pure oxygen should not be given except during artificial respiration. When breathing returns the victim should be turned on his side to lessen the work of breathing. The right side should be uppermost as this position lessens the risk of regurgitation. As soon as possible the patient should be removed to hospital. Some would use hypertonic saline in patients rescued from fresh water together with exchange transfusion to lower the potassium level. Isotonic solutions (dextrose 5 g/dl) should be given to those taken from the sea but a plasma expander is probably of more value.

When a person recovered from the water is obviously dead and an autopsy is held two important specimens should be obtained before they are spoiled. These are: (1) peripheral lung and stomach contents for algae, and (2) blood from the right and left ventricles to show differences in electrolyte concentrations.

'WINDING'

This is usually a footballer's injury when a blow in the epigastrium stimulates the solar plexus and causes inhibition of respiration, fall of blood pressure and perhaps loss of consciousness. Recovery has usually occurred before a doctor is called, but if it is slow the limbs should be raised and massaged towards the heart. Atropine 0·6 mg should be injected and failing this Nikethamide Injection BP 2 ml.

More often a blow on the lower chest causes spasm of the diaphragm and inability to breathe properly so the victim struggles to get air. If normal breathing is not quickly established artificial respiration should be used.

FAT EMBOLISM

This is a major cause of death following soon after fractures but it is probably often masked by an anaesthetic or the signs of injury. The mechanism of death is hypoxia secondary to the effects of pulmonary fat emboli. Fat emboli are found in the lungs of over 90 per cent of patients dying after a recent fracture but in most cases these histological emboli are silent. A suggested cause is the pressure rise in the femoral shaft caused by packing in of acrylic bone cement after reaming without release holes.

In the classical case the patient is admitted to hospital after a rough journey with his fracture not fully immobilised. About 24 hours later he shows symptoms of cerebral damage—confusion and restlessness going on to coma. In some cases the main feature is failure to recover from the anaesthetic. Fat globules enter the veins and so reach the lungs (pulmonary type) where they cause dyspnoea, cyanosis, cough with frothy sputum and moist sounds. Although some fat globules may pass through the lungs and reach the systemic circulation it seems that the main cause of cerebral symptoms is hypoxia caused by fat in the lungs. X-ray films show a ' snowstorm ' lung. Frozen sections of clotted blood may show neutral fat. Blood gas analysis will show low PaO_2. Skin, conjunctival and retinal petchiae occur later. Fat globules may appear in the urine. Since they float only the last drops may show them (on a stained slide). A platinum loopful of urine is said to sizzle in a Bunsen flame. These are all late signs and the diagnosis should be suspected earlier. Sometimes only a partial syndrome occurs without respiratory signs and shows pyrexia with cerebral symptoms or a few petechiae.

Treatment

Preventive measures are the use of a tourniquet during operations on bones, complete immobilisation of fractures and elevation of limbs. The aim of treatment is to prevent cerebral damage from hypoxia. Tracheostomy and intermittent positive pressure respiration may be needed. Cerebral oxygen need may be reduced and cerebral oedema prevented by hypothermia and the use of a ' lytic cocktail ' (p. 729). Dextran and phenoxybenzamine (Dibenyline) (p. 240) should be considered to combat poor tissue perfusion from shock.

Treatment of two other aspects of fat embolism deserve consideration. There is evidence that some fat embolic globules arise not from the bone marrow but from altered stability of blood lipids after injury. Clofibrate (Atromid-S) 250 mg capsules, six daily, will reduce lipaemia. To reduce the exudative reaction to fat in the lungs i v hydrocortisone should be used.

FROSTBITE

This only happens when the part is dry and the air temperature is well below zero. Unless precautions are taken frostbite can easily occur during flight as the temperature falls 2°C for every 305 metres above sea level until a temperature of minus 55°C is reached, when it remains constant. An early stage is ' frost nip ' which shows as a hard white patch on the skin detected in ' making a face '. Normal colour will soon return if the part is protected from the wind and warmed by the hand. When ice crystals form in the tissues the condition is frostbite. The nose, ears and hands are the common sites affected (Fig. 30.11). At minus 35°C contact of the skin with a metal surface in the presence of moisture produces instantaneous frostbite of a severity comparable with that of a second degree burn of similar extent. Frostbite has occurred when a little N_2O has remained in an open frosted cylinder and has rapidly expanded and cooled when the cylinder was inverted in handling.

Prevention

In cold climates adequate protective clothing and gloves must always be worn. Beards and moustaches should be kept short. In aircraft prevention depends on efficient cabin heating or upon electrically heated clothing and oxygen administration. The face can be protected by lanoline and the lips by colourless lipstick, both of which lower the freezing point of the skin. Metal studs and fittings must not be allowed to touch the skin.

Treatment

The first-aid treatment now recommended is rapid warming in water at 44°C for up to 20 minutes at a time. The part after gentle drying is then elevated and exposed at room temperature. It must never be warmed in front of the fire as the tissues are anaesthetized and could easily burn. Rubbing is ill advised. Oxygen can be given in the ordinary way at high concentration (p. 741) but it is much

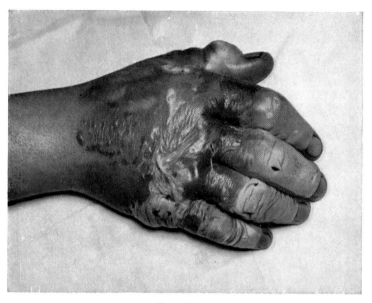

FIG. 30.11
Frostbite.

Table 30.1. *Some 'second grade' emergencies*

CLINICAL FINDING	POSSIBLE SEQUEL OF INACTION	COURSE OF ACTION
Temporal arteritis	Retinal involvement with blindness	Steroids
Oliguria	Stroke Fits	Stop water intake
Depression	Suicide	Antidepressants ECT
?Pulmonary TB	Infection of others	Sputum, chest X-ray
Rose spots	Confused evidence of typhoid	Ring with Biro to identify crops
Geographic history suggesting malaria (falciparum)	Coma	Blood film. Treat at once (p. 449). Don't wait
Deep vein thrombosis	Pulmonary embolism	Anticoagulants
Purpura	Massive haemorrhage ?intracranial	Withdraw drugs, steroids
Tremor and mood changes in cirrhosis	Hepatic coma	Protein free diet, neomycin
Throat exudate	Delay in giving serum for diphtheria	Swab
Salicylate overdose but patient looks well	Death	Gastric lavage
?Drug effects (e.g. phenothiazine rigidity)	Loss of evidence because drug eliminated	Blood and urine samples
Acute renal failure with overhydration and hypernatraemia	Pulmonary oedema Convulsions	Stop all fluids Dehydrate with diuretics or peritoneal dialysis
Oral thrush in patients in renal failure	Monilial colitis with diarrhoea	Oral nystatin
Renal colic in patients on cytotoxic anti-tumour treatment	Obstructive anuria	Increased fluid intake Sodium bicarbonate Allopurinol
Unusual injury in a child	Further battery	Admission and social investigation

better to use hyperbaric oxygen (p. 814). When persistent lividity and induration are present eventual tissue loss is probable.

'SECOND GRADE' EMERGENCIES

Certain conditions which, while not emergencies when found, demand immediate attention if disaster is to be avoided. Table 30.1 gives some examples.

It should not be forgotten that the prescription of certain drugs, e.g. methyl dopa, may place a patient in the second grade emergency category since if they should be withdrawn abruptly urgent symptoms of a first grade emergency could develop.

C. ALLAN BIRCH

CHAPTER 31

Medico-legal and other Non-clinical Emergencies

ALMOST all forms of treatment and investigation we use may, on occasion, be harmful to the patient and so lead to legal action. Every practitioner should, therefore, belong to a defence society (preferably the same one as his partner) and report to it *at once* when involved in a situation likely to lead to a claim for damages. Special medico-legal emergencies arising on board ship are described on p. 478 and the question of responsibility for advice given by wireless in an emergency is dealt with on p. 695.

ACCIDENTS IN HOSPITAL

Should an accident befall any patient or member of the staff go promptly when summoned. Enquire into the circumstances, examine the patient fully and order any necessary X ray examination. Make a full, frank and factual report preferably on a special form and send it to the hospital secretary. Include a note of the exact place where the accident occurred. It is often helpful to note the condition of the shoes. The report is a confidential statement for the use of the solicitor of the governing body in case any claim is made. So do not make any copy or tell its contents to others for this would destroy its status as a privileged document. 'Privileged' in this context means that in any action the other side cannot compel disclosure as evidence in Court. You should, of course, take all steps to reverse the consequences of the accident. If it seems that you may be involved as a cause inform you medical defence society at once.

LIABILITY FOR NEGLIGENCE

Since a charge of negligence may follow a doctor's attention to his patient, a clear statement of what negligence means is desirable. In law negligence is judged by the standard of prudence of an ordinary reasonable man but a person who undertakes something requiring special knowledge or skill is negligent if, by reason of not possessing that knowledge or skill he bungles, although he does his best. The negligence does not consist in the lack of skill but in undertaking the work without skill. The doctor must exercise such a degree of care as a normally skilful member of his profession may reasonably be expected to take in the actual circumstances of the case in question. This principle applies even though the doctor undertakes to do the work gratuitously. Extraordinary skill, however, is not required and erroneous judgment in a difficult case does not constitute negligence.

A doctor who does not adopt some line of treatment because he was not aware of it is not necessarily negligent. Whilst he must take reasonable steps to keep abreast of modern developments he is not negligent because he is not aware of some special publication though he might be deemed so if he had not heeded a series of advisory statements.

RESPONSIBILITY FOR ACTION IN AN EMERGENCY
(For responsibility for advice at sea see p. 695)

An emergency may justify a doctor in taking some action for which he had not been trained and which was beyond his competence. He would be then judged only by what in the circumstances was reasonable to expect of him. A doctor because of lack of skill should never deal with an emergency by transferring the patient to another hospital unless that is the quickest way of getting him the help he needs or if only thus will the necessary facilities be available. Nor should a patient presenting in Casualty or otherwise as an emergency be sent home without being seen by a doctor. The Department of Health and Social Security now accepts that every patient presenting at an NHS hospital should be seen by a doctor.

When a junior hospital doctor engages in a procedure which is well within his competence and skill and which is within the general delegation which he enjoys he can be held responsible for all that flows from that procedure. So long as he restricts his activities to the orbit within which it is usual for him to act then his chief can rightly repudiate responsibility for any mishap (though he might be involved because of his general responsibility for the supervision of the work of his staff). When a house officer, not being in charge of the case, carries out other treatment, in an emergency or otherwise, on the direct instruction of a consultant rather than on his own initiative and this treatment is found to be faulty or inadequate the house officer will not be liable unless the instructions had been manifestly wrong.

(This is a statement in general terms on a complicated subject. For more detail and discussion the reader is referred to *Law of Doctor and Patient* by S. R. Speller, 1973.)

CONTRIBUTORY NEGLIGENCE

If a patient alleges that he has been injured through the negligence of a doctor and brings an action in which it is established that the patient's own negligence was a contributory cause or had worsened its effect any damages may be reduced accordingly. Should the patient refuse to obey instructions following a medical accident the practitioner would be wise to seek a second opinion. If this supports the action of the doctor and is also refused the doctor should cease treatment. But he should give the patient full warning of his intention and his reasons and also give him ample opportunity to follow his instructions. He should, in fact, endeavour to provide what the Court would be likely to regard as clear and ample evidence that he had done everything that an ordinary and reasonably skilful practictioner would be expected to do.

PERMISSION TO ACT IN AN EMERGENCY

Consent is implied for any treatment which the patient willingly accepts. Without his expressed or implied consent treatment constitutes an assault in law and so when an operation seems likely it is as well to have a consent form signed. If the patient is incapable of speaking for himself those treating him act as his ' agents of necessity ' and do for him what any ordinary reasonable man would wish to have done for him. No more should be done than is necessary to deal with the emergency. For anaesthesia and any operative procedure and for some examinations (pp. 670 and 675) consent should be obtained after explanation of what it is proposed to do *in terms which the patient can understand.* Consent must be full and free. Unless a patient understands the nature and purpose of a proposed operation his consent is not ' real '. For example, to describe angiocardiography as putting a tube into an arm vein without saying that the tube would reach the heart would be ' consent by trickery ' and invalid. Although consent by word of mouth is just as valid in law as written consent it is preferable to have it in writing for witnesses may die and memories fade. It is generally felt that a maternity patient need not give written consent to any operative or manipulative procedure to do with childbirth. It can be assumed that she consents to this.

Age of consent

The Family Law Reform Act, 1969 reduced the age of ' majority ' from 21 to 18. The age when adolescents become registrable in the National Health Service is 16 and this is the age when they can give consent to operation. Under 16 the consent of a parent or guardian is needed. Even so the life of a minor should not be jeopardised by waiting for consent if operation or other treatment is immediately necessary. The consent of whoever stands *in loco parentis* should be sought and a full statement sent to the parents as soon as possible. A friend, however intimate, has no authority to give permission. A mentally defective person is in the same position as a minor.

Jehovah's witnesses. An emergency situation necessitating blood transfusion may arise in a patient who refuses it because he belongs to the religious sect called Jehovah's Witnesses, of whom there are about 50 000 in Britain. They sincerely believe that the words in the Bible (Genesis 9, 34) ' Flesh with the life thereof, which is the blood thereof, shall ye not eat ' means that blood transfusion, being i v ' feeding ' is forbidden. Immediate autotransfusion and diversion of the blood to bypass an organ is biblically permissible but not if the blood is stored, however briefly.

Some would regard this as hair-splitting nonsense and then, because the patient's disability is religious as well as physical, may approach the problem in an emotional and intolerant way. Because of this risk the following statement of the doctor's duty and the patient's rights is made.

Religious freedom embraces two concepts: (1) freedom to believe which is absolute and (2) freedom to act. This is not absolute, for a person's conduct is subject to regulation for the protection of others.

When the patient refuses blood transfusion it is for the doctor to use his own judgment in deciding how to act. If the position has been made clear to the patient and he dies untransfused no action can be taken against the doctor for no patient is obliged to preserve his life by the use of special or extraordinary measures. If a patient lays down a condition of no transfusion the doctor may prefer to refuse the case but whether avoiding the responsibility in this way is justified is a moral issue for him to decide, bearing in mind that it is his duty to do all he can to preserve the patient's life and health. An alternative approach is to regard the problem as akin to other situations in which ideal treatment is for some reason impracticable and while remaining responsible for the patient to get round the difficulty in some other way such as by using a plasma expander instead of blood. Whatever he does the doctor should make full records including a note as to whether the patient was in full possession of his faculties.

In the case of a baby suffering from haemolytic disease of the newborn the risk of death if not transfused should be clearly put to the parents in words which they understand and a record made of what was said. If the parents then refuse transfusion for their child the law presumes they intended the child's death and however conscientious their refusal they would be guilty of manslaughter. No one can escape criminal responsibility by being conscientiously wrong-headed, for in law he is presumed to intend what, if he were otherwise minded, he would know to be the result of his actions. If despite refusal a transfusion is given the doctor would be wise to obtain a written opinion supporting his action from a colleague and also an acknowledgment from the parent or guardian that consent was refused despite explanation of the danger. The procedure of bringing a magistrate to the bedside in order to transfer custody of the child to the Children's Officer who would then grant permission for transfusion is a stratagem to be discouraged. It is not approved by the Department of Health and its legality would be doubtful for the order could not be subject to appeal as other legal decisions are. No doctor would stand by and let a child die for want of a transfusion and if in the emergency he acted in good faith albeit without legal sanction the defence societies have guaranteed to support him in any action for assault. Even if this was sustained the damages would probably be minimal particularly if the child's life had been saved.

EMERGENCY TREATMENT BY LAY PERSONS

A lay person faced with an emergency and without medical help should render such emergency treatment as he thinks best and would not be deemed negligent if he did the wrong thing. He might be thought morally (albeit not legally) culpable if he did nothing. Occasionally injection of morphine for painful crises of incurable disease has been delegated to relatives. Although it would be difficult to devise safeguards to cover all possible legal consequences of this procedure, the doctor could arrange it at his discretion. He should make sure that the relative is competent to inject morphine without supervision. Supplies of drugs left with relatives should be small.

PATIENTS' STATEMENTS AS EVIDENCE AND DYING DECLARATIONS

Although there is no legal obligation on a doctor to take down the statement of a dying patient, he is usually the best person to do this in an emergency. Two situations must be clearly distinguished:
1. When the doctor thinks the patient is unlikely to recover but

the patient is unaware of the imminence of death and makes a statement this is a *deposition*. It is made on oath and taken down in writing by a Justice of the Peace (the local police station can supply the names of Justices of the Peace) or, in Scotland, by a Sheriff, within his area of jurisdiction, from a patient who has information he is prepared to give about a serious criminal offence, but who, in the opinion of the doctor attending him, is not likely to recover. The person against whom it may be used should be given reasonable notice of the proposal to take a deposition. If he chooses to attend he may cross-examine the deponent, either personally or through his solicitor. The deposition should be signed by the J.P. who should state his reason for taking it and the names of any persons present at the time.

2. When the patient is in settled hopeless expectation of death he may make a statement about the circumstance which caused his condition. Although it is only hearsay evidence and as such normally unacceptable in Court, it is admissible when it takes this form i.e. a *dying declaration*. It is a statement made by a dying person whose death results in a charge of murder or manslaughter, and is only admissible in evidence about his death and if when he made it he believed he was about to die. It is not for the doctor to decide on admissibility and he is not necessarily the best person to take it down. It might be better for a police officer to do it. To be in this position the patient would in most cases have to be told he was dying, and the doctor might not be certain enough of the imminence of death to deprive his patient of hope. A declaration differs from a deposition in that it need not be on oath or in writing. The accused need not be informed or present. Even so it is wise to write down the statement and have it signed by the dying person if possible and by whoever writes it down. A useful form of words is:

I, A. B., being in settled expectation of death and without hope of recovery make the following statement. (*Here follow the actual words used without alteration even of grammar and anything else that is said in the way of question and answer.*) *The following certificate should be written at the end of the declaration:*

The above declaration was taken down by me, X. Y. at .... on .... day of .... Signed by (declarant) after having been read over to him by me.
(*The signatures of any persons present should be added.*)

Before it is admitted in evidence the judge must be satisfied that the declarant was about to die and realised it, and that the cause of death was the subject of the dying declaration. If there was any hope of recovery, however slight, in the mind of the declarant when he made the declaration, this would render it inadmissible. But it would not do so if hope arose subsequently or if the doctor thought recovery possible.

HOW TO BEQUEATH A BODY FOR DISSECTION

This is hardly an emergency but I have known information to be sought urgently on behalf of a patient who intended his body to go to a medical school for the benefit of medical education but took no steps until he knew he was soon to die. As the procedure is little known it is described here. It may be stated at once that it is quite unnecessary for the donor or anyone else to pay money to have the arrangements made or to make any donation. It is not possible for a person to bequeath his body in a legal sense for in law there is no property in a body. The legal right to dispose of a body rests with the next of kin, executor or other person who has custody of the body. Even he cannot send the body for dissection if any relative objects. The Jews have no ruling as to the permissibility or otherwise of dissection. If there is doubt the Chief Rabbi should be consulted. He will consider each case individually in the light of all the circumstances. The Roman Catholic Church does not oppose dissection provided the remains are reverently disposed of.

A person who wishes his body to be used for dissection should make sure that near relatives do not object and then make a written and preferably witnessed statement of his intention. This should not be put with the will as this is not usually looked at until after the funeral. It is best to mention it to the next of kin.

When death occurs the relatives or the doctor should, in the London area (i.e. Surrey, Sussex, Middlesex, part of Essex, all of Kent and parts of Hampshire and Berkshire) telephone HM Inspector of Anatomy, 16 to 19 Gresse Street, London W1P 1PB (01-636 6811 Ext. 3572 or 3576, or after hours, DHSS Headquarters 01-407 5522 Ext. 7407). Full instructions will be given. The doctor will be questioned and a decision whether to accept or not will be given at once. An ordinary death certificate is necessary and on taking this to the Registrar a green Disposal Certificate will be issued. This must be given to the undertaker instructed by HMIA. Forms AA1 and AA4 are provided for completion by the doctor. No forms are sent to the donor. In Scotland a telephone message should be sent to HMIA, Anatomy Office Division IIIB/B2, Room 235, St Andrew's House, Edinburgh EH1 3DE (031-556 8501 Ext. 2936) or directly to the nearest medical school. In Wales and

Northern Ireland the Professor of Anatomy should be contacted. Bequeathing a body is probably not a practical proposition in the Isle of Man, the Scilly Isles or the Channel Islands.

It is not possible to guarantee acceptance of a body because there may be reasons such as diffuse disease or deep bed sores which make it unsuitable for demonstrating normal anatomy. A post-mortem examination would preclude the necessary embalming. There might be a lack of demand for bodies at the time. Some medical schools will refuse a body if the eyes have been removed. It is best not to bequeath a body to a particular medical school but to let it go to whichever is convenient. Within a week or so of death the next of kin or executor will receive a special form asking the wishes for final disposal of the remains. Normally the medical school will arrange burial or cremation (at Streatham Park cemetery in the case of London) within two years of death and will pay all expenses. It will also send details of the funeral to HMIA. A private funeral may be arranged at the expense of the next of kin or executor.

If the relatives do not wish to know of or take part in any burial or cremation ceremony they may ask the Licensed Teacher of Anatomy to proceed without their knowledge. Only one certificate is needed for cremation of anatomical remains and this is given by the Teacher of Anatomy. In most cases where the expense of final disposal is borne by a medical school a claim is made for the Death Grant.

EYES AND OTHER ORGANS BEQUEATHED FOR THERAPEUTIC PURPOSES

The regulations concerning bequest of parts of the body (including eyes) for therapeutic purposes or for medical education or research are given in the Human Tissue Act 1969 (no corresponding Act has been passed in the Isle of Man) the relevant parts of which read:

1. If any person, either in writing at any time or orally in the presence of two or more witnesses during his last illness, has expressed a request that his body or any specified part of it be used after his death for therapeutic purposes or for purposes of medical education or research, the person lawfully in possession of his body after his death may, unless he has reason to believe that the request was subsequently withdrawn, authorise the removal from the body of any part or, as the case may be, the specified part, for use in accordance with the request.

2. Without prejudice to the foregoing subsection, the person lawfully in possession of the body of a deceased person may authorise the removal of any part of the body for use for the said purposes if, having made such reasonable enquiry as may be practicable, he has no reason to believe (a) that the deceased expressed an objection to his body being so dealt with after his death and had not withdrawn it; or (b) that a surviving relative of the deceased objects to the body being so dealt with.

When a patient asks how his eyes may be donated for surgical purposes he should be told to sign a statement (preferably witnessed) of his wishes. It need not be in the Will but the executor should be told. Ideally a copy should be sent to the next of kin, the executor of the will, the family doctor and the appropriate hospital (p. 811). If the request is only oral the person to whom it is made should chose two witnesses who would not be upset by the request and ask the patient to repeat it before them. The request should be written down and signed by the witnesses in the presence of the patient and of each other. It is noteworthy that the eyes of old people tend to make better grafts than those of younger persons and so a would-be donor should not be discouraged because he is old.

When the doctor attending a dying patient is told of such wishes he should, after obtaining the consent of the relatives, promptly inform the nearest Eye Bank (see Appendix 10, p. 811) of the impending demise of the patient or should do so as soon as possible after death. The Eye Bank will, unless an inquest is likely, send out someone to collect the eyes or will make arrangements (e.g., through the local branch of the British Red Cross Society) for this to be done if the eyes are needed. Pending removal Chloramphenicol Eye-drops 0·5 per cent should be instilled into each eye. Close the lids lest the cornea dries. The eyes are enucleated under aseptic precautions within, at most, six hours after death and transferred immediately into a sterile screw capped bottle containing sterile liquid paraffin. The bottle is put into cracked ice or kept at 4°C. Enucleation is less urgent if the body is kept in the mortuary cool chamber. Steps should be taken to see that there is no obvious disfigurement of the body. Provided there is no disease the age of the patient does not matter but children's eyes are unsuitable. The eyes of any adult if externally healthy are suitable provided he is not suffering from syphilis and has not died from a generalised infection.

Bottles containing eyes must be sent by road or rail and *never by post*. (For details of transport by air see p. 825). The following particulars should be supplied : —

Name or number, age and sex of patient.
Place where eyes were removed.
Date, time and cause of death.
Length of time after death eyes were removed.
Details of any ocular abnormality.
Details of any systemic infection.

Note. 1. In the case of Roman Catholics, the Pope has said that there is no moral or religious objection to the removal of eyes for grafting purposes.

2. Jewish religious law raises no objection in principle to the bequest of eyes for corneal transplants provided certain conditions are met. In the case of Jewish donors it is advisable to consult a competent rabbi or the Office of the Chief Rabbi, Alder House, Tavistock Square, London WC1 9HN (01-387 1066).

3. If an inquest or coroner's post-mortem examination is likely the coroner's consent is necessary before the eyes are removed.

4. Removal of eyes does not involve the relatives in any extra expense.

DONATED (CADAVER) KIDNEYS

The problem of transplantation has medical, legal and technical-administrative aspects. It may arise urgently when a doctor, for example in Casualty, finds his very ill and possibly moribund patient carries a card on which he has expressed his wish to donate his kidneys for transplantation. There may be time to accede to his wish. Kidneys may be medically acceptable if the donor is between the ages of 2 and 65 years and is not suffering from cancer outside the central nervous system, diabetes, collagen diseases, established renal infection or severe septicaemia. Kidneys are probably unsuitable if there has been hypotension for more than 12 hours leading to oliguria or if the patient has been on a noradrenaline drip. (Most donors have suffered a head injury or a subarachnoid haemorrhage.)

From the technical aspect it would not be possible to proceed from Casualty and so the patient should be admitted to the ward or intensive care unit where his breathing should be kept going by IPPV if need be. If you don't know where tissue typing is done telephone the transplant team (p. 808) or the Regional Blood Transfusion Centre (p. 802) or the National Organ Matching Service at Bristol (0272 628021) and ask where blood should be sent for this. Take 20 ml of blood into 2·0 ml of 3·8 per cent trisodium citrate and also 10 ml of clotted blood. The sample will also be tested for hepatitis B (Australia) antigen.

The Human Tissue Act 1961 enables the person lawfully in possession of the body, such as someone in a post designated by the Hospital Authority, to allow the kidneys to be removed. Actual possession of a body is not the same as the right to possession of it. If a person with this right appears the Hospital Authority cannot dispose of the body. It can only do so if, having made such reasonable inquiry as may be practicable, no surviving relative objects. Specific consent is not necessary but merely lack of objection. When the deceased (to express his wishes) and the next of kin (to indicate their consent) have signed a kidney donation card this is sufficient. (It has been suggested* that objection should be recorded on a computerised register for rapid consultation.) The doctor may be relieved by the transplant team of the delicate task of asking the relatives. If a moribund potential donor's condition is deteriorating rapidly it would be wise to identify relatives quickly and bring them to hospital by police car.

If the relatives do not object or if it is decided to go ahead without asking them there are certain circumstances in which the coroner's permission to proceed must be obtained. The Human Tissues Act 1961 states that tissue shall not be removed without the coroner's consent if there is reason to believe that an inquest or post-mortem examination may be required by the coroner (p. 685). When criminal proceedings are contemplated removal of the kidneys should not even be considered. The coroner must be sure that, in a case likely to come before him, donor nephrectomy will not mask any evidence. If nephrectomy might destroy evidence of unsuspected abdominal trauma the operation to take the kidneys must stop. In a ' coroner's case ' the coroner's pathologist must be allowed to be present and should be sent a report including the negative findings. In cases of possible alcoholic intoxication he must be given a sample of blood.

It is advised that two doctors (one of whom should be at least five years registered and both independent of the transplant team) should be jointly responsible for establishing that the patient has died. In the case of a potential donor whose vital functions are mechanically assisted the doctor(s) must be satisfied that there has been irreversible brain damage and that the patient, being in a state of coma dépassé, could not live an adequate existence without artificial means (i.e. that he is, in current jargon, a ' heart-beating cadaver '). The findings should include such points as complete arreflexia and mydriasis, absence of spontaneous respiration after cession of IPPV for three minutes and, if available, a flat EEG. While

---

* The MacLennan Group. Cmnd. 4106.

awaiting nephrectomies the donor's blood volume should be maintained. Heparin 5 000 units, frusemide 250 mg and mannitol 100 g as a 5 to 20 per cent solution should be given to resuscitate border-line kidneys. Under no circumstances must the dying donor be moved to the recipient's hospital. The doctors removing the kidneys must be able to say that life was extinct before they started the operation. The kidneys should preferably be removed by the transplant team and in a way that makes them suitable for transplantation. They must be cooled to 4°C within one hour of the donor's death. They are perfused through the renal arteries with 500 ml of rheomacrodex (Perfudex) first at room temperature and then at 4°C. Successful perfusion is shown by complete blanching. This usually takes 15 minutes. Each kidney is put in a sterile plastic bag containing 100 ml of cold perfusate which is then put in another sterile bag. They are kept in a large polystyrene-lined box with ice cubes and kept there until used. Kidneys must be carefully labelled left and right. Under these conditions kidneys can be stored for 12 hours. A lymph node and a piece of spleen are sent in a separate container.

The recipient

Once the transplant team has been warned the recipient, if not already in hospital, is brought there. Ideally kidneys should be transplanted within 12 hours of donor nephrectomy unless they are put on a perfusion machine which will keep them in good condition for 36 hours. What follows is the same as in the case of non-urgent donations and is stated as a matter of interest and for completeness. The tissue typing results will have been phoned to the National Organ Matching Service at Southmead Hospital, Bristol, where details of some 800 patients in the UK who are awaiting transplants are kept. From these the names of possible recipients in varying categories of suitability and in order or priority and geographical position are produced by the computer of the South West Regional Health Authority in a matter of minutes. The Service arranges the transport of kidneys by Securicor or the St John Ambulance Air Wing (p. 826) to the appropriate transplant team (p. 808). Should there be no well-matched (so-called 'full house') recipient in Britain the kidneys may be offered via Telex to Eurotransplant in Leiden, Holland, Francetransplant in Paris or Scandiatransplant in Denmark. It is very rare for a structurally sound kidney to remain unused. Neither the relatives nor the recipients have any information as to the identity of each other or the whereabouts of the kidneys or donor though the donor's identity may have to be revealed at an inquest on him. The relatives may, if they wish, be informed of the result of the donation.

CRIMINAL ABORTION

If a doctor contemplates giving information to the police about an abortion he should seek expert legal advice, since there is no certainty that he will be protected against subsequent litigation for defamation.

If the patient knows she is dying the doctor may urge her to make a statement but this must meet the requirements of dying declarations (p. 662) for it to have legal value. He should not put leading questions. When she dies the coroner must be informed (p. 685). If criminal abortion is only suspected and the patient recovers, there is no obligation to make any report.

Especially during wartime it sometimes happens that the returning husband finds his wife ill. When this illness is caused by abortion and it is clear that the husband could not have been responsible for the pregnancy, the doctor should be careful of his replies to the husband's questions. The making of a defamatory statement to a husband about his wife is ' publication ' and could render the person making it liable to an action for slander. Such an action could not, of course, succeed if the statement giving rise to it were true, but if the doctor is not sure of his facts he should not say anything and would be wise to let the wife tell the husband herself. In general no spouse or relation should ever be given information about a patient either contrary to the patient's express wishes or when it is not plain what these wishes are.

WHAT TO DO IN A CASE OF ALLEGED RAPE

While it is probable that many raped women make no complaint of it because they wish to escape court proceedings and the attendant notoriety an occasional victim may go at once to the police or her family doctor. Sometimes she may arrive at hospital where she would best be seen by a senior doctor. Remember that evidence obtained may have to be disclosed in court later and so careful notes should be made and kept. There is no clear boundary between seduction and rape and in about 4 per cent of cases the problem will turn out to be rape fantasy. It may be preferable to exclude relatives and friends and let the woman tell her own story but if she is very distressed it is helpful for a woman friend to stay with her. This presents no legal difficulty. The questions should be the necessary ones to find out about the date of the last menstrual period and of the last intercourse, if any; the obstetrical and gynaecological

23

history and whether on the pill. It is not really the doctor's job to make a probing inquiry which is best left to the police. In any case the psychological aspects call for expert handling.

Since conclusive evidence soon disappears examine the woman in the lithotomy position when first seen and in a good light. Look for scratches and bruises and take charge of underclothing for examination for seminal stains. Note the state of and take specimens of pubic hair. Look for bleeding and for bruising of the vagina and tearing of the hymen. There may be little or no damage in a woman accustomed to intercourse and more evidence is needed in such a case than in a frightened virgin who would be more likely to struggle. Try with a syringe and tube to get some semen from the vagina. It may be helpful if its group can be shown to differ from that of the blood of the alleged assailant. Scrapings from beneath the finger nails and a specimen of pubic hair may provide useful evidence.

Make thin smears on new clean glass slides from any material aspirated. Put a high vaginal swab in transport medium for culture for gonococci. Take blood for a VDRL test. Gonorrhoea cannot be detected less than a week after the rape and syphilis less than six so arrange for the woman to be seen in the VD clinic later by direct referral or via her family doctor. If she is unwilling to attend treat her by probenecid 1 g by mouth followed by ampicillin 3·5 g or preferably Procaine penicillin G 2·4 g i m into each buttock. If the possibility of pregnancy exists tell her of the courses she may take. She may wish for some action to terminate a possible early pregnancy if the next period becomes overdue (' menstrual extraction '). Arrange to get the woman home where she should not be left unattended. The long-term psychosexual effects of rape, unless dealt with, may last for many years and wreck pre-existing relationships including marriage. The husband may need referral too for skilled help in coming to terms with the event.

If asked to examine a male accused of rape only do so with his full consent preferably written and witnessed. Tell him of his right to refuse. Look for scratches and bruises and examine the penis for recent turgescence and tears of the frenum. Make smears from any meatal moisture and take a specimen of pubic hair. Note signs of a struggle such as facial and genital scratches. Send blood for grouping.

Sodomy

Examination of the victim of alleged sodomy should be on similar lines to that in a case of rape. Written consent must be obtained and a third party must be present. The object is to find out whether there was a penetration of the anus. The only proof is the presence of semen. Examination of the accused should be for evidence of trauma to the penis, recent emission of semen and traces of lubricant. Contaminated clothing should be kept.

DEATH-BED WILLS

We have to distinguish between witnessing a death-bed will and helping to make it.

Anyone who understands what witnessing a signature means may witness a will. It is not necessary that the witness should know that the document is a will. He or she need not be of full age. A minor may witness a signature provided he or she has reached such a stage of education as to appreciate fully what is signified by the action of witnessing a signature. The witness is only ' attesting ' the signature, and is not concerned with the patient's mental state or how the patient disposes of his property. The doctor who attested a will may, of course, be called as an expert witness and asked if he thought the patient was sane when he signed his will. So he would be wise to make a note at the time of his impression of the patient's mental state.

The practitioner should only help the patient to *make* his will in a real emergency, and when a solicitor or administrative officer cannot be found. It is illegal for anyone other than a practising solicitor to draft a will for reward. The law requires that (1) the person is ' of sound disposing mind ' and knows he is making a will, (2) he knows the extent of his property and (3) knows ' the natural object of his bounty ', A doctor would be unwise to help a patient to *make* a will except in the simplest terms as in the example below.

All names and addresses of possible devisees and legatees, and descriptions of bequests, should be full and accurate and any possibly ambiguous words such as ' money ' should be avoided. Illegitimate children now have, in the main, the same property rights as their fellows born in wedlock.

The testator should sign the will if possible, or make a mark. If he cannot read or write, then someone may sign in his place but the testator should, if possible, acknowledge in some way as by nodding his head, that he understands what is being done. If a third person does sign on the testator's behalf, he *must* sign in the presence of the testator, and the testator must be shown to have seen the signature. Two witnesses must have seen the testator sign the will and then, in his presence and in the presence of each other, sign as witnesses of his signature.

A simple form of words is

> I, A.B., of —————— leave everything I have to
> my dear wife and appoint her my executrix.

Signed A.B.

Witness

Witness   Date

THE FAILED SUICIDE

By the Suicide Act 1961 there is no longer an indictable offence of attempted suicide. There is therefore now no legal obligation upon the doctor to report the matter to the police. In all cases the doctor should do what he thinks best. This will often be to seek consultation with the psychiatrist. If the patient refuses treatment and is deemed to be in need of it for the protection of himself and others, the procedure for compulsion is set out below.

PATIENTS WHO REFUSE TREATMENT

If after clear explanation a patient refuses to stay in hospital or to have treatment as advised the fact should be recorded in the notes. Before he leaves he should be asked to sign a statement that he is taking his own discharge against medical advice. You cannot compel him to sign. If he refuses you should record this fact also in the notes. If you feel that the patient is mentally ill, and particularly if he has made a suicidal attempt, you should seek the psychiatrist's opinion. Failing this you could act under Section 30 of the Mental Health Act 1959 (p. 674).

ADMISSION TO A PSYCHIATRIC HOSPITAL

INFORMAL ADMISSION. When admission to a psychiatric hospital is advised and the patient is not unwilling to go you may send him there in the ordinary way as to any other hospital. No special forms are needed. This should be the usual procedure for admission. (In this matter of informal admission the wishes of a patient of 16 or more override those of his parent or guardian.)

COMPULSORY ADMISSION. If a patient refuses to go to a psychiatric hospital and you are satisfied that he ought to be detained ' in the interest of his own health and safety or with a view to the protection of others ', there are now three courses of action under Sections 25, 29 and 26 of Part 4 of the Mental Health Act 1959 and one under Section 30.

1. Under Section 25 of the Mental Health Act 1959 by an Observation order. This is the procedure of preference and should be used if at all possible.

Ask a psychiatrist to see the patient. If there is no psychiatrist on the staff of your hospital telephone the Local Authority Social Worker (LASW) and he will tell you which psychiatric hospital to ask for one. (Any psychiatrist approved by the Local Health Authority can be asked but it is best if he is the one who will deal with the patient in hospital.) The necessary forms (obtainable from Shaw & Sons Ltd., Shaway House, Sydenham, London, SE26 5AE) Tel. 01-778 0192) are:

Forms 3A and 3B. These are for medical recommendations. The psychiatrist will sign form 3A or 3B. Form 3B must be signed also by the patient's own doctor though you could sign it yourself. If neither signatory has known the patient previously the reason why the patient's own doctor could not sign must be stated by the applicant in Form 1.

Form 1. This is the application for admission for observation and must be signed by the LASW or the nearest relative.

The LASW cannot be compelled to sign the form against his judgment and so if he does not think that admission is necessary he has the right to refuse to apply for it but it is very unlikely that he will do so. He need not consult the patient's relatives though he is expected to do so and he generally takes their views into account. He can, with the doctor's agreement, reverse their objection. Transport is arranged by the LASW. A patient admitted under Section 25 cannot be discharged by a relative.

This procedure allows the patient to be detained in a psychiatric hospital or observation ward for not more than 28 days beginning with the day on which he was admitted. Under this section he could even be detained in the general hospital for there is now no essential difference between a general hospital and a psychiatric hospital as far as detention is concerned. If such an exceptional procedure had to be used you should deliver the necessary forms to the Secretary of the Area Health Authority.

2. Under Section 29 of the Mental Health Act by an Emergency order.

If the case is urgent and cannot await a psychiatrist's opinion the patient may be admitted to a psychiatric hospital or observation ward (or exceptionally detained in your own hospital) on a single recommendation.

Call the LASW. He should (unless it is obviously impracticable) be the one for the area where the patient lives. He will get in touch with the relatives and provide the necessary forms. These are:

Form 2. Application for admission for observation. This must be signed *either* by a relative (it does not have to be the nearest) or the LASW, who may disregard a relative's objection.

Form 3A. The medical recommendation. A doctor who has known the patient previously should sign this. If he is not available a junior doctor should ask one of his senior colleagues, but in an emergency he could sign it himself. In either of these cases the reason why the doctor, who knows the patient, did not sign must be stated on Form 2. The LASW will arrange transport.

This method enables a patient to be compulsorily detained for up to 72 hours when a second recommendation is made (under Section 25) within this time. A patient admitted under this section cannot be discharged by a relative.

3. Under Section 26 of the Mental Health Act.

This is used when prolonged treatment is needed. Two forms must be completed—one by an approved doctor.

Admission under Section 30 of the Mental Health Act 1959 by a Treament Order is occasionally used when an informal patient is determined to leave before a relative or the LASW could arrive and the responsible medical officer thinks he would be a danger to himself and to others.

The 'medical practitioner in charge of treatment' may make a recommendation on Form 6 and this enables him to detain the patient in his own hospital for three days pending application for admission to a mental hospital. It is not necessary to call the LASW. The form is obtained from the hospital secretary and should be returned to him. A junior member of the staff would be wise to ask a senior colleague to sign it. Form 6 is not a transfer order and is mainly used to prevent an informal patient in a psychiatric hospital from taking his own discharge.

The procedure under the Mental Health (Scotland) Act is basically the same but differs in detail from that in England and Wales. Transport is arranged by the Scottish Hospital Service and not by the Social Worker. Compulsory admission involves approval by the Sheriff. In Northern Ireland admissions to psychiatric hospitals are effected under the Mental Health Act (Northern Ireland) 1961. The procedures differ only in detail from those which obtain in England, Wales and Scotland. An application for admission need be founded on the recommendation of only one medical practitioner.

The disturbed patient in the casualty department who refuses to accept treatment and leaves hospital presents an urgent problem. The simplest procedure is to ask the police to use their powers under Section 136 of the Act to remove the patient from a ' place to which the public have access' to a ' place of safety ', e.g. a hospital, for examination. He can then be dealt with as already outlined. Alternatively the police may themselves call the LASW to see the patient outside the hospital, e.g. in the police station. The police do not have power under Section 136 to enter private premises unless a magistrate issues a warrant.

NOTE. Completion of forms does not mean that admission will necessarily follow. The Area Health Authority through its senior medical staff always retains the right to control admissions.

EMERGENCY EXAMINATION AT POLICE REQUEST

An apprehended but unconvicted person may only be examined and the findings disclosed with his expressed consent. As the person is not being examined for his own welfare implied consent cannot be assumed. He should be told of his rights and also that the report of the examination may be given in evidence at trial. He may request the attendance of another doctor on his behalf. As a rule he is not formally charged until after a medical examination has been made or refused but there is no general rule about this. The police have no power to order an examination. Even if asked by the police to decide only whether symptoms are due to disease and whether the prisoner is fit to be detained the doctor should not be persuaded that an examination is unnecessary. Although from the legal standpoint it is immaterial whether the doctor knows the person to be examined or not he will be wise to refuse the examination if he had private information likely to affect the issue. If there is reason to suspect addiction to certain drugs the provisions of the Notification and Supply Regulations must be complied with (p. 43).

After conviction Prison Authorities may order the examination of a prisoner. Rule 19 of The Prison Rules 1949 provides that ' every prisoner shall, on the day of his reception, as soon as possible after his reception, be separately examined by the Medical Officer, who shall record the state of health of the prisoner'. The free cooperation of the prisoner will be required particularly for special tests such as those for venereal disease. If the prisoner objected the medical officer would not examine him but would take any necessary steps such as isolation to secure the safety of others. Magistrates may remand an accused person for medical examination before or after conviction or before referring him to a superior court.

WHAT SHOULD THE DOCTOR SAY IN AN EMERGENCY?

A doctor may be called on suddenly by the police and asked for evidence which might help in the arrest of an alleged criminal. Has he seen a patient with a cut hand or can he lead the police to a young woman who has just had an abortion? Similarly, information may be sought by an employer about an employee in circumstances which may appear to justify an urgent request.

Even though the police can act ' on information received ' without disclosing the doctor's name, he should never be stampeded by the emergency atmosphere and ' official ' environment into saying anything he would later regret. If he does speak, however, and tells the truth, he need not fear prosecution for he will be legally correct. But he may be ethically wrong and on this conflict between law and ethics he must make his own decision. If he can consult the person about whom information is sought and get permission to disclose the facts he is clearly in the right. But this would be difficult. What lawbreaker would agree to disclosure? In other circumstances he would be wise to regard his knowledge as confidential and only to disclose it if refusal or failure to do so might be contrary to the public interest or might render him liable to be charged as an accessory.

A doctor has neither a duty nor a right to assist the police if doing so would involve a breach of secrecy and the British Medical Association advises its members not to disclose voluntarily any information about a patient. But this does not cover a situation where a doctor is legally required to give information such as answering questions from the police after an accident. Even though information was obtained by a doctor solely from his doctor-patient relationship he might resolve the conflict of duty in favour of giving information if he felt that failure to do so might bring harm to an innocent third party or cause future risk to the community.

It is sometimes thought that a clergyman's request for urgent information about a patient must be complied with but this is not so. A clergyman or indeed any third party has no more right to information about a patient than anyone else. In each case disclosure should only be made when it is in the best interests of the patient and preferably with his consent. It is usual to give information to a spouse about the wife or husband but this might be inadvisable if a hostile relationship existed. It would then be wrong to discuss a patient even with his or her spouse.

If a doctor knows that there has been unlawful sexual intercourse with a person who is severely mentally handicapped the Department of Health advises that the police should be informed.

ALCOHOLIC INTOXICATION
(For facilities for treatment of alcoholism see Appendix 20, p. 828.)

A situation with urgent aspects arises when a doctor is called upon to examine an alleged drunk in charge of the police. The evidence is fleeting and so examination should be made promptly and recorded at the time. If you are called on behalf of the police tell the patient that he has a right to have his own doctor's opinion. Do not examine him without his consent (preferably obtained before witnesses) for without this the examination would be technically an assault. If consent is refused make notes about the behaviour of the accused and of what he says. If he is unconscious or inaccessible there is no objection to your examining him as an ' agent of necessity ' on the ground that he cannot consent, though it would be unwise to take a specimen of blood or to use a needle for a similar purpose. When a head injury is suspected in a drunken patient it is helpful to hasten the removal of the effects of alcohol. Laevulose can enhance the rate of fall of the blood ethanol level by approximately 25 per cent (Brown et al., 1972) and so a ' sobering up ' technique is to give 100 g of laevulose in 20 g per 100 ml solution i v. As there is hypoxia when severe ethanol overdosage depresses respiration the resulting acidosis could be dangerously increased by lactic acidosis produced by fructose. Intensive treatment with fructose should not be undertaken without full laboratory facilities to monitor blood lactate levels. ' Sobering up ' cocktail injections, containing nikethamide and insulin, are less desirable but frusemide (Lasix) by causing a diuresis will lessen cerebral oedema which is sometimes in part responsible for the clinical picture. It will also cause the blood alcohol level to fall at about twice the normal rate. Consent to any reasonable examination may be presumed in order to establish whether the person is ill or injured. In England the presence of a police officer (but not more than two) at the examination is obligatory to maintain the state of ' arrest '. In Scotland this is forbidden except in the case of a woman prisoner when a woman police officer is allowed to be present to protect a male examiner against accusations of improper conduct. For the benefit of the doctor the following headings are given as a guide to ensure that important points which may be needed in court are not overlooked.

History

Name, age, address and occupation of the person examined.
Date and all relevant times.
Patient's story including details of food and drink.
Past medical history (recent illness, drugs, injury).

Examination

Ask the patient to write his name and address. See that he wears his glasses and keep what he writes or make a note of his refusal.
General demeanour (hilarious, abusive, truculent, etc.).
State of dress. Any vomit or incontinence?
Insight into nature of the situation.
Smell of breath.
Evidence of vomiting.
Evidence of head injury.
Condition of eyes (pupils, ocular movements).
Condition of face (flushed, pale, cyanosed, sweating).
Note the findings in a general examination. Take the blood pressure and record the pulse rate at the beginning and end of the examination.

The accused person's consent for the collection of a specimen of urine must be obtained. The specimen should be passed in the presence of a witness and put into three bottles which must be sealed in the presence of the accused. One is for him, one for the police, and the third is retained for use in court.

Special tests of co-ordination

Ask the patient to read a newspaper and use a telephone directory.
Finger to nose test.
Walking on a chalked line.
Speech (but don't ask tongue-twisters).
Spelling test.
Counting money.

After the examination the doctor should tell the patient his opinion and record any reply. The private doctor who examines the patient may consult with the doctor called by the police as he thinks fit but as he is making the examination at the patient's request he should not discusss the matter with police officers. If invited to write something in the police station's book he should make a non-committal statement such as ' I have examined A. B. on . . .'

The doctor who examines the accused on behalf of the police should give a certificate stating his opinion that at the time of the examination the accused was or was not under the influence of alcohol to such an extent as to be incapable of having proper control of a motor vehicle. He should also state whether the accused is fit or not to be detained.

Opinion

Three questions about the patient should arise in the doctor's mind:

1. Is he ill? i.e. could his present state be brought on by illness or by drugs or insulin?

2. Is he ' drunk '? i.e. is alcohol responsible for his state?

3. How ' drunk ' is he? i.e. is his ability to perform some special act, such as driving a car, impaired?

Since individuals react differently to alcohol according to their make-up and state of health, it is difficult to draw a sharp line between the sober and the ' drunk.' It is best not to say whether a person is ' drunk ' but merely whether he is under the influence of alcohol to such an extent as to be incapable of performing the act in question. It must not be forgotten that the drink may have contained other toxic substances, e.g., methylated spirit (p. 34). Absinthe (banned in U.S.A.) contains extract of wormwood, an active narcotic poison which may cause convulsions.

Concussed or drunk? is often the problem if there has been an accident. The car driver may have been drunk before he was concussed or, though sober but concussed, he may smell of drink because of liquid ' first aid.' The history from onlookers may help. The patient, if concussed, has no clear recollection of what happened, but the alcoholic, though confused at first, becomes clearer on questioning.

In a person under the influence of alcohol the temperature is subnormal; the pulse rapid and bounding (in shock following an accident it is rapid but thin and thready). The pupils are dilated and sluggish. In alcoholic coma they may become small but will often dilate when the patient is stimulated sharply (Macewen's sign). The tongue is dry. The patient's breath smells of alcohol, and his speech is slurred. The patient tends to gesticulate wildly and breaks down emotionally during conversation. Hiccup, salivation, drowsiness and confusion are also significant signs.

In assessing the results of special tests it must be remembered that alcohol may dangerously impair judgment before it spoils the performance of these tests and occasionally it seems to improve the response to one of them. Several tests should therefore be used and allowance made for the fact that sober but nervous patients may perform them badly. Too much reliance should not be placed on any of the tests and particularly on the more acrobatic ones. It is a good plan if possible to repeat the tests after the patient has become sober.

Blood alcohol

Although the term ' drunk ' refers to a clinical condition and not to the amount of alcohol in the blood, the Road Safety Act (1967), now incorporated in the Road Traffic Act (1972), fixes 80 mg per 100 ml (17·4 m mol/l) as the level of alcohol (ethanol) at which legal sanctions are automatically applied. (The figure for mmol/l is roughly one quarter of that in mg per 100 ml.) This does not mean that lower levels are safe, for even small amounts of alcohol can impair judgment and manipulative skill. Hence prosecutions can be brought under the Road Traffic Act 1962 for driving under the influence of drink, regardless of the amount of alcohol taken. The alcohol content of expired air is the same as that of the blood and is measured by the Breathalyser.* The use of this is not author-ised under the Road Safety Act 1967 for it is only a screening test to assist the police to decide whether the driver can be required to give a specimen of blood. At the police station the driver must be offered a further breath test 20 minutes or more later. If this indicates a blood test 5 ml of blood should be taken into each of two fluoride-oxalate tubes (less if micro methods are used). Only non-alcoholic cleansers must be used on the skin. When a blood test is refused two specimens of urine must be provided one hour apart, and within one hour of the request, the second being sent for analysis (in duplicate). It is an offence not to provide a specimen of blood or urine. No excuse can be adjudged reasonable unless the person is physically (as from a tracheostomy) or mentally (as from extreme genuine fear of needles) unable to provide a specimen of breath or blood. The law, however, expects adults to overcome their fears, rational or irrational, in order to comply. Inability to provide urine at the appropriate time would probably invalidate the test on it. A less cumbersome procedure using a machine based on a fuel cell (The Alcometer) which gives an immediate and accurate reading is being developed. A urine concentration of 100 mg per ml (21·8 mmol/l) is deemed equivalent to a blood alcohol content of 80 mg per

---

* Alcotest 80 (not used in the Isle of Man).

100 ml (17·4 m mol/l). Blood can be taken from an unconscious person without waiting for anyone's approval other than that of the doctor if it is for diagnostic purposes, e.g: to look for and measure barbiturates as well as alcohol. Necropsy blood alcohol levels are satisfactory within 48 hours of death but are only as reliable as the conditions surrounding their collection. What use could be made of them would be usually for the coroner to decide. The police may test a driver at hospital if he is taken there but hospital staff are not required to take part in the obtaining of specimens or in getting consent for the police to do so. They should cooperate with the police and provide facilities but should do nothing that would significantly interfere with the patient's treatment.

Treatment

This is not usually an urgent matter for the patient will recover in time though, if methylated spirit has been drunk, special measures are indicated (p. 34). If there is doubt about head injury watch the patient for, as Osler said, ' Better admit a patient to hospital dead drunk than turn him away to be discharged from the jail dead but sober a little later.' An alcoholic who genuinely desires to give up drinking can be helped by Alcoholics Anonymous, P.O. Box 514 (11 Redcliffe Gardens, London SW10 9BG (01-352 9669) for London enquiries; 01-352 9779 for enquiries outside London) who will put him in touch with persons in many parts of the country and the world who will stand by him during the emergency period of urgent craving. A booklet *Where to find AA* is issued three times a year. (See also Appendix 20, p. 828).

Alcohol and flying

The Civil Aviation Authority in Circular 112/1973 states that even in simple aircraft blood alcohol concentrations of 40 mg per 100 ml (i.e. half the legal driving limit) are associated with highly significant errors by both experienced and inexperienced pilots. Even a single alcoholic drink can lead to a significant loss of performance which lasts for a considerable time. Pilots should not fly for at least eight hours after taking alcohol.

EMERGENCY ASPECTS OF DEATH

Signs of death

(For signs of brain death see p. 729).

While the fact of death is usually easily recognised there are cases where a decision is difficult and has certain emergency aspects such as whether to summon special aid and appliances.

In drowning and electrocution we should not too readily assume that biological death has occurred. Artificial respiration should go on for two hours after all signs of life have ceased or until an ECG can be done and shows, over a period of five minutes, no evidence of cardiac activity. In other cases, e.g., sudden coronary occlusion, it is possible to decide earlier that the patient has passed *flammantia moenia mundi* because there is evidence (silence on auscultation) that the circulation has ceased. Even so, death cannot be considered as certain, in these cases, unless the heart has stopped beating for at least five minutes. To be sure by palpation that the pulse is absent or that the nail bed changes colour on the application and release of pressure is difficult in a doubtful case. Fragmentation of the column of blood in the retinal vessels is a more useful sign. It is called ' cattle trucking ' or ' rail roading ' because the fragmented blood column resembles the wagons of a train. It is not always a conclusive sign of death and does not even always signify cardiac arrest. When the heart beat is very feeble ' rail roading ' may occur but then it moves along in one direction in a faintly pulsative fashion. It usually indicates a bad prognosis. The sign may also occur in leukaemia during life. When relatives request special confirmation of death the radial artery should be opened at the wrist to demonstrate that the circulation has ceased. A strip of plaster should be applied afterwards and it is best to place the arm on the abdomen, since if left at the side blood may seep out and cause an unsightly pool. Jewish law does not permit this test. (In case of doubt phone the office of the Chief Rabbi, p. 666.)

The time of death

It is wise when called to a patient whom you don't know and who has died suddenly and unexpectedly, to make observations on which an opinion may be given by you or someone else as to the time of death. (This is not necessarily the time of the injury which caused it.) The rectal, or failing this, the liver temperature (via a small incision under the right costal margin) should be taken. If the person has been dead for more than an hour or two a special low-reading thermometer may be needed. The rate of fall of body temperature after death is approximately $0.7°C$ per hour. Hence the number of hours since death is given by the formula

$$\frac{36.8°C \text{ minus rectal temperature.}}{0.7}$$

Temperature readings should be taken hourly for a few hours.

The elderly and the young cool relatively quickly after death and the obese relatively slowly. So it is difficult to be exact and the result must be interpreted with caution. A more accurate method is to use instead of the actual fall of temperature the percentage of the total fall from that of the body to that of the surroundings which has occurred in a given time. Space does not allow a full description. All the doctor need do is to supply the expert with two temperatures over a given period (four hours) and the temperature of the surroundings. From these the time of death can be calculated (Fiddes and Patten, 1958).

Rigor mortis should be noted. A rough timetable is that it starts on the face in six hours and reaches the hands and feet at 12 hours; it stays 12 hours and takes 12 hours to pass off.

Sometimes stiffness appears immediately on death and is shown by firm gripping of objects in the hands. This rare ' cadaveric spasm ' occurs in cases of violent death.

Post-mortem lividity due to movement of blood to dependent parts (hypostasis) begins within one or two hours of death and becomes fixed between six and eight hours later.

DEATH IN THE CONSULTING ROOM

This is an emergency situation for the corpse must be promptly removed. The police may not agree to take it from private premises and the ambulance service may refuse to transport a dead body. Probably the undertaker would be the most likely to help particularly if the doctor knew the patient and was able to certify the cause of death. In any event the coroner should be informed and preferably before the removal if the cause of death is unknown.

DEATH IN THE AMBULANCE

You may see the patient (BID—' Brought in dead ' or DOA— ' Dead on arrival ') in the ambulance to verify the fact of death. If this is uncertain you will see the patient in the casualty room. Consider the feelings of waiting patients in deciding how to act. Depending on where the patient lived you may accept the body in the hospital mortuary and tell the police or you may ask the driver to take it elsewhere, when he will notify the police. If the patient breathes his last in the receiving room while you are trying to save him this will not entitle you to sign the death certificate (see p. 684).

DEATH CERTIFICATES
(See note on p. 687.)

The issue of a death certificate (strictly a Medical Certificate of the Cause of Death) is not an emergency procedure though it often takes place in an atmosphere of stress. It is well to be familiar with the procedure beforehand.

The ' Notes and suggestions to certifying medical practitioners ' in the front of the certificate book and the ' list of indefinite and undesirable terms ' should be carefully studied, remembering that the reliability of statistics of the causes of death depends on the care with which these certificates are completed. The certificate now in use conforms to the recommendations of WHO and so allows international comparability.

Under the Births, Deaths and Marriages Regulations 1968 all deaths must be certified if a doctor has attended the patient during his last illness irrespective of whether the doctor or someone else has reported the case to the coroner. The doctor who certifies must be the registered (or for hospital deaths provisionally registered) medical practitioner who has been in attendance during the deceased's last illness. He must also have seen the deceased within fourteen days before death or his body after death (but not necessarily both). Unless it is for cremation there is at present (but see note on p. 687) no legal obligation on the doctor to see the body after death but he must be satisfied, e.g., from the ward sister's report that the patient is dead. What the doctor certifies is not the fact of death but its cause. The section:

$$' \frac{\text{seen}}{\text{not seen}} \text{ after death by me '}$$

on the certificate is included to help the registrar to decide whether to report the death to the coroner.

The procedure should therefore be as follows. Carefully observe the rules of your hospital about the time and place for signing death certificates. Fill in the cause of death and sign the certificate (giving your *registered* qualification) and also the Notice to Informant (for handing to the informant) and the counterfoil (for retention). In England and Wales the doctor is provided with a stamped addressed envelope in which to send the certificate, in confidence, to the Registrar. He does not have this privilege in Scotland or Northern Ireland. Be careful not to enter as a cause of death, albeit secondary, some condition such as an old and irrelevant fracture which would make the Registrar notify the Coroner for this would only cause distress to the relatives. Initial the back at A if the Coroner has been informed and at B if fuller information is offered later. When you are new to a hospital your signature will be unknown to the Registrar so it will help him if you also print it when you sign for the first time. In most hospitals it is usual when a death has been reported to the Coroner not to issue a death certificate. But the doctor has a statutory duty to certify and if the relatives desire it this must be done. In the rare instance of a Coroner deciding that there was no case for him to investigate the doctor's certificate would be needed. In the case of a cremation it is best to complete certificate B after necropsy since the cause of death has to be certified ' definitely ' and not just to the best of one's knowledge and belief.

If you see a patient for the first time who is moribund and who dies in the receiving room you are probably not the best person to give a death certificate since it has been held that one attendance may not be sufficient to justify your stating that you attended during the last illness. You should ring up the home doctor and if he cannot or will not give a certificate then you should ask the coroner's advice.

In Scotland the same (international) form of death certificate is used as in England and Wales in which the condition directly leading to death is stated first. The Scottish certificate records deaths during pregnancy or within six weeks thereafter. In Wales certificates in the Welsh language can be used.

NOTIFICATION OF THE CORONER

The Registrar of Deaths is the chief person whose statutory duty it is to report to the coroner (or in Scotland the Procurator Fiscal) deaths which seem to him to come within the coroner's jurisdiction. There is no similar statutory duty laid on a doctor as such. The head of a prison must report to the coroner the death of anyone dying there (whether a prisoner or not, but see p. 686). It may be that the coroner has a social or moral claim on the doctor as on anyone else to report an unnatural death to him but as such a claim would have no statutory basis and as in any case the test of enforcement could not be applied, no claim of this sort is exercised. The doctor and, indeed, anyone else should be careful that he could not, by any intended act or omission, be held to be obstructing the coroner in his duties. A system of cordial cooperation has grown up whereby ' coroner's cases ' are reported direct to the coroner and this is very convenient to all concerned. If you are in doubt as to whether the coroner should be informed, consult your chief or the records officer or have a word with the coroner's officer himself.

Deaths which a registrar has a statutory duty to report to the coroner are given in Regulation 51 (1) as follows:

Where a registrar is informed of the death of any person before the expiration of 12 months from the date of the death, he shall report the death to the coroner on a form provided by the Registrar General if the death is one—

(a) in respect of which the deceased was not attended during his last illness by a medical practitioner;

(b) in respect of which the registrar has been unable to obtain a duly completed certificate of cause of death;

(c) with respect to which it appears to the registrar, from the particulars contained in such a certificate or otherwise, that the deceased was seen by the certifying medical practitioner neither after death nor within 14 days before death; or

(d) the cause of which appears to be unknown; or

(e) which the registrar has reason to believe to have been unnatural or to have been caused by violence or neglect, or by abortion, or to have been attended by suspicious circumstances; or

(f) which appears to the registrar to have occurred during an operation or before recovery from the effect of an anaesthetic; or

(g) which appears to the registrar from the contents of any medical certificate to have been due to industrial disease or industrial poisoning.

Regulation 51 (2) says ' Where the registrar has reason to believe, with respect to any death of which he is informed or in respect of which a certificate of cause of death has been delivered to him, that the circumstances of the death were such that it is the duty of some person or authority other than himself to report the death to the coroner, he shall satisfy himself that it has been reported '. It is no longer necessary, however, for the death of a patient in a psychiatric hospital to be reported to the coroner for the reason of mental illness alone. Stillbirths must be reported if no doctor or midwife was in attendance. Deaths from any cause are reportable if the body is removed from the United Kingdom. This includes burial at sea because the limit of the Registrar's district is low water and not the three mile limit. An exception is an area of sea less than 12 miles across which is regarded as British territory.

Deaths of foster children have no longer to be reported but the possibility of the ' battered baby ' syndrome must not be forgotten.

Any doctor involved in an inquest is advised to get in touch with his medical protection society early rather than late. He can then be advised on any reports he has to make and can have legal representation if necessary.

Even in the mortuary, emergency situations may arise. An attendant once raised the alarm because he found blood dripping from the head of a corpse. Investigation showed that bleeding originated in the severed jugular veins following a partial necropsy (brain only).

For removal of kidneys for transplantation see p. 687.

Some coroners ask that all deaths within 24 hours of admission to hospital should be notified to them, but this is a purely private local arrangement.

INDUSTRIAL DISEASES AND POISONS

The current list of terms describing industrial disease or poisoning is:

1. INDUSTRIAL DISEASE OF THE LUNGS

   Anthracosilicosis, Anthracosis, Asbestosis, Bagassosis, Berylliosis, Dust Reticulation, Pneumoconiosis, Siderosis, Silicosis. Any lung disease qualified by an occupational term, e.g. Grinder's Phthisis, Farmer's Lung.

2. OTHER INDUSTRIAL DISEASES (except poisonings covered by 3 below).

   Anthrax, Caisson Disease, Compressed Air Illness. Decompression Sickness, Diver's Palsy, Farcy, Glanders, Leptospirosis ictero-haemorrhagica or canicola, Malignant Pustule, Mesothelioma of Pleura or Peritoneum, Spirochaetal Jaundice, Weil's Disease, Malignant Disease (Cancer or Sarcoma) or Leukaemia or Anaemia attributed to X-rays or Radio-Active Substances or Radiations. Any form of cancer of industrial origin due to a specific substance such as: Cancer of the Skin (Epitheliomatous Ulceration, Epithelioma, Squamous-celled Carcinoma) due to tar, mineral oil, arsenic pitch, bitumen, soot etc. Cancer of the Nose (Nasopharynx, Nasal Sinuses) or Cancer of the Lung (Bronchus or Bronchial) due to nickel fumes or vapour. Cancer of the Bladder or Renal Pelvis or Ureter (Papilloma of the Bladder) due to industrial chemical or dye-stuff preparations or processes. Any other disease qualified by an occupational term, e.g. Woolsorter's Disease.

3. INDUSTRIAL POISONING

   Toxic Jaundice and Toxic Anaemia unless the medical certificate clearly indicates that the condition is due to natural causes. Plumbism, Saturnism.

   Any condition certified as . . . poisoning or poisoning by . . .

NOTE.—The report of the Home Office Interdepartmental Committee on Death Certification and Coroners 1971 (The Brodrick Report) has been accepted in principal but the necessary legislation is awaited. When it is made the information given above about death certificates and coroners will be altered as follows. The doctor will be required to have seen the patient within seven days before death and must view the body after death. If he cannot certify he must notify the coroner who will decide whether to hold an inquest or not. Only in cases of homicide, deaths of persons in custody and unidentified bodies will the coroner be obliged to hold an inquest. The coroner will be able to accept documentary evidence and so reduce the need for doctors to attend court. There will be no medical coroners unless they are legally qualified also. Cremation certificates after death in hospital will be things of the past but outside hospital a second certificate from a member of a special panel will be needed. The certificate of the crematorium's medical referee will be abolished.

WHAT TO TELL THE PATIENT WHO HAS A FATAL DISEASE

The doctor is often faced with a very ill patient who asks what is really the matter and whether he will get better. This can be an emergency situation and much harm can be done and mental suffering caused by inexpert handling of it. It is well to be prepared, therefore, for sudden questions of this kind. It is always wise to avoid being trapped into giving an immediate answer unless this can be unmistakenly reassuring. When it would be otherwise consult the clergyman and the relatives first and find out the patient's religious views. These may be such that he would prefer to know that death is near and then it should be the priest who should tell him. Apart from this situation it is well to assume that where there is life there is hope and a good rule is never to tell a patient, and particularly a young patient, the hopeless truth for as Sir Frederick Treves advised, ' In the face of misfortune it is merciless to blot out hope '. Do not consider whether you will be thought clever or not but remember Sir Alfred Fripp's words ' If we cannot be clever we can always be kind '. The criterion to be satisfied should always be—what is best for the patient from the medical point of view? In most cases it is possible to give some fairly plausible and partially true explanation of the symptoms and to offer some hope that in the course of time things will be put right. Often disease and drugs dull the senses and there are few patients who when seriously ill can say with Dr. Johnson ' I have prayed that I may render up my soul to God unclouded '. The relatives should be told the true position but care should be taken that they do not by word or attitude convey anything but hope to the patient.

There are occasions when a patient who is likely to die soon should be given an opportunity to wind up his worldly as distinct from his spiritual affairs but this can usually be done in circumstances other than those of an emergency. When a patient wishes to make a death-bed will (p. 671) or a dying declaration (p. 662) he will know that he is about to die and his plight need not be hidden from him. Whether it is ever justifiable to tell a patient he is dying in order to extract a dying declaration is doubtful (p. 662).

ON WHAT TO DO WHEN THERE IS LITTLE TO BE DONE

One is sometimes called urgently by the relatives to the bedside of a patient dying a lingering death from advanced carcinoma. In such patients who have developed a high tolerance for morphine. A euphoriant linctus of the old ' Brompton cocktail ' type is recommended such as Morphine, Cocaine and Chlorpromazine Elixir BPC, Diamorphine and Cocaine Elixir BPC or Diamorphine, Cocaine and Chlorpromazine Elixir BPC. They all contain 5 mg of morphine or diamorphine and 5 mg of cocaine hydrochloride to each 5 ml.

There is no objection to the use of such preparations. Lord Horder said: ' It is the duty of a doctor to prolong life. It is not his duty to prolong the act of dying '. The Roman Catholic Church requires that nothing should be done with intention to hasten death even when it is imminent. There is no objection to using drugs to relieve suffering even if they will indirectly hasten death but if the patient's spiritual affairs are not in order his faculties should not be dimmed by drugs.

EMERGENCY BAPTISM

Any child which shows signs of life is qualified to be baptised even if it is not viable. It is not usual to baptise prematurely delivered products of conception which do not show signs of life. In deciding whether to baptise or not the wishes of the parents should be carried out.

Baptism constitutes reception as a Christian and not as a member of a particular church. It may be administered by anyone, male or female, having the use of reason whether baptised or not and irrespective of religious belief provided he intends to do what the Church does. Two things are necessary, (1) Invocation of the Holy Trinity and (2) the use of water. Lay baptism should be performed only in the case of necessity, but the reality of the necessity is for the person performing it to decide. Even if the urgency is not great the validity of the baptism is not affected provided the proper matter (i.e., water) and form of words are used. Godparents are not necessary for private or emergency baptisms.

The doctor's fingers moistened with water should touch the child's forehead while he says:— 'A. . . B. . . ., I baptise thee in the Name of the Father, and of the Son, and of the Holy Ghost.' This simple form is valid for Roman Catholics as for others, and is not afterwards to be repeated. It is valid and final whether the child lives or dies. A name is not necessary for emergency baptism. If there is any doubt particularly in the mother's mind as to whether baptism has been already performed or whether the child is alive, the baptism should be made conditional by prefacing the above words with ' If you can be baptised . . . .' The clergyman of the parents' denomination should be informed.

In the case of a moribund nameless foundling, it is for the doctor to decide whether to baptise or not. If he does administer baptism it should be conditional and a surname should be chosen afterwards. A clergyman of the Church of England should be informed unless the circumstances strongly suggest alternative procedures, such as the discovery of the child in a Roman Catholic church. It is well to choose names which would not handicap or embarrass him should he survive. The Local Authority who is his guardian has the right to choose names but will usually accept those given at an emergency baptism. The birth is registered by the Children's Officer of the Local Authority after application to the Registrar General.

Special points applicable to Roman Catholics

Roman Catholics require the water to run and therefore prefer pouring to sprinkling. Other points are expressed in the Code of Canon Law 1918, from which the following translation is made:

Canon 746, §1. No human being enclosed in the mother's womb may be baptised so long as there is probable hope of administering baptism after birth.

§2. If the head presents and there is danger of death it must be baptised on the head; if born alive it must not be baptised again conditionally.

§3. If other parts present and there is danger of death, the presented part must be baptised conditionally; if born alive baptism must again be administered conditionally.

§4. If a pregnant mother dies, the fetus must be extracted by those whose duty it is, and if certainly alive baptised absolutely; if doubtfully alive baptised conditionally.

§5. A fetus baptised in the womb must be baptised again conditionally after birth.

Canon 747. Care should be taken that every fetus born prematurely, no matter at what stage of growth, shall be baptised absolutely if certainly alive, conditionally if doubtfully alive.

Canon 748. Monstrous and unusual forms should always be baptised at least conditionally; if it is doubtful whether there is more than one individual, one must be baptised absolutely and the others conditionally.

Canon 749. Foundlings must be baptised conditionally, unless after careful investigation their certain baptism has been established.

C. ALLAN BIRCH

Note on rape

Women victims of rape (recent or remote) can get sympathetic advice and a companion to accompany them to the doctor, police or court hearing from The Rape Crisis Centre whose address is

PO Box 42, London N6 5BU

01.340 6913 (1000 to 1800 hours)

01.340 6145 (outside normal hours).

REFERENCES

FIDDES, F. S. & PATTEN, T. D. (1958). A percentage method for representing the fall in body temperature after death. *Journal of Forensic Medicine,* **5,** 2.

BROWN, S. S., FORREST, J. A. H. & ROSCOE, P. (1972). A controlled trial of fructose in the treatment of acute alcoholic intoxication. *Lancet,* **2,** 898.

CHAPTER 32

Some Practical Procedures

DOSES FOR CHILDREN

A system which expresses children's doses as a percentage of adult ones has been devised by Catzell. It gets over the difficulty that factors like lean body mass and extracellular fluid which really determine dosage are more closely related to surface area than to weight and uses the relationship between weight and surface area

Table 32.1 *Doses for children*

AGE	WEIGHT kg	PERCENTAGE OF ADULT DOSE
Premature	1·1	2·5 to 5
Premature	1·8	4 to 8
Premature	2·5	5 to 10
Term	3·2	12·5
2 months	4·5	15
4 months	6·5	20
12 months	10	25
18 months	11	30
3 years	15	33
5 years	18	40
7 years	23	50
10 years	30	60
11 years	36	70
12 years	40	75
14 years	45	80
16 years	65	90

to construct a table showing the percentage of an adult dose needed by a child. Table 32.1 is unreliable for newborn and premature infants who should only be given two thirds of the dose shown in the absence of special instructions from the manufacturers. It is also unreliable for narcotic drugs. Very fat children should only have about three quarters of the dose indicated.

The Alder Hey Book of Children's Doses (Liverpool, 1973) lists some 120 drugs and gives their dose calculated by the percentage method at birth to two weeks, from two weeks to one year, seven years and for an adult. This saves trouble in working out the percentage dose.

IDENTIFICATION OF TABLETS

Many doctors prescribe tablets which they rarely see and with whose appearance they are unfamiliar. Loose tablets have sometimes to be identified in an emergency and so a study of what various tablets look like is worthwhile. The addition of colouring to BP tablets other than those specified is not official and pharmacists generally disapprove of recognising tablets by colour. Although colour is not added to proprietary tablets for any scientific reason such as identification or to mask a mottled appearance it can help in its recognition. The doctor, for his own convenience, may consider it advisable to select for his bag brands of tablets of distinctive marking and colour as this may lessen (but not eliminate) any chance of confusion in an emergency. It must not be forgotten that colouring can make tablets dangerously attractive to children. Some tablets such as Gantrisin and Negram, have their full names impressed on them. Others have distinctive markings, often an abbreviation of the chemical name, e.g. SMZ (Sulphamerazine). *Imprex* (Index of Imprints used on Tablets and Capsules) by W. A. L. Collier, 5th edition 1975 (price 40p from Imprex, 19 Earl Street, Cambridge) facilitates recognition of imprinted tablets and other solid dose forms including Co-tabs (tablets with a code number stamped on them). Until an imprint system is generally adopted for all solid forms of medication other aids to identification will have to be used, such as the Colour Identification Chart published in *MIMS Annual Compendium* and a system of punched feature cards (*Lancet,* 1975, 1, 552). Help may also be obtained through the Poisons Information Service (p. 813).

THE TELEPHONE AND NEWSPAPER IN EMERGENCIES

In order to call the police or an ambulance the telephone should be used in accordance with the instructions issued by the Post Office. With the automatic (dial) telephones of London and certain other places, 999 should be dialled. This does not call the police or ambulance direct but makes a special signal at the telephone exchange. The call is then passed to the appropriate emergency authority by the operator according to the request of the caller. In some areas emergency calls are made by dialling ' 0 ' or ' 01 ' or by pressing an emergency button.

The *Daily Mail* will print in its Continental Edition emergency messages recalling relatives of urgently ill patients. The request must be made through the Automobile Association (Tel. 01-964 7373).

EXTRACT FROM RULES FOR THE BROADCASTING OF SOS AND SIMILAR MESSAGES

1. For relatives of sick persons

The British Broadcasting Corporation (Broadcasting House, London, W1A 4WW, Tel. 01-580 4468) will broadcast messages requesting relatives to go to a sick person only when the hospital authority or the medical attendant certifies that the patient is *dangerously ill,* and if all other means of communication have failed. In the normal course of events messages will be broadcast only when the full name of the person wanted is available.

Note. When the person sought is known to be on board a ship at sea, a message can only be broadcast if the ship is not equipped to receive messages by wireless telegraphy. Further, there must be a possibility that the return of the person sought can be hastened by the reception of such a message. This is not considered to be so when the ship is on its way to a known port. In such cases, enquirers are advised to communicate with the owners or agents of the ship or with the port authorities.

In no case can an S O S be broadcast requesting the attendance of relatives *after death has occurred.*

2. Appeals for special apparatus, foods or medicines

(See also Appendix 16, p. 822).

These appeals will be broadcast only at the request of major hospitals, and after every other means of obtaining the required item has failed. There is no charge for broadcasting S O S messages.

No message can be broadcast regarding lost animals or property, except where there is real danger to life, as from the theft of dangerous drugs or from escaped wild animals, and then only at the request of the police. If a doctor loses his bag he should emphasise the fact that it contained dangerous drugs. This may expedite measures to recover it. The police and the Family Practitioner Committee should be informed if an EC10 prescription pad is lost or stolen as it could be used for forged prescriptions.

MEDICAL ADVICE TO SHIPS AT SEA

Requests for medical advice by ships without a doctor are usually sent by radio as set out under Medical Advice by Radio in the Admiralty List of Radio Signals. Ships in convoy may use visual signals or a loud hailer. The Master of a ship seeking advice should indicate the range of medicines carried. This is prescribed in the Merchant Shipping Medical Scales Order 1968. The Captain has with him the *Ship Captain's Medical Guide* (20th edition 1967, reprinted 1973) or the *International Ships' Medical Guide* (1967, WHO, Geneva). Reference to this will show how details of a case should be given to the doctor. *The Medical Code of International Signals* is now rarely used except to overcome language difficulties. Whenever possible the doctor should reply with the diagnosis, directing the Master to the treatment in his book; he should make sure that any drug ordered is actually on board. The doctor may have to advise whether a ship should continue on her course or make for the nearest port. Often the best way of dealing with a medical emergency at sea is to make an all-ship broadcast asking for help. If the doctor has to see the patient and cannot deal with the situation by advice alone then it is best for the patient to be transferred to the doctor's ship rather than for the doctor to go to the patient. The facilities will be better and there is no risk of losing the doctor. If the doctor cannot examine his patient, instructions by radio do not involve him in any legal responsibility either through errors in transmission or from any other cause.

THE 'MEDICO' SERVICE OF THE GENERAL POST OFFICE

Ships of all nationalities can get free medical advice by radio through the 12 Post Office radio stations in Great Britain detailed in Table 32.2.

Although medical aid by radio is mostly sought when there is no ship's surgeon, advice may be asked by a ship carrying a doctor and so details of the available services are given.

The 'Medico' service is free of charge and is conducted by either exchange of radio telegrams using morse or by radio telephony between ship and shore if within approximately 350 miles. In addition, a world-wide service similar to CIRM is available through Portishead radio. Messages can be sent to CIRM but then a charge is made. Messages go onward by telephone or, increasingly, by direct radio telephone communication between the ship and the doctor or hospital via the coast radio station. Requests by ships for this service are normally prefixed MEDICO XXX or MEDICO PAN by radio telephone. When it is feasible and desirable to land the patient this is arranged by the coast station through the Port Medical Officer or the Coast Guard.

CENTRO INTERNAZIONALE RADIO-MEDICO (CIRM)
(via dell' Architettura 41 (EUR) Rome Tel. 593331-2)

The International Radio-Medical Centre, founded in 1935 by Professor Guido Guida, provides free continuous medical service

Table 32.2. *Radio Stations in Great Britain which will transmit medical advice to ships*

RADIO STATION	MEDICAL AUTHORITY	PHONE NUMBER
Wick	Public Health Department, Rhind House, Wick, Caithness.	Wick 2247 (STD 0955)
	Bignold Hospital, Wick, Caithness.	Wick 2434 (STD 0955)
	After office hours—	Wick 2742 (STD 0955) or 2539 (STD 0955)
	or Central Hospital, Wick	Wick 2261 (STD 0955)
	or Medical Centre, Wick	Wick 3477 (STD 0955)
Stonehaven	The Royal Infirmary, Casualty Department, Woolmanhill, Aberdeen.	Aberdeen 23423 (STD 0224)
Cullercoats	The Ingham Infirmary, South Shields	South Shields 60221 (STD 08943)
	or, the Royal Victoria Infirmary, Newcastle-on-Tyne.	Newcastle 25131 (STD 0632)
Humber	Grimsby General Hospital, West Marsh, Grimsby.	Grimsby 59051 (STD 0472)
North Foreland	The Medical Officer on Duty, Hulk ' Hygeia ', off Gravesend.	Gravesend 2325 (STD 0474)
Niton	The House Surgeon (or the Resident Medical Officer), Royal Isle of Wight County Hospital, Ryde, Isle of Wight.	Ryde 3311 (STD 0983)
Land's End	The West Cornwall Hospital, Penzance.	Penzance 2382 (STD 0736)
	or Port Medical Officer— Office—	Penzance 3866 (STD 0736)
	Home—	Penzance 3015 (STD 0736) and 2503 (STD 0736)
Ilfracombe	Ilfracombe and District Tyrrel Hospital, Marlborough Road, Ilfracombe.	Ilfracombe 3448 (STD 027 16)
Portishead	Weston-Super-Mare General Hospital, Boulevard, Weston-Super-Mare.	Weston-Super-Mare 25211 (STD 0934)
Anglesey	The Caernarvon and Anglesey General Hospital, Bangor.	Bangor 3321 (STD 0248)
Portpatrick	The Garrick Hospital, Stranraer.	Stranraer 2323 (STD 0776)
	or Health Centre, Stranraer (Weekdays 0800 to 1800 hours)	Stranraer 2666 (STD 0776)
Oban	The West Highland Hospital, Glencruitten Road, Oban.	Oban 2544 (STD 0631)

for patients of any nationality on ships sailing under any flag in any sea. Communications are made in English, French or Italian. The advice of specialists can be called for. It can arrange for transfer of a patient to a ship with a doctor on board. It also serves the small Italian islands in the Mediterranean.

Messages can be sent to IRM (the centre's radio station) or to IAR (Rome radio). A large network of radio stations can be used when direct contact with IRM and IAR is impossible.

The publication *Radio-Medical Assistance* (CIRM, via dell' Architettura 41, Rome) containing also a code for medical communications, gives instructions for the compiling of radio-medical messages.

The frequencies on which IRM operates during the 24 hours are chosen from among the following:

FREQUENCY	CALL-SIGN	SERVICE
KHz 4342	IRM	On request and in order to answer ships using the medium frequencies.
KHz 4350	IRM	Available when necessary.
KHz 6365	IRM	Winter night service.
KHz 6420	IRM	Available when necessary.
KHz 8685	IRM	Replaces the 12760 kHz frequency when this is used for other services, and on request.
KHz 12760	IRM	Continuous. When used for other services it is replaced by 8685 or 12748 kHz.
KHz 12748	IRM	Available when necessary.
KHz 17105	IRM	Continuous during the summer season; daytime during the winter.
KHz 22525	IRM	Available when necessary.

At 0200, 0800, 1 400 and 2 000 hours GMT, the list of outstanding traffic is transmitted on the particular frequencies being used at that moment. Ships are recommended to listen in to this list in case of any possible request for transmission of a message.

In order to facilitate and speed up the handling of the radio-medical traffic, Radio Officers are advised to observe the following rules, as far as possible:

(a) always to attempt to communicate directly with the CIRM station, requesting, in case of difficulty, to be linked through other Italian coastal radio-stations. This is particularly necessary when first-aid messages are concerned;

(b) always to indicate their position and the frequency that offers the best reception, in order to enable the frequency or frequencies most suitable for subsequent communications to be established;

(c) bear in mind that, in the event of urgent necessity and of difficulty in communicating with the CIRM radio station, messages can be sent, free of charge, through other stations. The reply messages will be transmitted through the same stations unless, in the meantime, direct communication has been established.

PATHOLOGICAL SPECIMENS BY POST

Very precise regulations govern the packing of pathological specimens for the post, including specimens from patients who have been given radioactive isotopes. These allow them to be sent by first class letter post but *on no account by parcel post* provided that they (1) are enclosed in a securely sealed receptacle, which is itself contained in a strong wooden or metal case and (2) are surrounded by sufficient absorbent material to prevent any leakage. The package must be conspicuously marked ' Fragile With Care ' and must bear the words ' Pathological Specimen '. It must be addressed to a recognised medical authority or laboratory or to a medical or dental practitioner or veterinary surgeon. It is well to add other words describing the contents, e.g. 'Agricultural Poison '. The Railex system (transfer by the Post Office to the next available train and collection and delivery by messenger) could be used. Outfits for sending specimens are supplied by the Public Health Laboratory Service and though they do not conform strictly to the regulations, they have been approved by the postal authorities. Postage is less if specimens are sent in lightweight sealed plastic tubes.

INFECTIOUS DISEASES IN GENERAL WARDS
(See also Isolation and Quarantine, p. 445.)

The occurrence of an infectious fever in a general ward creates an urgent situation for the doctor in that action and advice are needed at once. There is no rule of thumb plan about isolation and quarantine. Our aim should be to prevent spread of disease to susceptible patients, and at the same time, not to interrupt the work of the ward unnecessarily. Surveillance often achieves this object better than quarantine, but the nursing staff should be told what to look for, e.g., slight coryza and rise of temperature. Chicken-pox and mumps can be regarded as almost inevitable and it is a good thing if healthy children can get over them before they grow up. Elaborate measures to escape them are not to be encouraged except in special cases. Any members of the staff who have not had the disease in question or been vaccinated against it should be carefully watched.

It is best to let them leave the children's or maternity ward for an adult ward. In the case of certain diseases the Community Physician must be notified. In some areas he wishes to know about rubella also and other diseases may be made notifiable in special circumstances, e.g chicken-pox during an epidemic of smallpox.

The current (1968) list of infectious diseases notifiable in England and Wales is:

Acute encephalitis	Ophthalmia neonatorum
Acute meningitis	Paratyphoid fever
Acute poliomyelitis	Plague
Anthrax	Relapsing fever
Cholera	Scarlet fever
Diphtheria	Smallpox
Dysentery (amoebic or bacillary)	Tetanus
Infective jaundice	Tuberculosis
Leprosy	Typhoid fever
Leptospirosis	Typhus
Malaria	Whooping cough
Measles	Yellow fever

Food poisoning and suspected food poisoning is also notifiable (see p. 134).

These diseases, and food poisoning, are also notifiable in Scotland, with the addition of cerebrospinal fever, encephalitis lethargica, erysipelas, pneumonia (acute influenzal and acute primary), poliomyelitis, puerperal fever and puerperal pyrexia, and in Northern Ireland with the addition of gastroenteritis (under 2 years of age only).

Notification is no longer required in England and Wales in the case of pneumonia, acute rheumatism, erysipelas, membranous croup and puerperal pyrexia. The action to be taken in the ward is indicated in Table 32.3.

LABORATORY DIAGNOSIS OF SMALLPOX

When smallpox is suspected the local Community Physician should be informed. He will examine the patient and if necessary call a member of a panel of practitioners in each Regional Health Authority's area designated to assist in the diagnosis (see Diagnosis of Smallpox Medical Memorandum of the Department of Health and Social Security and the Scottish Home and Health Department, 1972).

Material should be collected as follows:

MACULO-PAPULAR RASH. Clean the skin with ether or spirit. Scrape at least six lesions with the needle and make six smears on four glass sides. Allow the smears to dry in the air. *Do not heat.* Place each pair of slides face to face but separated so that they will not stick together. Mark the side of the slide on which the smear is and return slides to the box. Replace needle in tube.

	DISPOSAL OF PATIENTS	IMMUNISATION OF CONTACTS	ADMISSIONS	DISINFEC-TION
Amoebic dysentery	O	O	O	D
Anthrax	R	O	O	D
Bacillary dysentery	H	O	O	D
Chickenpox	H	O	R	D
Cholera	R	O	O	D
Diphtheria	R	P+A. 1.	O	D
Encephalitis	R	O	O	D
Enteric fever (typhoid and para-typhoid)	R	O	O	D
Epidemic pleurodynia (Bornholm disease)	R	O	O	D
Erysipelas	H	O	O	D
Food poisoning	R	O	O	D
Gastroenteritis	R	O	O	D
Herpes simplex	H	O	O	D
Herpes zoster	H	O	O	D
Impetigo	H	O	O	D
Infective hepatitis (virus A & B)	R	O (? P)	O	D
Leprosy	S	O	O	D
Measles	H	O (? P)	O	D
Meningitis				
aseptic	R	O	O	D
meningococcal	R	O. 2	O	D
pneumococcal	O or R	O	O	O
tuberculous	O or R	O or A	O	O
Mumps	H	O	O	D
Mycoplasma pneumonia	R	O	O	D
Paratyphoid (*see* Enteric)				
Poliomyelitis	R	A	O	D
Psittacosis	R	O	O	D
Q fever	R	O	O	D
Roseola infantum	H	O	O	O
Rubella	H	O	O	D
Salmonella infections	H	O	O	D
Scarlet fever	R	O	O	D
Smallpox	S	A (? +P)	S	S
Staphylococcal infections	H	O	O	D
Typhoid (*see* Enteric)	R	O	O	D
Vaccinia	R	O	O	D
Whooping cough	R	O	O	D

Table 32.3. *Policy for infectious fevers in general wards*

1. Send nose and throat swabs from staff and patients in the ward.
2. Prophylactic sulphonamides to close contacts for 24 hours.

DISPOSAL OF PATIENTS
    O No action
    R Remove to infectious diseases unit.
    H Remove to infectious diseases unit or home as appropriate.
    S Special procedure. Notify Infectious Disease Consultant and
      Community Physician at once.

IMMUNISATION OF CONTACTS
    O No action.
    A Active immunisation.
    P Passive immunisation.

ADMISSION POLICY
    O No action.
    R Restrict admission to immunes.
    S Special precautions. No admissions or discharges.

DISINFECTION
    O No action.
    D Disinfect bed, mattress and bed table.
    S Special precautions. Destroy bedding.

Note
    Living measles virus vaccine is effective within the first few days
of the incubation period.
    A history of chickenpox is doubtful is there are not pockmarks
anywhere.
    Smallpox. You must not move the patient until he has been seen
by the Community Physician.

VESICULAR AND PUSTULAR STAGE. Remove the tops of 6 to 10 lesions and place in the small bottle. Collect fluid in capillary tubes and replace in large bottle. Scrape bases of lesions 4, 5 and 6 and make smears as above.

CRUSTING STAGE. Remove as many scabs as possible up to 12 and place in small bottle.

Samples of blood taken early and late in the illness may help to confirm the diagnosis when tested for rising antibody titres. Ten ml of clotted blood is sufficient. During the febrile stage of illness in a patient or contact there is the possibility of viraemia so that a blood sample sent then may be tested for the presence of virus. Give the patient's name and age and also his previous vaccination history. The whole outfit whether used or not should be packed up and sent by hand to the laboratory. Otherwise send it as indicated on p. 698. Always warn the receiving laboratory by telephone of the despatch of specimens.

RESULTS. The most sensitive test is egg culture and so, if material

24

is scanty, it must be used for this even though it takes 48 to 72 hours. The complement fixation test can be read the same day but it is only diagnostic of the variola-vaccinia-cowpox group. If there are sufficient slides one may be stained and can yield a presumptive diagnosis within an hour. Egg cultures from febrile controls may show a diagnostic growth by the time the patient's rash appears.

EMERGENCY TRAVEL ABROAD
(For details of removal of patients by air
see Appendix 18, p. 825.)

Note. A British Visitor's Passport valid without visa for short visits to most European countries may be obtained 'over the counter' at main post offices. Evidence of identification (birth certificate, pension book or NHS card), two photographs and a fee of £2 are needed.

Air attendants

Advice on the suitability of air travel should be sought from the medical department of the air line concerned. Most invalids can be accepted for air travel but may be refused if not accompanied by a doctor or a nurse. This requirement can be met quickly by the St John Association and Brigade who will provide Air Attendants free of charge. Travelling and other expenses such as the cost of displacing seats to accommodate a stretcher are the responsibility of the person requesting the service. Apply from Monday to Friday 0930 to 1730 hours to The Registrar, St John Ambulance Association, 1 Grosvenor Crescent, London SW1X 7EF (01-235 5231 and out of hours 01-650 4489). The escort service is world wide. Within the U.K. all means of transport are used. A patient fitted with a pacemaker (p. 74) or any metal prosthesis should disclose this as it would show on electro-magnetic screening now used to prevent sky-jacking. This momentary procedure would not affect the working of the pacemaker.

The Invalid Travel Section of the British Red Cross Society will provide help with the movement of invalids by expediting documentation and obtaining passports, visas and tickets. The Panel of Overseas Escorts provides nurses for those requiring constant care. Foreign nationals who fall ill in Britain are eligible for these services. The National Headquarters, 9 Grosvenor Crescent, London SW1 7EJ, will accept calls day and night and at weekends (01-235 5454).

VACCINATIONS FOR FOREIGN TRAVEL

Although most countries are now signatories to the International Health Regulations (1969) of the World Health Organisation, the requirements for certificates of immunisation may vary and are apt to be changed at short notice. The Department of Health's Notice to Travellers advises every person going abroad to contact the representatives in the United Kingdom of the country or countries to which he is going, asking for the precise requirements of each country as to vaccination and the validity of vaccination certificates. He should also state whether he intends to travel by air or otherwise. The Passport Office, Clive House, 70-78 Petty France, London SW1H 9HD (01-222 8010) gives a list of representatives in the booklet *Essential Information.* Advice can also be obtained from the reservations department of the air line or shipping company concerned or its accredited agents. A booklet, *Vaccination Certificate Requirements for International Travel,* published by the World Health Organisation, Geneva, gives details of the variations in requirements in 184 countries. Purchasers are kept informed yearly of changes. The present booklet is correct up to 1 January 1972. Amendments are also published in the *Weekly Epidemiological Record* of the World Health Organisation. A summarised version is provided in the Wellcome booklet *Traveller's Guide to Disease Protection.*

In addition to the specific requirements of particular countries all persons going overseas are advised to be effectively vaccinated against typhoid giving, for milder reactions, 0·1 ml of TABT intradermally. (The addition of tetanus toxoid seems to lessen any reaction.) Effective immunity develops after ten days but a further dose four to six weeks later is generally given. It is advisable for all travellers to Africa, Asia and America (except Canada and U.S.A.) to be vaccinated against poliomyelitis by one drop of Sabin vaccine on a sugar lump once every three weeks for three doses and a booster every three years. Travellers to West, Central and East Africa who are likely to be exposed to infection with *Trypanosoma gambiense* should be given pentamidine 300 mg i m which will give protection for three to six months. It is well to carry an ordinary certificate of vaccination against diseases for which protection has been given but for which there is no international requirement.

International Certificates of Vaccination

These are only necessary in the case of smallpox and yellow fever. A smallpox vaccination certificate is now only required from those entrants to the UK who, in the previous 14 days, have been in a country (hopefully now only Ethiopia) any part of which is infected.

Travellers from the UK should find the current requirements re smallpox from the relevant embassy or the DHSS 01-407 5522 Ext. 6711/6749 during normal working hours. Since 1 January 1974 there has been no legal requirement for international cholera vaccination certificates but as some countries may still require evidence of vaccination inquiries should always be made about the current requirements of the country concerned. Babies under 12 months no longer need smallpox vaccination certificates unless they are being brought from infected areas. If the first attempt at primary vaccination against smallpox fails at least two attempts with different batches of lymph should be made and the results recorded (p. 761). Any doctor can vaccinate against smallpox and cholera and certify but yellow fever vaccination and certification can only be done at special centres (p. 782). International Certificate forms for smallpox vaccination can be obtained from the transport company, travel agents or the Government Health Department (Appendix 1, p. 764). International certificates of vaccination against yellow fever are only supplied at special vaccination centres. An international smallpox vaccination certificate must be signed by the vaccinated person and the person doing the vaccination. A rubber-stamped signature is not acceptable. The vaccine batch number and maker must be stated. Certificates must be completed in English or French but another language may be added. Amendments and erasures make a certificate invalid. Strictly vaccination against smallpox and yellow fever is free in the NHS and it is the certificate for which a fee is charged. Other vaccinations attract fees whether certified or not. It is wise to obtain an international certificate of smallpox vaccination if there is any possibility of needing it in the next three years since if the doctor concerned was not available his deputy or successor strictly could not certify later. Nevertheless, the Health Authority's doctor might be prepared to certify vaccination from practice records if he knew the vaccinating doctor.

The doctor's written signature must be authenticated in a way prescribed by the Health Authority of the territory where the vaccination was done. Certificates by practitioners in Eire will be authenticated if sent to the Deparment of Health, Custom House, Dublin.

Difficulty sometimes arises when a person wishes to travel urgently by air and has only just been vaccinated against smallpox for the first time so that his certificate is not valid. The air line might accept him if he completes a form of indemnity against liability for expenses and delays. He would have to risk being refused admission or of being placed under surveillance at his destination though he might be accepted on compassionate grounds. The decision rests solely with the health authority on arrival. Emergency travel would not be by sea and in any case a sea journey would allow time for vaccination by the ship's surgeon. Occasionally a port medical officer has demanded two signatures on certificates before allowing passengers ashore. The overcautious passenger may meet this requirement before leaving home in case of need. The signature of the ship's surgeon might be regarded as invalid if he could not stamp it with the words ' National Maritime Board of the United Kingdom ' which it has been agreed should be used throughout the shipping industry.

The periods of validity of certificates are : —

Smallpox.—from eight days after primary vaccination for three years (Pakistan two years). From the day of revaccination for three years. Persons who have been abroad for long periods should be careful that the validity of the smallpox vaccination certificate has not expired before they arrive here.

Yellow fever.—From 10 days after primary vaccination for 10 years. From the day of revaccination for 10 years if vaccinated within the previous 10 year period.

DAY	VACCINE
First	Yellow fever 0·5 ml. Preferably using Arlivax Yellow Fever Vaccine BP (17D strain) (Wellcome) which can be stored at any temperature up to 15°C but not frozen. Cholera 1·0 ml (8 000 × 10⁶ vibrios). TABC first dose 0·25 ml.
Fourth	Vaccine lymph against smallpox.
Seventh to tenth	TABC second dose 0·5 ml. Read result of primary vaccination against smallpox and enter on International Certificate whether it is successful or not. The fact of revaccination against smallpox has to be recorded but not the result.

Sequence of vaccinations

When time permits an interval of at least three weeks should elapse between the giving of any two live virus vaccines whichever is given first. If this is against yellow fever some would proceed with primary vaccination against smallpox four days later. It is immunologically more sound to give vaccines separately but the concurrent use of smallpox and yellow fever vaccines is now practised in the U.S.A. and recommended in the United Kingdom where there is evidence of previous successful vaccination against smallpox. Vaccinations may have to be given as quickly as possible and intervals reduced or abolished in order to allow certificates to become valid before departure. The following sequence of the usual vaccinations is convenient.

Infants should not be vaccinated against yellow fever until nine months old unless the parent or guardian requests it in writing. A period of three weeks should separate vaccination against poliomyelitis from other vaccinations (four weeks in the case of BCG). It would be best to give polio vaccine before the others to obviate the very slight risk of poliomyelitis developing after other vaccinations.

RECIPROCAL HEALTH AND WELFARE ARRANGEMENTS WITH OTHER COUNTRIES

Reciprocal arrangements for medical treatment existing between the U.K. and certain foreign countries fall into the following categories. (Those ineligible for treatment on grounds of nationality should take out insurance. This is not usually available after age 75 and it does not apply to pre-existing conditions.)

1. Bulgaria, Norway, Sweden, Poland and Yugoslavia. These countries give treatment under their own schemes to British people including visitors. New Zealand gives treatment under its own legislation and not under a reciprocal agreement.

2. Countries of the European Economic Community (Belgium, Denmark, France, The Federal Republic of Germany, The Irish Republic, Italy, Luxembourg, The Netherlands). British nationals visiting these EEC countries and ' Stateless persons and refugees permanently resident in the United Kingdom ' and who work for an employer there are entitled to medical treatment for urgent illness on the same basis as the insured people of the country in question. Self-employed and non-employed persons are not so entitled (except in Germany) because nationals of the EEC countries in these categories are themselves not eligible for benefit. There is no upper age limit. National Insurance pensioners and their dependants and widows are eligible for treatment except that a retired person not receiving a National Insurance pension is not entitled to benefit. Reciprocal Health Agreements under EEC regulations do not apply to non-EEC nationals. Difficulties about nationality should be referred to the Home Office, Immigrations and Nationality Dept., Lunar House, Wellesley Road, Croydon CR9 2BY.

Form CM1 obtainable from the local office of the Department of Health and Social Security or from employment exchanges must be completed not more than six months before departure. A certificate of entitlement (E111) is then given or sent which entitles the holder to free treatment in some countries and full or partial reimbursement of fees in others. It is valid for one month after the intended date of return. Reimbursements must be applied for while still in the country concerned. It must not be assumed that because treatment is free here it will be entirely so abroad. Further details of exactly what to do in the various countries are given in Leaflet SA 28 January 1973 obtainable from local offices of the Department of Health. An article 'Patients and the Common Market' appeared in *Health Trends,* Vol. 5, No. 2, May 1973. Although Denmark and Western Germany are EEC countries form E111 is not needed there but simply a British passport. All visitors whether employed or not are eligible for treatment. In Denmark a doctor emergency service is obtainable by dialling Copenhagen 0041. In the Irish Republic you can consult any doctor who is in the Health Service and you only have to complete the form which he supplies. Drugs have to be paid for in Denmark but are free in Ireland. A visitor may feel that, except in Denmark and the Republic of Ireland, the arrangements are too complicated, especially if travelling alone. He may prefer to take out private insurance.

3. In Switzerland treatment is given to British residents if they belong to an insurance scheme. This generally means that they are employed in Switzerland and the temporary visitor is advised to take out his own insurance.

4. Australia, Israel and Malta provide treatment for certain beneficiaries under the British insurance scheme. In Israel everybody is given medical first aid provided for by the Magen David Adom (the Israeli equivalent of the Red Cross Society), including victims of terrorist attacks whatever their nationality. Further arrangements are not yet completed.

5. The U.S.S.R. A reciprocal arrangement now exists between the N.H.S. of the U.K. and the U.S.S.R. and all visitors are covered.

6. There are also agreements with the Isle of Man providing services similar to those in the U.K. and with the Channel Islands which provide for treatment for visitors from the U.K. who spend less than three months in the islands in any one year. In Jersey hospital treatment is free. In Guernsey and Alderney general practitioner and hospital treatment are free but there is no out-patient or casualty department in Guernsey. Drugs are not free except in Alderney. There is no free service in Sark. Form E111 is not needed in the Isle of Man and the Channel Islands.

7. Austria. A recent agreement with Austria allows visitors to obtain urgent in-patient hospital treatment free of charge but other medical expenses are still chargeable.

8. Roumania. British visitors to Roumania who become ill during their stay are entitled to free medical treatment on production of a United Kingdom passport valid for entry into the Socialist Republic of Roumania.

9. Albania. There is no officially announced arrangement as there are no diplomatic relations between Albania and the U.K., but the author found that treatment was free but that drugs had to be paid for.

10. Gibraltar. A reciprocal health service agreement exists between the United Kingdom and Gibraltar. U.K. citizens holding valid passports visiting Gibraltar will be entitled to any necessary health care. (There is special provision to admit up to 40 patients a year from Gibraltar for National Health Service hospital treatment in the U.K. if adequate facilities for this do not exist in Gibraltar.)

LUMBAR PUNCTURE
(For hazards see p. 57.)
(For risks with spinal tumour see p. 314.)

As a needle coming from behind can be very worrying plentiful reassurance is wise. A very nervous adult patient should be given diazepam (Valium) 5 to 10 mg i v. A smaller oral dose should be given to a child (p. 692).

Position

The secret of success is to start with the patient in the correct position. If the operator is right-handed the patient should lie on his left side with his buttocks and shoulders on the hard edge of the bed. If the mattress sags put fracture boards under it but if possible an operating table should be used (Fig. 32.1). The long axis of the spine should be horizontal and the plane of the iliac crests vertical. The spine must be fully but not forcibly flexed and the patient should be asked to get his chin as near to his knees as possible. Tell him to arch his back like a cat. A roller towel placed round the neck and knees and tightened by twisting with a rod sometimes helps to obtain and maintain the flexed position. A pillow between the legs will prevent the patient from rolling over. When landmarks are uncertain the sitting position can make entry easier.

Site of puncture

The usual site is the space between the spines of the third and fourth lumbar vertebrae. This space is on Tuffier's line passing through the highest points of both iliac crests. It crosses the spine just above the fourth lumbar vertebral spine. Never tap higher than the space between the second and third vertebrae or the cord will be damaged. Fig. 32.2 shows the correct position of the vertebrae.

The puncture

The operator should position himself on a stool so that he can look along the line of the needle. A stout needle can be used if the spine is stiff and difficulty is expected. The stilette must fit flush to the end of the needle. Otherwise a fine No. 12 needle (23 SWG $\times$ 1$\frac{1}{4}$ inches; 0.6×31 mm) is to be preferred. As this is apt to bend it is a good plan to introduce a needle director or even an i v cannula first. This is inserted as far as the ligamentum flavum and the puncture is made by a fine needle passed down it. Dattner's double needle achieves the same result.

Clean the skin and apply 70 per cent alcohol. Let it dry and then apply Weak Solution of Iodine BP. Everything should be dry including the operator's hands. Gloves are not essential and instead of them a sterile towel may be used through which the needle is held and the skin palpated. A wheal of 2 per cent lignocaine is raised in the skin over the junction of the lower and middle thirds of the interspace. The skin is pierced through the wheal by giving the lumbar puncture needle a rolling motion. The direction of the needle is then readjusted so that while in the horizontal plane it is inclined about five degrees towards the head. It is then parallel to the slope of the vertebral spines. No resistance is felt until the ligament is reached. This is pierced with the bevel in the spinal axis (p. 58). A ' give ' as the dura is penetrated is not always experienced with the modern ultra-sharp needle. Withdrawal of the stilette allows the CSF to flow. Its pressure cannot be measured by the rate of drip so attach a manometer to measure it. With a very sharp needle there is a danger of going too far and puncturing the veins in the vertebral epidural space rather than of not going deep enough. It is well therefore to remove the stilette a few times as the needle is advanced. Be careful to replace the stilette each time. A refinement to prevent over-penetration is to remove the stilette when the ligament is reached and to put a drop of saline in the butt of the needle. When the tip enters the extradural space the saline is drawn inwards by negative pressure.

Difficulties

1. No fluid flows. Replace the stilette. Advance the needle a few millimetres and rotate in case a nerve root is obstructing it. Never try aspiration by a syringe.

2. Bone is encountered. This usually means that flexion is incomplete. Withdraw the needle and adjust the position.

3. Blood appears. If it is only a few drops and then nothing more it means that the needle has not gone far enough but is in the subdural space. Over enthusiastic insertion may encounter the anterior subdural space. A 'bloody tap' may be due to trauma or subarachnoid haemorrhage. Traumatic bleeding often shows as a swirl and clears as the fluid drains. If in doubt, take specimens into three numbered tubes and have red cell counts done on all three. A lightening colour or a diminishing count indicates traumatic blood. Clotting in the fluid may occur if bleeding was due to trauma and, if centrifugalised, the supernatant fluid will be colourless. In subarachnoid haemorrhage clotting does not occur and the supernatant fluid becomes yellow after a few hours for about a week. Red cells disappear in 5 to 10 days. While simple measurement of pressure is acceptable, ritual testing of its response to compression of the jugular veins (Queckenstedt's test) is to be discouraged. It is sufficient to show the normal response of a brisk rise of 10 mm or so when a patient breathing quietly, gives a cough.

Post-puncture headache

Measures to avoid this are : —

1. To use as small a bore of needle as possible.
2. To keep the bevel in the spinal axis (p. 58).
3. To make the patient lie down, preferably prone, for one to four hours after puncture.

Lumbar puncture should be avoided in the ward if there is any suspicion of papilloedema on ophthalmoscopy and even if the history is suggestive of raised intracranial pressure although there is not yet any swelling of the disc. Lumbar puncture in such cases should only be done where there are full neurosurgical facilities.

CISTERNAL PUNCTURE

(For hazards see p. 58.)

Position

The patient should lie on his left side with his head at the foot of the bed so that the bedpost is not in the way. The head is supported on a small sandbag and flexed. The spine should be horizontal (Fig. 32.3). The sitting position may be used in the conscious patient.

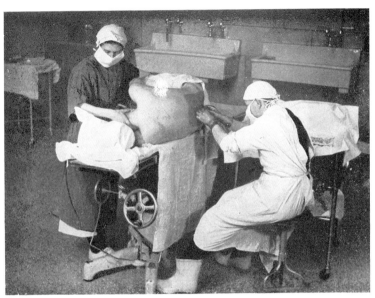

FIG. 32.1

Position for lumbar puncture. The operator's eyes are behind the hub of the
needle so that he can look along the line of the shaft.

(*Lumbar puncture and spinal analgesia. Macintosh & Lee.*)

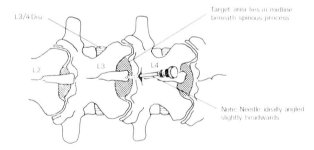

L3/4 Disc

Target area lies in midline
beneath spinous process

L2   L3   L4

Note: Needle ideally angled
slightly headwards

FIG. 32.2

Vertebral position with patient correctly placed.
(Courtesy of Teach-in and Dr John Patten.)

Facing p. 710

Site of puncture

This is determined by the fact that a horizontal plane through the tips of the mastoid processes bisects the atlanto-occipital space (Fig. 32.4). The tips of the mastoid processes are marked, and a horizontal line joining them is drawn using a tape measure and a skin pencil. The point where this line crosses the vertical midline of the neck is marked. This is the entry point.

The puncture

A Purves-Stewart graduated needle (Fig. 32.6) is convenient but a lumbar puncture needle may be used. A scratch made on it 5 cm from the tip is a useful guide.

The needle is directed slightly upwards so that the occipital bone is touched (Fig. 32.5). It is then worked down tapping the bone periodically until the atlanto-occipital ligament is reached. The needle is then advanced cautiously, removing the stylet at intervals until fluid appears. Some prefer to mount the needle on a syringe and apply slight suction when the atlanto-occipital ligament is pierced.

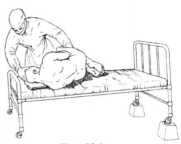

Fig. 32.3

Position for cisternal puncture in a comatose patient.

A rough idea of the depth at which the ligament will be reached is given by the neck circumference at the level of the upper border of the thyroid cartilage divided by nine. In an adult the cistern is about 5 cm from the skin and the medulla is about 1 cm further on.

STELLATE GANGLION BLOCK
(For indication see p. 535.)

The object is to infiltrate with local anaesthetic the region of the stellate ganglion on the side of the affected cerebral hemisphere (i.e., the opposite side to the paralysed arm and leg). The anterior route is the safest since the needle is above the dome of the pleura and there is little danger of pneumothorax. The injection is aimed at the upper part of the ganglion and we rely on the procaine seeping down to the part of the ganglion which overlies the neck of the first rib. The patient lies flat with his neck extended over a small pillow and this position is maintained throughout the operation. The entry point for the needle is a centimetre below the level

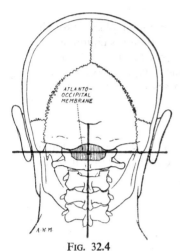

FIG. 32.4

The point of entry of the needle
at the intersection of a line joining the tips of the mastoids and
the vertical midline of the neck.
(Pye's Surgical Handicraft.)

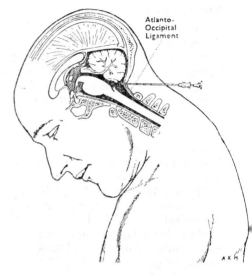

FIG. 32.5

Showing the direction of the needle which
has reached the atlanto-occipital ligament.
(Surgery of Modern Warfare.)

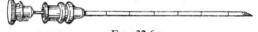

FIG. 32.6

Purves-Stewart's cisternal puncture needle.
(Pye's Surgical Handicraft.)

of the lower border of the body of the sixth cervical vertebra
close to the lateral border of the trachea. Two landmarks indicate
the sixth cervical vertebra. The cricoid cartilage lies opposite the
body and the large anterior tubercle of its transverse process (Chas-
saignac's tubercle) is fairly easy to feel. The entry point can also
be marked from below being about 4 cm above the inner end of
the clavicle at the median border of the sterno-mastoid muscle.
Raise a wheal of 1 per cent lignocaine at this point. Press the left
middle finger deeply on the inner border of the sterno-mastoid
muscle and palpate and displace laterally the carotid artery. Insert
a 10 cm needle along the finger and through the wheal straight
backwards between the carotid artery and the trachea until bone
(the body of the seventh cervical vertebra) is felt. These relationships are shown in Fig. 32.7. The stellate ganglion does not lie on

the periosteum but on the longus colli muscle and so the needle should be withdrawn 0·5 to 1·0 cm and a negative aspiration test obtained before injecting 5 ml of 1 per cent lignocaine. After withdrawing the needle a further 1 cm, 5 ml more are injected. The patient should be told to resist the desire to cough. Pain may be

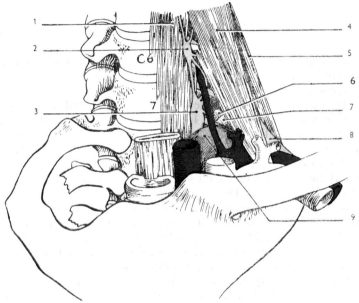

Fig. 32.7

The relations of the stellate ganglion.
1. Longus colli muscle. 2. Middle cervical ganglion. 3. Stellate ganglion.
4. Scalenus anterior muscle. 5. Scalenus medius muscle. 6. Transverse process of first thoracic vertebra. 7. Tubercle of first rib. 8. Brachial plexus. 9 Dome of pleura.

felt in the chest and arm but will pass off when the lignocaine is injected.

A successful injection is followed in about 10 minutes by Horner's syndrome (ptosis, miosis, enophthalmos, flushing of the face and conjunctiva and possibly unilateral blocking of the nose from engorgement). When performed for cerebral thrombosis or embolism the injection should be repeated every six hours during the first day and then daily for up to 15 days according to progress. It is possible to thread a fine polythene tube down the needle and to leave it in place for subsequent injections.

INTRA-CARDIAC INJECTION

Use a Langton Hewer cardiac puncture needle or a lumbar puncture needle and enter it in the third right interspace at the upper border of the fourth rib close to the sternum. Pass it downwards and towards the midline for two to four inches to enter the right atrium.

PERICARDIAL PUNCTURE
(For risks see p. 56.)

Circulatory arrest may complicate this procedure and so it is as well to insert fracture boards in the bed in case cardiac ' massage ' is called for.

The best place to insert the needle is 1 cm medial to the apex beat or if this cannot be felt, 1 cm medial to the left border of the cardiac dulness. The patient should be lying down so that the heart lies posteriorly. Infiltrate the site with 2 per cent lignocaine. (It is best not to include adrenaline lest any should enter the heart.) Use a very fine needle and if fluid is found replace it with a larger one to do the aspiration. Direct it towards the right sternoclavicular joint. If there is no fluid the fine needle will touch and may penetrate the left ventricle but will not damage it. It is helpful to use the needle as a lead and to attach it to the ECG machine. It will indicate when the ventricle is touched by showing marked ST elevation. When the atrium is touched PR elevation is shown.

Other routes may be used if fluid is loculated and it is necessary to obtain some but it would be wise to use diagnostic technical aids (radio-isotope scanning and ultrasound) first. The epigastric or Marfan route in which the needle is inserted in the costo-xiphoid notch is not advised. If there was no fluid the thin-walled atrium would be entered—a more serious complication than puncture of the left ventricle would be. If intercostal routes are used (5th or 6th left or 4th or 5th right) the needle should enter at least 2 cm from the sternal edge to avoid the internal mammary vessels. The 7th or 8th space in the mid-scapular line is particularly suitable in children.

CAROTID SINUS MASSAGE

When properly applied this is a very effective method of vagal stimulation, especially in patients with long narrow necks. It often fails because *pressure* only, rather than *massage,* is used. Give a sedative. The patient should lie flat (but when testing for hypersensitivity of the sinus (p. 228) he may stand). The head should be extended by a pillow under the neck and turned to one side. Face the patient and place the fingers of the left hand behind the neck and the thumb over the carotid sinus just below the angle of the jaw. The sinus may be felt as a bulge on the artery. Make firm strokes with the thumb up and down the artery for 3 or 4 cm while the patient counts aloud. Listen with a stethoscope all the time, letting the patient hold the bell over his apex. Massage for five seconds in the first instance. If ineffective try the other side but never massage both sides together. Some operators prefer to place the fingers in front and the thumb behind. As fatal ventricular fibrillation has occasionally resulted ECG monitoring is desirable so that stimulation can be stopped promptly if ventricular premature beats (especially ' R on T ' extrasystoles) occur. In all cases facilities for cardiac resuscitation should be at hand.

REMOVAL OF ASCITIC FLUID

Give a sedative if the patient is anxious (e.g. diazepam (Valium) 2 to 5 mg) an hour before. Make sure that the bladder is empty. Put a many-tailed bandage or binder under the patient. The puncture site may be in the mid-line between the umbilicus and the symphysis pubis or just above McBurney's point (midway between the anterior superior iliac spine and the umbilicus). Cleanse the skin and put sterile towels over the abdomen. Infiltrate the puncture site with 2 per cent lignocaine. Make a tiny nick with a scalpel and push in the trocar and cannula. The best instrument is Kerr's paracentesis trocar and cannula (Willen Bros. Ltd., 57 Dudden Hill Lane, London NW10 1BD). It has a blunt-ended cannula with side holes; is of narrow bore (2 mm outside diameter); has a wide flange to allow easy fixation and is quickly connected to the drainage tube by a Luer lock. Some prefer to insert first a wider cannula and to remove it after threading a plastic tube down it. If a Southey's cannula is used its little unattached silver guard must not be forgotten. The fine tubing is attached to the cannula at the start and the pointed trocar pushed through it to enter the cannula. Remove the fluid slowly into a Winchester bottle, and tighten the bandage as it drains. Inject 500 000 units of penicillin dissolved in 2 ml of isosmotic sodium chloride solution down the cannula before removal. Seal the puncture with a sprayed dressing. Send two samples of fluid to the laboratory (or all of it if requested). One sample should have citrate added to it. If there is doubt as to whether the fluid removed is ascitic fluid or urine have its urea content estimated. Urine contains about 300 mmol/litre of urea whereas ascitic fluid contains only about 5·0 mmol/l.

PNEUMO-PERITONEUM INDUCTION

A pneumoperitoneum may be induced in preparation for peritoneal dialysis (p. 718) and peritoneoscopy and to help in the diagnosis of liver abscess. It is no longer used as collapse therapy in pulmonary tuberculosis. The most convenient site for the intraperitoneal injection of air is near the left subcostal margin just external to the rectus abdominis muscle.

With aseptic precautions a wheal of 2 per cent lignocaine is raised in the skin with a small hypodermic needle. The syringe (2 ml) is recharged and, using a long serum needle, the abdominal wall is infiltrated down to the peritoneum. When this is punctured the sense of resistance to the piston disappears. Sudden penetration should be avoided. The piston should be withdrawn to make sure that the needle point is not in a blood vessel. A pneumothorax apparatus is then attached to the needle by an adaptor. Air is slowly injected in amounts up to 1 000 ml.

A manometer is unnecessary, but if available provides a useful indication that the needle is in the correct space by showing a rapid fall in pressure when the air flow is stopped. This procedure should be used at intervals during the induction. Other confirmatory signs that the needle is correctly placed are respiratory excursions and also a rise in pressure when the abdomen is pressed on. If before the air is run in the clips are suddenly opened and closed, the fluid in the manometer will rise and fall rapidly to almost zero if the peritoneal space has been entered. If the needle is outside the peritoneum, the pressure will remain high.

A Veress needle has certain advantages. It consists of a sharp needle in which runs a hollow, blunt-ended trocar with a lateral hole. The trocar is made to project slightly from the needle by a spring, thus ensuring that the gut is pushed away by the blunt end rather than the sharp needle point.

Clinical evidence that air has entered the peritoneal space is provided by pain in the shoulder regions and disappearance of liver dulness.

The most frequent cause of failure to induce a pneumoperitoneum is that the needle is not inserted far enough.

PERITONEAL DIALYSIS
(For hazards see p. 72.)

Indications

Peritoneal dialysis (PD) may be indicated in all types of acute and acute on chronic renal failure and occasionally to treat poisoning by dialysable agents. Its advantages are that the patient does not have to be bled, his veins remain untouched and there is no need for fluid and protein restriction. It is, however, about four times slower than haemodialysis and may prove technically impossible on account of ileus or adhesions. Relative contraindications are advanced pregnancy, large hernias, abdominal injury and recent surgery which has opened up the retroperitoneal space or disturbed the continuity of the peritoneum.

Dialysis fluid

The basic composition is : —

Na	140·5	mmol/litre
Ca	1·75	mmol/litre
Mg	0·75	mmol/litre
Cl	101·0	mmol/litre
Lactate	44·5	mmol/litre
Dextrose	13·6	g/litre

As this solution contains no potassium it may be used for the treatment of hyperkalaemia. The potassium level should be reduced with caution in digitalised patients lest digitalis toxicity be precipitated. When removal of potassium is considered inadvisable a solution containing potassium chloride 3 to 4 mEq/litre (mmol/litre) should be used. Commercial solutions are generally supplied with two concentrations of sodium and two of dextrose in 1 or 10 litre containers. The high dextrose solution is used for the rapid removal of oedema fluid. Normally the low sodium fluid is recommended except in hypotensive patients. Heparin 1 000 units per litre should be added to the first few exchanges to prevent occlusion of the cannula by fibrin. Gentamicin 4 to 6 mg per litre can be added but is best reserved for the treatment of established peritoneal infection. This is suggested by abdominal pain, tenderness, fever and a cloudy effluent and is confirmed by culture. Rarely monilial peritonitis ensues and is best treated by the addition of amphotericin B one mg per litre of dialysis fluid. Occasionally the same symptom complex is observed during PD from chemical peritonitis.

Apparatus

The plastic catheter of the Trocath (Chas. F. Thackray) fits over a long stilette introducer which makes a trocar unnecessary. The puncture is slightly smaller than the catheter diameter and this

25

ensures a tight fit and minimises leakage into the abdominal wall. Warming the bag of fluid to 40°C in a water bath makes for comfort and favours ionic exchange.

Technique

Shave the skin of the lower abdomen but leave the pubic hair. Prepare the abdominal wall with Betadine (which is subsequently removed with spirit) and place towels as for laparotomy. Let the patient empty his bladder or else catheterise him. Infiltrate 5 ml of one per cent lignocaine down to the peritoneum in either iliac fossa and introduce 1·5 to 2·0 litres of warmed dialysis fluid through the anaesthetised area by means of a plastic i v type of needle (Medi-cut 16 SWG × 1·8 inches; 1·7 × 45mm) and then withdraw the needle. Some operators induce a small pneumoperitoneum instead. Next choose a place in the midline one third of the way from the umbilicus to the symphysis but avoid any scars. Infiltrate down to the linea alba with one per cent lignocaine. Nick the skin with a small scalpel and pass it down till it grates on the linea alba. There will be very little bleeding in the midline. The Trocath is more easily inserted with the abdominal muscles contracted, so ask the patient to take a deep breath and raise his shoulders off the bed. Considerable force is needed to insert the Trocath and a ' give ' will indicate that it has entered the peritoneal space. Withdraw the stilette 4 cm and gently advance the catheter aiming for the true pelvis. If it meets resistance withdraw slightly and change the direction. It is normal for some fluid to come up the catheter even when the preliminary injection into the iliac fossa has been omitted. All the fenestrations of the catheter must be within the peritoneal space. Trim all but 4 cm of the projecting catheter. Securing of the catheter by adhesive and the metal disc provided is best delayed until a free flow is established. When fixing the fluid line to the chest or thigh this should be separate from the abdominal gamgee and elastoplast dressing to avoid accidental drag on the cannula. Use a bed cradle to keep the bed clothes off the catheter.

Connect the catheter to the main fluid container and run in one litre quickly (in about 10 minutes). Warn the patient against sudden movements such as sitting up in bed. Allow the fluid to remain for a dwell time of 20 to 40 minutes and then drain it off into a sterile bag by gravity. A non-return valve in the bag lessens the risk of retrograde infection. Slight initial blood staining of the fluid is unimportant. Always leave a few ml of PD fluid in the drainage bag to serve as an air lock. Normally one to two litres of fluid should be cycled hourly depending on the metabolic needs. The aim should be to keep the plasma urea below 180 mg per 100 ml (30 mmol/l) and the creatinine below 10 mg per 100 ml (884 μmol/l).

The dialysate should be cultured every 24 hours and the tip of the catheter after removal. Every time any part of the circuit is opened spray the connection with Betadine. Disconnections are fewer if a 10 litre container (Difusor, Boots) is used with a smaller bag between it and the patient. The Trocath can normally be kept in place for two to three weeks, i.e during the whole of an episode of acute renal failure. For long-term dialysis a Silastic catheter is to be preferred (Heal, M. R., England, A. G. & Goldsmith, H. J. (1973). Four years' experience with indwelling Silastic Cannulae for long-term Peritoneal Dialysis. *British Medical Journal, 4,* 596-600).

Difficulties

These are rarely encountered. If insertion proves too difficult try a site in the iliac fossa. It sometimes helps full insertion to have fluid running whilst introducing the catheter. A viscus may be perforated. Should this be the bladder your patient will be gratified by a sudden two litre ' diuresis '. Reinsert the Trocath elsewhere and put an indwelling catheter in the bladder. If faecal material is obtained ask a surgeon to come but leave the catheter *in situ* as it may help him to find the perforation. If he decides against operation remove the Trocath and insert a fresh one elsewhere adding genta-micin 6 mg/litre to the fluid. The commonest difficulty is failure to obtain an adequate outflow because of kinking, clinging omen-tum, fibrin clots or an air lock. If this happens withdraw the catheter a little but do not push it lest you introduce infection. If outflow remains poor or if the fluid contains much blood try forcible syringing with isosmotic sodium chloride solution. Large patients may need a large input before good drainage is established. Re-insertion in a second place may cause leakage into the abdominal wall from the first attempt. Discontinuance of PD for 24 hours will allow the first puncture to heal. If high dextrose fluid is used the blood sugar must be estimated daily and insulin given if need be to keep it below 250 mg/100 ml (13·7 mmol/l). Too hypertonic a solution may cause pain and then 10 ml of procaine 1 g/dl may be added to two litres of infused fluid. During dialysis the sodium and fluid balance needs careful watching. To treat uncon-trollable hypertension use one litre of pure dextrose 5 g/dl to four litres of 130 mmol sodium dialysis fluid. To treat fluid retention or pulmonary oedema a mixture of high and low dextrose fluid in the proportion of 1 : 3 to 1 : 4 should be used with short dwell times.

CATHETERISATION

Warning

The indication is acute retention of urine. Urethral (as opposed to suprapubic) catheterisation should be avoided in chronic retention particularly if there is also overflow. Since bacteria are normally present in the distal urethra, it is impossible to pass a catheter in a completely sterile manner, but, even so, secondary cystitis is rare after catheterisation except when there is residual urine. Catheterisation then ensures infection and often precipitates acute retention when the bladder refills.

Premedication

Give a sedative, diazepam (Valium) 2 to 5 mg by mouth or pethidine 100 mg by injection, according to circumstances.

Which catheter to use

Don't be appalled by the display of catheters which a surgeon can choose from. It is best to try a small one first and, preferably, a Gibbon catheter. This is a long (150 cm) tube of polyvinyl chloride with a diameter of only 1·5 mm. The tip is rounded and there are side holes and 30 cm down, there is a collar with flaps for attachment to the penis or, in a female, the thighs. The tubing is non-irritant and its small size allows urine and mucus to escape alongside it. A Gibbon catheter may be left in place but if a disturbed patient pulls it out, then a Foley catheter with a latex balloon should be used, but never let a nurse persuade you to commit ' Foley folly ' by catheterisation just to ensure a dry bed. If, when it has to be removed the balloon won't deflate, pass a ureteric catheter up the side channel to let the water off. It is dangerous to try to burst it by overdistension.

Technique of passage

Observe strict aseptic precautions and wear a mask. A catheter should preferably be used only once so choose one from a presterilised pack. Wash the penis with soap and water and then dab it with 1 in 2 000 chlorhexidine (Hibitane) solution. Isolate the area with sterile towels—preferably using one with a central hole for the penis. At this stage the operator should wash and put on sterile rubber gloves. Inject into the urethra with a urethral syringe up to 10 ml of sterile jelly containing lignocaine 1 g/dl and chlorhexidine (Hibitane) 0·1 g/dl. Retain it by using a penile clamp for 4 to 5 minutes and massage some into the posterior urethra via the perineum—a towel intervening. If the specimen is being sent for poison tests warn the pathologist that there may be lignocaine in it. Lubricate the catheter with the same jelly. Hold the penis between the finger and thumb of the left hand. With the right hand grasp the catheter with a sterile haemostat or a special catheter-holding forceps and pass the tip into the urethra; then advance the catheter using the haemostat to hold it, if necessary. If it is held in the fingers, see that the part which is touched does not enter. If the catheter sticks, withdraw it a little and twist it round before trying again. Having entered the bladder, connect the catheter to a sterile, closed drainage bag.

Suprapubic puncture and catheterisation

To avoid the risk of introducing organisms by a catheter the bladder may be entered suprapubically. For this it is essential that the bladder is full. If this cannot be confirmed by palpation and percussion give a drink and wait an hour or so until there is a strong urge to micturate. Clean the suprapubic skin with an antiseptic. Infiltrate one per cent lignocaine 5 cm above the symphysis and make a 5 mm incision there. Any long needle may be used. It should be entered in the mid-line and at right angles to the abdominal wall. 10 ml of urine is sufficient for bacteriological examination. If a trocar and cannula is used a polythene catheter can be passed down the cannula which is then withdrawn to leave the catheter *in situ*. But it is better to use the three way Argyle Ingram trocar catheter (Sherwood Medical Industries Ltd., Crawley, England).

GASTRIC LAVAGE
(For risks, see p. 72.)

This should only be done in a properly equipped department. It is not a bedside procedure.

Indications

The stomach should be washed out:

1. If the patient is seen within four hours of swallowing tablets (unless your are sure that only a few were taken).

2. If the patient is unconscious and the time of taking the tablets is unknown.

3. In all cases of salicylate poisoning.

Gastric lavage is generally contraindicated if corrosive poison has been swallowed though its risk has to be weighed against that of absorption of the poison (see p. 26).

In the unconscious patient

Preliminary insertion of a cuffed endotracheal tube by an anaesthetist is essential. If, however, lavage is deemed necessary without
this safeguard it must be done with the head low and the patient
preferably prone over the end of a table. If an operating table
is available the Trendelenburg position with the patient supine
can be used. Some prefer to have the patient in the left lateral
position with the head low. Struggling is less likely in the prone
position but the patient may have to be immobilised by straps or
by wrapping him tightly in a blanket. Two assistants are
necessary in most cases. Remove the dentures and open the
mouth with a gag or boxwood wedge with a central hole (Fig.
32.8). Use a fairly stiff oesophageal tube preferably 3·75 metres long

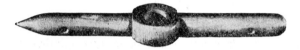

FIG. 32.8
Boxwood wedge with central hole to take oesophageal tube.

and about 1 cm in diameter (for an adult) with several large holes
cut into it near the end. Lubricate the tube and pass it through the
hole in the wedge if this is used or over the tongue and quickly
down the oesophagus. It is virtually impossible to enter the larynx.
The end of the tube should be 50 cm from the incisor teeth in an
adult and 25 cm in a child. It is an advantage to mark these distances on the tube by a safety pin in its wall (but not in its lumen).
A Ryle's tube should not be used except when it is impossible to
open the mouth. It could then be passed through the nose.

When the tube enters the stomach attach a Senorans's evacuator
(Fig. 32.9) or use an Aakin's syringe to withdraw stomach contents
by suction. In cases of poisoning the stomach contents should be
kept. Then attach a funnel and pour in warm water. Bicarbonate
solution can be used but not in barbiturate poisoning (p. 33). After
about 300 ml of fluid has entered (less in children) but with the
level of fluid still visible in it, lower the funnel over a pail on the
floor and siphon off the fluid. A total amount of nine and a half
litres should be used but the temptation to pour a lot at a time
should be resisted as this might force the pylorus and defeat the
object of lavage. The first washings should be kept.

In the conscious patient

This is a different proposition for the patient's consent must be
obtained. He usually gives it. If he will not and you think his life

would be in danger without lavage seek advice of the Local Authority Social Worker (p. 674) in order to act under Section 29 of the
Mental Health Act 1959.

Try to reassure the patient by explanation. Use the prone position and let someone hold his hands. Hold the mouth open with a
gag and proceed as in the unconscious patient. If the patient vomits
there is danger of inhalation. Remove the tube (he will probably
shoot it out anyway) and clear the pharynx by a sucker before
reinsertion. Occasionally laryngeal spasm occurs. The tube should
be removed and reinserted when struggling has ceased. If, despite
precautions, stomach contents are inhaled treat as described on
p. 527.

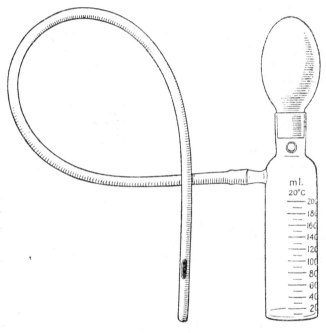

Fig. 32.9
Senorans's evacuator.

GASTRIC COOLING

Two plastic tubes are passed into the stomach, one through each
nostril. One is for gravity or low suction drainage; the other delivers
into the stomach an electrolyte solution consisting of dextrose
5 g/dl of water with KCl 0·745 g per litre, NH_4Cl 2·0 g per litre

and buffered with NaH CO_3 to pH 7·4. This solution is cooled to a temperature between 5 and 16°C by running it over a flask containing crushed ice. Failing this, ice may be added to the flask containing the fluid.

About 4 000 ml of fluid are used in four hours. Gastric distension must be avoided by seeing that the drip, however fast, is never faster than the fluid return.

OESOPHAGEAL TAMPONADE
(For risks see p. 75.)

Test the tri-lumen Sengstaken-Blakemore tube (Fig. 32.10) for puncture of its balloons. Spray the pharynx with 2 per cent ligno-caine (see p. 61). With the patient on his left side pass the tube, lubricated with glycerine, into the stomach using firm pressure. When the end is in the stomach inject 120 to 150 ml of water containing about 10 per cent of Hypaque into the gastric balloon. Pull on the tube to engage the gastric balloon in the cardia and tape its end to the face. (It is inadvisable to apply traction to the tube as formerly advocated.) If the patient is not bleeding at the time the position of the tube may be checked radiologically. This step should be omitted if the patient is bleeding and the oesophageal balloon should be inflated to a pressure of 40 mm of water on the Tycos gauge. A Ryle's tube attached to the oesophageal tube allows for pharyngeal aspiration. The oesophageal balloon may be left inflated for two hours but should be let down for three minutes every hour. The tube may be used for periods of up to 48 hours but after this there is a risk of pressure necrosis of the oesophageal mucosa. Gastric aspiration should be used between feeds given down the tube. A soft rubber disposable tube may be introduced through the nose using an attached Ryle's tube to facilitate passage (Fig. 32.11).

CIRCULATORY ARREST

Stopping of the heart beat is, of course, a terminal event in fatal illnesses and the following measures do not apply to such cases. Once it seems that the heart beat has stopped confirm that the pulse in the carotid artery (or other major artery) is absent, note the time and act at once. Do not delay to see if other pulses can be felt or to listen wonderingly for heart sounds or to wait for the pupils to dilate (a late, 90 seconds, sign). These measures would waste some of the precious minutes during which the brain may be saved. If it is known that there have been no heart beats for three minutes

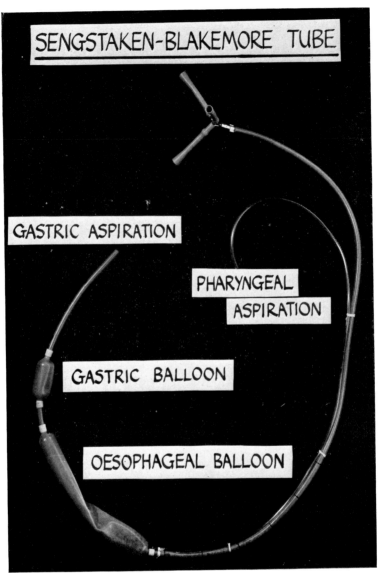

SENGSTAKEN-BLAKEMORE TUBE

GASTRIC ASPIRATION

PHARYNGEAL ASPIRATION

GASTRIC BALLOON

OESOPHAGEAL BALLOON

Fᴉɢ. 32.10
Red rubber trilumen Sengstaken-Blakemore tube with attached
pharyngeal drainage tube.

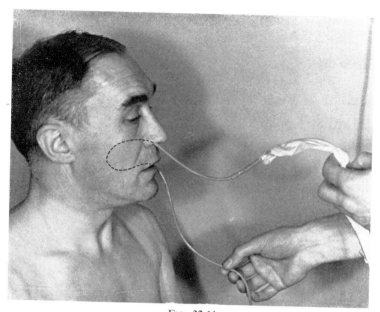

FIG. 32.11
Use of Ryle's tube to facilitate passage of oesophageal balloon through the nose.

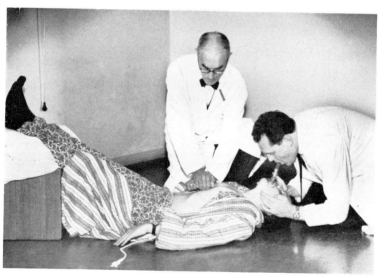

FIG. 32.12

the brain will have suffered irreparable damage for three minutes is the length of time the brain will stand total anoxia at normal temperatures. When the patient is already connected to a monitoring device cardiac arrest and its type will be apparent at once but even without this evidence the correct treatment is to give a defibrillating shock (400 joules for a 50 kg person) at once with the likelihood that other measures will not be needed. So sound the 'May Day' alarm and while awaiting the defibrillator give a sharp blow over the heart. This may start a heart arrested from simple asystole. There is no need for an ECG as there is no evidence that 'blind' defibrillation will harm a heart stopped in simple asystole. Indeed in such cases it may have the same effect as a blow on the chest. While awaiting re-establishment of the heart beat our task is to keep oxygenated blood going to the brain but even a flow of unoxygenated blood will help as it will remove lactic acid.

External cardiac compression (' cardiac massage ')

This should be started by whoever reaches the patient first. When combined with artificial respiration (mouth-to-mouth in the first instance) as it always must be, it can keep the the brain oxygenated and so give time to prepare for the next step.

Circulatory arrest in venous air embolism (p. 65) or in a patient with a severely deformed chest calls for the surgeon as the chest may have to be opened. Arrest after a severe haemorrhage calls for a large intra-arterial transfusion and 10 ml of calcium gluconate 10 g/dl i v (to counter the hyperkalaemia from transfused blood and the fall in ionised calcium caused by the formation of a calcium-citrate complex). In pulmonary embolism it is possible that compression may fragment the clot but there is no proof of this.

Technique

Slip the hard resuscitation board under the patient since it is useless to try compression on a bed which would yield. Failing this put the patient on the floor. (Although an advantageous position for compression it makes intubation difficult.) Provide an airway by extending the neck and pulling up the jaw or by putting in a Brook airway (p. 734). Press vertically downwards on the lower sternum using your whole weight and push it in and then release it. Do this about 60 times a minute (Fig. 32.12). Compression can be achieved mechanically by a machine. It is best to start cardiac compression before inflation as the brain's need for blood is paramount. Preferably an assistant should perform artificial respiration by manual intermittent positive pressure using an intratracheal tube.

Failing this if you are alone you will have to stop to inflate the lungs twice by the mouth-to-mouth method every 15 compressions. A pause must be made occasionally to see if spontaneous heart beating has returned.

In children cardiac compression may easily be excessive and cause damage and for them a modified technique is best. Stand on one side of the supine child, put one hand underneath his chest and two or three fingers of the other hand on the lower sternum. Then compress the hands together with a rapid rhythm of 80 to 100 per minute.

Note on defibrillation

An effective shock will make the trunk muscles contract. There is a risk of giving a shock to bystanders so no one should be touching the patient when the shock is given. Cardiac compression and artificial respiration must continue between the shocks if more than one is needed. Avoidable reasons for defibrillation failure are:—

1. Broken wires, wrong adaptors, etc. These should be avoided by regular checking and maintenance. They are avoided by a battery set but the batteries must be regularly checked.

2. Incorrect placement of electrodes. Since defibrillation depends on an adequate amount of current traversing the heart one electrode should be on the right sternal border and the other on the left side of the chest.

3. Short circuiting by excess of electrode paste.

4. Insufficient energy. For persons over 50 kg 400 joules (watt seconds) are needed. The energy output of the defibrillator must be checked regularly.

Acidosis

Tissue anoxia during circulatory arrest quickly causes a metabolic acidosis (Stewart, 1964; Smith and Anthonisen, 1965) and this lowers the threshold for ventricular fibrillation. But the acid-base status following cardiac arrest is very variable. If an Astrup device is available the correct dose may be calculated from the base deficit as shown on p. 11. Failing this Gilston's formula (Gilston, A. (1965). Clinical and biochemical aspects of cardiac resuscitation. *Lancet*, 2, 1039) may be used. This is:

dose of $NaHCO_3$ mmol (mEq)=
weight of patient in kg $\times$ duration of
cardiac arrest in minutes $\times$ $^1/_{10}$.

Alternatively, 100 mmol (mEq) (100 ml of an 8·4 g/dl solution) should be given followed by 40 mEq every 15 minutes until cardiac action is satisfactory but it is best to decide further doses by blood gas analysis.

Note. Sodium Bicarbonate Injection BP is 8·4 g/dl (1 mmol (mEq) per ml) (i.e. saturated) and can be obtained from The Boots Company in half litre Polyfusor containers. These, unlike glass containers, do not allow precipitates to form. If an ordinary glass bottle or flask has to be used the addition of 0·02 per cent sodium edetate will prevent precipitation.

Failure to restart the heart beat

If the heart beat does not return fairly soon after compression and defibrillation a reassessment of the situation must be made while compression is continuing. The ECG will distinguish between simple asystole and ventricular fibrillation. Asystole is the more serious but less common type of arrest.

SIMPLE ASYSTOLE. The object is to induce fibrillation so that DC shock can be used effectively. Give 10 ml of calcium chloride 5 g/dl and 10 ml of 1 in 10 000 adrenaline into the heart (p. 714). Otherwise a large vein, e.g. the subclavian vein (p. 747) or even an arm vein could be used. If these methods fail arrange for a transvenous pacemaker.

VENTRICULAR FIBRILLATION. When the heart beat is not maintained because of recurring bouts of ventricular fibrillation a continuous lignocaine drip giving 1 to 2 mg per minute is often effective.

The aim is to achieve full oxygenation (without hyperventilation) and correct any acidosis. When it is clear that external methods have failed open chest cardiac massage should be considered and a surgeon called. A mechanical complication such as tension pneumothorax or haemopericardium may be preventing recovery.

How long to go on?

Ten minutes is about one's limit of endurance and an assistant or machine should be ready to take over then or earlier. But the circulation must be kept going until skilled help including a defibrillator arrives. After the slightest flicker of encouragement rhythmic compression should continue for an hour or until the heart beat is established. If there has been no suggestion of a heart beat or an effective return of circulation as shown by improvement in colour, constriction of the pupils and a carotid pulse for an hour despite treatment the situation is probably hopeless. If circulation is maintained but the patient remains comatose and needs artificial respiration, treatment should go on for four to eight hours before being abandoned. More prolonged resuscitation is indicated for arrest in ventricular fibrillation than in simple asystole since its outlook is more hopeful. On the other hand, worsening of any underlying disease argues against prolonged resuscitation.

Brain damage

Brain damage with oedema is probable if the pupils remain fixed, if temperature control is lost and if there is no spontaneous breathing. It is vitally important to prevent cerebral oedema after a period of anoxia *from any cause*. Even if consciousness returns quickly after cardiac arrest prophylactic measures must be used because cerebral oedema may come on after several hours.

1. *Cerebral dehydration.* Normal renal function is necessary and may be assumed if the patient is otherwise healthy and if his urine specific gravity is 1 020. When there is doubt a catheter should be passed and a timed specimen taken over about an hour and its urea content measured. With a flow rate of 0·5 ml per minute the urea content should be 1·59 mg per 100 ml (0·26 mmol/l). If renal function is good mannitol should be given i v. The speed of infusion is important since its effectiveness depends on a good osmotic gradient between the brain and blood. 500 ml of mannitol 25 g/dl should be given in 20 minutes and repeated in 12 hours. The total duration of treatment should not exceed 48 hours. Failing mannitol, frusemide 2 ml (Lasix 20 mg) should be given i v and may be preferable after acute myocardial infarction.

(A less effective method of causing cerebral dehydration is to give 200 ml of magnesium sulphate 50 g/dl into the rectum and keep it there for 30 minutes. A vessel if half filled with Epsom salts will yield a 50 g/dl solution when the crystals are dissolved and the vessel is topped up with tap water.)

2. *Induced hypothermia.* By deliberately cooling the skin to 30 to 33°C the oxygen requirement of the body is lowered and hypoxia can be tolerated. (At 35°C or higher there is no benefit and below 30°C there is a risk of ventricular fibrillation.) The main indication to reduce oxygen consumption is failure to maintain oxygen saturation of the blood even with IPPV using 100 per cent oxygen. This sometimes occurs when the ventilation perfusion relationship is abnormal following cardiac infarction and pulmonary embolism. Other indications are the strong probability of brain damage because of the duration of cardiac arrest and the presence of papilloedema.

The simplest method is to put a wet sheet over the patient and to pack ice chips around him. Care should be taken not to let ice touch the skin. An electric fan should blow air over the patient. Promethazine (Phenergan) 100 mg and chlorpromazine (Largactil) 50 mg may be given i v over a period of 20 minutes. This ' lytic cocktail ' enhances the effect of cooling and prevents shivering. Cooling should be stopped when consciousness returns and should not last longer than seven days.

3. *Intravenous vitamins.* Paired ampoules of Parentrovite (Bencard), vitamins B and C, should be given i v.

Diagnosis of brain death

While action on a decision that a patient is in a state of ' coma depassé ' (brain dead but heart beating) is never urgent it is necessary in a patient maintained on artificial respiration to gather the evidence on which to make a diagnosis of brain death. Some guide lines on the consequent ' switch off ' are given on p. 22. The clinical diagnosis of a permanently non-functioning brain is based on a summation of many findings. These are:

1. Absence of spontaneous movement and breathing over a period of three minutes after breathing room air or oxygen enriched air for at least ten minutes.

2. Widely dilated fixed pupils persisting for more than 24 hours (except when the iris is bound down by adhesions or the patient is poisoned by drugs causing mydriasis).

3. No response to firm supra-orbital pressure.

4. Absence of the normal ' doll's head ' eye movements whereby ocular fixation is maintained despite movement of the head so that normally the eyes lag behind when the head is moved.

5. No ocular movements after ice cold water is syringed into one ear.

6. The cilio-spinal reflex (dilatation of the pupil on painful stimulation of the skin of the neck on the ipsi-lateral side) must be absent. This will be hard to detect as the pupils will be already dilated so look for it in a dim light using the plus 15 lens of the ophthalmoscope in order to detect the slightest movement.

These signs must be demonstrable at two examinations 12 hours apart. The diagnosis of brain death may be supported by a completely flat EEG record over a period of at least 10 minutes but even this is not infallible. The possibility that brain death is being simulated by the effects of depressant drugs, hypothermia or a metabolic disorder must be borne in mind.

STEP BY STEP PROGRAMME FOR CIRCULATORY ARREST

1. Feel for the carotid pulse. If it is absent there is circulatory arrest. Cessation of breathing and wide dilatation of the pupils are confirmatory signs. Note the time.

2. Send someone to sound the ' May Day ' alarm.

3. Thump the sternum.

4. Commence cardiac compression on a hard surface (board or floor).

5. Use the defibrillator.

6. Lower the head and raise the legs.

7. Clear the upper airways and use mouth-to-mouth artificial respiration. Two ventilations for every 15 compressions.

8. Take an ECG. If asystole give 10 ml 1 in 10 000 adrenaline and 10 ml calcium chloride 5 g/dl into the right atrium (see p. 714). If sinus rhythm with ectopics give 50 mg lignocaine i v. If ventricular fibrillation give a further shock.

9. Check pH, $PaCO_2$ and PaO_2. Start measures to combat cerebral oedema and for post-resuscitation care.

RESPIRATORS FOR RESCUE WORK

Three types are available. At least two models appropriate to the industry should always be provided and workmen should be practised in their use.

1. *Canister types* such as **Purethra** (Fig. 32.13) can be relied on for short periods in low concentrations of gas. Many canisters of distinctive colours are provided to give protection against different gases. Appropriate canisters should be available in any given industry.

2. *Fresh air apparatus.* The **Antipoys** has the same facepiece as the Puretha and is connected to an air pipe nine metres long the end of which must be in fresh air.

3. *Self-contained oxygen apparatus.* The **Mark 5 Proto** apparatus is completely self-contained and provides oxygen for one or two hours. It has a CO_2 absorber and a cooling canister. Breathing is via a mouthpiece or a full face mask. A warning whistle indicates approaching cylinder exhaustion. The **Aerolox** liquid oxygen breathing apparatus has no moving parts and provides oxygen for $2\frac{1}{2}$ hours. A cooling device is not needed.

MECHANICAL AIDS TO BREATHING FOR EMERGENCY USE

1. MACHINES SUITABLE FOR SHORT PERIODS
a. Using oxygen or air:

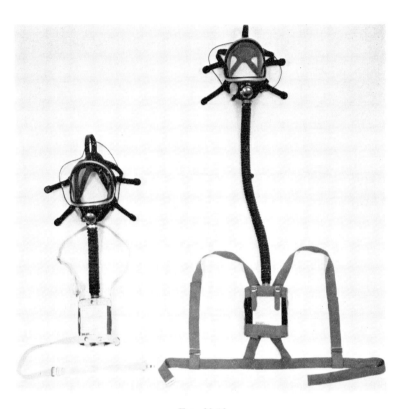

FIG. 32.13
Puretha gas respirator with Vistarama mask
(*Siebe Gorman & Co. Ltd.*)

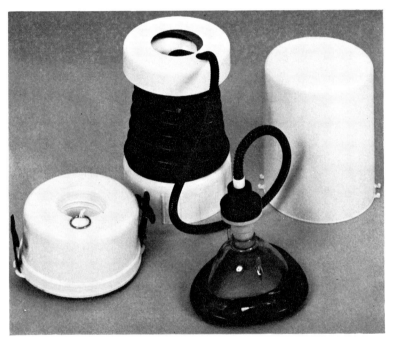

FIG. 32.14
The Handyman Emergency Oxygen Pack.

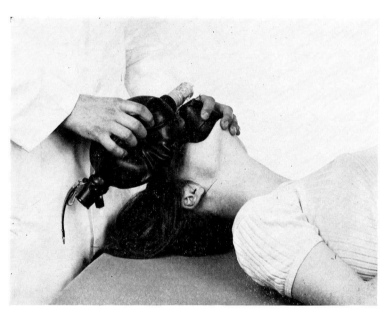

Fig. 32.15
The Ambu Bag.

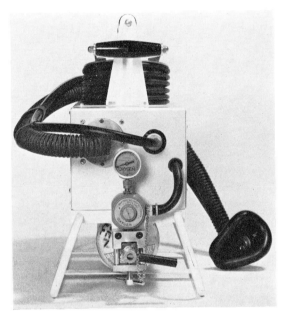

Fig. 32.16
Automan Mk 2 resuscitator.

The **Handyman Emergency Oxygen Pack** (Fig. 32.14). This provides instantly available oxygen. All that has to be done is to remove the lid and unscrew the plastic base in which oxygen is stored in a tube. On pulling the ring oxygen is released. There is a 20 minute supply but resuscitation can be continued by using the bellows to pump air into the lungs.

The **Respirex HK 300 oxygen dispenser** stores up to 300 litres of oxygen in a circular drum and delivers it to a face mask. Its Respirex Ball Resuscitator fits into the operator's hand and when incorporated in the line allows positive pressure to be given. The patient can also breathe spontaneously through the equipment.

b. Using air and automatically self-filling:

The **Ambu bag** (Fig. 32.15) is a simple apparatus which acts like mouth-to-mouth respiration. When the bag is squeezed air is driven into the patient's lungs via a face mask. On release of pressure a self-restoring foam rubber insert causes the bag to inflate automatically. The recoil of the chest causes air to leave the lungs by an expiratory valve protected by wire gauze. Bags without this filter are dangerous since they allow bits of deteriorated rubber sponge to enter the lungs. The **Laerdal Resuscibag** is similar and constructed from transparent plastic material.

2. MACHINES SUITABLE FOR LONGER PERIODS

a. Positive-negative respirators use air and are operated by an electric pump or by hand. The rate and the stroke volume can be varied.

b. Automatically cycled machines operated by time, pressure or volume. They can be fully automatic, acting irrespective of the patient's efforts to breathe or triggered so that they assist any breathing effort the patient makes They cannot be used through a face piece for long because of the leakage and the tendency to inflate the stomach. They could be used for up to 12 hours via a cuffed endotracheal tube, but after that a tracheostomy would be necessary. A good example is the **Bird respirator.** It is very versatile and enables oxygen to be given when the frequency of breathing and the inspiratory and expiratory pressure vary widely. An expiratory negative pressure of 10 cm of water can be obtained, the gas mixture can be varied and aerosol medication can be included. During phases of apnoea the respirator works automatically but follows the slightest attempt at spontaneous breathing. Humidification, preferably by an ultrasonic device, is essential if any breathing machine is used for more than a few hours. An apparatus which is simpler to operate is the **Automan Mk 2 Resuscitator** (Fig. 32.16) designed for first aid work. It automatically calculates the volumes, pressures and frequency of breaths required and so guards against over-inflation. It can be operated by hand.

(Tank respirators and breathing jackets are not included here as the other methods described are better for occasional use in an emergency. Tank respirators are quite unsuitable when there is any question of airway obstruction.)

ARTIFICIAL RESPIRATION

(For a method of artificial respiration in the apnoea of whooping cough see p. 435.)

If breathing has stopped for 10 minutes death is almost certain and it may occur after a two minute stoppage. So when breathing fails artificial respiration must be started *on the spot* at once. *There is literally not one second to lose.* Don't stop to remove dentures, to loosen clothing or drain the lungs (a doubtful possibility). All these can be attended to later.

The best method is direct insufflation of the patient's lungs with your expired air, an ancient method of mouth-to-mouth resuscitation mentioned in the Bible (II Kings IV, 34) and therefore called Elisha breathing. It is also used by many animals to inflate the lungs of their offspring.

Technique

Some prefer mouth-to-*nose* technique since it can be used with the patient on his side and carries less risk of inflating the stomach and subsequent trouble from vomiting. If the mouth-to-mouth method is used the patient must be on his back. If external cardiac massage has to be done at the same time, it is an advantage to have the patient off the ground on a hard surface. This position also facilitates laryngeal intubation should it become necessary. It is very important to align the pharynx and larynx correctly (Fig. 32.17). Using both hands lift the head (A) and tilt it back (B). You may put your thumb in the victim's mouth to grasp the jaw if need be. Put your lips over the patient's mouth or nose (or mouth and nose in a child) so as to make a good seal. With the thumb and forefinger of one hand close the patient's nostrils or lips gently (a nose clip may be used). Take a deep breath and exhale into the patient (with a little force in an adult, gently in a child and with a few puffs in the new-born) (c). It is essential to see and feel the chest rise. Then remove your lips and let the chest deflate (D).

Those who have used this method say that in the thrill of the emergency they do not find it repulsive but some are happier if they avoid contact with the patient and breathe into the hole of an oro-nasal mask or a simple new device, the Resusciade, a nylon mouthpiece with a valve set in a small sheet of plastic. A Brook airway (Fig. 32.18) is the best appliance to use. During expiration a

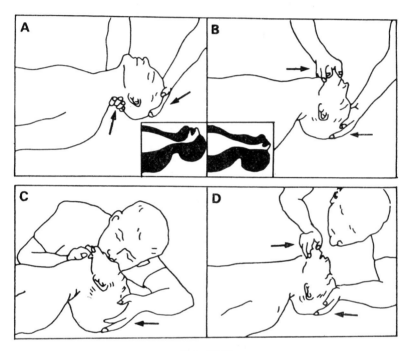

FIG. 32.17

Head-tilt oral method. A, neck is lifted; B, head is fully tilted back; C, lungs are inflated via nose or mouth and D, victim exhales by himself, if necessary, through his mouth. (By courtesy of the Editor of the *Journal of the American Medical Association*.)

valve closes the blow tube and allows air to escape by a side vent. The tube prevents the tongue from falling back. Air blown into the stomach may cause an explosive vomit which will threaten the air passages. Be ready to clear the pharynx by suction. A similar but simpler (valveless) resuscitating tube is the SALAD airway.* Its long end is inserted in adults and its short end in children. Repeat

* Save A Life A Day campaign, 9 Whitecliffe Road, Parkstone, Poole, Dorset BH14 8DU.

the cycle 12 times a minute (i.e. once every five or six chest compressions) turning your head away as you breathe in so as not to fill your lungs with the patient's expired air. Continue inflation and deflation of the lungs until spontaneous breathing is maintained.

Over vigorous use of artificial respiration may wash out CO_2 from the blood (acapnia) and so remove the normal stimulus to breathing. This may account for those cases in which recovery of breathing has been delayed for many hours although the pulse has returned and the colour is good. In none of the methods should the

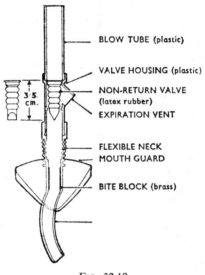

FIG. 32.18
The Brook Airway.

frequency be more than 12 per minute. Another risk is gastric inflation followed by vomiting and inhalation of stomach contents. It can be avoided by seeing that inflation is unhurried and not too forceful. Excessive pressure sufficient to inflate the stomach is less likely in mouth-to-nose than in mouth-to-mouth inflation.

The advantages of this method are that it is universally applicable and that it leaves both hands free to control the jaw and maintain an airway. A possible disadvantage is that the 4 to 5 per cent of CO_2 in the operator's expired air may be deleterious to the anoxic and hypercapnic patient. This would only be important if artificial respiration was prolonged and could be avoided by interposing a CO_2 absorber between the operator and the victim.

General measures

Recovery depends on the circulation of warm oxygenated blood to the brain. Artificial respiration is not, therefore, merely a question of getting air in and out of the lungs but is a triad of warmth, circulation and ventilation. Therefore, without interrupting the rhythm of whichever method is used, steps should be taken by assistants to make the shocked and cold patient warm, and to give him an analeptic (Nikethamide Injection BP 2 ml).

How long to go on?

Artificial respiration must be kept up until natural breathing is permanently restored or death occurs. In drowning and electrocution death may be presumed when there have been no signs of life (breathing, heart beats or movements) at all for two hours or until an ECG has shown absence of all cardiac activity over a period of five minutes.

POLIOMYELITIS—EMERGENCY MEASURES
(For Respiratory Units see p. 790.)

Poliomyelitis is always an emergency if only in the sense that it causes anxiety and makes relatives seek advice urgently. Paralysis of limbs does not call for urgent treatment unless complicated by retention of urine, but when swallowing and breathing are affected, the case is an emergency. The patient should then be transported as rapidly as possible to the nearest respiratory unit (p. 790). The practitioner should, however, have a clear idea of the dangers which threaten his patient for he may have to improvise treatment to keep him alive. Patients with dangerous poliomyelitis can be placed in three groups.

1. *With paralysis of swallowing.* Here the patient is able to breathe but is in danger from his inability to swallow. If he is on his back secretions accumulate in the pharynx, and in order to avoid inhaling them, he adopts rapid shallow breathing. This may raise the suspicion of respiratory paralysis. As an emergency measure he should be turned on to his face, and the foot of the bed raised so that the angle of tip is 40 degrees. This means that the foot of the bed must be 1 metre higher than the head. Bandages or a special harness will prevent slipping. An efficient sucker is essential and a polythene tube should be passed via the nose into the stomach for feeding purposes. When encephalitis complicates the picture, sedation is necessary to control restlessness, so that posture and feeding can be maintained.

2. *With paralysis of respiration.* Here the tank respirator is ideal *provided that swallowing is satisfactory.* Artificial respiration may be needed until the patient can be got to hospital. Because of the risk of gastric dilatation and aspiration of vomited material (p. 601) it is best to keep a Ryle's tube in the stomach in the early days of the illness. Tipping the tank respirator is a wise precaution.

3. *Bulbo-spinal paralysis.* When both breathing and swallowing are paralysed the ideal management is by intermittent positive pressure ventilation (IPPV) through a tracheostomy opening. One of several machines may be used, the cycle being controlled by pressure or volume changes or simply by time (p. 731). While this is being arranged, suction and artificial respiration should be used to keep the patient alive. (It may be added in case there is a tank respirator in the hospital that a patient who cannot swallow must on no account be put in it.)

LARYNGEAL INTUBATION

This is usually best done by an anaesthetist. To introduce a laryngoscope successfully the long axes of the mouth, pharynx and larynx must be brought into line. This is done by flexing the neck at its lower end (by a pillow under the occiput) and extending it manually at its upper end. Having achieved this position hold the laryngoscope in the left hand and introduce its blade along the tongue until the tip of the epiglottis is seen. Advance it a little more and then lift the tongue and epiglottis upwards taking the weight of the head with the instrument. It is important not to use any levering action. A relaxant such as suxamethonium chloride (Scoline) 50 mg i v is sometimes needed. As the intubated patient is always in danger of obstruction a skilled assistant must always be at hand.

LARYNGOTOMY

Nearly always laryngeal or supraglottic obstruction threatens before it becomes complete and so preparations for tracheostomy may be made. Occasionally a foreign body such as an aniseed ball in a child causes sudden respiratory obstruction. There is no inspired air so it cannot be coughed out. The patient strains to breathe and quickly becomes cyanosed and unconscious (see p. 225). Unless the airway is restored within four minutes irreversible damage will be done to the brain. Up-ending the patient and a sharp blow between the shoulder blades may dislodge a foreign body. Failing this the simplest procedure for the non-surgeon is the ' stab laryngotomy' or cricothyrotomy. Identify by palpation the crico-thyroid membrane between the thyroid and cricoid cartilages and puncture it with a sharp knife or large i v needle (' mini-tracheos-tomy '). In contrast with the trachea the cricothyroid membrane can be easily palpated no matter how fat the neck may be. A tube can then be inserted but must be removed within 12 hours. In the interval a tracheostomy must be done. A suitable instrument for emergency laryngotomy was described by Sir Terence Cawthorne (1964, *Lancet, 1,* 1081) (Fig. 32.19) and should be at hand in the casualty department.

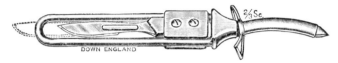

FIG. 32.19
The Cawthorne laryngotomy instrument.

EMERGENCY TRACHEOSTOMY

Tracheostomy is preferable to intubation as it is far less likely to cause permanent damage. A planned operation is best but if there is no time as in sudden laryngeal obstruction the operation can be done with a knife alone. Artery forceps and a piece of stout rubber tubing are a great help. (Red rubber is rendered irritant by ethylene oxide used to sterilise it and must be avoided.)

With the patient lying flat put a pillow under his shoulders to extend the head. Tilt the feet downwards a little. An assistant must hold the head firmly in the mid-line. Local anaesthesia may be used if there is time. An i v anaesthetic is dangerous and must not be used. On the other hand it is a help to use an inhaled non-explosive anaesthetic (halothane and oxygen). If right handed, stand on the patient's right and grasp the larynx with the left thumb and middle finger so that the index finger is on the cricoid. Make a skin incision vertically about 2·5 cm below the cricoid cartilage and incise the deeper tissues from the thyroid cartilage to the supra-sternal notch. The wound fills with blood but ignore bleeding and deepen the incision until the rings of the trachea are felt. There is no need to divide the thyroid isthmus as the trachea can be suitably exposed below it. Incise the trachea through the second and third or third and fourth rings and twist the scalpel to make an opening. This controls the immediate emergency. Steps can now be taken to improve the incision and to make a good-sized hole in the trachea. Before the incision is lost the wound should be opened by using artery forceps and the rubber tube pushed in. Opening through the first ring of the trachea should be avoided as it leads to stenosis. Suturing is unnecessary until the patient reaches hospital, but a stitch to fix the tube is wise. Gross bleeding should be controlled lest blood is aspirated. Go with the patient in the ambulance. Those nursing tracheostomised patients should always wear gloves since the herpetic whitlow (p. 551) is an occupational hazard.

In acute inflammatory conditions (laryngo-tracheo-bronchitis pp. 225 and 419) some surgeons prefer to perform tracheostomy with a bronchoscope in position.

When intermittent positive pressure respiration is to be used via a tracheostomy a cuffed tracheostomy tube should always be used to prevent leakage.

OXYGEN THERAPY

Some confusion still exists about the indications for the use of (isobaric) oxygen and what may be expected from it. Our aim is to maintain sufficient arterial saturation to prevent tissue hypoxia but not to remove the hypoxaemic drive. In a normal subject (Hb 15 g/dl) breathing air, the arterial blood will be 97 per cent saturated with oxygen. It will carry 19·8 ml O_2 per 100 ml, of which 19·5 ml is bound to Hb and 0·3 ml is in solution. The PaO_2 will be about 100 mm Hg (1·33 kPa). When pure oxygen is breathed through a well-fitting face mask, the arterial PaO_2 will rise six fold to 600 mm Hg (79·8 kPa) and 100 ml blood will then carry 22 ml O_2 (20·1 ml combined and 1·9 ml dissolved).

A brief statement follows on the use of oxygen in the various conditions causing hypoxia.

Hypoxia in Subjects with Normal Heart and Lungs

When the heart and lungs are normal hypoxia can result from airways obstruction, hypoventilation and low oxygen content of inspired air (e.g. at high altitude).

In airways obstruction hypoxia is accompanied by hypercapnia because there is alveolar hypoventilation. While oxygen will relieve the anoxia it will not lower the $PaCO_2$. Treatment to clear the airways is imperative.

Deficiency of oxygen in the air causes a low PaO_2 and $PaCO_2$ also falls because respiration is stimulated by hypoxia. When rapidly induced such hypoxia causes coma but symptoms are delayed when hypoxia is gradual because of compensatory polycythaemia and increased cardiac output.

Hypoventilation as in poisoning or after a stroke, or when due to muscular weakness as in poliomyelitis, also causes hypoxia, with CO_2 retention. The essential treatment of respiratory failure is artificial respiration but whether to use air or oxygen is immaterial.

HYPOXIA IN LUNG DISEASE

Pneumonia, pulmonary embolism and collapse all cause PaO_2 to fall and the resulting hyperventilation usually prevents a rise in $PaCO_2$. But, since the blood in the unaffected lung is fully saturated with oxygen, the hyperventilation cannot increase the oxygen content. Breathing oxygen can improve matters, however, by increasing the oxygen dissolved in the plasma.

In obstructive airways disease (bronchitis, asthma) there is gross hypoxaemia and hypercapnia. This is because uneven ventilation means that many alveoli receive little air though they are perfused with plenty of blood, while a few alveoli get most of the air but only a little blood. Oxygen therapy is beneficial but carries the risk of causing CO_2 narcosis. This is because the raised $PaCO_2$ when between 60 and 90 mm Hg depresses the respiratory centre and when oxygen therapy removes the hypoxic drive, the further rise in $PaCO_2$ results in coma. Nevertheless the dangers of giving oxygen must not be overstressed. It is better to be pink and sleepy than blue and awake. Oxygen should, therefore, be given at a concentration insufficient to remove the hypoxic drive and so prevent $PaCO_2$ from rising too high.

Various infiltrative lesions in the lungs interfere with the transfer of oxygen between the alveolar gas and the blood. There is no CO_2 retention, firstly because the gas is very soluble in the lung tissue, secondly because the hypoxia causes hyperventilation and washes it out. The hypoxia is greatly improved by giving oxygen.

HYPOXIA IN HEART DISEASE

The heart conditions causing hypoxia are pulmonary oedema, low cardiac output and congenital lesions.

The pulmonary oedema transudate in the alveoli obstructs ventilation and diffusion. Blood is shunted away to the normal lung but at the periphery of the oedematous area some diffusion, albeit impaired, occurs. PaO_2 is reduced but $PaCO_2$ is normal. Oxygen in high concentration is helpful (but it will not improve the dyspnoea as this is due to increased stiffness of the lungs). When low cardiac output and shock result in tissue hypoxia, the cause is poor blood flow to the tissues. Oxygen does not help greatly, because blood which does pass the alveoli is fully saturated. Therapy may, however, increase the oxygen dissolved in the plasma. Intracardiac shunts in congenital heart disease may allow blood entering the heart to by-pass the lungs. Blood which comes from the lungs is fully saturated and so oxygen has little place in this type of hypoxaemia.

METHODS OF GIVING OXYGEN

Oxygen, like any other medicament, should always be prescribed. It is given at atmospheric pressure in high and low dosage and also at increased pressure. Its use should be continuous and not intermittent. Adequate ventilation is important and oxygen by itself is no substitute for it.

Low dosage

Concentrations of 25 to 40 per cent are used for patients with hypoxaemia due to poor ventilation or uneven lung function, the aim being to prevent tissue hypoxia and hypercapnia while not removing the hypoxic drive.

In the MC (Mary Catterall) small close-fitting leak-proof mask the effect of a valve is obtained by the shape and volume of the mask. A cone of inflowing oxygen is delivered direct to the nostrils and mouth. A small hole enables CO_2 to escape. A flow of 2 l/min gives a concentration of 35 per cent.

Plastic nasal tubes are satisfactory but even when the flow is three to six litres/minute a concentration of oxygen in the inspired air of 30 to 60 per cent can only be achieved if the patient breathes through the nose. The oxygen should be humidified preferably by an ultrasonic machine. A single tube should be placed so that its end is visible below the soft palate but when both nostrils are used the tubes need not pass so far. A T-piece with a tube dipping under 5 cm of water is advisable as a safety blow-off in case the tube slips into the oesophagus. Various disposable oxygen masks deliver oxygen in the same concentrations.

The Ventimask (Fig. 32.21) works on the Venturi principle whereby a jet of oxygen entrains air from holes in the side of the mask at a fixed ratio of 1:10. The concentration of oxygen is constant because if its flow rate is increased to rates up to 8 l/min so is the amount of air entrained. A flow rate of 2 l/min is needed to deliver 24 per cent oxygen. Extra oxygen used to be added by a jet but it is found better to use a range of masks giving oxygen at fixed concentrations (24, 28, 35 and 40 per cent). The flow of oxygen flushes away the expired CO_2. The Hudson Multi-Vent disposable mask allows a choice of oxygen concentration from 24 to 50 per cent.

Humidification is not necessary with masks as it takes place in the nose. The Ventimask with a 1 360 litre cylinder of oxygen can be prescribed on form EC10 in the NHS but not the smaller portable (100 l) sets. In the Edinburgh mask air is breathed through a large hole in its front and oxygen is added by a jet. There is no reservoir. The concentration of oxygen inspired is varied by the flow rate but the concentration reaching the lungs varies inversely with ventilation. Hence there is a risk when respiration is depressed of abolishing the hypoxic drive. For a patient who will not tolerate tubes or close-fitting masks an improvised method of giving oxygen in low concentration is to use an X-ray film 375×300 mm as shown in Fig. 32.20.

Oxygen tents (p. 743) are mainly of value for children (Croupette, p. 417) and very disturbed patients. They do not provide higher concentrations of oxygen than simpler methods and there is a risk of accumulation of CO_2. The HAFOE (High Air Flow with Oxygen Enrichment) head and shoulders tent provides oxygen by the Venturi principle. Leakage is freely allowed and there is no need for cooling. The air flow is set at 8 l/min and the oxygen concentration regulated by varying the entrainment ratio of the Venturi.

High dosage

The main clinical indications for this are CO poisoning and cardiac infarction. All masks delivering oxygen in high concentration use a high flow rate equalling the minute volume (5 to 7 l/min) and store it in a bag during expiration from which it is inspired via a one-way valve. There is no rebreathing. Aviation oxygen masks are of this type. Expiration is also via a one-way valve. In the Portagen mask the expiratory valve is replaced by a hole. The BLB and similar masks use a partial rebreathing system. There is no inspiratory valve and expired gas goes into a reservoir to be rebreathed. There is no absorption of CO_2. Even with a high flow rate of 8 l/min it is hard to achieve an oxygen concentration of over 60 per cent and close fitting of the mask is essential. In masks using a T piece the patient breathes in from a stream of oxygen and out down the other limb of the T piece. When the oxygen flow is low the inspired gas is diluted with air and expired gas. It is hard to achieve a predetermined oxygen level with such masks. (For dangers of oxygen therapy see pp. 71 and 79.)

Hyperbaric oxygen

Here the patient is placed for two hours at a time in a special tank in which the pressure is built up (p. 814). In the few hyperbaric *rooms* which exist it is the pressure of *air* which is built up. Since the pressure of oxygen does not improve ventilation hyperbaric apparatus is not used in respiratory failure.

It is scarcely necessary to add that to try to give oxygen by a tube and funnel held near the face is futile. A small rubber funnel with a flimsy edge and expiratory hole may, however, be held closely over the face of an infant as a temporary measure.

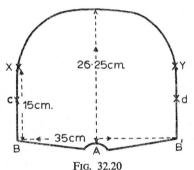

FIG. 32.20
Pattern for improvised mask

AB and AB[1] are sewn together with about 2·5 cm overlap; the perforated rubber tube is attached along this junction for about 10 cm; XBB[1]Y is reinforced with copper wire and bound with lint, and the tapes are attached at X, Y, c and d. When the mask is applied to the patient, the wire reinforced edge has to be moulded to give close contact with the skin under the chin and up to the level of the ears, and the mask should be adjusted to leave a space of about 6·25 cm between its upper part and the patient's forehead. All seams should be made air-tight with strapping. A simpler mask can be quickly made from a 30 × 37 cm film. Form a cone by bringing the corners of a long side together so that they overlap by about 5 cm. Stitch or clip the margins together, and into the apex of the cone fix a rubber tube with adhesive strapping. Pad with gauze the edges that touch the patient's face.

Size of cylinder and rate of flow

Note. The British Standard marking for medical oxygen cylinders is black with a white shoulder. Oxygen is obtainable from most pharmacists and from British Oxygen Company Ltd., Great West Road, Brentford, Middlesex TW8 9AL (01-560 3123) and branches.

Oxygen used in industry comes in cylinders at 1 987 p s i and 2 005 p s i and is of the same purity as oxygen in medical cylinders though it need not meet the strict controls imposed by the Medicines Act. The humidity at 1 987 p s i may be higher than that of medical oxygen. The cylinder at 1 987 p s i could be used in an emergency in place of a medical one if it could be connected to the medical apparatus.

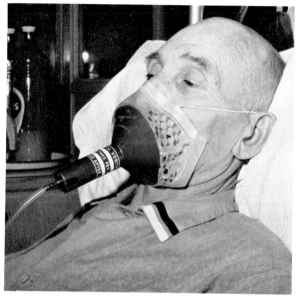

FIG. 32.21
Fixed concentration Venturi mask (Ventimask).

Facing p. 742

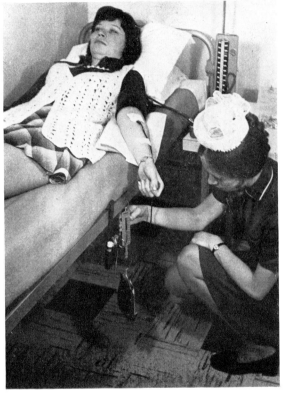

FIG. 32.22
Bleeding a blood donor. The amount taken is measured
by the spring balance, one unit weighing 500 g.

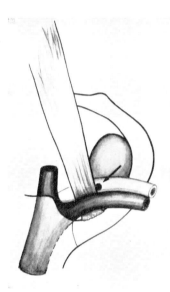

FIG. 32.23

Deep relations of subclavian vein.
Black dot indicates ' clavisternomastoid angle '.

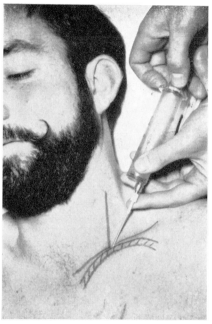

FIG. 32.24

To show the 45° direction of the needle
in the sagittal and transverse planes.

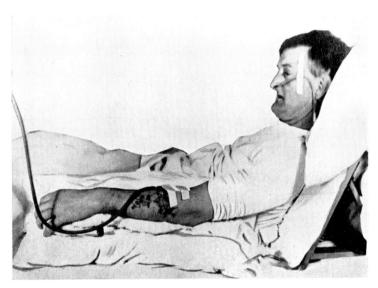

FIG. 32.25

Position of hand, tubing and clamp for i v drip.

Note : 1. Hand in pronation (more comfortable than in supination).
2. Loop of tubing below level of needle.
3. Clamp near needle rather than near bottle.

Medical oxygen is normally supplied in cylinders of 100, 170, 340, 680, 1 360, 3 400 and 6 800 litres.

A full oxygen cylinder gives a definite ' ring ' when tapped but a pressure gauge is the only reliable means of finding out how full it is. Gasses like nitrous oxide, which are liquid in the cylinder, maintain full pressure until empty. (The cylinder must be weighed to determine its content.) Oxygen, however, does not liquefy at the maximum pressure in cylinders of 137 bars (1 bar is 100 kPa, 0·9869 atmospheres, 1·020 kg/cm^2 or 14·50 lb/in^2) and so the volume is proportional to the pressure. A half-full cylinder will therefore register 68·5 bars. Oxygen should always be delivered through a reducing valve.

Oxygen tents

Tents and other oxygen equipment for all types of patient including the newborn will be delivered by the shortest possible route and at all hours if a phone call is made to Vickers Medical (previously Oxygenaire) (Telephones: London, 01-965 7635; Bristol, 77677 (STD 0272); Dublin, 975755; Belfast, 669266 (STD 0232); Birmingham, 021-373 1653; Glasgow, 041-339 2945; Leeds 700344 (STD 0532); Manchester, 061-928 8118; Newcastle, 810071 (STD 0632).

An experienced operator will bring the tent and set it up. The tent should be flushed through with oxygen for 10 to 15 minutes after installing it over the patient and then a flow of at least 4 litres per minute kept up. After use the tent should be washed with Savlon Liquid Antiseptic. Soda lime to remove CO_2 is not necessary in most tents because CO_2 is lost by unavoidable leakage, especially at a high rate of flow. If leakage is prevented and CO_2 absorbed, much more supervision is necessary. The oxygen content inside the tent is easily measured by a simple analyser and, if leakage is prevented, should be tested every three or four hours.

Precautions. Oil and grease must not be used on flowmeters, regulators or cylinder attachments (p. 70). Electrical apparatus of all kinds, and anything liable to spark should be kept well away from the oxygen tent. Static sparks from nylon sheets are very unlikely to cause trouble in the absence of anaesthetic gases and substances of low flash point. It is wise to avoid the use of oxygen (and ether) when the diathermy or electric cautery is used in the mouth and to interrupt it during an X-ray examination. Smoking and the use of matches must be absolutely forbidden near an oxygen tent. They are the commonest cause of fire in tents. Oxygen boxes for infants should not be wiped with spirit as this reacts with the plastic material and yields small amounts of formaldehyde. (For risks of oxygen therapy in premature infants see p. 79.)

BLANKETING A STRETCHER

The method of the St John Ambulance Association, of which Fig. 32.26 is sufficiently descriptive, is recommended.

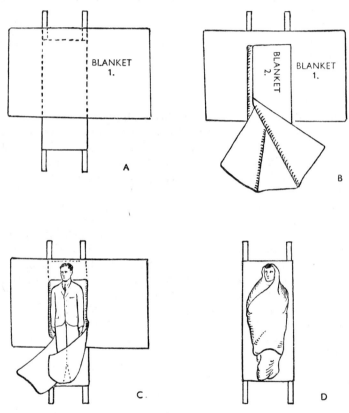

FIG. 32.26
How to wrap a patient in a blanket.
(The St John Ambulance Association.)

Note. If a shocked patient has to be carried down an incline, he should be moved head first, i.e. with the head lower than the feet. If carried feet first, blood supply to the brain may be impaired and shock increased.

SERUM BY INJECTION

Always keep the batch number of any serum injected, particularly if it is derived from a horse or other animal. If there is a history of infantile eczema or asthma, serum should be avoided unless it is absolutely necessary. Always start with a preliminary i m injection of 0·2 ml of serum and wait at least half an hour. If there is no reaction the whole dose should be warmed and given very slowly. The patient should receive this injection lying down and should remain so for one hour. If serum must be given to a known asthmatic it is best to give first 0·2 ml of a 1 in 10 dilution subcutaneously. If nothing happens after watching for half an hour 0·2 ml of undiluted serum should be given i m and a further watch kept. If nothing develops the full dose of serum can then be given. Reactions call for graduated doses in slow sequence.

An **anaphylaxis tray** should always be ready when serum is being given (see p. 81). It should have on it:

Adrenaline 1 in 1 000 in ampoules
Aminophylline 250 mg in 10 ml ampoules
Hydrocortisone sodium succinate (Efcortelan Glaxo 100 mg ampoules with 2 ml water for injection)

as well as the necessary syringes and needles, an airway (p. 733), tracheostomy instruments (p. 731) and a cutting down set. Oxygen and suction apparatus should be at hand. Antihistamines by injection are best avoided particularly if there is much bronchial spasm lest the added respiratory depression makes matters worse.

ARTERIAL PUNCTURE
(See also Aortography, p. 17.)
(For risks see p. 51.)
(Cole, P. & Lumley, J. (1966). Arterial puncture.
British Medical Journal, 1, 1277.)

With the elbow extended determine the course of the brachial artery by palpation as it lies on the inner side of the lower end of the humerus. Local analgesia is not really necessary and may make puncture difficult. If for special reasons it is desired a wheal should be raised with 2 per cent lignocaine and the tissues down to the artery infiltrated. Use a 21 SWG needle 0·81 inch outside diameter, $1\frac{1}{2}$ inches long (40 mm $\times$ 8/10) and a siliconed all glass syringe. Fill the dead space of the needle with heparin injection BP (1 000 international units per ml). Introduce the needle at an angle of 45 degrees and approach the artery. Keep the left index finger over the artery just above where it is to be punctured. When the needle touches the artery wall pulsations are transmitted to it and when the lumen is entered blood rises easily into the syringe without the need to pull on the piston. Remove 8 to 10 ml of blood to minimise the heparin dead space effect. The nurse or the patient himself should press on the artery for five minutes. Remove the needle from the syringe and expel any air bubbles. Draw up a little mercury to act as a seal and then plug the nozzle with a match stick. Alternatively the blood may be put into a bijou bottle so as to fill it and then centrifuged for an hour. The plasma is then drawn off and placed in the refrigerator if not used at once. The radial or femoral arteries may be used instead of the brachial.

VENEPUNCTURE

Either arm may be used for blood sampling but for infusion it is best to use the left arm in a right-handed person and vice versa. Apply a tourniquet or sphygmomanometer cuff above the elbow tightly enough to obstruct the venuous return while not obliterating the radial pulse. A pressure of 80 mm Hg is sufficient. For methods of making the vein prominent see p. 50. Take the blood as soon as possible after applying the tourniquet. If an i v infusion is running take the blood from the other arm. See that the piston of the syringe moves freely. Cleanse the skin, put it on tension and insert the needle at an angle of 30° just to one side of the vein. Advance it a few mm so that its point is just over the distended vein and then push it on for 2 or 3 mm into the lumen. (For position of the bevel see p. 52.)

When the blood is taken for transfusion (Fig. 32.22) the needle is attached to a plastic tube about 375 cm long leading to a blood transfusion bottle or bag (see p. 754). The 35 mm 1·9 mm external diameter Luer needle 15 SWG×1⅜ inch is used in the transfusion service for bleeding donors. Blood is admitted through a rubber disc under the screw top by a needle which pierces it. The place for the donor inlet needle is depressed and thinned to aid easy insertion of the needle. The opposite quadrant marked 2 is for the air vent. Quadrants 1 and 1 are for the giving set needles. This arrangement ensures against puncturing the same place twice.

If the flow of blood becomes feeble the following points should be considered. (1) The air inlet may be blocked. (2) The angle at which the needle enters the vein may need changing. (3) Clasping and unclasping the hand may increase the flow. (4) Clotting in the tubing may necessitate its withdrawal.

Much blood is now transfused from plastic bags sometimes called 'blood packs' (not to be confused with bags of packed cells). No air vent is needed. A sampling tube is provided. Plastic packs have the advantage that withdrawal of blood can be assisted by applying negative pressure to the outside as with the Fenwal Hemolator. The giving of blood can be accelerated by applying pressure to the bag.

SUBCLAVIAN VENEPUNCTURE
(Yaffa, D. (1965). *Lancet, 2,* 614.)

This may be used when, because of obesity or venospasm, an arm vein cannot be entered. The technique must be precise and accurate. It must succeed at the first attempt and no poking about to seek the vein is allowable. The supraclavicular approach is easier than the infraclavicular. The subclavian vein is separated from the skin by the clavicle and rises to the upper border of the bone just medial to the centre. The landmark is the 'clavisternomastoid angle' (Fig. 32.23) at the junction of the lateral margin of the sternomastoid muscle with the upper border of the clavicle and this is where the needle is introduced.

Technique

The patient must lie flat with no pillow. This is to obviate the risk of air embolism. A right-handed operator should use the left subclavian vein. Tense the sternomastoid by making the patient raise his head against resistance and so see and feel its outer edge. It is useful to mark the entry point in the clavisternomastoid angle with the finger nail or by raising a wheal of local anaesthetic there. Use a 4 cm 22 SWG × $1\frac{1}{2}$ inch (40 mm × 7/10) needle and, preferably, a Luer syringe. Having pierced the skin, direct the needle at an angle of 45 degrees to the sagittal plane (Fig. 32.24) and 15 degrees forwards in the coronal plane. Advance the needle through the deep cervical fascia until it enters the subclavian vein with a slight 'give' at a depth of 1·5 cm. Blood will then enter the syringe freely. If the syringe has to be disconnected don't leave it for so long.

FEMORAL VENEPUNCTURE
(For risks in infants see p. 50.)

With the patient lying supine palpate the femoral artery just below the inguinal ligament. If right handed approach the right side. Use a short bevelled needle attached to a syringe and enter the vein just medial to the femoral artery and at right angles to the skin. Blood is easily and quickly aspirated.

INTRAVENOUS INJECTION AND INFUSION

Choice of vein

An easily palpable and visible forearm vein may be used but not at the bend of the elbow as this would mean immobilising the joint. The arm should be pronated after insertion as this position is more comfortable than supination (Fig. 32.25). A leg vein may be used in a restless patient as the leg is easier to splint than the arm but its veins are more liable to spasm and thrombosis (p. 50). A convenient leg vein is the anterior saphenous as it lies on the anterior surface of the tibia midway between the internal malleolus and the tendon of the tibialis anticus. This vein can often be seen and invariably felt there. In children a scalp vein is usually the best choice.

Needle and cannula technique

For a single injection the same technique is used to introduce the needle as in sampling. For multiple injections or samples the needle can be fitted with a rubber diaphragm. For continuous infusion and for multiple sampling cannulation is necessary. Teflon over-the-needle catheters such as the Quik-Cath (Travenol) have made the cut-down technique less necessary. They are introduced in the same way as is the needle for venepuncture. It is important to fix them by criss-crossed strapping and then Elastoplast and to make a loop before the tube goes to the bottle. It is well to seal the entry point with an antiseptic seal skin (Nobecutane). If there is a hold-up in the passage of a catheter (from impinging on a valve) twist it, move the arm and let the infusion flow gently but do not use force. Never withdraw a catheter with its introducing needle in place (see p. 54).

Cut down technique

This may be necessary if a vein is collapsed or inaccessible through the skin but light-hearted cutting down is to be deprecated.

First check all the instruments in the set. Make sure the cannula is not blocked and that all fittings are of the same type. After infiltration with lignocaine 2 g/dl make a 2·5 cm incision along or transversely across the vein and divide the superficial fascia (longitudinal cut down incisions heal better than transverse ones in the leg; in the arm there is little difference). Free 2·5 cm of vein by inserting closed sharp-pointed scissors or a small haemostat and opening the blades longitudinally. Free the vein similarly from its deeper attachments. Using an aneurysm needle draw a loop of ligature material (0 catgut or 3N nylon) under it (Fig. 32.27) and then by cutting the loop leave two ligatures *in situ*. Tie each loop loosely with a single knot and secure both ends of each piece by artery forceps. Hold the artery forceps between the index, middle, ring and little fingers respectively, so that by traction on the catgut the vein is held taught (Fig. 32.28). Make a nick, preferably vertical, in the vein with a small knife or scissors and relax the tension on the vein to

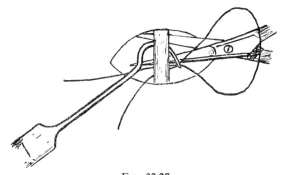

FIG. 32.27
Insertion of catgut under vein by aneurysm needle.
(*J. H. Kirkham.*)

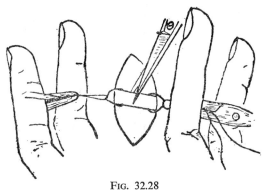

FIG. 32.28
Vein rendered taut by traction on catgut.
(*J. H. Kirkham.*)

see that blood flows. Insert the cannula and connect the drip. If the vein is small it is an advantage to put the finger tip under it, so that the end of the cannula can be pressed against it.

There should be as little delay as possible in letting fluid run from the container once the vein is entered since otherwise blood will enter the cannula and clot.

26

Warning

Infusion solution may be supplied in double plastic bags, the outer one being for protection only. Examine in bright transmitted light and reject if the inner bag is damaged, if the solution is not absolutely clear and if there are droplets between the bags.

Failure to flow and other difficulties

The causes of failure to flow are:

1. Forgetting to release the tourniquet.
2. Tight bandaging.
3. Kinked tubing.
4. Point of needle or tube against side of vein.
5. Blocked air inlet.
6. Filter blocked with clot.
7. Clot in needle. Detach the tubing and try to clear the needle by suction with a syringe.
8. Venous spasm. Pinch the tube with one hand and milk its contents towards the needle. Place hot water bottles on the arm. Inject a few ml of 2 per cent procaine around the vein.
9. An air lock. This is liable to form if the drip chamber is not vertical, particularly when bottles are being changed. Once it forms it is necessary to disconnect the needle and expel the air. Clamp the tube distally and suspend the bottle at its full height. Bring the end of the tube up to just below the level of the fluid in the bottle and slowly open the clip. Air will then be expelled.

Drip chamber full of fluid.

When the air column in the drip bulb is lost the rate of flow cannot be observed. Unhook and lower the container. Squeeze the contents of the drip chamber back into it. On raising the container there will be a fluid level in the bulb.

Rate of drip (see p. 107)

Taking down the drip

This must be done carefully with proper closure of the wound. The ligatures under the vein may be removed after cutting down, so that its patency is maintained just as it is after needling. Simple pressure is applied and the skin sutured accurately. Alternatively the loops can be brought out through the skin and tied as shown in Fig. 32.29. This ensures that the catgut or nylon can be removed and not left round the vein.

Air embolism

For methods of avoiding this risk see p. 63.

Thrombophlebitis after infusions (see p. 53)

CENTRAL (R. ATRIAL) VENOUS PRESSURE
(For contraindication see p. 54.)

Choose the basilic vein at the elbow or the right external jugular vein in the neck. (Avoid the cephalic vein because of its valves and the kink at the delto-pectoral groove.)

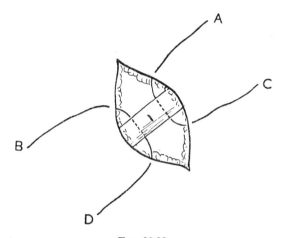

FIG. 32.29

Showing technique for maintaining patency after cutting down on a vein. Tie A to B and C to D and place an extra suture in the skin if necessary.

Use an Argyle 8F 10 cm infant feeding tube and cut off its end obliquely to avoid stagnation and clotting near the tip. (The smaller 6F tube is liable to blockage.) Measure the distance from the elbow to the superior vena cava (35 to 45 cm). The tube is marked at 25 cm intervals and this enables you to avoid overinsertion. Fill the tube with sterile isosmotic sodium chloride solution. Infiltrate the skin with 2 per cent lignocaine and isolate the vein through a 1 cm incision. Make a small opening in it with scissors and pass the tube till its end is judged to be in the right auricle. Next demonstrate a free respiratory rise and fall of blood. To do this remove the cap over the end of the tube and let blood flow till it can be seen at the elbow. Ask the patient to take a few deep breaths and note the movements of the column of blood. If there is pulsation withdraw the tube a bit. Tie in the tube by proximal and distal ligatures of Dexon 3/0. Connect the tube to a venous pressure manometer set. (Travenol Laboratories FKCO 121, formerly Baxter BR-5). Fill its tubes with fluid from the bottle by use of a flow clamp and tap.

Make an indelible X mark on the patient's chest in the mid-axillary line. This is midway between the spine and the sternum and corresponds to the level of the right auricle. Put the self-adhesive centimetre scale on the drip stand and level 0 cm to be opposite the X mark on the chest wall. Turn the tap to connect the mano-meter line and read the CVP in cm of saline. A rise and fall of 1 cm with respiration is easily seen. A little methylene blue in the manometer arm is a help. If the patient moves or sits up 0 cm must be levelled to X before reading the pressure.

The CVP measures the balance between the return of blood to the heart and the heart's capacity to expel it. While it is a valuable guide in hypovolaemic shock it is not the sole criterion of the necessity for fluid replacement (p. 606). Normally a tube whose end is in the right atrium shows a pressure of 6·2 cm $\pm$ 1·5 cm saline but some authorities give somewhat lower figures (see also p. 59). At the sternal angle it is up to 3 cm. When the CVP is low (-2 to 4 cm) it indicates the need for fluid replacement. When it is high ($>$15 cm) the patient is either in cardiac failure or is being overloaded. Airways obstruction and IPPV raise the CVP.

FRESH BLOOD FOR EMERGENCY TRANSFUSION

Failing a suitable relative fresh blood may be taken into a con-tainer from a donor sent by The Greater London Red Cross Blood Transfusion Service, 4 Collington Road, London S.W.5 (01-373 1506/7). The Department of Health advises that only blood which is negative for hepatitis B (Australia) antigen (HBsAg) should be used for transfusion. Red Cross donors are tested for Australia antigen on enrolment and after the tenth donation. The user hospital is advised to test each donation used. In the National Blood Trans-fusion Service all blood is tested for Australia antigen on the occa-sion of each donation.

CROSS MATCHING OF BLOOD

Except in grave emergencies away from hospital all blood grouping and cross matching must be done unhurriedly by a pathologist or experienced technician familiar with the many difficulties which may arise. The simplest cross matching procedure is described here since in an emergency this might have to suffice. Take a sample of blood for cross matching before giving a dextran infusion as this substance in the blood may interfere with the test. Methyldopa (Aldomet) may interfere with cross matching in some patients (p. 96).

The grossest ABO incompatibilities could be detected by simply mixing on a slide one drop of the recipient's and one drop of the donor's blood suitably anticoagulated. The slide is rocked for two minutes and then examined with the naked eye or preferably with the aid of a lens. A better alternative for emergency grouping and cross matching is the use of Eldon cards (available for ABO and Rh grouping and also for cross matching from Nordisk Diagnostics Ltd., 17 Halkingcroft Road, Langley, Bucks. (Slough, 27767 (STD 0753)). Full instructions are provided with the cards and they can be stored satisfactorily for long periods. Those doctors in remote areas who may be faced with the entire responsibility for blood transfusion are advised to contact the Director of Regional Transfusion Service who can supply reagents for emergency use and give training facilities. If it is proposed to use Eldon cards the doctor should study the instruction leaflet in advance and practice using the cards as there is no doubt that this requires some skill.

The Rh negative patient

If a patient is Rh negative, pregnancy with a Rh positive fetus or transfusion of Rh positive blood may stimulate the production of Rh antibodies. Subsequent transfusions may be followed by haemolytic reactions. If a patient, therefore, has been pregnant, has had previous transfusions, or is likely to need further transfusions it is wise to determine the Rh group in the laboratory.

If the patient is Rh negative then only Rh negative blood should be transfused. Eldon cards or special emergency slides produced by the Regional Blood Transfusion Service can be used to obtain the correct ABO and Rh group of the patient. To use entirely group 0 Rh negative blood in emergencies puts a strain on the supply of this blood and every effort should be made to identify those recipients who are group A or AB Rh negative so that they can be transfused with group A Rh negative blood.

A woman should never be transfused with her husband's blood, even if the ABO and Rh groups are identical and cross matching shows no agglutination. This is because of rare factors which, although not very potent antigenically, do carry a small risk of causing trouble in subsequent pregnancies (p. 99).

BLOOD TRANSFUSION

Blood is taken into a bottle or plastic bag as described under Venesection (p. 746) and used fresh or after storage. If a vacuum type bottle is used there is a risk to the donor of air embolism if the vacuum is lost (p. 64).

The technique of entering a vein is exactly as described under i v transfusion but there are certain special points in the use of blood as opposed to other fluids.

The bottle must not be shaken or allowed to warm. It should merely be inverted several times. A filter should always be used and is normally built into the giving set. Any bottle which has been opened for cross matching must be used within 24 hours. A small pilot bottle enables tests to be made without the risk of contamination and wastage. If a 'concentrated red cell suspension' is prepared for a 'packed cell transfusion' by drawing off the plasma it should be used within 12 hours of preparation. The viscosity of the packed cells will depend on the amount of plasma removed. Little difficulty should be encountered during administration if not more than 200 ml of plasma is removed at the time of concentrating. Blood should be rejected if it has been frozen or if there are signs of haemolysis (red tinge in the supernatant plasma) or infection (turbidity of plasma). After transfusion the bottle should be returned to the laboratory *unwashed*. Calcium gluconate, 10 ml of a 10 g/dl solution, may be slowly injected i v (never i m) for every 1 000 ml of blood transfused to counteract the effect of citrate in binding ionised calcium (p. 105). It must not be added to the bottle unless this is first heparinised to maintain anticoagulation.

Printed instructions are supplied with these sets and may vary with slight differences in design. The batch number of a set should be recorded in the patient's notes for future reference as it is not unknown for certain batches of plastic to cause febrile reactions. If these occur full details including the manufacturer and batch number of the set should be given to the Regional Transfusion Director.

Disposable plastic bags

Many transfusion services have changed completely from the use of glass bottles to disposable plastic bags which incorporate a taking tube and needle. The whole kit is already sterilised and the bag contains acid citrate dextrose. This reduces the risk of infection and allows fractionation of the blood by aseptic techniques in the preparation of cryoprecipitate (anti-haemophilic factor concentrate) and platelet concentrates. The amount of blood taken has to be determined by weight (see Fig. 32.23). More than one patient may, therefore, be transfused safely with different blood products from a single donation.

When transfusing blood from a plastic bag, the usual disposable giving set is used by inserting its piercing needle through a port in the bag. No air vent is required and if one is built into the giving set, it should be sealed off by means of a clip before the set is introduced into the bag. Rapid transfusions may be given by simply squeezing the bag or, if preferred, a roller pump can be used on the giving set line. After use care should be taken to seal the outlet port effectively with a small cork or other device to prevent leakage while awaiting incineration.

PARALDEHYDE
(For risks see p. 85.)

This is a valuable sedative (but poor analgesic) in emergencies because it causes very little respiratory depression. Apart from causing confusion in some elderly patients and occasionally addiction in alcoholics its only disadvantage is its undisguised though not unpleasant smell. This permeates the ward as the drug is excreted unchanged by the lungs (and kidneys).

By mouth. The adult oral dose is 2 to 8 ml and is best given as Paraldehyde Draught BPC (paraldehyde 4 ml, syrup 8 ml, liquid extract of liquorice 3 ml, water to 45 ml).

Intramuscularly. Paraldehyde can be given in doses up to 10 ml straight from the bottle (though preferably from an autoclaved ampoule as, like alcohol, it is not self sterilising until diluted). The rapidity of its effect can be much increased by mixing it with hyaluronidase (1 500 international units) before injection. Paraldehyde dissolves plastics so use an all glass syringe.

Intravenously. See pp. 86 and 311.

By rectum. The dose can be calculated as 0·5 ml per kg BW. It should be dissolved in warm water (solubility in water 1 in 8, i.e roughly 4 ml in 30 ml or, when cold, 1 in 10).

VITAMIN K THERAPY

One of the two naturally occurring forms of vitamin K_1 (phytomenadione) is available as Konakion (Roche). It is supplied as 10 mg tablets and as 1 ml (10 mg) ampoules for i v and i m injection. Absorption of Vitamin K_1 is enhanced by diluting it in an aqueous medium. Fruit juice is suggested to disguise the taste. 10 mg will increase prothrombin activity in four hours and cause an 'anticoagulant fast' state for 24 hours. Larger doses may be needed if the response is slow. (For risks in infants see p. 80.)

Vitamin K analogues (e.g. Synkavit) are less effective than vitamin K_1 in correcting hypoprothrombinaemia caused by anticoagulant drugs. They can cause haemolysis and kernicterus if given to premature babies in excessive doses. Vitamin K_1 does not do this. A daily dose of Synkavit of up to 2 mg is sufficient to restore the plasma prothrombin of the newborn to normal levels and this dose should not be exceeded.

CORTICOSTEROIDS IN THE EMERGENCY OF SEVERE INFECTIONS

Whether to use corticosteroids in severe infections is a very difficult question to answer. While they are certainly indicated when there is evidence of suprarenal damage (Waterhouse-Friderichsen syndrome) some doctors think that they may be of benefit in other acute infections. There is no doubt that they can depress the body's defence mechanism and it would seem wrong to use them unless the objective is clearly defined. This may be:

1. Antitoxic—to avoid death from early toxaemia before antibiotics have had time to act.

2. Anti-inflammatory—to lessen local inflammatory swelling which is endangering life (as in acute laryngo-tracheo-bronchitis) or causing pain (as in ophthalmic herpes zoster) or is in an unyielding space (otitis externa and mumps orchitis).

3. Anti-allergic—to lessen an allergic reaction as in the acute encephalomyelitis following specific fevers.

There is no easy way of making the decision. Clinical judgment is the only guide. If used they should be discontinued after say 48 hours and antibiotics should always be given at the same time.

Equivalence of corticosteroids

There is no real equivalence of dosage of corticosteroids as therapeutic potency varies from one patient to another. It may be useful however to know that the following doses correspond roughly to 25 mg cortisone: hydrocortisone 20 mg, prednisone 5 mg, prednisolone 5 mg, methylprednisolone 4 mg, triamcinolone 4 mg, dexamethasone 0·75 mg, betamethasone 0·5 mg, paramethasone 2 mg.

SMALLPOX VACCINATION

(Risks, pp. 83 and 551; refusal of vaccination, p. 761;
international certificate, pp. 703 and 760; emergency
diagnosis, p. 699.)

Vaccine lymph is obtainable from the various laboratories of
the Public Health Laboratory Service (p. 780) and also by private
purchase through Vestric Ltd. 01-253 9377, or Bell and Croyden
01-935 5555, Martindale 01-580 2441 or Allen and Hanburys
01-499 7571. Glycerinated vaccine lymph remains potent for two
weeks if kept in a domestic refrigerator continuously below
10°C. At room temperature in temperate climates it lasts a week.
It should never be used in the tropics. Dried smallpox vaccine
remains potent for at least two years if kept below 10°C (normal
domestic refrigerator temperature) and for a year at room temperature (one month in the tropics). These figures allow a good margin
of safety.

CONTRAINDICATIONS

In non-endemic areas these are:—

1. *Constitutional disturbance.* Vaccination may be contraindicated by constitutional disturbance or, in early childhood, failure to
thrive. When primary vaccination has caused an allergic rash
revaccination is contraindicated unless and until the patient is a
smallpox contact.

2. *Pregnancy.* Vaccination in pregnancy may, in rare instances,
endanger the fetus. Routine vaccination should, therefore, be postponed.

3. *Infantile eczema* (p. 551). Children with eczema or other
generalised skin lesions may develop eczema vaccinatum, a severe
generalised vaccinia which may be fatal. Careful consideration
should be given to the desirability of routine vaccination of any
person with a history of eczema or other allergic condition. Unless
protection against smallpox is essential the members of the household of an eczematous child should not be vaccinated because of
the risk of cross-infection with vaccinia virus. When the vaccination
of the child or its family is indicated because of risk of exposure to
smallpox, a minimal trauma technique (say 8 pressures) should be
used. Human specific immunoglobulin (p. 801) (250 mg up to 1
year, 500 mg from 1 to 6 years, 750 mg from 7 to 15 years, and
1 000 mg over 15 years) may protect the eczematous child against
the risk of generalised vaccinia. It should be injected into the other
arm at the same time or next day.

4. *Septic skin lesions.*
5. *Hypogammaglobulinaemia.*
6. *Corticosteroid and immuno-suppressive treatment.*
7. *Leukaemia.*
8. *Age.* It is generally accepted that primary smallpox vaccination except in endemic areas (see below) should be deferred until the second year of life when the risk of complications is less. A vaccine of reduced virulence but which causes a good antibody response is not yet generally available.

IN ENDEMIC AREAS

Contraindications do not apply in the few endemic areas remaining in 1976 for the risk of smallpox is far greater than the risk of complications of vaccination. Only those who are obviously seriously ill should be exempted. This is really because if they die people will say death was due to vaccination and will refuse it.

Techniques

The best site is on the outer aspect of the upper arm over the insertion of the deltoid muscle. The sole of the foot is sometimes recommended in an infant but vaccination here may be followed by keloid formation. Vaccination on the thigh or buttock is often accompanied by a more severe local and general reaction than vaccination on the arm but it may be used if an arm scar is unwanted. Revaccination is more likely to succeed if done on the volar surface of the forearm if, from faulty technique or low potency of the vaccine, it has failed elsewhere. This site should be avoided for primary vaccination, though in mass vaccination it is the easiest to get at.

Do not cleanse the skin unless it is obviously dirty. Never use a non-volatile antiseptic. Place a drop of lymph on the skin.

MULTIPLE PRESSURE TECHNIQUE

Grip the arm with the left hand to make the skin taut. Smear the lymph over an area the size of a new penny piece with a sharp sterile needle and through this area make 30 pressures with the side (not the point) of the needle held tangentially to the skin. There should be no movement of the needle in its long axis.

MULTIPLE PUNCTURE TECHNIQUE

This is the best method for the amateur. Proceed as above but make 15 perpendicular stabs rather than pressures with the needle.

A special bifurcated needle may be used which when dipped in lymph holds a droplet of 0·002 ml in its fork.

SCRATCH METHOD

Make a single linear scratch 6 mm long through the vaccine. Rub it into the scratch with the side of the needle.

The object of all techniques is to put the virus into the deeper layers of the skin. The area should redden and some prefer a little blood to appear. This does not prevent a successful ' take '. If the patient is terrified of the needle the tip of a sharpened match or a wooden cocktail cherry stick may be moistened with lymph and then rubbed on the area for a few seconds.

No dressing is necessary until a vesicle forms, but it should certainly be applied then in children lest they scratch the site and then inoculate their eyes by rubbing with contaminated fingers. For the same reason it is wise in children to wipe off excess lymph and then spray with a plastic dressing (Nobecutane).

Vaccine lymph is now supplied by the Department of Health as individual doses coloured green in a plastic tubing pack. The end of a section should be snipped off with scissors and the lymph squeezed out. There is no need to squeeze it all out. To be sure of avoiding ' vaccinator's thumb ' it is well to wear a glove. A simpler method is to pierce the plastic tube section with a needle, squeeze out the lymph on to the arm and then use the needle on the skin. If scissors are used they are bound to be contaminated so they should be boiled or soaked in spirit afterwards. It is a good plan to keep a pair solely for use in vaccination. Spirit should be got rid of by burning. The hands should be washed after vaccinating. Accidental infection of the eyes by contaminated fingers can cause corneal scarring.

Dried vaccine is reconstituted by breaking off the ampoule end, inserting the opened end of the ampoule of reconstituting fluid and then opening its other end. The fluid then enters and the vaccine is rapidly suspended. With dried vaccine it is sufficient to dip the (cold) needle into it after reconstitution.

The remains of the plastic tube of vaccine lymph or the top of the ampoule of dried vaccine should be discarded into disinfectant and the needle disposed of safely.

Successful vaccination in the first six days of the incubation period will probably prevent smallpox; in the next three days it will modify the attack but after the ninth day it will be ineffective. In comparison with an unvaccinated person vaccination within a year of contact reduces the attack rate to 1 in 1 000; within 3 years to 1 in 200 and within 10 years to 1 in 8.

It is thought that primary vaccination is ineffective in conferring immunity in less than three weeks unless a vesicle more than 12·7 mm in diameter is produced.

Certification (see also p. 703)

The international certificate simply requires the doctor to say whether vaccination was primary or a revaccination and if primary whether it was successful at the first or second attempt. The type of vaccine used—freeze-dried or liquid—must be indicated. The result of revaccination need not be certified since its proper interpretation would require frequent inspection which is often impracticable. Other certificates (e.g. for local authorities) ask for the type of result. The vaccination site should be inspected about the seventh day. Vaccination or revaccination is considered to have been successful if a ' major reaction ' has occurred. A ' major reaction ' after primary vaccination is a typical Jennerian vesicle; after revaccination it is a vesicle or pustule, or an area of definite palpable induration or congestion surrounding a central lesion, which may be a scab or an ulcer.

Any other reaction is termed an ' equivocal reaction '. An equivocal reaction or no local reaction may be regarded as an indication that vaccination has been unsuccessful and should be repeated.

Failure to obtain a local reaction should not be interpreted too readily as showing immunity. A further attempt should be made for it has been found that most ' failed ' revaccinations ' take ' at the second attempt. If there is complete insusceptibility this should be stated on the certificate. In recording the date arabic numerals should be used for the day and year and letters for the month, e.g. 30 Oct. 1970. The new international certificate of vaccination is printed in English and French. It must be signed by the person who has been vaccinated as well as by the doctor who gave the vaccination. A rubber stamp signature is no longer acceptable. The vaccine maker and batch number must be stated. Amendments, erasures and failure to complete the certificate may make it invalid. If a certificate is lost a duplicate should not be given but a new certificate bearing the original dates issued by the doctor who did the original vaccination. It should be marked ' copy '. This is to avoid doubt as to which figure refers to the month when the date is expressed in numbers only (e.g. 12 6 74 could mean 12 June '74 or 6 Dec. '74). But there would be no objection to adopting the logical recommendation of the International Standards Organisation, accepted by all major countries, which is to write the year, month and day in this order, allowing two digits for each, so that 12 June 1974 would be written 74 06 12.

Failure to ' take '

Primary vaccination may fail to ' take ' in very young infants because of placentally transmitted maternal antibodies. In such cases vaccination should be repeated at about 8 months. Failure to ' take ' in adults suggests an error in technique. In revaccination it should not be interpreted as indicating immunity for anyone who has ever had primary vaccinia will show at least an immediate allergic response. This may go on to a vaccinoid reaction in those partially immune. Revaccination properly done with potent lymph will cause a demonstrable lesion even after recent vaccination. If primary vaccination fails at least two more attempts should be made, preferably on new sites. All should be classed as primary.

To reduce the risk of failure when vaccinating in the face of possible exposure to smallpox the Department of Health recommends employing the multiple pressure or puncture and the scratch techniques in two separate areas 2·5 cm apart.

Refusal of Smallpox Vaccination

A passenger is liable to be detained in quarantine if his smallpox vaccination certificate is not in order. Conscientious objectors are treated similarly. Passengers from endemic or locally infected areas are offered vaccination. If this is refused they are placed under surveillance (endemic area) or isolation (locally infected area) but there is no question of compulsory vaccination. If for medical reasons (p. 757) the doctor decides that smallpox vaccination is inadvisable he should certify this and have the ' certificate of contra-indication ' authenticated by stamping in the same way as a vaccination certificate. It is not, however, a substitute for a certificate of vaccination and is no guarantee against the passenger being quarantined. This is solely a matter for the health authority at the place of arrival. The position of persons returning from an infected as distinct from an endemic area must be clearly understood. On arrival back from a country where smallpox is endemic a ' certificate of contra-indication ', would probably be as acceptable as a certificate of vaccination. But on return from a smallpox infected area the position is different. Apart from the risk of the unvaccinated traveller getting smallpox he would be in difficulty on return home and would probably have to spend 14 days in quarantine. A person who refused smallpox vaccination could be given temporary protection by specific immunoglobulin (p. 801) but this would not excuse him from the immigration requirements. A doctor whose patient refused vaccination would be wise to get a signed release from him.

EMBALMING

(For embalming of corpses containing radioactive isotopes see p. 595.)

If a person dies when far from home or aboard ship, the doctor may be called upon, particularly in a hot climate, to preserve the body, and steps may have to be taken quickly to do this.

1. If no embalming materials are available, ice or solid CO_2 should be packed around the body which should be kept in the coolest available place.

2. In the absence of ice or instruments other than a syringe, any available antiseptic (preferably formalin) should be poured into the mouth and injected into the chest and abdomen. The coffin should then be packed with a mixture of ashes or sand with chloride of lime (bleaching powder). This will delay decomposition but is of no value if the relatives wish to view the body later. Stench may be mitigated by damp sawdust and bleach powder 5 to 1 or an aerosol air freshner.

3. The Lear Embalming Service Ltd. recommends that formalin solutions stronger than 5 to 8 per cent of formalin should not be used as they may damage vessels and prevent onward flow. A good one contains 1 part of formalin (40 per cent formaldehyde) in 20 parts of water with crystalline carbolic acid 50 g (about three table-spoonsful) to the litre.

There are many excellent proprietary solutions (Arandee and 20th Century). For obvious medico-legal reasons arsenic should never be used. In most cases, two gallons of solution will be needed for an adult.

Technique

To avoid fixation in awkward positions the body should be horizontal and the eyes and mouth closed. If necessary a thread may be inserted round the lower jaw and through the nasal septum and tied. A small pad of wool lubricated with petroleum jelly under the eyelids improves the facial appearance. Rigor mortis should be broken down by moving all joints. Any necessary shaving should be done before injecting. The lips should be smeared with petroleum jelly to protect them against preserving fluid regurgitated from the lungs.

Injections by Higginson's syringe or by gravity should be made within a few hours of death before the blood loses its fluidity. Expose the axillary artery and vein. Tie the vein and insert a glass —or metal-ended wide-bore rubber tube into the proximal part and clamp it. Then open the artery and put a tube into its distal end and inject one or two litres of formalin embalming fluid. Drain off the first fluid injected by making an opening into the distal part of the vein. Tie it later and inject more fluid. Clamp the artery and inject the proximal end putting in up to 5 litres of fluid. Then unclamp the vein and drain off the fluid. It will be thick at first and manipulation of the tube and massage of the limbs will be needed to get it out. Inject two to two and a half more litres and drain, repeating this operation until the fluid returned is thin. The total amount of fluid to leave in is about 80 ml per kilogram body weight. Arterial injection is insufficient to preserve the viscera. Make a small incision near the umbilicus and insert a 30 cm long wide-bore pointed metal tube. Suck out fluids from the viscera with a pump or aspiration bottle and then inject one or two litres of embalming fluid. Properly injected tissues assume a definite firmness and any part which does not ' firm up ' must be separately injected. Oedematous tissues present a difficult problem. Weak formalin (1 per cent) should be used first so that the oedema fluid is not coagulated *in situ*. Excess fluid may be removed by incisions posteriorly and the application of rubber bandages.

If a post-mortem examination has been performed, then the ' 12 point' method must be used. This consists of injecting in both directions each carotid, axillary and femoral artery. In addition, the wall of the abdomen and chest must be infiltrated by needle and syringe. The soft viscera are best destroyed; otherwise they should be soaked for 24 hours in the solution and then returned. If autopsy is performed after embalming it should be delayed 24 hours.

Although it is difficult to compete with the professional mortician the cosmetic aspect should not be ignored. The body should be smeared with petroleum jelly (preferably containing 10 per cent paradichlorbenzene) to prevent the growth of moulds.

Should stench become a problem, as it might on board ship, damp sawdust and bleach powder 5 to 1 will render the atmosphere tolerable. If available a scented aerosol would be preferable. It is usual to pack paraformaldehyde around the body.

C. ALLAN BIRCH

Note on Telephone Numbers:

The word Tel. is not printed before the telephone number in every case. The following cities use All-Figure Numbers; they do not have exchange names. Numbers in London begin 01, in Birmingham 021, in Edinburgh 031, in Glasgow 041, in Liverpool 051, in Manchester 061. The 'city' code (01 for London etc.) is not dialled when the call is made within the city itself. Elsewhere telephone numbers may still have exchange names. The Subscriber Trunk Dialling code is also given in most cases although all do not yet have STD access to the exchange concerned. Trunk calls to these exchanges can be obtained via the operator by first dialling the code 100. For Directory inquiries dial 142 in London and 192 elsewhere.

APPENDIX 1

Government Health Departments

England	Department of Health and Social Security,
	Alexander Fleming House,
	Elephant and Castle,
	London, SE1 6BY.
	    Tel. 01-407 5522.
	    Telegraphic address, Healthmin, London SE1 6BY.
	    Telex 22106.

Scotland	The Scottish Home and Health Department, St Andrew's House, Edinburgh EH1 3DE. Tel. 031-556 8501. Telegraphic address, Health, Edinburgh.

Wales	The Welsh Office,
	Health Department, Pearl Assurance House,
	Greyfriars Road, Cardiff CF1 3RT.
	    Tel. 0222 44 151.
	    Telegraphic address, Health, Cardiff.

Northern Ireland	The Department of Health and Social Services (Northern Ireland),
	Dundonald House,
	Upper Newtownards Road,
	Belfast, BT4 3SF.
	    Tel. Belfast 650 111 (STD 0232).
	    Telex 74547.

Ireland (Eire)	The Department of Health,
	Custom House,
	Dublin.
	    Tel. Dublin 42961.
	    Telegraphic address, Health, Dublin 1.

Channel
Islands: **Jersey**
Public Health Offices,
Pier Road,
St Helier,
Jersey.
     Tel. Jersey Central 22541 (STD 0534).
     No telegraphic address.
Guernsey and Alderney
States of Guernsey Board of Health,
Lukis House,
Grange,
Guernsey.
     Tel. Guernsey 24316 (STD 0534).
     No telegraphic address.

Isle of Man Isle of Man Health Services Board,
3 Harris Terrace,
Douglas,
Isle of Man.
     Tel. Douglas 3303 (STD 0624).
     No telegraphic address.

Vaccines, Sera and Antivenines

Prophylaxis of rabies and tetanus, and treatment of anthrax, botulism, organo-phosphorus poisoning, snake-bite and tetanus

---

Preparations should be protected from the light and stored at a temperature between 2°C and 10°C. (Human antitetanus immunoglobulin (Humotet) at between 4°C and 6°C).

Anthrax antiserum. This is refined and concentrated and is supplied in 10 ml bottles each containing a full therapeutic dose (15 rabbit neutralising doses). Stocks after three years and time-expired ones are reprocessed.

Botulinum antitoxin. This is refined and concentrated so that two 25 ml vials constitute a full therapeutic dose. It may need to be repeated. Stocks are replaced after three years and time-expired ones reprocessed.

Human tetanus immunoglobulin. Supplies are available for prophylaxis if test doses of tetanus antitoxin of equine origin establish severe hypersensitivity to horse serum. (Dose 250 units=1 ampoule.)

Ovine antitetanus serum. Supplies are available for the prophylaxis and treatment of tetanus if test doses of tetanus antitoxin of equine origin establish severe hypersensitivity to horse serum.

P_2S *(pralidoxime mesylate).* P_2S is supplied for the treatment of certain types of organo-phosphorus poisoning. It is now supplied in ampoules of sterile solution.

Rabies vaccine and antiserum. Supplies of 'duck embryo' vaccine (DEV) and of Semple-type (rabbit brain) vaccine for active immunisation against rabies and of rabies antiserum for immediate passive protection are available as shown.

Adder-bite antivenom serum. A serum specifically for adder-bite poisoning is now available commercially from Regent Laboratories Ltd., Cunard Road (off Chase Road), Park Royal, London, NW10 6PN (01-965 3637/9). It is prepared by Imunoloski Zavod but is not held in the laboratories listed below. Kits contain one 5·4 ml ampoule with disposable syringe and needle. The initial dose is 20 ml (0·4 ml per kg for children). For hazards see p. 81 and precautions see p. 745.

LIST OF CENTRES HOLDING SUPPLIES OF CERTAIN PROPHYLACTIC AND THERAPEUTIC AGENTS IN ENGLAND AND WALES
(In alphabetical order of towns)

(a) anthrax antiserum *

(b) botulinus antitoxin

(c) human antitetanus immunoglobulin

(d) ovine antitetanus serum

(e) P2S

(f) rabies vaccine and antiserum

A 24 hour service is maintained at each Centre unless otherwise stated.

CENTRE	TELEPHONE NO.	SUPPLIES HELD OF:
The Group Pharmacist, Bronglais District General Hospital, Caradog Road, Aberystwyth.	Aberystwyth 3131 (STD 0970)	(b) (c) (d) (e)
Officer Commanding, Cambridge Military Hospital, Aldershot, Hants.	Aldershot 22521 (STD 0252)	(c)
The Chief Pharmacist, Caernarvon & Anglesey General Hospital, Bangor, Gwynedd.	Bangor 3321 (STD 024 8)	(a) (b) (c) (d) (e)
Group Pharmacist, Bedford General Hospital (S Wing), Kempston Road, Bedford.	Bedford 55122 (STD 0234)	(e)
The Group Pharmacist, Selly Oak Hospital, Raddlebarn Road, Selly Oak, Birmingham B29 6JD.	021 - 472 1361	(a) (b) (c) (d) (e)
The Group Pharmacist, Royal Victoria Hospital, Shelley Road, Boscombe, Hants.	Bournemouth 35201 (STD 0202)	(e)
The Chief Pharmacist, Ham Green Hospital, Pill, Bristol.	Pill 2661 (STD 0275 81)	(a) (b) (c) (d) (e)

* Some stocks which failed potency tests have been destroyed. Future availability is uncertain.

Centre	Telephone No.	Supplies held of :
The Director, Regional Transfusion and Immuno-Haematology Centre, Long Road, Cambridge.	Cambridge 45921 (STD 0223)	(a) (b) (c) (d) (e)
The Group Pharmacist, Kent & Canterbury Hospital, Eethelbert Road, Canterbury, Kent.	Canterbury 66877 (STD 0227)	(e)
The Director, Regional Public Health Laboratory, University Hospital of Wales, Heath Park, Cardiff CF4 4XW.	Cardiff 755944 (STD 0222)	(f)
The Chief Pharmacist, Cardiff Royal Infirmary, Newport Road, Cardiff, South Glamorgan LF2 1SZ.	Cardiff 33101 (STD 0222)	(a) (b) (c) (d) (e)
The Pathological Laboratory, Cumberland Infirmary, Carlisle, Cumbria.	Carlisle 23444 (STD 0228)	(a) (b) (c) (d) (e)
Officer Commanding, Military Hospital, Catterick Camp, North Yorkshire.	Catterick Camp 2521 (STD 07848 83)	(c)
The Group Pathologist, Chelmsford & Essex Hospital, London Road, Chelmsford, Essex.	Chelmsford 55139 (STD 0245)	(e)
Officer Commanding, Military Hospital, Circular Road, Colchester CO2 7UD, Essex.	Colchester 4215 (STD 020 6)	(c)
The Group Pharmacist, Darlington Memorial Hospital, Hollyhurst Road, Darlington, Durham.	Darlington 60100 (STD 0325)	(e)
The Director, Public Health Laboratory, Pathology Department, Glyde Path Road, Dorchester, Dorset.	Dorchester 3123 (STD 0305)	(c) (d)
The Dispensary, Guest Hospital, Dudley, West Midlands.	Dudley 54321 (STD 0384)	(g)

CENTRE	TELEPHONE NO.	SUPPLIES HELD OF :
The Chief Pharmacist, Edgware General Hospital, Edgware, Middlesex.	01-952 2381	(b) (c) (d) (e)
Group Pharmacist, Epsom District Hospital, Dorking Road, Epsom, Surrey.	Epsom 26100 (STD 39)	(e) (b)
Pathological Department, Royal Devon & Exeter Hospital, Southernhay East, Exeter, Devon.	Exeter (STD 0392) 72261 Exeter (STD 0392) 59261	(a) (b) (c) (d) (e)
The Group Pharmacist, West Wales General Hospital, Glangwili, Dyfed.	Carmarthen 5151 (STD 0267)	(c) (d) (e)
Accident & Emergency Dept., County Hospital, Hereford, Hereford and Worcester.	Hereford 2561 (STD 0432)	(e)
The Group Pharmacist, Castle Hill Hospital, Castle Road, Cottingham. Hull, North Humberside.	Hull 847372 (STD 0482)	(a) (b) (c) (d) (e)
Group Pharmacist, W. Norfolk and King's Lynn General Hospital, London Road, King's Lynn, Norfolk.	King's Lynn 61281 (STD 0553)	(e)
The Chief Pharmacist, Seacroft Hospital, York Road, Leeds, West Yorkshire.	Leeds 648164 (STD 0532)	(a) (b) (c) (d) (e)
Senior Casualty Officer, County Hospital, Lincoln.	Lincoln 29921 (STD 0522)	(e)
The Chief Pharmacist, Fazakerley Hospital, Longmoor Lane, Liverpool L9 7AL.	051 - 525 5980	(a) (b) (c) (d) (e)
The Director, Regional Public Health Laboratory, 126, Mount Pleasant, Liverpool, 3.	051 - 709 3636	(f)

Telephone no.	Centre	Supplies held of:
The Director, Central Public Health Labora- tory, Colindale Avenue, London, N.W.9.	01-205 7041	**(f)**
The Chief Pharmacist, Royal Northern Hospital, Holloway Road, London, N.7.	01-272 777	(a)
Chief Pathologist, North Middlesex Hospital, Silver Street, London, N.18.	01-807 3071	(a) (b) (c) (d) (e)
The Director, South London Transfusion Centre, Tooting Grove, Tooting, London SW17.	01-672 8501	(a) (b) (c) (d) (e)
Group Pharmacist, Luton and Dunstable Hospital, Dunstable Road, Luton, Beds.	Luton 53211 (STD 0582)	(e)
The Group Pharmacist, Manchester Royal Infirmary, Oxford Road, Manchester 13.	061 - 273 3300	(a) (b) (c) (d) (e)
The Director, Regional Public Health Laboratory, Institute of Pathology, Newcastle General Hospital, Westgate Road, Newcastle-upon-Tyne, NE4 6BE.	Newcastle 38811 (STD 0632)	(f)
The Group Pharmacist, Newcastle General Hospital, Westgate Road, Newcastle-upon-Tyne, NE4 6BE.	Newcastle 38811 (STD 0632)	(a) (b) (c) (d) (e)
Poisons Reference Service, New Cross Hospital, Avonley Road, London SE14.	01-407 7600	(e)
Department of Pathology, Northampton General Hospital, Billing Road, Northampton.	Northampton 34700 (STD 0604)	(a) (b) (c) (d) (e)

Telephone no.	Centre	Supplies held of :
Group Pharmacist, Norfolk & Norwich Hospital, St. Stephen's Road, Norwich, Norfolk, NOR 53A.	Norwich 28377 (STD 0603)	(e)
The Chief Pharmacist, Nottingham City Hospital, Hucknall Road, Nottingham.	Nottingham 63361 (STD 0602)	(a) (b) (c) (d) (e)
The Pharmacy, Churchill Hospital, Headington, Oxford.	Oxford 64841 (STD 865) Day only No night service	(c)
The Pharmacy, Radcliffe Infirmary, Oxford.	Oxford 49891 (STD 0865) Day only No night service	(d)
Officer in Charge, Accident & Emergency Dept., Plymouth General Hospital (Freedom Fields), Plymouth, Devon.	Plymouth 68080 (STD 0752)	(a) (b) (c) (d) (e)
The Group Pharmacist, Royal Portsmouth Hospital, Commercial Road, Portsmouth, Hants.	Portsmouth 22281 (STD 0705)	(c) (d) (e)
Group Pharmacist, Royal Infirmary, Deepdale Road, Preston PR1 6PS.	Preston 54747 (STD 0772)	(e)
The Group Pharmacist, Royal Berkshire Hospital, London Road, Reading, Berkshire.	Reading 85111 (STD 0734)	(a) (b) (c) (d) (e)
Officer i/c Accidents and Emergencies Department, Salisbury General Hospital, General Infirmary Branch, Fisherton Street, Salisbury, Wiltshire.	Salisbury 3231 (STD 0722)	(c) (d)
The Chief Pharmacist, Salisbury General Hospital, Odstock Branch, Salisbury, Wiltshire.	Salisbury 511 (STD 0722)	(a)
Group Pharmacist, Royal Hospital, West Street, Sheffield S1 3SR.	Sheffield 20063 (STD 0742)	(e)

Telephone no.	Centre	Supplies held of :
The Pharmacy, Royal Salop Infirmary, Shrewsbury, Shropshire.	Shrewsbury 53931 (STD 0743)	(a) (c) (d) (e)
Chief Pharmacist, Wexham Park Hospital, Slough, Bucks.	Slough 34567 (STD 75)	(e)
The Group Pharmacist, Royal South Hants Hospital, Fanshawe Street, Southampton.	Southampton 26211 (STD 0703)	(a) (b) (c) (d) (e)
The Dispensary, Staffordshire General Infirmary, Foregate Street, Stafford.	Stafford 4251 (STD 0785)	(e)
Chief Pharmacist, N. Staffordshire Royal Infirmary, Princes Road, Hartshill, Stoke-on-Trent ST4 7LN.	Stoke-on-Trent 44161 (STD 0782)	(a) (c) (d) (e)
Chief Pharmacist, Singleton Hospital, Sketly, Swansea, West Glamorgan.	Swansea 25666 (STD 0792)	(a) (b)
The Pharmacy, Royal Cornwall Hospital, Treliske Branch, Truro, Cornwall.	Truro 4242 (STD 0782)	(a) (b) (c) (d) (e)
The Director, South London Blood Transfusion Centre, South East Depot, David Salomon House, Southborough, Tunbridge Wells, Kent.	Day. Mon.-Fri. Sat. mng Tunbridge Wells 28172 (STD 0892) All other times Tunbridge Wells 29510 (STD 0892) 22631 (STD 0892) Tonbridge 5727 (STD 07322)	(a) (b) (c) (d) (e)
Chief Pharmacist, Worcester Royal Infirmary, Ronkswood Branch, Newton Road, Worcester.	Worcester 26971 (STD 0905)	(e)
The Dispensary, Worcester Royal Infirmary, Castle Street Branch, Worcester.	Worcester 27122 (STD 0905)	(e)

Telephone No.	Centre	Supplies held of :
The Chief Pharmacist, Maelor General Hospital, Croesnewdd Road, Wrexham, Clwyd.	Wrexham 3512/6 (STD 0978) Monday—Friday Day only Saturday—Morning only No night service	(a) (b) (c) (d) (e)

Prophylactic agents (a) to (f) inclusive are not held in the Channel Islands and would be obtained by plane from Colindale in case of need.

P_2S for organophosphorus poisoning is held at the Royal Victoria Belfast (Belfast 40503—STD 0232) and at Altnagelvin Hospital, Londonderry (Londonderry 65171/9—STD 0504).

SCOTLAND

The centres outlined below hold stocks of the materials indicated and hospitals requiring supplies should address their demands to the Chief Pharmacist at each hospital. Demands for vaccine lymph should not exceed the estimated consumption for three months.

Vaccine lymph **Anthrax vaccine**	Bridge of Earn Hospital, Bridge of Earn, Perthshire. 073 881 331. Law Hospital, Carluke. Wishaw (069 83) 72621. Peel Hospital, Galashiels, Selkirkshire. 0896-2295.
Rabies vaccine (rabbit brain) **Botulinus anti-toxin** **Anthrax antiserum**	Kings Cross Hospital, Clepington Road, Dundee. Dundee 85241 (STD 0382). Glasgow Royal Infirmary, 84 Castle Street, Glasgow, C.4. 041-552 3535. Ext 486. Central Microbiological Laboratories, Western General Hospital, Crewe Road South, Edinburgh EH4 2X0. 031-332 1311 (Ext 170 or 179). Raigmore Hospital, Inverness. Inverness 34543 (STD 0463).
Rabies (duck embryo) vaccine	Glasgow Royal Infirmary 84 Castle Street, Glasgow C4. 041-552 3535. Ext 486. King's Cross Hospital, Dundee. 85241 (STD 0382). Central Microbiological Laboratories, Western General Hospital, Edinburgh EH4 2XO. 031-332 1311. Ext 170 and 179.

Rabies antiserum

Glasgow Royal Infirmary.
Western General Hospital, Edinburgh.
—See above.

Ovine anti-tetanus serum

Raigmore Hospital, Inverness.
Western Infirmary, Glasgow.
Royal Infirmary, Glasgow.
Royal Infirmary, Edinburgh.
Bridge of Earn Hospital.
Royal Infirmary, Aberdeen.   —See above.
Blood Transfusion Centres at
    Raigmore Hospital, Inverness.
    Royal Infirmary, Aberdeen.
    Royal Infirmary, Dundee.
        23125 (STD 0382).
    Royal Infirmary, Edinburgh.
    Law Hospital, Carluke.   —See above.

Human anti-tetanus gamma globulin

Aberdeen Royal Infirmary,
Foresterhill, Aberdeen.
0224 23423.

Bridge of Earn Hospital,
Bridge of Earn, Perthshire.
073 881 331.

Edinburgh Royal Infirmary,
Lauriston Place, Edinburgh 3.
031-229 2477.

Glasgow Royal Infirmary,
84 Castle Street, Glasgow C.4.
041-552 3535.

Western Infirmary,
Dunbarton Road, Glasgow W.1.
041-339 8822.

P₂S (pralidoxime mesylate)

Law Hospital,
Carluke, Lanarkshire.
Wishaw (069 83) 72621.

Bridge of Earn Hospital,
Bridge of Earn, Perthshire.
073 881 331.

Scottish Poisons Information Bureau,
Edinburgh Royal Infirmary,
Lauriston Place, Edinburgh EH3 9YW.
031-229 2477.
Peel Hospital, Galashiels.
2295 (STD 0896).
Raigmore Hospital, Inverness.   —See above.
Aberdeen Royal Infirmary.   —See above.
Caithness General Hospital.
Wick 2261 (STD 0955).
Dumfries and Galloway Royal Infirmary,
Dumfries 5264 (STD 0387).
Gilbert Bain Hospital, Lerwick, Shetland.
Lerwick 751.
Maryfield Hospital, Dundee.
40011 (STD 0382).

Any hospital requiring supplies of diphtheria prophylactic, Schick test toxin, equine tetanus antitoxin, TABC, gas gangrene antitoxin, tetanus toxoid, dysentery vaccine, cholera vaccine or typhus vaccine should obtain them from ordinary trade sources.

For adder-bite antivenom serum see p. 766.

Northern Ireland

In Northern Ireland The Royal Victoria Hospital, Belfast, Tel. 30503 (STD 0232), holds supplies of botulinus antitoxin, gas gangrene antitoxin, tetanus antitoxin and tetanus toxoid. The Laboratories, Belfast City Hospital, Belfast 9 Tel. Belfast 32521 (STD 0232) (after hours Belfast 29241 (STD 0232) hold stocks of anti-anthrax serum, botulinus antitoxin, vaccine lymph, anti-rabies vaccine, typhus vaccine and immunoglobulin. Antileptospiral serum is not kept in Northern Ireland.

P_2S for oganophorphorus poisoning is held at the Royal Victoria Hospital, Belfast, and at Altnagelvin Hospital, Londonderry 5171/9 (STD 0504).

Republic of Ireland (Eire)

In Eire vaccines and sera may be obtained from drug firms and pharmacists. Vaccine lymph for use by doctors may be had on request to the Director, Vaccine Branch, Department of Health, University College, Dublin 2 (Tel. 752116) and Messrs Fannins, Grafton Street, Dublin (Tel. 774731). The advice of the local Chief Medical Officer or the Medical Officer in charge of the nearest Fever Hospital could be sought in any case of doubt or difficulty.

Ireland

Cherry Orchard Hospital, Dublin.
Tel. Dublin 364702.

Isle of Man

Supplies of anthrax antiserum, botulinus antitoxin, snakebite anti-venom and P_2S are not held in Isle of Man hospitals. They would be obtained from mainland regional centres in case of need.

Channel Islands

Guernsey

Tetanus toxoid and antitoxin and gas gangrene antitoxin are held at Princess Elizabeth Hospital. Tel. Guernsey 2100 (STD 0481).

Tetanus antitoxin and vaccine are held at St Peter Port Hospital. Tel. Guernsey 1606 (STD 0481).

Other materials including diphtheria antitoxin, immunoglobulin, triple antigen, calf lymph, B.C.G. and poliomyelitis vaccine are kept at Lukis House (p. 765).

Jersey

Sera for diphtheria, scarlatina, tetanus, gas gangrene, staphylococcal infections and leptospirosis are held at The General Hospital, St. Helier. Tel. Central 24242 (STD 0543).

Diphtheria antitoxin and tetanus antitoxins are held also at Overdale Hospital, Westmount, St. Helier. Tel. Central 31411 (STD 0543).

RABIES (p. 537)

Centres holding free supplies of rabies vaccine and serum and providing diagnostic facilities in animal material.

London
Central Public Health Laboratory, Colindale Avenue, NW9 5HT. 01-205 7041.

Newcastle
Public Health Laboratory, The Dispensary, Newcastle General Hospital, Westgate Road, Newcastle NE4 6BE. Newcastle 38811 (STD 0632).

Liverpool
Public Health Laboratory, 126 Mount Pleasant, Liverpool. 051-709 3636.

Wales
Public Health Laboratory, Institute of Preventive Medicine, The Parade, Cardiff. Cardiff 29110 and 23967 (STD 0222).

Ireland
An information service about rabies is provided by Cherry Orchard Fever Hospital, Dublin. 364702.

Vaccine and serum can also be obtained on payment from the Lister Institute, Elstree, Herts. 01-953 4301. Telegrams, Prevent, Elstree.

BLOOD DINITRO AND CHOLINESTERASE ESTIMATIONS

The names of laboratories able to estimate DNOC and ' dinoseb ' (DNBP) content can be obtained by telephoning the Regional Health Authority. Some of them can also measure cholinesterase activity on blood samples.

SUPPLIERS OF ANTI-VENINES FOR SNAKE-BITE POISONING OUTSIDE GREAT BRITAIN

(For adder-bite antivenom see p. 766.)

Supplies of antivenom in different areas can best be obtained from places numbered in this list as indicated below.

Americas: Polyvalent viper antivenom from 13; coral-snake antivenom from 3.

North Africa: Viper antivenom from 1, 4, or 5.

Mid Africa: Mamba antivenom from 10 (or 4); African cobra antivenom from 4, 5, or 10; viper antivenom from 4 (Bitis-Echis), 5 (Echis) or 10 (Echis).

South Africa: Mamba, cobra, and viper antivenom from 10.

Middle East: Viper-cobra antivenom from 4, 5, or 8.

Asia—Seasnake bite: Seasnake antivenom from 2. Also supplies see wasp antivenom (see p. 627).

Burma, India, and Pakistan: Cobra-krait-viper antivenom from 6 (a) or 6 (b).

Cambodia, Laos, Malaysia, Vietnam, Thailand: Viper and cobra antivenoms from 12.

Indonesia: Cobra-krait-viper antivenom from 7.

Japan: Viper antivenoms from 9.

Philippines and Taiwan: Cobra, krait, and viper antivenoms from 11.

Algeria

(1) Institut Pasteur d'Algerie, rue Docteur Laveran, Algiers. Also supplies scorpion antivenom.

Australia

(2) The principal manufacturer and supplier of antivenines in Australia is the Commonwealth Serum Laboratories, 45 Poplar Road, Parkville, Victoria 3052. Tel. Melbourne 387 1066. (Also serum for red back spider bite.)
The State branches are:—
Queensland—49-51 Gregory Terrace, Brisbane 4000.
New South Wales—212 Willoughby Road, Naremburn 2065.
Victoria—45 Poplar Road, Parkville 3052.
South Australia—282 Gilbert Street, Adelaide 5000.
Western Australia—416-418 Newcastle Street, Perth 6000.
Tasmania—123 Murray Street, Hobart 7000.
Any of the above should be contacted first and failing them the Director of Health, viz.:—
Head Office—Director-General of Health, PO Box 100, Woden. ACT 2600.
Australian Capital Territory—CML Building, Darwin Place, Canberra. ACT 2600.
Queensland—Anzac Square, Adelaide Street, Brisbane 4000.

New South Wales—Chifley Square, Cnr Philips & Hunter Streets, Sydney 2000.
Victoria—Cnr Spring & Latrobe Streets, Melbourne 3000.
South Australia—AMP Building, King William Street, Adelaide 5000.
Western Australia—Victoria Centre, 2-6 St George's Terrace, Perth 6000.
Tasmania—Kirksway House, Kirksway Place, Hobart 7000.
Northern Territory, PO Box 147, Darwin 5790.

Austria

Serotherapeutisches Institut Wien, Triesterstrasse, 50 (European vipers only).

Argentina

Instituto Nacional de Microbiologia, Avenida Velez Sarsfield, 563 Buenos Aires.

Brasil

(3) Instituto Butantan, Caixa Postal 65 Sao Paulo SP, Brasil. Also supplies spider and scorpion antivenom.
Instituto Butantan, Commercial Agents: C. Amaral & Cia, Rua da Gloria, 34 Sao Paulo SP, Brasil.
Instituto Pinheiros, Productos Terapeuticos, SA Rua Teodora Sampaio, 1860 Sao Paulo, Brasil.

Colombia

Instituto Nacional de Salad, Calle 57 Numero 8-35, Bogota DE, Colombia.

France

(4) Institut Pasteur, 36 rue du Docteur Roux, Paris XVe.
Institut Merieux, 17 rue Bourgelat, Lyon, Rhone.

Federal German Republic

(5) Farbwerke Hoechst AG, 6230 Frankfurt, Main 80.
Behringwerke AG, Postfach 167, 355 Marburg, Germany.

Holland

Rijksinstitut voor de Volksgezondheid, Utrecht, Sterrenbos I.

India

(6) Central Research Institute, Kasauli RI, Punjab, India.
(Bivalent antivenine against cobra and Russell's viper.)
Director, Haffkine Institute, Parel, Bombay.
(Lyophilised polyvalent serum against cobra, common krait, Russell's viper and saw scaled viper.)

Indonesia

(7) Perusahaan Negara Biopharma (Pasteur Institute), Djalan Pasteur No 9, PO Box 47, Bandung, Indonesia.

Iran

(8) Institut d'Etat des Serums et Vaccins Razi Boite Postal 656, Tehran.

Israel

Rogoff Institute, Beilinson Hash, Tel-Aviv University, Tel-Aviv.

Italy

Institut Sieroterapico Milanese, Serafino Belfanti, Ente Morale Aggregato Alla Universita di Milana, Milano, via Darwin 20.
Instituto Sieroterapico e Vaccinogeno Sclavo Via Fiorentine I, Siena, Italy.

Japan

(9) Institut for Infectious Diseases, University of Tokyo, Densenbyo-Kenkyusho, Shiba Shirokane-Daimachi, Minato-ku, Tokyo.
Laboratory of Chemotherapy and Serum Therapy, Kumamoto City, Kyashu, Japan.
Takeda Pharmaceutical Co., Osaka, Japan.

Mexico

Laboratory MYN, SA Avenue, Coyoacan 1717 Mexico 12 DF, Mexico.
Instituto Nacional de Higiene, Czda, M Escobedo No 20, Mexico 13 DF, Mexico.

Pakistan

The Bureau of Laboratories, Old Naval Isolation Camp, Napier Barracks, Karachi.

Phillipines

Bureau of Research and Laboratories, Department of Health, San Lazaro Hospital Compound, Manila, Phillipines.
Serum and Vaccine Laboratories, Alabang, Muntilupa, Rizal, Phillipines.

Poland

Warsaw Manufacturing Plant of Sera and Vaccines, Chelmska St 30/34, Warsaw.

Rhodesia.

CAPS, PO Box 2279, Salisbury, Rhodesia.

South Africa

(10) The South African Institute of Medical Research, PO Box 1038, Johannesburg.
Also supplies scorpion and spider antivenom.
There are branches at Buckingham Road, Port Elizabeth and 7 Roth Avenue, Bloemfontein.
The Institute also supplies serum to the Government Departments of Nigeria, Ghana, Zaïre, Central African Republic, Mozambique, Angola, Guinea Bissau, The Cameroun Republic and the numerous missionary stations in Central Africa.
Fitzsimon's Snake Park, PO Box 1, Snell Parade, Durban, Natal.

Taiwan (Formosa)

(11) Taiwan Serum Vaccine Laboratory, 130 Fuh-lin Road, Shilin, Taipei, Taiwan.

Thailand

(12) Queen Saovabha Memorial Institute, Rana 4 Road, Bangkok.

Union of Soviet Socialist Republics

Tashkent Institute of Vaccines and Serums, c/o Ministry of Health, Moscow.

United States of America
The sole producers of antivenines for snakebite in the USA are Wyeth Laboratories, Box 8299, Philadelphia, Pa.
Polyvalent serum supplied dry.

Vietnam
Pasteur Institute, Nha Trang, Vietnam.

Venezuela
Laboratorio Behrens, Ave Principal de Chapellin, Apartado 62, Caracas.

Yugoslavia
Imunoloski Zavod, PO Box 548 Rockefellerova, 2, Zagreb 1, Zagreb.

EMERGENCY PROPHYLAXIS

The laboratories of the Public Health Laboratory Service of England and Wales holds stocks of certain prophylactic materials not readily obtainable through trade sources. They also receive specimens for investigation. Addresses are given in telephone directories. There is no Public Health Laboratory Service in Scotland (see p. 773).

The prophylactics and places of supply are as follows:

Smallpox vaccine	Most P.H.L.S. laboratories.
Immunoglobulin	Most P.H.L.S. laboratories (limited stocks).
Anti-rabies vaccine	P.H.L.S. laboratories at London (Colindale), Liverpool, Newcastle and Cardiff only.
Anti-typhus vaccine	P.H.L.S. laboratories at Birmingham, Bristol, Cambridge, Cardiff, Exeter, Leeds, Liverpool, London, Manchester, Newcastle, Oxford, Sheffield.
Anthrax vaccine	P.H.L.S. laboratories in Bradford, Liverpool and London (Colindale).

Virus reference laboratory
Central Public Health Laboratory, Colindale Avenue, London, N.W.9. 01-205 7041.
Note: With the exception of smallpox and related virus diseases, rabies and the serology of typhus fever this laboratory does not receive specimens for routine diagnosis. Such specimens are received at all regional and most area laboratories and enquiries should be directed to the nearest P.H.L.S. laboratory.

REFERENCE EXPERTS

Reference experts normally receive specimens only from other laboratories within and without the Service. It should be added, however, that all regional and most area laboratories are undertaking the routine diagnosis of virus infections, and that several laboratories are undertaking the serological identification of members of the *Salmonella* group, the serological diagnosis of leptospiral infections, and the bacteriophage-typing of strains of *Staphylococcus aureus*. For this reason enquiries on these subjects should usually be addressed to the local public health laboratory.

There are reference experts for the following organisms and techniques. (Addresses and telephone numbers are to be found in *The Year Book of the Public Laboratory Service* (Headquarters Administrative Office, 24 Park Crescent, London W1N 4DA 01-636 2223).) Amoebiasis; Anaerobes; Anthrax; Arboviruses; Arizona group; Blood, tissues and intestinal parasites including malaria, Brucella, Cholera and related vibrios; Aeromonas and Plesiomonas; *Clostridium welchii*; Coxsackie A viruses; Cytomegaloviruses; Diphtheria bacilli; Disinfection; Drug resistance in Enterobacteria; Enteric fever; Entomological specimens; *Escherichia coli*; Farmer's lung; Food poisoning; Fungi (pathogenic); Helminthological specimens; Hydatid disease; Immunofluorescence; Influenza; Listeria typing; Meningococcal typing; Parasitic infestations; Plague; Pneumococci; Poliomyelitis; Protective cabinets; Psittacosis; Rabies; Rickettsia; Salmonella typing; *Shigella sonnei;* Shigella and related organisms; Smallpox (see p. 699); Staphylococcal enterotoxin; Streptococci of Group A; Toxoplasmosis; Trichinosis; Tubercle bacilli and other mycobacteria; Typhus fever; Venereal diseases (Treponemal immobilisation test); Vibrio parahaemolyticus; *Yersinia pseudotuberculosis* and *Yersinia enterocoltica*.

REFERENCE LABORATORIES IN NORTHERN IRELAND

Virus

Department of Microbiology, Queen's University of Belfast, Grosvenor Road, Belfast, BT12 6BN. Belfast 40503 (STD 0232) Ext. 408.

Bacteriology

The Laboratories, Belfast City Hospital, 51 Lisburn Road, Belfast BT9 7AD. Belfast 42521 (STD 0232).

Histopathology

Institute of Pathology, Grosvenor Road, Belfast BT12 6BN. Tel. Belfast 40503 (STD 0232) Ext. 346.

The Laboratories, Belfast City Hospital, 51 Lisburn Road, Belfast BT9 7AD. Tel. Belfast 29241 (STD 0232).

REFERENCE EXPERT IN SCOTLAND

Salmonella infections

Bacteriology Department, Stobhill Hospital, Glasgow N.1. 041-558 5042. Help in other infections should be sought at present from reference experts in England.

27

Notes on other immunological materials NOT obtainable through the Public Health Laboratory Service:

1. *Antisera for therapeutic use*
   Obtainable through the Hospital Pathological Service.
2. *Yellow fever vaccine*
   For a list of centres see p. 783.
3. *TABC, cholera and other vaccines*
   Most of these are available commercially.
4. *Smallpox Vaccine*
   Obtainable from Public Health Departments of Local Authorities (Counties, County Boroughs and London Boroughs).

YELLOW FEVER AND OTHER VACCINATIONS

Yellow fever vaccination can only be done at special centres and at some air terminals.

Vaccination at air terminals

London. Yellow fever vaccination is obtainable at the Air Corporations Joint Medical Service Unit at London Airport (01-759 5511) by appointment and at the ACJMS Immunisation unit, Air Terminal, Buckingham Palace Road, London S.W.1 (Tel. 01-834 2323) from 0900 to 1730 hours Monday to Friday and 0900 to 1100 hours on Saturday, preferably by appointment. Fee £1.40.

Smallpox, cholera and TAB vaccination can also be carried out. Fee £1.00 per injection.

Manchester. Yellow fever vaccination is not provided but vaccination against cholera and typhoid is available on Monday to Friday 0900 to 1715 hours. Fees £0·75 per injection. Telephone 061-437 5277. Emergency smallpox vaccination can be made at the same time except when the doctor is visiting out stations.

A 24 hour emergency service for immunisation against smallpox, cholera and yellow fever is provided (free of charge) at the Health Control Unit at Terminal 2 (Tel. 01-759 7212) and Terminal 3 (Tel. 01-759 7209) at London (Heathrow) Airport for outgoing passengers.

CENTRES FOR YELLOW FEVER VACCINATION

Important. 1. Every person requiring vaccination must make an appointment with the centre: at many centres this may be done by telephone at any time during normal office hours (usually 1000 to 1700 hours). Where times of attendance are shown, they are given for guidance only.

2. The centres marked * undertake other vaccinations as well as vaccination against yellow fever.

Town	Address	Telephone	Time of Attendance (see note 1 above)
	ENGLAND AND WALES		
London Borough of Camden	*Yellow Fever Vaccination Service, Hospital for Tropical Diseases, 4 St Pancras Way, London, N.W.1.	01-387 4411 Ext. 137	Mon. to Fri. morning By appointment
Corporation of London	Yellow Fever Vaccination Service, Medical Department, Unilever House, Blackfriars, London, E.C.4.	01-353 7474 Ext. 2841	Tues. & Fri. 1545 hrs
London	Cavendish Immunisation Centre, 99 New Cavendish Street, London, W.1.	01-637 8941	**Daily 0900** to 1730 hrs
Westminster City Council	*Yellow Fever Vaccination Service, 53 Great Cumberland Place, London W1H 7LH.	01-262 6456	*Yellow fever:* Mon. to Fri. 1000 to 1100 hrs Tues., Wed., Thurs.
	Yellow Fever Vaccination Centre, St George's Hospital Medical School, Hyde Park Corner, London, SW1.	01-235 8344	1400 to 1500 hrs *Other vaccinations:* Mon. to Fri. 1000 to 1700 hrs by appointment
London Borough of Kingston-upon-Thames	Health Centre, Grangewood, Kingston-upon-Thames.	01-546 7261	By appointment
Barnsley	*Medical Services Clinic, New Street, Barnsley.	Barnsley 3525, (STD 9226) Ext. 243	By appointment
Birmingham	*Birmingham Area Health Authority (T), Immunisation Section, Congreve Street, Birmingham, B3 3DH.	021-235 9944 Ext. 3428	**Wed.** 1400 to 1500 hrs 24 hrs notice if possible

Town	Address	Telephone	Time of Attendance (see note 1 above)
Blackburn	Health & Welfare Services Department, Larkhill Health Centre, Mount Pleasant, Blackburn.	Blackburn 63611 (STD 0254) Ext. 207	Mon. 1600 hrs By appointment
Bournemouth	*Avebury Clinic, 10 Madeira Road, Bournemouth.	Ferndown 6161 (STD 02017)	**Wed.** 1400 hrs By appointment
Bradford	*Edmund St Clinic, 26 Edmund St., Bradford, 5.	Bradford 28421 (STD 0274) Ext. 22	By appointment
Brighton	Health Dept., Royal York Buildings, Old Steine, Brighton BN1 1NP.	Brighton 29801 (STD 0273) Ext. 331	By appointment
Bristol	Control of Infection Unit, GPO Box No. 201, Tower Hill, Bristol BS99 7BQ.	Bristol 291010 (STD 0272) Ext. 231	By appointment
Cambridge	County M.O.H., Shire Hall Annexe, Gloucester St., Cambridge.	Cambridge 58811 (STD 0223)	**Mon.** 0930 hrs **Thurs.** 1630 hrs
Cardiff	*Vaccination Clinic, Occupational Health Services Consulting Suite, 54 Newport Road, Cardiff.	Cardiff 31033 (STD 0222) Ext. 365	Thurs. afternoon. In special circumstances at other times.
Carlisle	Central Health Clinic, Victoria Place, Carlisle.	Carlisle 23411 (STD 0228)	Mon. & Thurs. 1100 hrs
Chelmsford	Health Suite, Ground Floor, Block A, County Hall Extension, Chelmsford.	Chelmsford 53233 (STD 0245) Ext. 2751	**Tues. & Fri.** afternoon
Coventry	Room 132, Health Dept., New Council Offices, Earl St., Coventry.	Coventry 25555 (STD 0203) Ext. 2635.	**Wed.** 1400 hrs (24 hrs notice required)

Town	Address	Telephone	Time of Attendance (see note 1 above)
Derby	*Derbyshire County Council Clinic, Cathedral Rd., Derby.	Derby 45934 (STD 4332)	Mon. morning
Doncaster	*Health Offices, York House, Cleveland St., Doncaster.	Doncaster 67051/6 (STD 0302)	Mon. 1400 to 1600 hrs
Exeter	*School Health Dept., 1A Southernway West, Exeter.	Exeter 77888 (STD 0392) Ext. 220	By appointment
Gloucester	*Gloucestershire Royal Hospital, Southgate St., Gloucester.	Gloucester 23584 (STD 0452)	Tues. 1000 to 1200 hrs
Grimsby	Health Dept., Queen St., Grimsby.	Grimsby 580860 (STD 0472)	By appointment
Haverfordwest	County Health Dept., Merlins Hill, Haverfordwest.	Haverford-west 3345 (STD 0437)	By appointment 48 hrs notice
Kingston-upon-Hull	*Health Dept., Branch Office, Witham, Kingston-upon-Hull.	Hull 24364 (STD 0482) Ext. 65	Tues. & Fri. 1100 hrs
Lancaster	*Ashton Road Clinic, Lancaster.	Lancaster 2558/9 (STD 0524)	By appointment
Leeds	*8 Park Square, Leeds, 1.	Leeds 30661 (STD 0532)	Wed. & Fri. 1530 to 1600 hrs
Leicester	*Midland House, 52-54 Charles St., Leicester.	Leicester 25732 (STD 0533)	By appointment
Lincoln	*City Health Dept., Beaumont Fee, Lincoln.	Lincoln 27196 (STD 0522)	By appointment
Liverpool	*Vaccination Centre, Health Dept., Hatton Garden, Liverpool, 3.	051-227 3911 Ext. 389	Mon. to Fri. 1400 to 1630 hrs

Town	Address	Telephone	Time of Attendance (see note 1 above)
Liverpool (2nd Centre)	*School of Tropical Medicine, Pembroke Place, Liverpool, 3.	051-709 2298	Tues. & Fri. 1400 hrs. In special circumstances at other times by appointment
Maidstone	*Health & Welfare Dept., Springfield, Scandling Rd., Maidstone.	Maidstone 54371 (STD 0622)	By appointment
Manchester	*Health Dept., 3rd Floor, Town Hall Extension, Manchester, 2.	061-236 3377 Ext. 2528	By appointment
Middlesbrough	Cleveland Area Health Authority, 4th floor, Marton House, Borough Road, Middlesbrough.	Middlesbrough 49141 (STD 0642) Ext. 260	By appointment
	The Medical Centre, Warwick House, 17-19 Warwick Road, Old Trafford, Manchester, M16 0QQ.	061-872 7717/8	By appointment
Newcastle-upon-Tyne	Jesmond Clinic, 48 Osborne Rd., Newcastle-upon-Tyne, 2.	Newcastle-upon-Tyne 28520 (STD 0632) Ext. 92 or 558	By appointment
Newport	Public Health Dept., Civic Centre, Newport, Mon.	Newport 65491 (STD 0633) Ext. 12	By appointment
Northampton	County Offices, Guildhall Rd., Northampton.	Northampton 34833 (STD 0604) Ext. 115	Thurs. 1145 to 1215 hrs
Norwich	*Churchman House, 68 St Giles St.. Norwich NOR 22E.	Norwich 22233 (STD 0603) Ext. 99	By appointment
Nottingham	Radfield Welfare Centre, Grant Street, Nottingham NG7 3GS.	Nottingham 50551 or 55782 (STD 0602)	By appointment

Town	Address	Telephone	Time of Attendance (see note 1 above)
Oxford	Health Dept., Greyfriars, Paradise St., Oxford.	Oxford 47712 (STD 0865)	Tues. 1400 to 1430 hrs
Penzance	Health Clinic Bellair, Alverton, Penzance.	Penzance 2321 (STD 0736)	Wed. morning
Plymouth	Health Dept., Municipal Offices, Plymouth.	Plymouth 68000 (STD 0752) Ext. 2427	Tues. 1430 hrs
Sheffield	Central Health Clinic, Mulberry Street, Sheffield S1 2PJ.	Sheffield 731661 Ext. 24 or 26 (STD 0742)	Tues. 1600 to 1700 hrs
Shrewsbury	County Health Dept., (2nd Floor, North Block), Shirehall, Abbey Foregate. Shrewsbury.	Shrewsbury 52211 (STD 0743) Ext. 524	First & third Monday each month
Southampton	Central Health Clinic, East Park Terrace, Southampton.	Southampton 34321 (STD 0703)	Wed. 1430 hrs
Southend-on-Sea	*Municipal Health Centre, Warrior Sq., Southend-on-Sea.	Southend-on-Sea 49451 (STD 0702)	By appointment
Swansea	Public Health Dept., 21 Orchard St., Swansea.	Swansea 51501 (STD 0792)	By appointment
Taunton	Health Centre, Tower Lane, Taunton.	Taunton 82251 (STD 0823)	By appointment
Teesside	The Yelow Fever Centre, Carlow Street Clinic, Carlow St., Middlesbrough. (Request for appointments to Area Health Authority Offices, PO Box 92, Marton House, Borough Road, Middlesbrough. Tel. Middlesbrough 49141.)		

Town	Address	Telephone	Time of Attendance (see note 1 above)
Truro	Health Area Office, The Leats, Truro.	Truro 2202 (STD 0872)	Mon. 1100 hrs
York	*Health Services Centre, 33 Monkgate, York.	York 59881 (STD 0904) Ext. 241	By appointment

SCOTLAND

Aberdeen	Beach Boulevard Clinic. Beach Boulevard, Aberdeen AB2 1HB.	Aberdeen 29427 (STD 0224)	Thurs. 1630 to 1730 hrs
Dundee	Kings Cross Hospital, Clepington Road, Dundee DD3 8EA.	Dundee 85241 (STD 0382)	**Wed.** 1500 hrs
Edinburgh	Central Vaccination Clinic, 9 Johnston Terrace. Edinburgh EH1 2PP.	031-225 8474	Mon. & Wed. from 1500 hrs
Glasgow	*Public Health Clinic, 20 Cochrane St., Glasgow C1O1 1RN.	041-221 9600 Ext. 332	Tues. & Fri. 1430 hrs

ISLE OF MAN

Douglas	Noble's Hospital, Westmoreland Rd., Douglas.	Douglas 3661 (STD 0624)	By appointment

CHANNEL ISLANDS

Jersey	Pathological Laboratory, The Parade, Jersey.	Central 22695 (STD 0543)	By appointment (Fee £2)
Guernsey	Public Health Dept. Lukis House, Grange, Guernsey.	Guernsey 24541 (STD 0481)	By appointment (Fee £1 4s)

NORTHERN IRELAND

Belfast	Belfast Corporation Yellow Fever Vaccination Centre, Lincoln Avenue Clinic, Antrim Road, Belfast.	Belfast 41771 (STD 0232) Ext. 275	

Town	Address	Telephone	Time of Attendance (see note 1 above)
Ballymena	Ballymena Yellow Fever Vaccination Centre, 51 Castle Street, Ballymena.	Ballymena 6324 & 2108 (STD 0266)	
Omagh	Omagh Yellow Fever Vaccination Centre, The Health Centre, Mountjoy Rd., Omagh.	Omagh 3521 (STD 0063) Ext. 59	

REPUBLIC OF IRELAND (EIRE)

Town	Address	Telephone	Time of Attendance
Dublin	(Vaccination is not free of charge in Eire)		
	Dr J. F. Fleetwood, 11 Proby Sq., Blackrock, Co. Dublin.	Dublin 882683	
	Professor F. S. Stewart and Dr J. D. McKeever, Dept. of Bacteriology, Trinity College, Dublin.	Dublin 72941 Ext. 94	
	Dr Joseph Barnes, 47 Fitzwilliam Sq., Dublin.	Dublin 65267	
	Dr Ivor Hooper, 2 Mount Harold Terrace, Leinster Rd., Dublin, 6.	Dublin 972201 If not present phone Shannon 972458	
Drogheda	Our Lady's Hospital, Drogheda.	Drogheda 7601	
Ennis	Dr Michael Hanrahan, County Clinic, Bindon Street, Ennis, Co. Clare.	Ennis 21525	
Limerick	County Medical Officer, Limerick.	Limerick 46655	
Shannon Airport	Airport Medical Officer, Shannon Airport, Co. Clare.	Shannon Airport 61207	

APPENDIX 3

Regional Respiratory Units

THESE were set up when poliomyelitis was prevalent and are still necessary for other conditions, e.g. tetanus and toxic polyneuritis in which assisted respiration may be needed. The doctor is advised to find out from his Regional Health Authority which hospitals in his area can provide for patients needing these services. Arrangements for the provision of a portable respirator for use during the journey and any other details should be made with the hospital concerned. Centres with special experience of tetanus exist at The General Infirmary at Leeds (Leeds 32799—STD 0532); and at Addenbrooke's Hospital, Cambridge (Cambridge 55671—STD 0223).

Haemophilia

(For suppliers of coagulation factors see p. 795.)

A HAEMOPHILIC should carry a green explanatory card issued under the authority of The Department of Health and Social Security, The Welsh Office and the Scottish Home and Health Department. The patient is specially tested and then registered at one of the Haemophilia Reference Centres. His card informs the doctor of the clotting defect and thus protects the patient against the risk of operation. It also names the hospital to which the patient should be referred in an emergency. The patient may also wish to wear a Medic-Alert necklet (p. 822). Help other than medical treatment may be obtained through The Haemophilia Society, PO Box 9, 16 Trinity Street, London SE1 1DE (01-407 1010).

The following is the current list of Haemophilia Reference Centres for patients suffering from haemophilia and closely related diseases (e.g. Christmas disease).

Aberdeen
Department of Medicine, Royal Infirmary, Foresterhill, Aberdeen AB9 2ZB. 0224 23423. Ext 2823.

Alton
Treloar Haemophilia Centre, Lord Mayor Treloar Hospital, Alton. 0420 82811.

Belfast
Department of Clinical Pathology. Royal Victoria Hospital, Belfast BT12 6BA. 0232 40503.

Birmingham
Haematology Department, Queen Elizabeth Hospital, Edgbaston, Birmingham B15 2TH. 021-472 1311.
Department of Haematology, The Children's Hospital, Ladywood Middleway, Ladywood, Birmingham B16 8ET. 021-454 4851.

Bournemouth
Royal Victoria Hospital, Shelley Road, Boscombe, Bournemouth BH1 4JG. 0202 35201 Ext 323. (At night and at weekends please ask for the number of the doctor on call for haemophiliac control.)

Bradford
Royal Infirmary, Bradford BD9 6RJ. 0274 42200 Ext 289.

Bristol
Department of Medicine, The Royal Infirmary, Bristol BS2 8HW. 0272 22041.

Cambridge
Haematology Clinic, Addenbrooke's Hospital, Hills Road, Cambridge CB2 1QT. 0223 45151 Ext 7125. (At night and at weekends please telephone Addenbrooke's Hospital—Cambridge 55671—and ask for the Duty Haematologist to the Haematology Department).

Cardiff
Department of Haematology, University Hospital of Wales, Cardiff C4F 1XW. 0222 755944. (After 5 p.m. and at weekends please ask for the house physician to the Haematology Department.)

Carlisle
Department of Pathology, Cumberland Infirmary, Carlisle CA2 7HY. 0228 23444.

Coventry
Department of Haematology, Coventry and Warwickshire Hospital, Stoney, Stanton Road, Coventry CU1 4FH. 0203 24055.

Darlington
Memorial Hospital, Darlington. 0325 60100.

Derby
Royal Infirmary, Derby DE1 2QY. 0332 47141.

Dublin
National Haemophilia Treatment Centre, Meath Hospital, Heytesbury Street, Dublin, 8. 01-752983.

Dundee
Wards 5/6, Ninewells Hospital, Dundee DD1 9SY. 0382 60011 Ext 2574.

Edinburgh
Royal Infirmary, Edinburgh EH3 9YW. 031-229 2477. There are two centres. 1. University Dept. of Therapeutics (Prof. R. H. Girdwood. Ext 2523). 2. Dept. of Haematology (Dr S. H. Davies. Ext 2099).

Exeter
Department of Pathology, Royal Devon and Exeter Hospital, Exeter EX1 1PQ. 0392 72261, 59261.

Glasgow
Department of Medicine, Royal Infirmary, Glasgow G4 0SF. 041-552 3535. (If not available ask for the receiving physician.)

Hull
Department of Pathology, Kingston General Hospital, Beverley Road, Hull HU3 1UR. 0482 28631.

Inverness
Regional Blood Transfusion Centre, Raigmore Hospital, Perth Road, Inverness IV2 3UJ. 0463 34151.

Leeds
St James' Hospital, Leeds L59 7TF. 0532 33144.

Liverpool
Liverpool Royal Infirmary, Pembroke Place, Liverpool L35 PU. 051-709 5511.

London
Haematology Department, **St George's** Hospital, Blackshaw Road, Tooting, London SW17 0QT. 01-672 1255.
Department of Haematology, **Guy's** Hospital, London SE1 9RT. 01-407 7600.
Haematology Department, Royal Postgraduate Medical School, **Hammersmith** Hospital, Ducane Road, London W12 6HS. 01-743 2030 Ext 510. (At night and at weekends please ask operator for the haematology registrar on duty.)
Haematology Department, **King's** College Hospital, Denmark Hill, London SE5 8 AF. 01-274 6222.
Haematology Department, **Lewisham** Hospital, High Street, Lewisham, London SE13 6LH. 01-690 4311.
Haematology Department, The **London** Hospital, Whitechapel Road, London E1 1BB. 01-247 5454.

Haematology Department, St **Mary's** Hospital, Praed Street, Paddington, W2 1PG. 01-262 1280 Ext 37.

Bland-Sutton Institute of Pathology, The **Middlesex** Hospital, Mortimer Street, London W1PDB. 01-636 8333. (At night and at weekends please ask hospital telephone operator for the duty pathologist.)

Haematology Department, The Hospital for Sick Children, Great **Ormond** Street, London WC1N 3HJ. 01-405 9200 Ext 331. (At night and at weekends please ask hospital telephone operator for the resident assistant physician.)

The Haemophilia Centre, The **Royal Free** Hospital, Pond Street, London NW3 2QG. 01-794 0500. (After 5.30 p.m. and at weekends please ask for the resident pathologist on call for the Haemophilia Centre.)

Department of Haematology, **St Thomas'** Hospital, London SE1 7EH. 01-928 9292. Ext 2268. (At night and at weekends please ask hospital telephone operator for the doctor on duty for haemophilia.)

Haematology Department, **University College** Hospital, Gower Street, London WC1E 6AU. 01-387 9300.

Haematology Department, **Westminster** Hospital, Dean Ryle Street, London SW1P 2AP. 01-828 9811.

Manchester
Department of Clinical Haematology, The Royal Infirmary, Manchester M13 9WL. 061-273 3300.
Department of Haematology, Royal Manchester Children's Hospital, Pendlebury, Manchester M27 1HA. 061-794 4696.

Margate
Isle of Thanet District Hospital (Margate Wing), St Peter's Road, Margate CT9 4AN. 0843 20222.

Middlesbrough
Middlesbrough General Hospital, Ayresome Green Lane, Middlesbrough, Teesside TS1 5JE. 0642 83133.

Newcastle
Royal Victoria Infirmary, Newcastle-upon-Tyne NE1 4LP. 0632 25131 Ext 773.

Nottingham
Haematology Department, General Hospital, Nottingham NG1 6HA. 0602 46161 Ext 603 or 385.

Oxford
Oxford Haemophilia Centre, Churchill Hospital, Oxford OX3 7LJ. 0865 64841 Ext 575. (After 5 p.m. and at weekends please ask the hospital telephone operator for the doctor on call for the Haemophilia Centre.)

Portsmouth
Central Laboratory, St Mary's General Hospital (East Wing), Milton Road, Portsmouth PO3 6AG. 0705 22331.

Sheffield
The United Sheffield Hospitals, Department of Haematology, The Royal Infirmary, Sheffield S10 2TH. 0742 20977. (At night and weekends ask for the doctor on call for the Haemophilia Centre.)

Southampton
Royal South Hants Hospital, Fanshawe Street, Southampton SO9 4PE. 0703 26211.

Sunderland
Royal Infirmary, Durham Road, Sunderland, Co. Durham SR2 7JE. 0632 56256.

Whitehaven
West Cumberland Hospital, Hensingham, Whitehaven, Cumbria CA28 8JG 0946 3181.

Supply of Immunoglobulins and Other Blood Products

NORMAL IMMUNOGLOBULIN

England and Wales

(a) For protection against rubella (p. 799), measles (p. 798) and infective hepatitis (p. 798). Available from Laboratories of Public Health Laboratory Service.

For laboratory workers accidentally inoculated with hepatitis B antigen contact the Virus Reference Laboratory, Colindale Avenue, London NW9 5HT 01-205 7041 for a supply of immunoglobulin containing a high titre of antibodies. In Scotland this serum can be obtained through the Regional Blood Transfusion Centres.

(b) For treatment of hypogammaglobulinaemia. Available from the following centres which also provide a diagnostic and assessment service (see HM(70)56).

Immune Deficiency Referral Laboratory Clinical Research Centre, Northwick Park Hospital, Watford Road, Harrow, Middlesex. HA1 3UJ. 01-864 5311.

Immunological Laboratory, East Birmingham Hospital, Bordesley Green East, Birmingham. 021-772 4311.

(c) Specially prepared for use with measles vaccine is available from Area Health Authorities.

SPECIFIC IMMUNOGLOBULINS

Anti-tetanus immunoglobulin is kept at certain hospitals (p. 767).

Anti-D immunoglobulin is distributed by Regional Transfusion Centres (p. 802).

Anti-vaccinia immunoglobulin (p. 801) is obtainable from laboratories of the Public Health Laboratory Service (p. 780).

Scotland

The Community Medical Specialist should be approached.

Northern Ireland

Immunoglobulin is available at The Laboratories, Belfast City Hospital, Belfast, BT9 7AB. Tel. Belfast 29241 (STD 0232).

Anti-D immunoglobulin is available from Northern Ireland Blood Transfusion Service, 89 Durham St., Belfast BT12 4GE. Tel. Belfast 46464 (STD 0232).

Republic of Ireland (Eire)

The following Normal and Specific Immunoglobulins are available at the Blood Transfusion Service Board, 52 Leeson Street, Dublin, 2. Tel. (01) 66981.

Human Normal Immunoglobulin for prophylaxis of measles and infective hepatitis. Also made available for prophylaxis of rubella.

Human Immunoglobulin Anti-D (Rh_o).

Human Immunoglobulin Anti-vaccinia.

Other specific immunoglobulins may be available. Inquire from Blood Transfusion Service (p. 802).

COAGULATION FACTORS

England and Wales, Scotland

FRESH FROZEN PLASMA (FFP) and *cryoprecipitate* (*Factor VIII*) are provided by Regional Transfusion Centres to Haemophilia Centres (p. 791) and hospitals.

FACTOR VIII CONCENTRATE (HUMAN). This freeze-dried product is prepared for the Department of Health and Social Security at the Blood Products Laboratory, Elstree, and at its satellite Plasma Fractionation Laboratory, Haemophilia Centre, Oxford. The Oxford Product is used at the Haemophilia Centre, Oxford; the Elstree product is issued to Haemophilia Centres for treating named patients.

It is also available commercially as *Hemofil* from Travenol Laboratories, Caxton Way, Thetford, Norfolk IP24 3SE. Tel. Thetford (0842) 4851.

Kryobulin from Serological Products Ltd., Arctic House, Rye Lane, Dunton Green, near Sevenoaks, Kent TN1H 5HB. Tel. Sevenoaks (0732) 73 50342.

Profilate from Abbott Laboratories Ltd., Queenborough, Kent ME11 5EL. Tel. Sheerness (07956) 3371.

(Commercial products cost from 10 to 14 p per unit. A 70 kg man would need about 900 i u to cause a 30 per cent rise in his Factor VIII.)

FACTOR IX (CHRISTMAS FACTOR) concentrate is available through Haemophilia Centres and also from The Plasma Fractionation Laboratory, Churchill Hospital, Oxford. Tel. Oxford (0092) 64841.

COAGULATION FACTORS II, IX, AND X are available as *Prothromplex* from Serological Products Ltd. (see above).

Northern Ireland

Fresh frozen plasma containing AHG and antihaemophilic factor (Factor VIII) cryoprecipitate are supplied by the Northern Ireland Blood Transfusion Service, 89 Durham Street, Belfast BT12 4GE. Tel. Belfast 46464 (STD 0232).

Republic of Ireland (Eire)

The following products are available from the Blood Transfusion Service Board, 52 Lower Leeson St., Dublin 2. Tel. (01) 66981.

Antihaemophilic factor (Factor VIII) cryoprecipitate prepared according to the method of J. Pool.

Antihaemophilic factor (Factor VIII) concentrate fraction 10 prepared according to the method of M. Blomback.

Concentrate of factors II, IX and X.

Patients should be referred to the National Haemophilia Treatment Centre, Meath Hospital, Heytesbury St., Dublin 8. Tel. (01) 752983.

DRIED SMALL POOL PLASMA, ALBUMIN AND PLASMA PROTEIN FRACTION

In England, Wales, Scotland and Northern Ireland the Regional Transfusion Centres should be approached.

Plasma Protein Fraction BP (4·3 per cent) is also available from Serological Products Ltd. as Haemoderivate, price £18 per 400 ml (see above).

FIBRINOGEN

England and Wales, Scotland

For the treatment of acquired and congenital fibrinogenopenic states fibrinogen is obtainable through Regional Transfusion Centres (p. 802).

Northern Ireland

A limited amount of fibrinogen is held at the Royal Maternity Hospital, Grosvenor Road, Belfast BT12 6BA. Tel. Belfast 40503 (STD 0232).

Republic of Ireland (Eire)

Dried Human Fibrinogen (units of 1 g) available from Blood Transfusion Board, 52 Lower Leeson St., Dublin 2. Tel. (01) 66981.

ALBUMIN

Republic of Ireland (Eire)

Human Albumin in 20 per cent and 5 per cent solution is also available from Blood Transfusion Service Board; (see above).

PLASMA CONCENTRATES

In all countries the supply of platelet rich plasma and platelet concentrates are subject to local arrangements between hospitals and the Director of the Regional Blood Transfusion Service.

Risks of hepatitis from blood products

The manufacturing process renders immunoglobulin, plasma protein fraction and albumin free from Australian antigen. (For other risks see p. 71.)

Although the blood from which other blood products (plasma, fibrinogen and the various coagulation factors) are prepared is tested for Australia antigen they are not necessarily free from the risk of transmitting hepatitis. 'Hepatitis-free fibrinogen' for diagnostic use in deep venous thrombosis is made from 'accredited donors', i.e. those of long-standing who appear to be safe.

USE OF HUMAN IMMUNOGLOBULIN

Immunoglobulin should be injected i m. It is not suitable for i v use. Two or more sites (p. 54) should be used if the volume of the dose is large.

Immunoglobulin should be stored at between 2°C and 10°C and should not be frozen. Ampoules should not be kept in a warm atmosphere but it is unlikely that there would be an appreciable deterioration during a week at room temperature, or, for example, in the post over a weekend.

Normal Human Immunoglobulin

At present dispensed usually in ampoules containing 250 mg in 1·6 ml or 750 mg in 5·1 ml

INDICATION	EFFECTIVENESS	DOSAGE	COMMENT
Measles: prevention in contacts with no previous history of measles and who are at special risk, e.g. children with active tuberculosis, or malignant disease; immuno-suppressive therapy.	Effective. Given within five days of exposure.	Under 1 yr. 250 mg 1-2 yr. 500 mg 3 yr. and over 750 mg	Active immunisation should if possible be carried out three months later. To prevent side effects it may be necessary to inject a small dose of immunoglobulin with the vaccine but at a separate site—dose 0·6 mg per lb body weight. Low dose preparations are held for this purpose by Medical Officers of Health.
Measles: attenuation in those at special risk, e.g. children with chronic chest disease.	Effective. Given within five days exposure. A mild clinical infection should result with the development of active immunity.	All ages over 1 yr. 250 mg	Measles vaccines should reduce much of this requirement for immunoglobulin.
Infectious hepatitis: prophylaxis, e.g. travellers to countries where the disease is endemic; institutional outbreaks.	If given before exposure, or up to two weeks afterwards, should prevent clinical disease in about 85% of contacts. The prophylactic effect lasts about three to six months. Effect declines up to six weeks after exposure, after which time it is no longer believed to be of prophylactic value.	Children under 10 yr. 250 mg Adults and children of 10 yr. and over 500 mg	May allow the development of active immunity as a consequence of subclinical infection. No therapeutic activity has been found. Probably no activity against serum hepatitis.

Rubella: prevention in exposed pregnant women.	Probably does not prevent infection when given *after* exposure to a florid case of german measles, but may prevent clinical manifestations.	750 mg as early as possible after exposure.	Only recommended when the patient will not consider a therapeutic abortion. Serological tests for immunity should be done—over 80% of women possess antibodies and would not be at risk, and not all 'exposed' patients become infected.
Varicella: attenuation in persons at special risk, e.g. ill or eczematous children. (a) newborn; pregnant women; patients on low steroid doses. (b) blood dyscrasia; high steroid dosage: cytotoxic drug therapy. (c)	Attenuation of the disease should result when given within three days exposure.	Newborn 250 mg Under 1 yr. 500-750 mg 1-6 yr. 1 000-1 500 mg 7 yr. and over: 1 500 mg group (a) 2 250-4 000 mg group (b) 4 500-8 000 mg group (c) patients	Specific anti-varicella immunoglobulin is sometimes available for patients at special risk (see below).
Other conditions where immunity and resistance may be impaired—in order to prevent bacterial and/or virus infections generally, e.g. burns, immuno-suppression, prematurity.	Doubtful.	Speculative; possibly 1500 mg for adults, repeated if necessary.	The present evidence is not sufficient to recommend use of human IgG in these conditions. Further controlled experimental work is needed.

Specific Human Immunoglobulin

PREPARATION	INDICATION	EFFECTIVENESS	DOSAGE	COMMENT
Anti-Australian antigen (from plasma naturally containing antibody to the antigen).	Prophylaxis of hepatitis, e.g. medical staff accidentally injured by a needle contaminated with blood containing Au antigen.	Early studies suggest may be of some value.	Not certain	The material is under study and is not yet generally available.
Anti-mumps (at present from convalescent patients).	Prophylaxis in exposed high-risk patients, e.g. those with leukaemia.	Large doses may have some effect in preventing mumps, or in preventing orchitis in patients with parotitis, but evidence at present is conflicting.	Under 1 yr. 500 mg 1-6 yr. 1 000 mg 7 yr. and over 1 500 mg	More studies are needed. The material is in very short supply. Normal immunoglobulin is not believed to have any effect.
Anti-tetanus (from donors recently boosted with tetanus toxoid).	(1) Prophylaxis in wounded patients who have not been actively immunised.	Probably very effective.	250 units.	Not supplied by P.H.L.S. Obtained from special centres listed in the D.H.S.S. Memorandum HM(70)37. Certain of these centres are Public Health Laboratories. At present in short supply and therefore used mainly in patients hypersensitive to horse antitoxin.
	(2) Treatment of tetanus.	Possibly of value.	10 000 units.	Use restricted to patients susceptible to heterologous antiserum.

Product	Indication	Efficacy	Dosage	Notes
Anti-vaccinia (from recently re-vaccinated donors).	For prophylaxis: (1) To prevent complications when vaccination is necessary in the presence of contra-indications, e.g. eczema; steroid therapy; patients with marked allergic tendencies; elderly persons.	Probably effective.	Under 1 yr. 500 mg 1-6 yr. 1 000 mg 7-14 yr. 1 500 mg 15 yr. and over 2 000 mg	Given at the same time as vaccination, but in a different limb.
	(2) In unvaccinated persons exposed to smallpox.		As above.	Of most value in unvaccinated exposed persons who are first seen late in the incubation period, when vaccination alone would be insufficiently protective. Should be accompanied by vaccination.
	Treatment of: (3) Generalised vaccinia; progressive vaccinia; eczema vaccinatum.	Probably of value.	As above; repeat in two days if necessary.	No evidence of value in treatment of post-vaccinial encephalitis.
	(4) Vaccinial lesion of eye.	Probably effective.	As above, plus local installation of 1% solution in sterile saline half-hourly. (Dilute with 14 volumes of sterile saline.)	Note: Herpes simplex infection may cause similar manifestations.
Anti-varicella-zoster (from patients convalescent from either condition).	Prophylaxis in exposed high-risk persons, e.g. children on large doses of steroids.	Probably of value when given within 72 hours of exposure, but the information so far available is limited.	Under 1 yr. 500 mg 1-6 yr. 1 000 mg 7 yr. and over 1 500 mg	Rarely available at present. Normal immunoglobulin may be used (see above). Role in treatment of varicella-zoster (as in patients with Hodgkin's disease) requires study.

National Blood Transfusion Service

REGIONAL TRANSFUSION CENTRES

MANY hospitals in each region, too numerous to list, have 'night blood banks' and provide a 24 hour service for crossmatching and the provision of blood.

ENGLAND AND WALES

Northern Region

Regional Transfusion Centre, Westgate Road, Newcastle on Tyne, NE4 6QB. Newcastle 3-7804/5/6 (STD 0632).

Yorkshire region

Regional Transfusion Laboratory, Bridle Path, York Road, Seacroft, Leeds LS15 7TW. Leeds 64-5091 (STD 0532).

Trent region

Regional Transfusion Centre, Longley Lane, Sheffield, S5 7JN. Sheffield 6327-1-2-3-4 (STD 0742).

East Anglian region

Regional Transfusion and Immuno-haematology Centre, Long Road, Cambridge CB2 2PT. Mon. to Fri. 0830 to 1730 hours, Sat. 0830 to 1230 hours. Cambridge 45921 (STD 0223).

N.W. Thames region

North London Blood Transfusion Centre, Deansbrook Road, Edgware, Middlesex HA8 7BD. 01-952 5511.

N.E. Thames region

N.E. Met. Regional Blood Transfusion Centre, Crescent Drive, Brentwood, Essex. Brentwood 223545 (STD 0277).

S.E. and S.W. Thames region

South London Transfusion Centre, 75 Cranmer Terrace, London, SW17 0RB. 01-672 8501/7.
Sub-depot at No. 2 The Stables, David Salaman's House, Southborough. Tunbridge Wells 28172 (STD 0892).

Oxford region

Regional Transfusion Centre, Churchill Hospital, Headington, Oxford OX3 7LJ. Oxford 64841 (STD 0092).

South-western region

S.W. Regional Transfusion Centre, Southmead, Bristol BS10 5ND. Bristol 62-8021 (STD 0272).

Wessex region
Regional Transfusion Centre, Coxford Road, Southampton SO9 5UP. Southampton 776441 (STD 0703).

Welsh region
Regional Transfusion Centre, Rhud-Lafar, St Fagans, near Cardiff CF5 6XF. Pentyrch 302 (STD 044-725). (For south and mid Wales. North Wales service is supplied from Liverpool.)

W. Midlands region
Regional Transfusion Centre, Vincent Drive, Edgbaston, Birmingham B15 2SG. 021-472 3111.

N. Western region
Regional Transfusion Centre, Roby Street, Manchester M1 3BP. 061-236 8181.
Sub-regional centre, Queensmore Road. Lancaster 3456 (STD 0524).

Mersey region
Regional Transfusion Centre, West Derby Street, Mount Vernon, Liverpool L7 8TW. 051-709 7272. (Also serves North Wales.)

SCOTLAND

In Scotland the responsible body is a voluntary one, The Scottish National Blood Transfusion Association, which is in contract with the Secretary of State.

Northern region
Blood Transfusion Centre, Raigmore Hospital, Inverness. Inverness 34151 (STD 0463).

North-eastern region
Blood Transfusion Centre, Royal Infirmary, Foresterhill, Aberdeen. AB2 2ZB. Aberdeen 23423 (STD 0224) Ext. 2086.

Eastern region
Blood Transfusion Centre, Royal Infirmary, Dundee DD1 9ND. Dundee 26785 (STD 0382).

South-eastern region
Blood Transfusion Centre, Royal Infirmary, Edinburgh EH3 9YW. 031-229 2477.

Western region
Blood Transfusion Centre, Law Hospital, Carluke, Lanarkshire. Wishaw 73315 (STD 0552-3).
Blood Transfusion Centre, 82 West Regent Street, Glasgow, C.2. 041-332 8425.

ISLE OF MAN

Clegg Pathological Institute, Noble's Hospital, Douglas, I.O.M. Douglas 987 (STD 0624).

REPUBLIC OF IRELAND

The Blood Transfusion Service Board, Pelican House, P.O. Box 97, 52 Lower Leeson Street, Dublin, 2. Tel. 66981.
St John's Hospital, Limerick. Tel. 45913.
Blood Transfusion Service, 21 Leitrim Street, Cork. Tel. 51228.

NORTHERN IRELAND

Northern Ireland Blood Transfusion Service, 89 Durham Street, Belfast BT12 4GE. Belfast 46464 (STD 02232).
Donor Registration Bureau, 6-10 Howard Street, Belfast, 1. Belfast 40305 (STD 0232).

Haemo-Dialysis Units

Aberdeen
Royal Infirmary. Aberdeen 23423 (STD 0224).

Aylesbury
Princess Mary's R.A.F. Hospital, Halton, near Aylesbury, Bucks. Wendover 2241 (STD 0296-62).

Belfast
Belfast City Hospital, Lisburn Road, Belfast. Belfast 29241 (STD 0232) Ext. 226 (day), 669918 (night).

Birmingham
East Birmingham Hospital (general branch), Birmingham 9. 021-772 4311. Queen Elizabeth Hospital, Birmingham 16. 021-472 1311.

Brighton
Royal Sussex County Hospital. Brighton 66611 (STD 0273).

Bristol
Ham Green Hospital. Bristol 2661 (STD 0275 81).

Cambridge
Addenbrooke's Hospital Annexe, Douglas House, Trumpington Road. Cambridge 55671 (STD 0223).

Canterbury
Kent and Canterbury Hospital. Canterbury 66877 (STD 0227).

Cardiff
Royal Infirmary. Cardiff 33101 (STD 0222).

Carshalton, Surrey
St Helier Hospital. 01-644 4343.

Cork
Republic of Ireland. St Finbarr's Hospital. Cork 26721.

Coventry
Walsgrave Hospital. Coventry 323232 (STD 0203).

Derby
City Hospital. Derby 40131 (STD 0332).

Dundee
Maryfield Hospital, Dundee. Dundee 40011 (STD 0382).

Dublin
Jervis Street Hospital. Dublin 45812.

Edinburgh
The Royal Infirmary, Edinburgh. 031-229 2497.

Exeter
Royal Devon and Exeter Hospital. Exeter 59261 (STD 0392).

Galway
Republic of Ireland. Merlin Park Hospital. Galway 4021.

Glasgow
Department of Medicine, Royal Infirmary, Castle Street, Glasgow. 041-552 3535.
Western Infirmary, Dumbarton Road, Glasgow. 041-339 8822.
Stobhill General Hospital, Glasgow. 041-558 5042.

Hull
Royal Infirmary (Sutton), Hull. Hull 71711 (STD 0482).

Leeds
The General Infirmary, Leeds. Leeds 32799 (STD 0532).
St James' Hospital, Leeds. Leeds 33144 (STD 0532).

Liverpool
Sefton General Hospital, Smithdown Road, Liverpool L15 2HE. 051-733 4020.
Mossley Hill Hospital, Liverpool L18 8BU. 051-724 2335.

London
St Bartholomew's Hospital. 01-606-777.
Charing Cross Hospital. 01-836 7788.
Dulwich Hospital. 01-693 3377.
Fulham Hospital, Hammersmith. 01-748 2050.
Guy's Hospital. 01-407 7600.
Hammersmith Hospital. 01-743 2030.
King's College Hospital. 01-274 6222.
Lambeth Hospital. 01-735 8141.
London Hospital. 01-247 5454.
Middlesex Hospital. 01-636 8333.
St Leonard's Hospital. 01-739 3311.
St Mary's Hospital. 01-262 1280.
St Paul's Hospital. 01-836 9347.
Royal Free Hospital, Lawn Road Branch, Hampstead. 01-794 4561.
Westminster Hospital. 01-828 9811.

Manchester
Withington Hospital, Nell Lane, West Didsbury, Manchester. 061-445 8111.

Middlesbrough
North Ormesby Hospital. Middlesbrough 44641 (STD 0642).

Newcastle upon Tyne
Royal Victoria Infirmary. Newcastle 25131 (STD 0632).
Rye Hill Hospital. Newcastle 33131 (STD 0632).

Nottingham
City Hospital. Nottingham 63361 (STD 0602).

Oxford
   Churchill Hospital. Oxford 64841 (STD 0092).

Plymouth
   Plymouth General Hospital. Plymouth 68080 (STD 0752) Ext. 29.

Portsmouth
   St Mary's Hospital. Portsmouth 22331 (STD 0705).

Rhyl
   Royal Alexandra Hospital. Rhyl 4631 (STD 0745).

Romford, Essex
   Oldchurch Hospital. Romford 46090 (STD 70).

Sheffield
   Lodge Moor Hospital. Sheffield 306555 (STD 0742).

Stoke on Trent
   N. Staffordshire Royal Infirmary. Stoke on Trent 44161 (STD 0782).

Stourbridge
   Wordsley Hospital. Kingswinford 3341 (STD 038-44).

Sunderland
   Royal Infirmary. Sunderland 56256 (STD 0783).

Renal Transplant Teams

Place	Hospital	Telephone	STD
Brighton	Royal Sussex County	Brighton 66611	0273
Bristol	Southmead	Bristol 622821	0272
Cambridge	Addenbrooke's. New site	Cambridge 45151	0223
Canterbury	E. Kent & Canterbury	Canterbury 66877	0227
Cardiff	Royal Infirmary	Cardiff 33101	0222
Edinburgh	Western General	031-332 1311	
Exeter	Royal Devon & Exeter	Exeter 72261	0392
Glasgow	Western Infirmary	041-399 8822	
Leeds	St James	Leeds 33144	0532
Leicester	Royal Infirmary	Leicester 23281	0533
Liverpool	Royal Infirmary	051-5511 -709	
London	St Bartholomew's	01-606 7777	
	new Charing Cross	01-748 2050	
	Guy's	01-407 7600	
	Hammersmith. Royal Postgraduate	01-743 2030	
	King's College	01-274 6262	
	The London	01-247 5454	
	St Mary's	01-262 1280	
	Royal Free	01-837 6411	
	St Thomas's	01-928 9292	
Manchester	Royal Infirmary	061-273 3300	
Newcastle	Royal Victoria Infirmary	Newcastle 25131	0632
Oxford	Churchill	Oxford 64841	0865
Portsmouth	St Mary's	Portsmouth 22331	0705
Sheffield	Royal Hospital	Sheffield 20063	0742

The Emergency Bed Service (E. B. S.)

IF A doctor cannot secure a bed for an urgent case he may ask the E.B.S. to find one. Although it was originally intended that the E.B.S. should have no boundaries it now mainly confines its activities to the area of the Greater London Council. Its headquarters at Fielden House, 28 London Bridge Street, London, S.E.1., may be contacted at any hour by telephoning 01 - 407 7181. All acute cases except those of mental disease and tuberculosis (i.e., all cases suitable for general hospitals) will be dealt with. After office hours requests concerning emergencies in tuberculous patients will be accepted. Beds are not found for epileptics except those in status epilepticus. Admission of cases of urgent mental illness should be arranged through the Local Authority Social Worker (p. 672). Cases of sudden illness or accident occurring in a ' public place ', in the street, at work or in a doctor's surgery, but not in the home, will be taken to the nearest hospital if an ambulance is requested by dialling 999 in London (or 0 or 01 in other districts). Patients already under treatment should not be sent to hospital in this way. The E.B.S. can often provide useful information on various services needed in emergency situations.

Emergency Bed Bureaux exist in many other centres, some of which are:

Bath
The Royal Bath United Hospital, Bath. Bath 28331 (STD 0225).

Chelmsford
Essex Hospital Bed Service, St John's Hospital, Wood Street, Chelmsford, Essex. Chelmsford 54851 (STD 0245). 0800 to 1800 hours seven days a week, including bank holidays and Christmas Day.

Liverpool
The Liverpool Emergency Bed Bureau, Pearl Assurance House, 55 Castle Street, Liverpool, L2 9TU. 051-236 9431.

Luton
Luton and Dunstable Hospital, Dunstable Road, Luton, Bedfordshire. Luton 51810 (STD 0582). 0830 to 1700 hours Monday to Friday. 0800 to 1200 hours Saturday. Closed on Sundays, bank holidays and Christmas Day.

Redhill
Redhill County Hospital, Earlswood Common, Redhill, Surrey. Redhill 63883 (STD 0737). 0900 to 2130 hours Monday to Saturday inclusive. 0900 to 1700 hours Sundays and bank holidays. Closed on Christmas Day and Good Friday.

Shrewsbury

Shrewsbury Emergency Bed Bureau, Royal Salop Infirmary, Shrewsbury. Shrewsbury 2856 (STD 0743), 0900 to 2130 hours. From 2000 to 0830 hours Shrewsbury 53931 (STD 0743).

Watford

Watford General Hospital, Vicarage Road, Watford, Hertfordshire. Watford 22664 (STD 923), 0900 to 1700 hours Monday to Friday. Closed on bank holidays, Saturdays and Sundays.

Windsor

King Edward VII Hospital, Windsor, Berkshire. Windsor 60441 (STD 0753-5).

Edinburgh

The Emergency Bed Bureau, 11 Drumsheugh Gardens, Edinburgh. 031-225 2244.

Glasgow

Hospital Admissions Department, 23 Montrose Street, Glasgow, C.1. 041-221 9600.

Belfast

Emergency Bed Service, Central Ambulance Depot, Broadway, Belfast. Belfast 28555 (STD 0232).

Dublin

Dublin Hospitals Bureau. 52 Upper Mount Street, Dublin, 2. Tel. Dublin 65591.

APPENDIX 10

Corneal Grafting

(For technique of collecting eyes see p. 665.)

SINCE about half of all deaths occur in hospital, most enucleations for grafting and research are performed there. A hospital doctor, wishing to know where the nearest eye bank is, should ask his Regional Health Authority.

Domiciliary enucleations are carried out at present within a radius of about 30 miles of the following hospitals.

Queen Victoria Hospital, East Grinstead. East Grinstead 24111 (STD 0342).
Moorfields, Westminster and Central Eye Hospital, London. 01-253 3411.
Birmingham and Midland Eye Hospital. 021-236 4911.
Bristol Eye Hospital. Bristol 25535 (STD 0272).

A general practitioner wishing to know which hospital will send someone to enucleate eyes, should enquire from his General Practice Committee.

There are facilities for corneal grafting at The Royal Victoria Hospital, Belfast, 40503 (STD 0232).

There are no special centres in the Republic of Ireland but keratoplasty is undertaken at the Royal Victoria Eye and Ear Hospital, Adelaide Road, Dublin 2. Tel. 785500.

Anthrax

For clinical aspects see p. 549.
For hospitals holding anthrax anti-serum see p. 767.
For reference experts see *Year Book of the Public Health Laboratory Service* (p. 780).

ALL suspected cases of anthrax should be referred to one of the designated hospitals (names obtainable from the Regional Health Authority). These hospitals can give the names of factories and warehouses where there is a risk of anthrax. There are no specially designated centres in Northern Ireland or the Isle of Man.

APPENDIX 12

Poisons Information Service

THIS service consists of the following four official centres in the U.K. and a co-opted centre in Dublin.

London
> Poisons Reference Service, New Cross Hospital, Avonley Road, London, SE14 5ER. 01-407 7600.

Edinburgh
> Scottish Poisons Information Bureau, Royal Infirmary, Edinburgh EH3 9YW. 031-229 2477.

Cardiff
> Poisons Information Centre, Cardiff Royal Infirmary, Cardiff CF2 IS2. 33101 (STD 0222).

Belfast
> Poisons Information Centre, Royal Victoria Hospital, Belfast, 12. Belfast 40503 (STD 0232) Ext. 704.

Dublin
> The Poisons Information Centre, Jervis Street Hospital, Dublin. Dublin 0001 45588.

There are other (unofficial) centres:

Bristol
> Poisons Information Centre, Royal Infirmary, Bristol. Tel. Bristol (STD 0272) 22041.

Consett, Co. Durham
> There is an Adverse Drug Reaction Information Service at Shotley Bridge, Consett, Co. Durham DH8 0NB. Consett 3456 (STD 020 72) Ext. 57). Inquiries can be made throughout the 24 hours.

Leeds
> Poisons Information Centre, Casualty Department, General Infirmary, Leeds. Leeds 32799 (STD 0532). (Lay inquiries answered.)

Birmingham
> Only a capsule and tablet identification service is available at present between 0900 and 1730 hours (0900 to 1300 hours on Saturday) at the General Hospital, Birmingham. 021-368 8611, Ext 368.

Brandon, Suffolk
> U.K. Poisons Control Centre, 48th Tactical Hospital U.S.A.F., R.A.F. Lakenheath, Brandon, Suffolk. Eriswell 2666 (STD 0638 81).

Romford
> The Regional Barbiturate Unit, Oldchurch Hospital, Romford, Essex. Romford 46099 (STD 70). This unit has special facilities for treatment, including haemodialysis.

Manchester
> Booth Hall Children's Hospital, Charlestown Road, Blackley, Manchester M9 2AA. 061-740 2254.

Newcastle
> Regional Poisons Information Centre, Royal Victoria Infirmary, Newcastle upon Tyne 1. Newcastle 25131 (STD 06321).

Hyperbaric Oxygen

(For risks see p. 70.)

THE main present indications for hyperbaric oxygen therapy are severe carbon monoxide poisoning, gas gangrene, acute vascular injury, frostbite and burns. The following hospitals can provide it but those where it is used in radiotherapy and for neonates only are not included.

Aberdeen
The Royal Infirmary. Aberdeen 23423 (STD 0224). (Patients should be sent to the helicopter landing field.)

Ascot, Berks.
Heatherwood Hospital. Ascot 21515 (STD 0990).

Aylesford, Nr Maidstone, Kent
Preston Hall Hospital.
British Legion Village. Maidstone 77262 (STD 0622).

Belfast
Royal Victoria Hospital. Belfast 40503 (STD 0232).

Bristol
Frenchay Hospital. Bristol 656291 (STD 0272).

Bury, Lancs.
Fairfield General Hospital. 061-764 6081.

Cheltenham
General Hospital. Cheltenham 21344 (STD 0242).

Cottingham, North Humberside
Castle Hill Hospital. Hull 847371 (STD 0482).

Derby
Royal Derbyshire Infirmary. Derby 47141 (STD 0332).

East Grinstead
Queen Victoria Hospital. East Grinstead 24111.

Glasgow
The Western Infirmary. 041-339 8822.

Gosport, Hants.
Royal Naval Hospital, Haslar. Portsmouth 22351 (STD 0705).
Ext. 41370/41391.

London
The London Hospital, Whitechapel, E.1. 01-247 5454.
University College Hospital, Gower Street, London WC1E 6AU. 01-387 5050.
Westminster Hospital, S.W.1. 01-828 9811.
Whipps Cross Hospital, Leytonstone, E.11. 01-539 5522.

Maidstone
Preston Hall Hospital. Maidstone 77262 (STD 0622).

Manchester
Monsall Hospital. 061-205 2254.

Newport, Mon.
Royal Gwent Hospital. Newport, Gwent 52244 (STD 0633).

Northwood, Middx.
Mount Vernon Hospital. Northwood 26111 (STD 09274).

Peterborough
Peterborough and District Hospital. Peterborough 67451 (STD 0733).

Sutton Coldfield
Good Hope General Hospital. 021-354 7881.

Winchester
Royal Hampshire County Hospital. Winchester 5151 (STD 0962).

Wroughton, Swindon, Wilts.
R.A.F. Hospital. Wroughton 291 (STD 079 381).

There are no facilities for treatment by hyperbaric oxygen in the Republic of Ireland.

28*

Befrienders International (Samaritans Worldwide) and Similar Organisations

SAMARITANS now exist in many towns in the United Kingdom and as their addresses are given in telephone directories they are not listed here. The General Secretary, Rev. Basil Higginson, 17 Uxbridge Road, Slough, Bucks., Slough 32713 (STD 0753) will give addresses of Samaritans overseas in some ten countries. Samaritans do not give information about clients to any person or agency whatever without the client's express permission. They do not act as police spies.

The doctor may like to be able to provide a patient who is travelling abroad with addresses of services providing emergency telephonic help. Details may be obtained from the following affiliated organisations.

Life Line International
 Harold Henderson, General Secretary, Life Line International, Wesley Centre, 210 Pitt St., Sydney 2000, Australia.
Contact
 Robert Larson, Contact Teleministry Inc., Room 125, 900 S. Arlington Ave., Harrisburg, Pa. 17 109, USA.
Telecare Canada
 Rev. William Lamb, Box No. 1, Weston, Ontario, Canada.
 A directory of all Canadian crisis intervention centres is available from The Distress Centre, Ottawa, Ontario.
International Federation for Services of Emergency Telephonic Help
 20 rue du Marche, CH 1204, Geneva, Switzerland.

Details of other helpful organisations such as Cruse Clubs for widows can be obtained from the Social Worker.

The Friends Anonymous Service, Friendship House, 27 Hackney Grove, London E8 (O1-986 2233) provides a local 24-hour befriending service.

SAMARITANS OVERSEAS
Bombay
Bulawayo
 P.O. Box 806. Tel. Bulawayo 5000.

Open Line offers help to lonely people in time of crisis, depression or anxiety. It is run from St Martin in the Fields church in London. A phone call to 01-930 1732 (which can be anonymous) will bring expert advice. The service is an emergency one and acts as a referral rather than a therapeutic centre. It does not seek to convert people to any particular way of life.

Foreign Nationals

A MEDICAL emergency in a patient from a foreign country who speaks no English can present great difficulties.

INTERPRETERS

The London Hospital (01-247 5454) can readily provide interpreters in the following languages for hospitals in its own group.

Afgan	Hindi	Portuguese
Arabic	Hindustani	Singhalese
Benghali	Hungarian	Spanish
Dutch	Italian	Swahili
French	Kannada	Swedish
German	Kashmiri	Tamil
Ghanaian	Kiswhili	Telgu
Greek	Maltese	Urdu
Guiarati	Persian	Welsh
Hebrew	Polish	

For patients whose language is not listed it is usually possible to find an interpreter if sufficient notice is given.

Help may be sought through the appropriate Embassy or Legation or the Institute of Linguists, 91 Newington Causeway, London, S.E.1 (01-407 4755). If these fail, the Overseas Department of the B.B.C. could be tried (01-580 4468). The British Red Cross Society, 6 Grosvenor Crescent, London, S.W. 1 (01-235 7131) can often enlist the help of an interpreter through a local branch.

In Liverpool a language bank is related to the University Library for the translation of documents. In an emergency the library could be asked to provide an interpreter.

Language cards are provided free of charge by the British Red Cross Society. Standard cards are in 34 languages and maternity cards in 9 languages.

Standard

Arabic	Ethiopian	Hungarian	Maltese	Spanish
Bengali*	Finnish	Italian	Norwegian	Swedish
Chinese	French	Japanese	Persian	Turkish
Czech	German	Jugoslav	Polish	Ukrainian
Danish	Greek	Korean	Portuguese	Urdu*
Dutch	Gurkhali	Latvian	Roumanian	Swahili
Estonian	Hindi	Lithuanian	Russian	

Maternity

French	Greek	Hungarian	Polish	Urdu
German	Hindi	Italian	Spanish	

The University of Manchester International Society, 84 Plymouth Grove, Manchester M13 9LW (061-273 1372) keeps a record of people in its area who can act as interpreters.

University College Hospital, Gower St., London, WC1E 6AO (01-387 5050) has a list of over 60 languages for which an interpreter can be found on its staff.

There is a 'language bank' in Manchester. Details can be obtained from Mr P. J. Middlemiss, c/o The International Society, 84 Plymouth Grove, Manchester M13 9LW (061-273 1327).

Persons who have expressed willingness to act as interpreters in London are:

Jugoslav patients (Serbian language)

> Mr Djordje Pantelic,
> 1A Gertrude St.,
> London S.W.10 (01-352 2685).

Ukrainian patients

> Miss M. Wolosczanska or
> Mr Alex Marunchak,
> c/o Mychajlo Zacharczuk,
> Welfare Officer,
> Association of Ukranians in Great Britain Ltd,
> 49 Linden Gardens, Notting Hill Gate, W2 4HG
> (01-229 8392 and 01-229 0140).

* Pakistani patients speak Bengali or Urdu.

Roumanian patients

> Mrs Page,
> Flat 21, 1 Hyde Park Square,
> London, W.2. (01-262 1541).
> Rev. Lucian Gafton,
> 54 Tredegar Square,
> London, E.1. (01-980 7404).

Polish patients

More medical facilities exist for Polish patients than for any other national group. The Department of Health and Social Security administers directly the medical unit of 56 beds in the National Assistance Board's Polish Hostel at Ilford Park, Devon.

Other organisations which can help with Polish patients are:

Association of Friends of Polish Patients, Kolbe House, 18 Hanger Lane, Ealing, London, W.5. (No telephone.)

Marbledon Hospital, Dartford, Kent. (Contact through Department of Health, Room 223, 194 Euston Road, London, N.W.1. 01-387 4366. Ext. 287.)

Penley Hospital for Chronic Sick, Wrexham, Denbighshire. Hanmer 341.

The Polish Dispensary, 33 Weymouth Street, London W.1. 01-580 4693. (The physician superintendent of Marbledon Hospital holds a clinic here.)

Czech and Slovak patients

> Fr. Lang S. J. Velehrád,
> 22 Ladbroke Square,
> London, W.11.
> (01-727 7489).

Lithuanian patients

> Lithuanian House, 3 Ladbroke Gardens,
> London, W.11.
> (01-727 2470).

Slovene patients

> 62 Offley Road,
> London, S.W.9.
> (01-735 6655).

Serbo-Croat patients

    Fr I. Kunštelj,
    Serbian Community Centre,
    89 Lancaster Road, London, W.1.
    (01-727 9718).

White Russian and Byelo-Russian patients

    Fr A. Radson,
    Marian House, Holden Avenue,
    London, N.12.

Estonian patients

    Estonian House Ltd.,
    18 Chepstow Villas,
    London, W.11.
    (01-229 7196 and 6700).

Miss Laura Gurdikian of The School of Slavonic Studies, University of London, W.C.1 (01-636 9782) can act as an interpreter for patients who speak Armenian, Roumanian, Turkish and French.

Unofficial Emergency Services

1. The St John Ambulance Air Wing

This service will transport drugs and equipment as well as patients—see p. 826.

2. Radio Amateurs' Emergency Network (Raynet)

The rule that an amateur radio licence prohibits 'third party traffic', i.e. messages not intended for one of the two operators taking part in a conversation, can be expressly varied in times of disaster. In the unlikely event of failure of other communications, a 'ham' radio operator could be asked to send a message on behalf of the police, the British Red Cross Society and the St John Ambulance Brigade. Contact should be made with the Radio Society of Great Britain, 35 Doughty St., London WC1N 2AE (01-837 8688).

3. Medic-alert

This potentially world-wide service to protect patients against emergencies was started in 1956 by Dr Marion Collins of California after his daughter had nearly died following an injection of tetanus antitoxin given routinely after a minor accident. It is a non-profit-making organisation registered as a charity and it has the approval of the British Medical Association. Life membership to include the bracelet costs £3.50 plus 8 per cent VAT. Apply to Mrs J. M. Smith, Secretary General, 9 Hanover St., London W1R 9HF (01-499 2261). On joining a patient gives full details of his particular condition. Records are filed at the headquarters in Britain. Countries participating at present are: Australia and Fiji, Canada, Holland, New Zealand, Philippine Islands, South Africa, U.S.A., West Malaysia, Rhodesia, Mozambique and the United Kingdom.

The patient wears a bracelet or necklet with the serpent sign of Aesculapius engraved on it in red and the name of his allergy or condition and his number on the reverse. Details of blood groups should not be given. In an emergency when a patient cannot give information about himself the name of his condition on the bracelet is a 'flash warning' for the doctor. Further details may be obtained by telephoning Medic-alert (reversed charge) from anywhere in the world at any time.

The emergency telephone numbers in some other countries are: U.S.A. 209-634-4917; Canada 209-634-4917 (the same as U.S.A.); S. Africa 43-7003. Failing Medic-alert the word ' Allergy ' etc. could be written prominently on the passport.

SERVES
(South East Region Volunteer Emergency Service)

The owners of all kinds of transport constitute this service which carries drugs, blood, specimens and equipment as well as the handicapped, aged and infirm between 1800 and 0700 hours Monday to Friday and for 24 hours on Saturday and Sunday. Requests are only accepted from doctors and hospitals, and not from the public. It is not a free taxi service. It operates over the counties of Beds, Berks, Bucks, Essex, Herts, Kent, London, Middlesex, Surrey and Sussex. Emergency calls should be made to Erith (032 24) 49952. No charge is made for missions. Most volunteers live in and around Greater London but are willing to go outside London to start their missions.

Mobile emergency aid teams are provided by the South London Scout Centre, Grange Lane, London SE21.

Various other volunteer emergency services exist in many districts though not all have full facilities. Details should be sought from the Social Worker and the Area Health Authority concerned.

5 CHAR
The Campaign for the Homeless and Rootless, 27 Endell Street, London WC2 (01.240 2691) hopes to establish walk-in health centres for sick homeless people in many cities staffed by a rota of doctors admitted to medical lists for this limited purpose.

APPENDIX 17

International Medical Aid

Two bodies in the U.S.A. exist which can provide urgently required medical aid for groups rather than individuals in any part of the world.

Direct Relief Foundation

This is a non-governmental, non-profit, non-denominational organisation which donates pharmaceuticals, medical supplies and hospital equipment to needy hospitals and clinics in medically deprived areas. A doctor in need can apply to DRF, PO Box 1319, Santa Barbara, CA 93102. Tel Area Code (805) 966-9149.

Aesculapian International

This is a division of Direct Relief Foundation and operates from the same address. It arranges assignments for physicians, dentists and paramedical personnel to developing areas where their skills are acutely needed.

Removal of Patients by Air

HELICOPTER

Very occasionally in circumstances of special medical emergency it is necessary to move a patient by helicopter to another hospital. Requests for a helilift must be made to the Area Health Authority who should be asked to contact:

1. In Northern England and Wales
   The Northern Rescue Coordination Centre, R.A.F., Pitreavie Castle, Dunfermline, Fife. Tel. Dunfermline 23436 (STD 0383).
2. In Southern England and Wales
   The Southern Rescue Coordination Centre, R.A.F., Mount Batten, Plymouth, Devonshire. Tel. Plymouth 61201-4 (STD 0752).

The responsibility for deciding whether a service helicopter (or a fixed wing aircraft) can be used rests with the Rescue Coordination Centre who will discuss details of emergency landing sites, etc. The high cost (£77.00 per hourt for a Whirlwind) has to be met by the Area Health Authority.

In the Republic of Ireland requests for the helicopter service should be made to Air Corps Headquarters, Casement Aerodrome, Baldonnel, Co. Dublin. Tel. 592493. A helicopter is airborne within five minutes of a call and carries a medical team and resuscitation equipment. No part of Ireland is more than 90 minutes flying time from Dublin.

In Northern Ireland requests should be made to the Senior Administrative Medical Officer, Northern Ireland Hospitals Authority, 25 Adelaide Street, Belfast 2. Tel. Belfast 40321 (STD 0232).

In Scotland if the patient can be taken to an airfield ring BEA 041-887 1111 and ask for Air Ambulance. If a helicopter lift is needed the request must be made through the Regional Health Authority or through the doctor authorised to act on behalf of the Authority who will relay it to the Northern Rescue Coordination Centre.

SHIP TO HOSPITAL (' HELOCASEVAC ') see p. 486.

The progress of events is:

1. The doctor decides that the patient should be got ashore after possible medical consultation (see 5). If there is no doctor the

Master decides. The Board of Trade International Code of Signals 1969 should be used.

2. The Master initiates communications. This may mean a direct signal of the ship's owners or via the GPO or other Coast Radio or on Channel 16 VHF or by radio call to the Coastguard. In any case the Master should inform the owners.

3. In the U.K. the local coastguard coordinates the pick-up in his own area of activity where he has intimate local knowledge. This often involves a direct link to the ship for discussion of details.

4. On landing the patient is taken to the nearest convenient casualty department. Except in certain very limited areas such as round Dover there is more discussion of clinical matters than there is in the case of a casualty from a road accident.

5. For medical discussion or advice there is worldwide coverage maintained in Britain by the Post Office Medico Service and elsewhere by CIRM (see p. 695). On a request by the doctor or Master the ship's radio officer makes contact by radio telephone or morse with an appropriate station ashore depending upon the ship's position. The shore station links with a volunteer doctor or the casualty department of a hospital and coordinates the dialogue. This is facilitated if both parties refer to the *Ship Captain's Medical Guide,* which is held in all ships.

AIRCRAFT

The St John Ambulance Air Wing with a control headquarters at St Margaret's Hospital, Epping (Epping 5642 (STD 375)) offers transport by air of drugs, tissues (kidneys), medical equipment and patients in any circumstances in which the saving of time means the relief of suffering or the saving of life. Its motto is 'Anywhere, any time'. It operates throughout the United Kingdom, the Republic of Ireland, Scandinavia and Northwest Europe. The plane's radio call-sign prefixed 'Air Wing' gives it priority flight routing. Pilots and medical nursing air attendants give their time free and the only expense is that of running the aircraft.

Tropical Diseases: where to get Advice

London

The London School of Hygiene and Tropical Medicine,
Keppel Street, London WC1E 7HT. 01-636-8636.
    Ext 344 or 342. Professor W. H. R. Lumsden
      Re malaria and other protozoal diseases.
    Ext 201. Professor L. J. Bruce-Chwatt
      Re epidemiological matters.
    Ext 234 or 01-387-4411. Professor A. W. Woodruff
      Re clinical matters.
    Telegrams: Hygower, London, WC1.
Amoebiasis Diagnosis and Research Unit, St. Giles Hospital,
St Giles Road, London SE5 7RN. 01-703 0898. Ext 6091.
    Air Vice Marshall W. P. Stamm. Re problems of amoebiasis.

The Seamen's Hospital, Greenwich SE10 9LE. 01-858 3433.
    Dr P. E. C. Manson-Bahr attends at 1300 hours every Tuesday.

Hospital for Tropical Diseases, 4 St Pancras Way, London NW1.
    01-387 4411.

Liverpool

The Liverpool School of Tropical Medicine,
Pembroke Place, Liverpool L3 5QA. 051-709 7611.

Birmingham

Department of Communicable and Tropical Diseases,
East Birmingham Hospital, Bordesley Green East,
Birmingham B9 5ST. 021-722 4311.

The Department of Tropical Medicine in Edinburgh closed in 1972.
    Advice may also be obtained from the Department of Health and
Social Security (p. 764), the Welsh Office (p. 764) and The Health
Control Unit, Terminal 3, Heathrow Airport, Hounslow, Middlesex.
01-897 4361/4.

The Emergencies of Alcoholism

FEW units can accept acute alcoholic emergencies such as acute alcoholic hallucinosis and delirium tremens and these will have to be dealt with in general hospitals. Transfer to a special unit can be arranged later. The Medical Council on Alcoholism, 8 Bourdon Street, Davies Street, London W1X 9HY, 01-493 0081, has issued a booklet to all doctors listing facilities in Great Britain and Northern Ireland for the treatment of alcoholism.

The Drugs Branch of the Home Office

If you know or suspect that your patient is addicted to heroin or other opiate you must within 24 hours get in touch with the Drugs Branch of the Home Office, Romney House, Marsham Street, London, SW1P 3DY (Tel. *see below*) who will give you details of any known addict in the UK. When you think the symptoms are genuinely due to withdrawal of heroin you should contact the physician authorised under The Misuse of Drugs (Notification of and Supply to Addicts) Regulations 1973 and obtain his authority to give methadone 10 to 20 mg preferably as a linctus. This will relieve the symptoms for 12 hours or so. Then arrange to transfer the patient to a treatment centre of which there are 25 in Greater London and 50 elsewhere in Britain. The hospital administrator will have details of these. Failing him ask the Home Office. The treatment centre will want to be sure that treatment is not being already received elsewhere and so will ask the Home Office if they can identify the addict. When you ring the Drugs Branch (which is open during normal office hours)

dial 01-212 6337	for patients with surnames A to G
01-212 0838	for patients with surnames H to P
01-212 6564	for patients with surnames Q to Z
or 01-212 0335	for general inquiries.

Make a note of tattoos, birthmarks, scars, colour of eyes, hair and complexion and any special features. There is no reason to conceal the fact that these particulars may be used for an identity check.

General advice can be obtained from The Institute for the Study of Drug Dependence, Kingsbury House, 3 Blackburn Road, London, NW6 IXA. 01-328 5541.

Index

Reserpine (Serpasil), 254
in paroxysmal tachycardia, 254
Resistance vessels, 240
Resonium A (sodium polystyrene
sulphonate), 380
Respiration, in unconscious patient,
294
Respirators, 730
cabinet type, risks of, 430
Respiratory depression, 568
Respiratory distress syndrome
of newborn, 392
blood changes in, 393
in adults, 206
Respiratory failure, 193
Respiratory function tests, 195,
Table 8.1
and anaesthesia, 564
at bedside, 317
Respiratory insufficiency, post-trau-
matic, 207
Respiratory obstruction, 224
during anaesthesia, 567
in haemophilia, 280
Respiratory syncytial virus (RS), 416
Respiratory tract irritants, 463
Respiratory units, 790
Respirex oxygen dispenser, 731
Responsibility for emergency action,
658
Restlessness, post-operative, 579
Resuscitation, 6
when to abandon, 22
Resusciade, 733
Retention of urine, 319
Retina, detachment of, 528, 536
Retinopathy, diabetic, 536
Retrobulbar neuritis, 536
Retrolental fibroplasia, 79, 397
Retropharyngeal abscess, 419
tuberculous, 223
'Return trip', 42
Rewarming, danger of, 362
Rhabdomyolysis, 125, 323
Rheomacrodex, in peripheral embol-
ism, 245
Rh immunisation, 98
Rh negative patient, 753
Ribs, fractured in resuscitation, 70
Rickets, 368
Rifampicin in meningitis, 437
Rigidity, abdominal, 126
Rigor mortis, 683
and embalming, 762
Ring, fixed wedding, 640
Rinne's test, 216
Risk to doctor, 328
of kernicterus, 408
Road Traffic Act, 680
Roccal, in dog bites, 633, 635

Rodents, diseases carried by, 477
Rogitine (phentolamine), 233, 357
Roman Catholics
and baptism, 690
and bequeathed eyes, 666
and death of mother, 183
'Roof tile' appearance in pulmonary
collapse, 600
Roumania, treatment in, 708
Round ligaments, stretching of, 175
Route, wrong, 89
Rubella
antibody titres, 176
passive immunisation, 444
in pregnancy, 176
Ruptured aneurysm, 112
Ruptured aorta, 112
Rule of Nines, 555
Rust ring, 526
Ryle, 'Eyes without the microscope',
vi
Ryle's tube, 724, Fig. 32.11
swallowed, 73

S

St John Ambulance Air Wing, 826
Saccharine test, for punctured ven-
tricle, 57
Saddle embolus, 245
Safety in laboratories, 91
SALAD airway, 733
Salbutamol (Ventolin), 196
by injection, 198
in shock, 239
Saline emetics, risks of, 73
Saline, hypertonic, in fresh water
drowning, 652
Salicylate poisoning, 31
cf. diabetic coma, 341
Salmonellosis, 135
invasive, 439
Salpingitis, acute, 173
cf. appendicitis, 173, Table 7.1
medico-legal implications, 174
tuberculous, 174
'Salt losers', 412
Salt-losing nephritis, 353
Samaritans Worldwide, 335, 816
Sand-fly fever, 485
Sandocal (calcium gluconate), 369
Sarcoidosis, hypercalcaemia in, 368
Sausages, 137
Saventrine (isoprenaline), 264
Say (what to say in an emergency),
676
Scandiatransplant, 668
Scarlet fever, 432
passive immunisation, 444